The Back Pain Revolution

To Sandra, with love
who shared it all
and made it all worthwhile.

For Churchill Livingstone:

Publishing Director: Mary Law
Project Manager: Derek Robertson
Design Direction: Judith Wright

The Back Pain Revolution

Gordon Waddell CBE, DSc, FRCS
Orthopaedic Surgeon, Glasgow

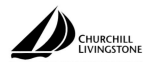
CHURCHILL
LIVINGSTONE

EDINBURGH LONDON NEW YORK OXFORD PHILADELPHIA ST LOUIS SYDNEY TORONTO 2004

CHURCHILL LIVINGSTONE
An imprint of Elsevier Limited

First published 1998

Second edition 2004

ISBN 0-4430-7227-2

British Library Cataloguing in Publication Data
A catalogue record for this book is available from the British Library

Library of Congress Cataloging in Publication Data
A catalog record for this book is available from the Library of Congress

Notice
Medical knowledge is constantly changing. Standard safety precautions must be
followed, but as new research and clinical experience broaden our knowledge,
changes in treatment and drug therapy may become necessary or appropriate.
Readers are advised to check the most current product information provided by
the manufacturer of each drug to be administered to verify the recommended
dose, the method and duration of administration, and contraindications. It is the
responsibility of the practitioner, relying on experience and knowledge of the
patient, to determine dosages and the best treatment for each individual patient.
Neither the publisher nor the author assumes any liability for any injury and/or
damage to persons or property arising from this publication.

The Publisher

your source for books,
journals and multimedia
in the health sciences

www.elsevierhealth.com

The
Publisher's
policy is to use
**paper manufactured
from sustainable forests**

Printed in China

Contents

Additional contributors

David B Allan MB ChB FRCS
Director, National Spinal Injuries Unit,
Glasgow, Scotland

A Kim Burton PhD DO
Director, Spinal Research Unit, University of
Huddersfield, UK

Chris J Main PhD FBPsS
Professor of Clinical and Occupational
Rehabilitation, University of Manchester, UK

Maurits van Tulder PhD
Associate Professor Health Technology
Assessment, VU University Medical Centre,
Institute for Research in Extramural Medicine
(EMGO) and Department of Clinical
Epidemiology & Biostatistics, Amsterdam,
The Netherlands

Paul J Watson PhD MCSP
Senior Lecturer in Pain Management and
Rehabilitation, University of Leicester, UK

Foreword

At the beginning of the 21st century the international epidemic of back pain and disability continues to exact a huge toll in terms of suffering and costs.

Scientists are searching far and wide for biomedical solutions to this crisis: new drugs, innovative surgical methods, and space-age technologies. Yet it is unlikely that medical advances alone can solve this terrible problem. The back pain epidemic does not revolve solely around medical issues.

Back pain is and always has been a common feature of human life. There is no evidence that its prevalence has increased over the past 50 years; what has changed is the way individuals, the medical community, and society have responded to back pain. Any solution to the back pain epidemic must address all these domains. Simple solutions, in other words, are unlikely to work.

But what if an innovative approach to low back pain could attack this epidemic at multiple levels: altering attitudes, rebutting fears, fine-tuning medical care, and speeding millions of employees back to work? This is the approach envisioned in *The Back Pain Revolution*.

The concepts and strategies described in this book have the potential to achieve the unthinkable: put an end to this spiraling problem. Indeed, there is emerging evidence that the back pain crisis may already have peaked in societies that have adopted some of these concepts (see Waddell et al 2002).

Scottish orthopedist Gordon Waddell needs no introduction to anyone familiar with back pain research. He is among the most influential researchers of this generation, with an impressive record of studies, guidelines, reviews, and reports to his credit. He has made major contributions to myriad fields, as evidenced by the scope of this book. He played a central role in deposing the traditional medical approach to low back pain and in creating a more productive alternative (see Waddell 1987).

Yet, for all his achievements, Waddell is not an ivory tower researcher. His main focus has always been the common man and woman with back pain, and the plight they face in the clinic, the workplace, and the social welfare system. In the UK, he was recently honored by the Queen with the title 'Commander of the British Empire' (CBE) for his contributions to disability research – for helping those teetering on the far edge of productive life.

A TRUE REVOLUTION

When the word 'revolution' appears in the title of a medical textbook, it usually signals hyperbole and exaggeration. But when applied to the back pain arena, 'revolution' is a perfectly accurate description.

Over the past quarter century, the traditional medical model of back pain management has been overthrown. In this model back pain was interpreted as a signal of disease or injury, often attributed to the stresses of work. The typical prescription was rest and inactivity until the 'injury' resolved and pain abated. This medical model let a common, benign and self-limiting symptom snowball into an avalanche of chronic pain and disability – and exorbitant costs across the industrialized world.

The outmoded medical model has given way to a more flexible and productive approach: the so-called 'biopsychosocial model' that forms the basis for modern back care. This label is a nod to the complexity of pain complaints and the rich diversity of factors which influence them.

CHANGING ATTITUDES ABOUT BACK PAIN

The back pain revolution begins with changing perceptions about the nature of back pain and its significance. It involves rebutting the idea that back pain typically stems from a discrete injury or disease – or that activity and work are to be feared.

This model prescribes a careful but streamlined approach to back pain in clinical settings. It allows the efficient identification of those with serious back problems – and encourages the rest to make a quick and confident return to normal life.

It involves using creative psychosocial approaches to identify and overcome barriers to recovery. It recommends a variety of interventions – whatever it takes, really – keep back pain sufferers at work. It also involves tinkering with social welfare and disability systems to ensure that an active life holds greater allure than disability and invalidity.

Prevention is a major thrust of this movement: prevention of back pain's all too frequent consequences – withdrawal from normal activity, physical deconditioning, work disability, and social dislocation. Early prevention is a key, since medicine has a poor track record of resolving the complex problems that accompany chronic disability.

AN INTENSIVE RESEARCH EFFORT

This revolution is not based on a single algorithm or management protocol. It is a fluid, broad-based movement that is strongly linked to an intensive research process. It will change over time with gains in knowledge.

That the approach described in *The Back Pain Revolution* can succeed is not really in doubt. There have been tantalizing glimpses of the kinds of progress than even modest interventions can produce. A multimedia information campaign in Victoria, Australia – modeled on many of the concepts that Waddell and colleagues developed – produced lasting changes in the attitudes and behavior of health care professionals and the general public (see Buchbinder et al 2001). The on-going 'Working Backs' campaign in Scotland appears to be having a similarly impressive effect (see Burton & Waddell 2004).

The concepts described in *The Back Pain Revolution* can also have a major impact on the culture of disability. The UK recently reported a 42% reduction in new awards of back pain-related disability benefits since the mid-1990s. In human terms, this is a spectacular achievement (see Waddell et al 2002).

OBSTACLES TO PROGRESS

Though the back pain revolution can succeed, it may not. There are cultural and institutional barriers to success. Important stakeholders – from governments to major industries – are still heavily invested in the back pain injury model and the back pain crisis itself. The back pain 'market' is a humming, economic machine that produces billions in revenue annually.

Some segments of the medical establishment have been slow to abandon the old ways. Some health care providers fear needlessly that modern approaches to non-specific back pain might erode their influence or limit their options in treating patients with specific spinal diseases.

The mass media, in terms of editorial content and advertising, may also be an impediment to progress. Patients have been conditioned to expect instant fixes and passive cures.

A BLUEPRINT FOR THE FUTURE

So who would benefit from reading *The Back Pain Revolution*? It is essential reading for everyone in the back pain field: medical and non-medical providers, patients, healthcare administrators, economists, lawyers, and leaders of government.

The Back Pain Revolution is a 'hands-on' manual for those involved in the provision of clinical back care. But it goes far beyond that; it is also a guide to the major social, economic, and political issues affecting the back pain crisis. It is a call to arms and a blueprint for the future.

Mark L. Schoene, 2004
Editor, *The BackLetter*
Newbury, Massachusetts, USA

References

Burton AK Waddell G 2004 Information and advice for patients. In: Waddell G (ed.) The Back Pain Revolution. Churchill Livingstone, Edinburgh, pp 331–341

Buchbinder R et al 2001 Population-based intervention to change back pain beliefs and disability: three-part evaluation. British Medical Journal 322:1516–1520

Waddell G 1987 A new clinical model for the treatment of low-back pain. Spine 12(7):632–644

Waddell G, Aylward M, Sawney P 2002 Back Pain, incapacity for work and social security benefits: an international literature review and analysis. Royal Society of Medicine Press, London

Acknowledgments

I claim this book as my own, and I did write it, but such as this could never be a solo effort.

Most of all, I am indebted to my patients with back pain who presented their needs and posed the questions. I am acutely aware that I owe them much more than my inadequate efforts for them could ever repay. I only hope this will help future health professionals to provide a better service for future patients.

The late John McCulloch and Ian Macnab introduced me to back pain, and I have never escaped their spell. Chris Main shared the first faltering steps and has remained a trusty companion on this journey. My fellows Emyr Morris, Mike Di Paolo, David Finlayson, Martin Bircher, Douglas Somerville, Mary Newton and Iain Henderson provided much-needed support at various stages along the way. In recent years, Kim Burton has taken over the task of soul-mate.

I have tried to acknowledge the source of ideas and material as far as possible. I am particularly grateful to The Royal College of General Practitioners, The Faculty of Occupational Medicine, The Stationery Office and Health Scotland in UK, COST B13 Management Committee in EU, and The National Advisory Committee on Health and Disability and The Accident Rehabilitation and Compensation Insurance Corporation in New Zealand, for permission to reproduce clinical guidelines and patient information material. Inevitably, I have gathered ideas from many papers and meetings over the years and adopted them as my own. I apologize if I have forgotten some of the original sources, and failed to acknowledge your pet idea. I can only say that imitation is the most sincere form of flattery.

I am especially grateful to my fellow contributors. In both editions, many friends and colleagues around the world have read draft chapters in their fields of expertise, and offered comments and suggestions: Alan Breen, Peter Croft, Rick Deyo, Scott Haldeman, Craig Liebenson, Chris Main, Carol McGivern, Roger Nelson, Reed Phillips, Malcolm Pope, Mark Schoene and Clive Standen. I thank them all for their useful advice and accept full responsibility where I chose to ignore it.

Last, and most of all, my deepest thanks go to my family. For the first edition, my wife Sandra spent many hours typing and pandering to my obsession. She and my daughters sacrificed much more family life than they should. Misty, my border collie, never could understand why I was not ready for her walk. After the first edition I promised I would mend my ways, but their scepticism was justified. At least the word processor relieved Sandra of typing the new edition, but little else has changed and my grandchildren now voice the same complaints. Once again, I can only thank you all, and hope the new edition makes it seem worthwhile.

GW, 2004

Chapter 1

The problem

Back pain was a 20th-century medical disaster and the legacy reverberates into the new millennium.

Medicine has made great advances over the past two centuries and especially since World War II. We have developed powerful tools to treat disease. Medical technology and resources reached a peak in solving the mystery of life itself in DNA, in our ability to replace hip joints and even transplant hearts. We now have cures that past generations would literally have thought were miracles. We have vaccines to prevent polio and drugs to cure tuberculosis. We have high-tech investigations that lay bare the anatomy and pathology of the spine. We can perform bigger and better operations. Yet we have no answer for ordinary backache. Modern medicine has been very successful in treating many serious spinal diseases, but this whole approach failed with back pain. For all our efforts and skill, for all our resources, low back disability got steadily worse (Fig. 1.1). Rising trends of work loss, early retirement, and state benefits all show our failure to solve the problem. By the end of the 20th century, simple back strains disabled many more people in western society than all the serious spinal diseases put together.

There are many paradoxes about back pain. Over the past few decades we have learned much about back pain, about pain itself, and about how people react and deal with pain. We should now be able to manage back pain better, even if we still cannot offer a cure. Chronic back pain and disability should be getting less, but for too long the opposite was true. Why? Why are we not delivering better and more

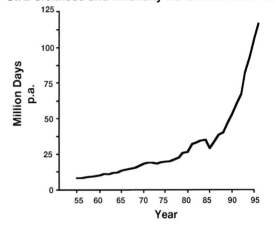

U.K. Sickness and Invalidity Benefit for Back Pain

Figure 1.1 The rising trend of low back disability from 1953–1954 to 1994–1995. Based on annual statistics from the UK Department of Social Security.

effective health care for back pain? There are, I believe, many reasons. We do not seem to put our better understanding of pain into clinical practice. We are poor at dealing with disability. Too often, we just ignore disability and assume it will get better if we treat the pain. There has also been a shift in social attitudes and behavior. It is now acceptable to stay off work, get workers' compensation or social security benefits, and retire early because of back pain. So we can already see that health care is only part of a larger story.

Much of this applies to all kinds of chronic pain. So why is back pain, in particular, such a problem?

What is different about it? Part of the trouble is that back pain is only a symptom, not a disease. Most of us get back pain at some time of our lives, but most of the time we deal with it ourselves and do not regard it as a medical condition. But back pain can also be the presenting symptom of serious spinal disease. The symptom of pain in the back is the common link between that everyday bodily symptom, serious disease, and chronic disability. We get into trouble when we confuse them. It is the health care system and health professionals who label ordinary backache as a serious spinal disease. We do not really understand the cause of most back pain and there is usually little or no serious pathology that we can demonstrate. We often regard back pain as an injury, but most episodes occur spontaneously with normal everyday activities. Our high-tech investigations for spinal disease tell us very little about back pain.

So back pain is a problem. It is a problem to patients, to health professionals, and to society. It is a problem to patients because they cannot get clear advice on its cause, how to deal with it, and its likely outcome. It is a problem to doctors and therapists because we cannot diagnose any definite disease or offer any real cure. So we are unsure and uncomfortable dealing with back pain. To society, back pain is one of the most common and fastest-growing reasons for work loss, health care use, and sickness benefits. And there is no good medical explanation.

Patients, therapists, and doctors are now more aware of the limitations of health care for back pain. The scientific evidence shows that most treatments in routine use are pretty ineffective. Indeed, many of the things we do may be worse than no treatment at all, especially if they divert attention from dealing with the real issues. The sheer range of treatments betrays our ignorance. The variation in clinical practice suggests that many patients receive care that is less than ideal. Much of the health care we give for back pain is inappropriate. Too often, the choice of treatment reflects the skills of the professional rather than the needs of the patient. To put it simply, what treatment you receive depends more on who you go to see than on what is wrong with your back. Many patients in the US and the UK are now so dissatisfied with orthodox medical treatment for back pain that they seek alternative health care instead.

There is much agreement on the need for change. There is growing demand from patients and family doctors for better health care services for back pain. Policy makers and those who fund health care are in a position to enforce this demand. But health professionals are conservative. We are slow to change our professional practice. Until recently, there was also lack of a clear direction for change. There are still many gaps in our knowledge, but there is now a growing body of scientific evidence from which we can begin to draw principles for better treatment. There is now the start of a consensus, and change is begun. There is still a long way to go, and a great deal of inertia and resistance to overcome. But I believe there is now the dawn of a revolution in the care of back pain.

Near the end of my training as an orthopedic surgeon, I was still unsure about treating spinal disorders. So I went to Toronto and worked for a year with the late Drs John McCulloch and Ian Macnab. I reviewed 103 Workmen's Compensation patients who had had repeat back operations (Waddell et al 1979). To a young surgeon at the start of my career, the results were frightening. A first operation made 70–80% of patients better, but 15% were worse after surgery and sooner or later had another operation. The results of repeat surgery got worse. By the third operation there was only a 25% chance of a good result and an equal chance it would make the patient worse. It was also obvious that the outcome of surgery depended only partly on physical factors. Sixty-five percent of these patients had psychological problems by the time I saw them. That year changed my thinking. Ian Macnab (one of the kings of spinal fusion!) taught me to "know as much about the patient who has the back pain as about the back pain the patient has." John McCulloch introduced me to the non-organic signs (Waddell et al 1980). Neville Doxey taught me, to my surprise, that doctors can learn something from clinical psychologists. I went to Toronto to learn about spinal surgery, but ever since I have been intrigued by back pain, how it affects people, and how they react. I learned that back pain is not simply a mechanical problem. Low back disability and how people react to pain and to treatment depend just as much on psychological and social factors as on the underlying physical problem.

Compare a patient with back pain with one who has a hip replacement for osteoarthritis (Figs 1.2 and 1.3). In back pain we often cannot find the cause or even the exact source of the pain. Patients do not understand what is wrong and cannot get clear answers to their questions. If back pain becomes chronic, patients soon realize that we do not know what is wrong. In contrast, with arthritis the problem is clear to both patient and surgeon and both can see it on X-ray. Treatment of arthritis is logical. Complications and failures do occur, but they are relatively uncommon and the reason for failure is usually obvious. Treatment for back pain is empiric and has a high failure rate. Understandably, many patients are reluctant to accept, and many doctors or therapists to admit, the limitations of treatment for back pain. So, when treatment for back pain fails, the professional may look for psychological reasons or other excuses. The patient is likely to become defensive. Both patient and professional may become angry and hostile. It should come as no surprise that some patients develop psychological problems.

When I came back to Glasgow, I started working with Chris Main, a clinical psychologist. Soon after we started, Chris confronted me. If we were going to work together, I would need to improve my clinical data to match his psychological data. I nearly punched the guy! He had no medical training and naively I thought he had little proper clinical experience, yet he was telling me how to do my job. The trouble, of course, was that he was right. Most clinical data and research are not very scientific. It was painful but instructive to apply Chris's scientific rigor. I learned a lot and that was the start of one of the closest and most productive collaborations of my career.

Another paradox is that the problem of back pain is greatest in western "civilization." In 1985,

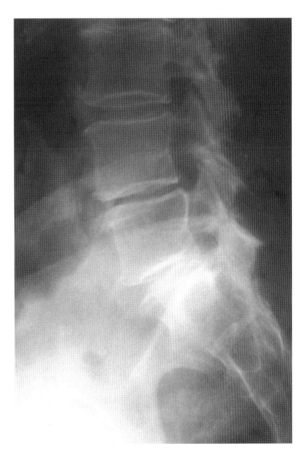

Figure 1.2 Osteoarthritic changes in the hip usually correspond reasonably well with clinical pain and disability.

Figure 1.3 Degenerative changes in the lumbar spine bear very little relationship to clinical symptoms.

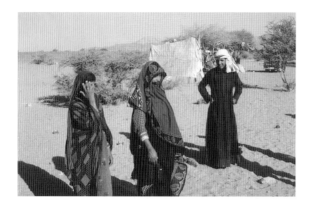

Figure 1.4   Back pain is just as common in Oman, but causes very little disability.

I visited Oman to advise on orthopedic services for back pain (Fig. 1.4). At that time, Oman was a rapidly developing Arab state. Within the previous 10 years, new oil wealth and political change had propelled it from a medieval state into the 20th century. In that short period, health care in Oman had become as good as in much of North America and Europe.

By 1985, health care was just reaching out to the more rural areas of Oman. We held one clinic in a desert town for children with polio, caught before vaccination started a few years earlier. In one day we saw nearly 40 severely crippled children. They had never seen a doctor nor had any treatment. That was one of the most moving experiences of my professional life. We could only offer palliative care with splints and reconstructive surgery, but despite that, the children and their parents were grateful and uncomplaining. They accepted their fate as the will of God: *insh'allah*. Yet we needed locks and guards on the clinic doors to keep out the noisy and demanding adults seeking a western "cure" for their back pain. Otherwise, we would never have been able to see the children with polio. Incidentally, in that society the demand was all from men, which reflects the power of social pressure on illness behavior.

Patients with back pain flood the new orthopedic clinics in Oman. Patients with back pain seem to crawl out from under the very stones of the desert. Or, to be more accurate, they walk out. Because the striking thing is that, although back pain is so common, it causes very little disability.

People in Oman may be crippled by polio, spinal tuberculosis, or spinal fractures, but no one becomes disabled by ordinary backache. Even the nurses do not stay off work with back pain. Two matrons in hospitals 650 km (400 miles) apart both said that in 10 years they had never had a nurse off work with back pain. More careful surveys confirm this. Anderson (1984) studied a peasant community in Nepal and "found a virtual epidemic of spinal pain." Forty-four percent of adults had back or neck pain at the time of interview, more or less the same as in western surveys. But it was usually an incidental finding. Anderson was "struck by the virtual absence of disability." People expected back or neck pain as part of their lives and did very little about it.

People in less developed societies get much the same back pain as we do, but they have much less disability. Only with the introduction of western medicine does chronic back disability become common. Indeed, the new back cripples in Oman are those who have had the "advantage" of surgery in India, Europe, or the USA. Similarly, in North America and in Europe, 25–50% of patients in most pain clinics are the failures of modern treatment for back pain (Fig. 1.5). Perhaps it is time to stop and ask ourselves what we think we are doing to our patients with back pain.

For 17 years I ran a Problem Back Clinic for the west of Scotland. Most of these patients had a long history of chronic pain and disability. They had seen many specialists and therapists, and had many investigations and treatments. They had tried complementary and alternative medicine. Everyone they saw gave them a different story, but none gave lasting relief. These patients were frustrated and depressed by our failure. As you would expect, I was rarely able to make any new diagnosis or offer any miracle cure. These patients were highly selected and are not representative of all patients with back pain, but they can teach us a lot about the limitations and failures of our system. Listening to them, I became convinced that most of the problems are to do with our basic approach to management. Most patients with back pain do get better, but the failures of treatment may be worse than no treatment at all. Too often, I wondered if a patient might have been better if he or she had never seen a doctor, and especially not a surgeon. It would

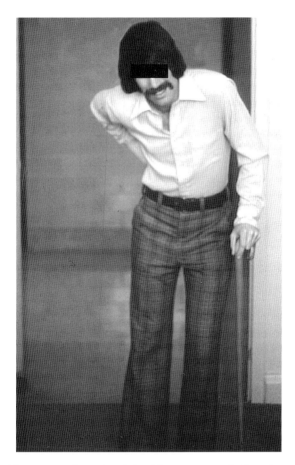

Figure 1.5   A previously healthy young man in Canada, permanently disabled by a simple back strain.

clearly be better to prevent these people ever developing chronic pain and disability, rather than trying to treat their intractable pain.

Once again, the problem is that back pain is only a symptom, not a disease. Western medicine works best for acute physical diseases with clearly understood anatomy and pathology. Then, we can demonstrate and deal with the problem. It is much less successful in chronic and poorly understood conditions, particularly if there are psychosomatic features, like back pain. Most back pain is simply a mechanical disturbance of the musculoskeletal structures or function of the back. We cannot diagnose any specific pathology. We cannot even localize the exact source of most soft-tissue pain. Some doctors and therapists claim to be able to diagnose the site and nature of the lesion, but that often tells

us more about the health professional than about the patient's back. And it is striking how these professionals disagree! To confuse the issue further, back pain is often a recurrent problem and patients are often distressed.

So perhaps it is not surprising that diagnosis and health care are not nearly as logical as they appear in textbooks. This is particularly obvious in patients with failed back surgery, even when we look at a clear-cut condition like an acute disk prolapse. We all know how to diagnose the nerve that needs surgical decompression. It is a logical decision based on well-known criteria. We can all produce the right answer in an exam. However, experience in the Problem Back Clinic shows that practice can be different from theory. Morris et al (1986) confirmed this in a prospective study of routine spinal surgery. They found that surgical decisions depend on the severity and duration of the patient's symptoms, their distress and failed conservative treatment, more than on objective evidence of a surgically treatable lesion. "Because the pain is so severe and has not got better with bed rest it must be a disk prolapse." That is a direct quote from the record of a patient with nonspecific low back pain who never had any symptoms or signs of a disk prolapse. Depending on how strongly the patient demands and the surgeon feels that "something must be done," there is a strong temptation to proceed to investigations. We rationalize this by saying that we "want to make sure we are not missing anything." Or when the clinical picture is not clear, we use tests as a short cut to diagnosis. We order a magnetic resonance imaging (MRI) instead of taking a more careful history or physical exam and using time to clarify the picture. If these sensitive tests show even minor changes, we forget about false-positives and the lack of matching clinical features. The trap is then complete. The patient has genuine needs and demands, we have run out of options, and we want to help. It is then difficult to withhold the knife. Too often, in such a case, the surgical findings are unimpressive. Despite our best intentions, the brutal reality is that the patient has had an unnecessary operation. Surprise, surprise, it does not help. But more important, and often forgotten, even when there are no complications failed surgery may make the patient's pain, disability, and distress worse. (And do not fall into the trap of thinking this patient's condition is so bad you cannot make it any worse. You can, always!)

All my clinical experience and research have convinced me that our treatment of back pain has failed because we have lost sight of basic principles. What matters is not the technical detail but our whole strategy of clinical management. We need to rethink our whole approach. If we get the basic principles right, the detail can follow. So this book is about basic clinical principles:

- Why and how do some people become chronic back cripples due to ordinary backache?
- Why have their numbers increased?
- What went wrong with our management of back pain?
- How can we stop this epidemic?
- How can we improve health care for patients with back pain?

We all agree in principle that we should treat people, not spines. Plato taught in ancient Greece: "So neither ought you to attempt to cure the body without the soul." All health care still has its roots in Hippocratic concepts of caring. We cannot separate the doctor's role as healer from the more ancient role as personal adviser and comforter in illness. Chiropractic and osteopathy share similar philosophy. Physical therapists spend their whole working life helping people to regain function and get back to normal life. The problem is that in busy modern practice we too often forget about such ideals and get on with treating pain and physical disease. We all agree on the ideals – the challenge is to put them into routine clinical practice.

This book presents what I have learned from nearly 30 years of research, but it is not about academic research or scientific results. My interest has always been in the clinical care of patients with back pain, and we must apply the lessons of research to daily practice in the clinic or the office. So this is a clinical text. It starts with, concentrates on, and is all about the clinical problem of back pain. Some teachers claim that anatomy, biomechanics, and pathology are the basis for clinical practice. In one sense that is true: of course we need to know that basic science. But we must also

remember these are only tools to serve our patients' needs. They cannot and must not drive our clinical practice. If we build our theories upwards from the foundation of these basic sciences, then it is too easy to select or bend the clinical facts to fit our theories. It is no surprise that approach to back pain failed. The real study of medicine and the foundation of clinical practice is human illness. Only if we start from clinical reality can we select and use those basic sciences that help us to understand and explain our clinical observations.

The fascination and challenge of health care are the variety of ways in which human beings react to illness. You cannot learn this by reading a book. You can only learn by working with patients. There is a wonderful quote from Sir Isaac Newton:

> I seem to have been only a boy playing on the seashore, and diverting myself in now and then finding a smoother pebble or a prettier shell than ordinary, whilst the great ocean of truth lay all undiscovered before me.

This does not do justice to a great scientist's approach to knowledge. In health care as in science, there comes a time when you have to plunge into the ocean and enter that world of experience that you cannot imagine standing on the shore watching the waves. So you can only truly learn about back pain from your patients. This book aims to serve as a companion that helps you to think about and learn from your clinical experience.

We are at the dawn of a revolution in back pain. Dawn is a time of light, of hope, of new beginnings. This book is my contribution to the new approach to back pain. It tries to develop the basic principles and describe how to put them into clinical practice. It looks at how we might improve the health care system. If you are happy with how you treat back pain and have not thought about these issues, then I hope this book will disturb you. I hope that after reading it and thinking about these questions, it will change forever how you think about back pain and how you deal with your patients. This book will not give you all the answers, but I hope it will help to focus the questions and stimulate you to join the search for answers. For our patients and society rightly demand that there must be a better way of treating back pain.

References

Anderson R T 1984 An orthopaedic ethnography in rural Nepal. Medical Anthropology 8: 46–59

Morris E W, Di Paola M P, Vallance R, Waddell G 1986 Diagnosis and decision-making in lumbar disc prolapse and nerve entrapment. Spine 11: 436–439

Waddell G, Kummel E G, Lotto W N, Graham J D, Hall H, McCulloch J A 1979 Failed lumbar disc surgery and repeat surgery following industrial injuries. Journal of Bone and Joint Surgery 61A: 201–207

Waddell G, McCulloch J A, Kummel E, Venner R M 1980 Non-organic physical signs in low back pain. Spine 5: 117–125

Chapter 2

Diagnostic triage

Diagnosis is the foundation of management and is based on clinical assessment. A careful history and examination also help to build rapport with the patient. These are basic principles of clinical practice, but difficult to apply to back pain. We can only diagnose definite pathology in about 15% of patients with back pain. Patients want an answer (Table 2.1), but we must be honest and they must be realistic about what is possible. However, we should not be too pessimistic. We can exclude serious disease, predict likely progress, and provide a rational basis for management, all of which are positive and helpful. We should also present as good news the fact that we cannot find anything serious. We should be able to allay these fears. That is a long way towards providing a diagnosis and it is then more a matter of how we put this into words.

This chapter offers a reliable approach to diagnosis that will let you offer this reassurance with

Table 2.1   Concerns of US patients in primary care

The wrong movement might cause a serious problem with my back	64%
My body is indicating that something is dangerously wrong	50%
I might become disabled for a long time due to my back pain	47%
My back pain may be due to a serious disease	19%

Data from Von Korff & Moore (2001).

very little risk of error. It is basic diagnostic triage:

- ordinary backache
- nerve root pain
- possible serious spinal pathology.

At first sight, this may seem too simple. For many years I taught this approach to my medical students and they loved it. My residents and fellows tested it and found that it worked in practice. At academic meetings, however, experienced doctors dismissed it because "we all know and do that." Unfortunately, experience in the Problem Back Clinic shows that is not true. It is the fundamentals that are most important but most difficult to get right. The Quebec Task Force first emphasized the value of such an approach (Spitzer et al 1987). Those involved in primary care are very aware of the need to deal with basics, and both American (AHCPR 1994) and British (RCGP 1999) clinical guidelines use this approach.

DIFFERENTIAL DIAGNOSIS

Textbooks often present diagnosis as a forced choice between different diseases. They describe each disease in detail. We teach students to ask: "Which of the diseases in my textbook most closely resembles this patient's clinical picture?" To ease the task, we hunt for pathognomonic symptoms and signs. We then select tests to confirm our diagnosis. Medical teaching has used this approach for nearly three centuries. But it is a very inefficient way of thinking and a poor approach to clinical practice.

Most textbooks give long lists of diseases that cause back pain, but they are all rare. Indeed, some books apologize that these diseases are "rare but important." Non-specific low back pain is at the end of the list, almost an afterthought, and diagnosis is by exclusion. Such lists do not reflect the incidence or importance of these conditions. I freely confess that I cannot think of every possible disease in my busy clinic. Also, most patients do not read medical textbooks and their symptoms and signs never quite fit the classic descriptions. In practice, it is almost impossible to match each patient against a long list of half-forgotten thumbnail sketches. So it should be no surprise this approach often results in misleading investigations and bad management.

Instead, I want to suggest a simple diagnostic triage. The concept of triage comes from battle casualties. In a busy casualty clearing station, a senior doctor briefly assesses each casualty on arrival. He or she divides them into three categories. Some have major but salvageable injuries and they receive first priority for treatment. Some have more minor injuries that need treatment, but will not come to any harm by waiting. The third group have such major injuries that death is inevitable and they do not receive limited and overpressed resources. That senior doctor does not attempt any more precise diagnosis or carry out any treatment, yet makes the single most important decision in management. Everything follows from that first step. Triage decides who receives what treatment and the final outcome. In battle casualties, triage literally decides who lives or dies.

Diagnosis determines management. Whether we make the decision consciously, or do it without thinking, diagnostic triage of back pain is just as vital. It sets the pattern for referral, investigation, and management. It very much determines the further course and often the final outcome of treatment. If we get it right, the rest follows almost automatically. If we get it wrong, the whole strategy of management goes wrong, often with a poor outcome. This is one of the basic decisions that is hardest to make but most important to get right.

I first developed this approach in a series of 900 patients with back pain (Waddell 1982). Half were routine referrals from family doctors to an orthopedic outpatient clinic and the others were at my Problem Back Clinic. The series included 35 patients with tumors, 15 with infection, 25 with osteoporosis, and 23 with other pathologies. Let me hasten to say that serious spinal pathology is not nearly as common as that. This was a highly selected series that we used simply to work out the system of diagnostic triage. Deyo et al (1992) independently produced very similar findings. Bogduk (1999) and Bogduk & Govind (1999) provide an extensive and critical review of the evidence base.

Diagnostic triage

Ordinary backache

This is common or garden, non-specific, low back pain (Box 2.1). It is "mechanical" pain of

---

Box 2.1   Ordinary backache

- Clinical presentation usually at age 20–55 years
- Lumbosacral region, buttocks, and thighs
- Pain is mechanical in nature
  - varies with physical activity
  - varies with time
- Patient well

Box 2.2   Nerve root pain

- Unilateral leg pain is worse than back pain
- Pain generally radiates to foot or toes
- Numbness or paresthesia in the same distribution
- Nerve irritation signs
  - reduced straight leg raising which reproduces leg pain
- Motor, sensory, or reflex changes
  - limited to one nerve root

---

musculoskeletal origin in which symptoms vary with physical activities. Backache may be related to mechanical strain or dysfunction, although it often develops spontaneously. Backache may be very painful, but severity of pain does not tell us anything about the diagnosis. Backache often spreads to one or both buttocks or thighs. We previously called this "simple" backache to reassure patients there was no damage to the nerves or any more serious spinal pathology. Critics point out that failed to acknowledge that backache can be very painful and disabling, and is not always "simple" to treat. I will come back to the use of labels later, but the important thing is that this is common or ordinary backache and there is no serious disease.

Of course, I realize that non-specific low back pain includes a variety of different conditions. There have been many attempts to identify subtypes (Binkley et al 1993, Delitto et al 1993, Merskey & Bogduk 1994, Moffroid et al 1994) but unfortunately the distinction is unclear. There is little correlation between the anatomic identification of pain generators, actual pathology, and clinical syndromes. Most of these classifications have not been replicated and different specialists cannot agree. Obviously, this is an important future goal, but at present we have no reliable way of subclassifying non-specific low back pain (Abraham et al 2002).

We will consider more detailed assessment of back pain in later chapters. At this stage, the first priority is simply to be clear that the problem is ordinary backache.

Nerve root pain

Nerve root pain is a better term than sciatica, as it stresses the pathologic basis and specific clinical features. Nerve root pain can arise from a disk prolapse, spinal stenosis, or surgical scarring. In most patients with a low back problem, nerve root pain stems from a single nerve root. Involvement of more than one nerve root raises the possibility of a more widespread neurologic disorder. Nerve root pain is sharp, well-localized pain down one leg that at least approximates to a dermatomal pattern. It radiates below the knee and often into the foot or toes. There may be numbness or pins and needles in the same distribution. There may be signs of nerve irritation or neurologic signs of nerve compression, though these are not essential for the diagnosis (Box 2.2). When present, nerve root pain is often the patient's main complaint and is usually greater than back pain.

Serious spinal pathology

Serious spinal pathology includes diseases such as spinal tumor and infection, and inflammatory disease such as ankylosing spondylitis (Box 2.3). Serious spinal pathology may give back pain or, less commonly, nerve root pain. The clinical presentation, diagnosis, and management concern the underlying pathology.

Most back pain is ordinary backache. Less than 1% is due to serious spinal disease such as tumor or infection that needs urgent specialist investigation and treatment. Less than 1% is inflammatory disease that needs rheumatologic investigation and treatment. Less than 5% is true nerve root pain, and only a small proportion of that ever needs surgery.

Diagnosis should be a clear and logical process. A clinical history and physical exam should not be a mindless gathering of facts. Nor can you wait for

---

Box 2.3   Serious spinal pathology

Red flags
- Presentation age <20 years or onset >55 years
- Violent trauma, e.g., fall from a height, road traffic accident
- Constant, progressive, non-mechanical pain
- Thoracic pain
- Previous history
  - carcinoma
  - systemic steroids
  - drug abuse, human immunodeficiency virus (HIV)
- Systemically unwell
  - weight loss
- Persisting severe restriction of lumbar flexion
- Widespread neurology
- Structural deformity
- Investigations when required
  - erythrocyte sedimentation rate (ESR) >25 mm
  - plain X-ray: vertebral collapse or bone destruction

Warning signs in children (after A Crawford, personal communication)
- Age less than 11
- Constant pain lasting more than a few weeks

- Pain interfering with daily activities and play – inactive, listless
- Spontaneous night pain
- Fever or raised ESR
- Spinal deformity because of severe muscle spasm

Cauda equina syndrome/widespread neurologic disorder
- Difficulty with micturition
- Loss of anal sphincter tone or fecal incontinence
- Saddle anesthesia about the anus, perineum, or genitals
- Widespread (>one nerve root) or progressive motor weakness in the legs or gait disturbance
- Sensory level

Inflammatory disorders (ankylosing spondylitis and related disorders)
- Gradual onset before age 40 years
- Marked morning stiffness
- Persisting limitation of spinal movements in all directions
- Peripheral joint involvement
- Iritis, skin rashes (psoriasis), colitis, urethral discharge
- Family history

---

these facts to fuse into a clear picture in some blinding flash of intuition. It is simpler, faster, and more efficient to start from the main presenting symptoms. Your history should focus on the key items of information required for triage, and brief examination should supplement these key items. You may then need a few investigations to confirm or refute the diagnosis. At each step you use symptoms, signs, or investigations to confirm or modify the diagnostic process. Triage is the logical outcome from clearly identified clinical evidence. Provided you focus on the key issues, you can easily cover everything that matters within the average family doctor's consultation of 10–15 minutes. And still have time left over to listen and talk to the patient.

Diagnosis also depends on combining all the key facts into the decision. Single symptoms and signs may be unreliable. Diagnosis based on a combination of key symptoms and signs is more accurate and much safer.

I will present diagnostic triage as it should occur in the first clinical consultation. This is the ideal, but it is not always possible, and sometimes time may assist the diagnostic process. Consistent or progressive findings on several occasions may be more reliable and assume more significance. Failure to improve with time may raise the need for reassessment. The ideal is diagnostic triage on the first consultation, but there is still the opportunity to review this on further visits.

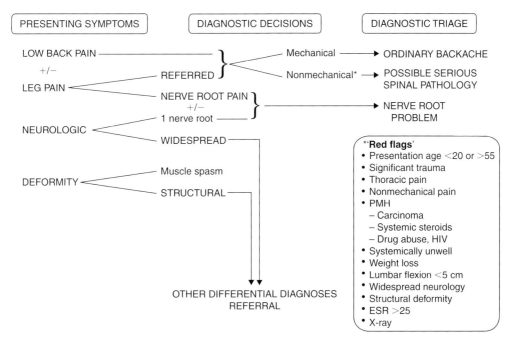

| PRESENTING SYMPTOMS | DIAGNOSTIC DECISIONS | DIAGNOSTIC TRIAGE |

Figure 2.1 Differential diagnosis flow chart. PMH, previous medical history; HIV, human immunodeficiency virus; ESR, erythrocyte sedimentation rate.

PRESENTING SYMPTOMS

Patients with low back disorders present with four key symptoms:

1. back pain
2. leg pain
3. neurologic symptoms
4. spinal deformity.

More than 99% of low back problems present with back pain and it is rare to see a low back problem with no back pain. Pain always tends to radiate distally and 70% of patients with back pain also have some pain down one or both legs. Neurologic symptoms and spinal deformity are much less common but crucial to diagnosis.

These four presenting symptoms lead us on to four questions:

1. Is this a low back problem and can we exclude disease elsewhere?
2. Is there any major spinal deformity or widespread neurologic disorder?
3. Is there any question of serious spinal pathology?
4. Is there nerve root involvement?

We should direct our history and examination to answer these questions. The answers automatically lead to triage into the three broad diagnostic groups (Fig. 2.1).

Is the pain coming from the back?

The first step is to be sure that back pain is due to a musculoskeletal problem in the back. This is obvious, but we often take it for granted and sometimes forget other possibilities. We must exclude back pain due to disease elsewhere in the body.

Back pain usually dominates the clinical picture of a low back problem and the patient often has other low back symptoms such as stiffness and tenderness.

Occasionally, back pain comes from the abdominal or pelvic organs, but these rarely present as back pain alone. There are nearly always some gastrointestinal, urinary, or gynecologic symptoms. Renal lesions may give loin pain with classic radiation. If the history raises suspicion, you should palpate the abdomen and perform a rectal exam, but you do not need to do so in every patient with backache.

Back pain may be only one part of a systemic musculoskeletal or rheumatologic problem, but this should be clear from the history. Low back pain often spreads to the buttocks and hips and you should then exclude a hip problem. The patient may describe problems with walking and hip movements. Your examination of the back should always include the range of hip movement and gait pattern. Leg symptoms may be due to peripheral vascular disease. Symptoms of vascular claudication usually affect muscle groups of the leg rather than dermatomes. There are circulatory symptoms rather than sensory symptoms, and peripheral pulses and circulation may be poor.

You should usually be able to distinguish gastrointestinal, genitourinary, hip, or vascular disease, *if you think about them.* We miss them when we do not think, but just assume that every patient who presents with back pain must have a spinal problem. We must allow patients time to describe their symptoms and hear what they tell us. But not just hear: we must make the effort to listen and to understand. Above all, we must not focus too quickly on leading questions about the back.

Major spinal deformity and widespread neurologic disorders

Major spinal deformity and widespread neurologic disorders are rare but should be obvious – again, provided you are aware.

You should not miss a major deformity such as a kyphosis or structural scoliosis *providing you get the patient to undress.* This may seem obvious, but one recent survey found that more than 50% of patients with back pain said their doctor had never examined them. In backache the common deformity is a list (Fig. 2.2). Muscle spasm pulls the spine to one side when the patient is standing and may also cause loss of the lumbar lordosis. In true scoliosis there is a fixed deformity with compensatory curves above and below (Fig. 2.2). A spinal list usually, but not always, improves when the patient lies prone and the muscles relax, but true scoliosis never changes. You can see early scoliosis as a rib hump when the patient reaches down to his or her toes.

You should not miss a widespread neurologic disorder provided you think how the patient's

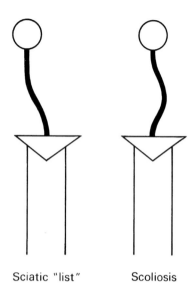

Sciatic "list"   Scoliosis

Figure 2.2   List due to muscle spasm vs structural scoliosis. With muscle spasm the trunk is offset on the pelvis when erect, but this often corrects when the patient is prone. A structural scoliosis usually has compensatory curves above and below, so the trunk is still centered on the pelvis. A structural deformity persists at all times, even when the patient is anesthetized, and there is a rib hump when bending forward.

symptoms fit anatomy. Most local problems in the lower back affect a single nerve root, with dermatomal numbness or paresthesia, or muscle weakness in a single myotome. If neurologic symptoms or signs affect several nerve roots or both legs, then there may be a more widespread neurologic disorder. You should look for a few key symptoms. There may be unsteadiness or gait disturbance. Urinary retention is an emergency. If there is loss of bladder sensation, the patient may instead complain of difficulty passing urine or overflow incontinence. Some neurologic diseases may also give symptoms in the arms or cranial nerves. If you have any suspicion, you should do a more thorough neurologic exam, although you can still pick up the key features in a few minutes (Box 2.4).

The detection of serious spinal pathology

Serious spinal pathology accounts for less than 1% of all back pain. Serious pathology is rare, but one of our most important jobs is to detect it or to

Box 2.4   General neurologic examination when there is a question of widespread neurology

- Brief sensory testing of the arms, the trunk dermatomes, and the saddle area
- Palpate the bladder
- Upper motor neurone signs in the legs include increased muscle tone, brisk reflexes, clonus, upgoing plantar reflexes, loss of position sense in the toes and loss of coordination in the heel–shin test

exclude it and reassure the patient. Indeed, some patients say this is their only reason for coming to see a doctor. If we can assure them there is nothing serious, then they can deal with their backache themselves. That depends on confident reassurance. Bringing the patient back "to check" raises doubt that you are not sure or, worse, that there may be something serious you are hiding. All we need at this point is a simple yet reliable screen to decide if there is any risk of serious spinal pathology. Diagnosis of the pathology can come later. Triage simply decides if there is a need for further investigation and referral, or if we can rule out serious spinal pathology.

Most backache affects the lower back or neck. It varies with time and physical activity. It presents in the early to middle years of adult life. It does not affect general health. Serious spinal pathology presents the opposite features. In our series of 900 patients, we found that a few key features detected all 73 patients with serious spinal pathology. Deyo et al (1992) produced a similar list. AHCPR (1994) and RCGP (1999) called these "red flags" for possible serious spinal pathology (Box 2.3).

The concepts of triage and red flags seem to have caught people's imagination and helped to sell this approach.

Age

Most backache presents in the early or middle years of adult life. Patients who present for health care before the age of 20 are more likely to have serious pathology or a structural problem such as

spondylolisthesis. Patients who develop new or different back pain after the age of 55 are more likely to have serious pathology, particularly spinal metastases or osteoporosis.

Non-mechanical back pain

Ordinary backache is mechanical in the sense that it varies with physical activity. Certain postures or movements may make the pain worse. A comfortable position, change of position, stretching, or certain exercises may make the pain better. The pain varies over the course of the day or weeks in response to different activities or treatment.

In contrast, non-mechanical back pain is unrelated to time or activity. It may start spontaneously and gradually. It often becomes gradually worse. Rest or exercises do not relieve it and the patient may not be able to find any position of comfort. Pain may be worse in bed at night when the patient has no distractions.

Thoracic pain

Most mechanical problems affect the lower back or the neck. Pain in the thoracic spine or between the shoulder blades is less common but when it does occur is more likely to be due to serious pathology. In our selected series, 30% of patients referred to hospital with thoracic pain had either spinal pathology or osteoporotic collapse of a vertebra.

Violent trauma

Only violent trauma, such as a fall from a height or a road traffic accident, is likely to fracture the normal spine. Postmenopausal women with osteoporosis or patients on systemic steroids may suffer collapsed vertebrae as a result of more minor injury.

Previous medical history

Many systemic diseases can affect the back. A history of carcinoma is most important, however long ago. A history of rheumatologic disorders, tuberculosis, and any recent infection may be relevant. Drug abuse, immune suppression and human immunodeficiency virus (HIV) may predispose to infection. Systemic steroids may cause osteoporosis.

Systemic symptoms

Patients with ordinary backache are generally healthy. If a patient with back pain is unwell, there is more likely to be some serious disease. The most significant symptom is weight loss. General malaise, fever, or simple clinical impression may all raise suspicion. However, many patients with a spinal infection do not have fever, so the absence of fever does not exclude infection. If the clinical history raises your suspicions, your examination should include the common tumor sites – thyroid, breasts, lymph nodes, abdomen, and prostate. You may also order urine testing, an erythrocyte sedimentation rate (ESR), and a chest X-ray.

Limited lumbar flexion

Clinical examination of the spine is not very good for detecting spinal pathology, apart from major spinal deformities and widespread neurologic disorders. So a normal examination does not exclude serious pathology, particularly metastases.

The most important physical sign in the back itself is persistent severe restriction of lumbar flexion. In our series, 50% of patients with limited lumbar flexion had either serious spinal pathology or an acute disk prolapse. Lumbar flexion was severely restricted in 70% of patients with spinal infection. However, flexion was normal in 30% of patients with spinal infection, in 81% with inflammatory disease, and in 91% with spinal metastases. Spinal pathology can be present in the thoracic spine without any restriction of lumbar movement. *Remember that a normal physical exam does not exclude serious spinal pathology.*

We must also improve how we measure lumbar flexion. How close you can reach towards your toes does not test spinal movement, but depends on a combination of lumbar and hip flexion, hamstring tightness, and motivation. Some patients with ankylosing spondylitis and a fused lumbar spine can still touch their toes (Fig. 2.3). So if we want to measure spinal movement we must measure the back itself. The simplest method is the Schober technique. Make two marks on the skin and see how much they move apart as the patient bends forward (Fig. 2.4). This gives a reliable measure of lumbar flexion. We will discuss more precise

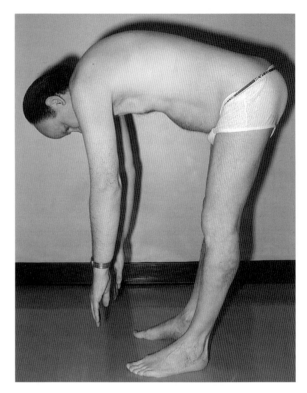

Figure 2.3   The distance from the fingers to the ground does not measure lumbar flexion. Look at the shadow on the wall showing no loss of lumbar lordosis in this patient with ankylosing spondylitis.

methods using an inclinometer when we look at the evaluation of physical impairment in Chapter 8, but this simple method is sufficient for routine clinical use.

Summary: possible serious spinal pathology

- The most important screen for serious spinal pathology is a careful clinical history of red flags.
- A normal physical exam does not exclude serious spinal pathology.
- A normal X-ray does not rule out spinal pathology.

Triage is based on red flags, but the problem is that individual red flags are not very accurate for diagnosing pathology (van den Hoogen et al 1995). There are too many false-negatives and false-positives. So it is a question of clinical judgment,

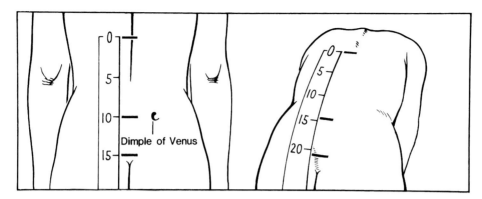

Figure 2.4   The Schober technique of measuring lumbar flexion. Make a mark at the level of the dimples of Venus, which approximates to the lumbosacral junction. Make a second mark 10 cm higher, and a third mark 5 cm lower. Ask patients to reach down as far as they can towards their toes, and measure the increase in the distance between the top and bottom marks. The normal is at least 5 cm. From Waddell (1982), with permission.

combining all the clinical features. If there are no red flags on careful clinical assessment, you can be 99% confident that you have not missed any serious spinal pathology. If there are some red flags, it still depends on clinical judgment. With typical, mechanical low back pain after a minor lifting injury in an 18-year-old, it would be reasonable to wait and see how the patient gets on before considering any referral or investigation. A 60-year-old who presents with several months' gradual onset of new thoracic pain and weight loss needs urgent investigation, even if clinical exam and plain X-rays are completely normal.

The aim of triage is to decide if there is any question of possible serious spinal pathology. Exact diagnosis will come later. Triage is only to decide which patients need further investigation.

The interpretation of leg pain

One of the most common mistakes is to assume that all leg pain is sciatica, and must be due to a disk prolapse pressing on a nerve. That is false logic. Leg pain *may* be nerve root pain due to a disk prolapse pressing on a root, but more often it is not. Most leg pain is not nerve root pain, and has nothing to do with a disk prolapse. There is so much confusion about the term "sciatica" that it is better not to use it. Sciatica is pain in the distribution of the sciatic nerve, but different doctors and therapists use the term differently, varying from any leg pain

to a precise definition of nerve root pain. We will think and communicate more clearly if we talk about referred leg pain and nerve root pain.

It is nearly 60 years since Kellgren (1939) showed that stimulation of any of the tissues of the back can cause pain down one or both legs. Seventy percent of patients with back pain have some radiation of pain to their legs. This referred pain can come from the fascia, muscles, ligaments, periosteum, facet joints, disk, or epidural structures. It is usually a dull, poorly localized ache that spreads into the buttocks and thighs (Fig. 2.5). It may affect both legs. It usually does not go much below the knee. Referred pain is not due to anything pressing on a nerve. It is not sciatica.

Stimulation of the nerve root gives a quite different pain, which is sharp and well localized (Fig. 2.6). At the common L5 or S1 levels, nerve root pain usually radiates to the foot or toes. It at least approximates to a dermatomal distribution. Patients often describe the pain with sensory qualities such as pins and needles, or numbness. It usually affects one leg only and is greater than back pain. Nerve root pain is much less common than referred leg pain.

Triage should distinguish referred leg pain from nerve root pain. You can usually make a provisional decision from the patient's description of the pain. If a patient presents with back pain alone and no leg pain or neurologic symptoms, a nerve root problem is very unlikely. There is then no need for any neurologic exam. If the patient does have leg

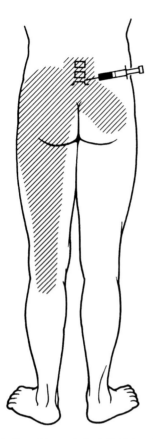
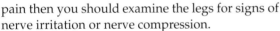

Figure 2.5   Referred leg pain is dull, ill-localized, and usually does not radiate much below the knee(s). From Waddell (1982), with permission.

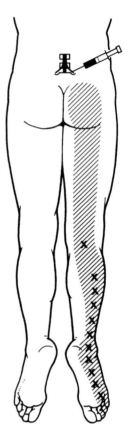

Figure 2.6   Nerve root pain usually radiates to the foot or toes and at least approximates to a dermatome. From Waddell (1982), with permission.

pain then you should examine the legs for signs of nerve irritation or nerve compression.

Nerve irritation and compression signs help to confirm the diagnosis of nerve root pain. Ninety-eight percent of disk prolapses are at L4/L5 or L5/S1 and affect the L5 or S1 roots, and most clinical tests look at these levels. Textbooks emphasize motor, sensory, and reflex signs, but these only occur when there is actual compromise of nerve function. Nerve irritation signs are earlier and more common, and just as important for diagnosis.

Root irritation signs

Nerve irritation signs depend on tests that stretch or press on an irritable nerve root to cause root pain. The diagnostic finding is this *reproduction of symptomatic nerve pain*. Straight leg raising is the most

widely used test for nerve irritation (Deville et al 2000) but many doctors and therapists still misinterpret it. Limited straight leg raising in itself is not a sign of nerve irritation. The key finding is not the limitation, but the reason for it. Limitation due to back pain or hamstring spasm probably has nothing to do with irritation of a nerve. The specific sign of nerve irritation is limited straight leg raising due to reproduction of nerve pain down the leg (Edgar & Park 1974; Fig. 2.7). Pain may only radiate to the thigh and not down the full length of the dermatome. Passive dorsiflexion of the foot at the limit of straight leg raising may increase the leg pain or make it radiate more distally.

Other signs of nerve irritation also depend on reproducing nerve pain. A positive cough impulse is pain down the leg, not back pain alone. The well-leg raising test or cross-over sign uses passive straight

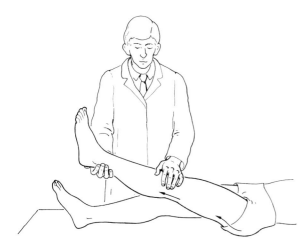

Figure 2.7   The diagnostic feature of straight leg raising is reproduction of the symptomatic root pain.

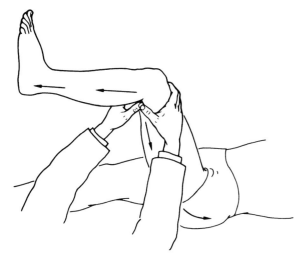

Figure 2.8   The diagnostic feature of the bowstring test is reproduction of the symptomatic root pain or paresthesia.

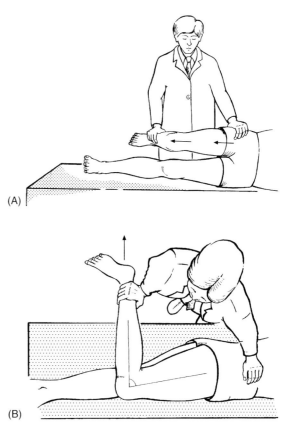

(A)

(B)

Figure 2.9 (A, B)   The diagnostic feature of the femoral stretch test is reproduction of the symptomatic root pain.

stretch test (Fig. 2.9). The diagnostic finding of nerve irritation is again radiating nerve pain in the anterior thigh and not back pain. You should distinguish that from hip disease or a tight quadriceps muscle.

Nerve compression signs

Neurologic signs include muscle wasting, motor weakness, sensory change, or a depressed tendon reflex. These are traditionally called nerve compression signs, though that is perhaps simplistic. Whatever the exact mechanism, they show that nerve function is compromised. Most low back problems affect a single nerve root, although they occasionally affect the same nerve root to both legs. Nerve function is usually only depressed because of overlap from adjacent roots. Complete anesthesia or paralysis is rare, so you must look for minor neurologic changes. You should check each

leg raising of the painfree leg to give nerve pain in the symptomatic leg. The bowstring test is better known in North America than in Europe (Fig. 2.8). At the end of the straight leg raising test, slightly flex the knee to relieve pain. Then press your thumb on the nerve where it is bowstrung across the popliteal fossa. With an irritable nerve, you may produce pain or paresthesia radiating up or down the leg. Local pain beneath your thumb is not diagnostic.

If the pattern of pain suggests an upper lumbar nerve root, then you should also do the femoral

Table 2.2   The nerve supply of the L4–S1 nerve roots

	L4	L5	S1
Distribution of pain and sensory disturbance	Anterior thigh	Dorsum of foot Great toe	Lateral border of foot Sole
Motor weakness	Quadriceps (Dorsiflexion ankle)	Dorsiflexion ankle Eversion ankle Dorsiflexion toes[a]	Plantar flexion ankle (Dorsiflexion great toe)
Reflex	Knee jerk	(Ankle jerk)	Ankle jerk

[a]An L5 lesion usually only affects some of these muscles.

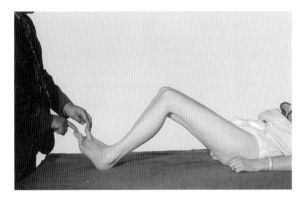

Figure 2.10   Clinical exam for motor weakness should test each myotome in turn, comparing the two legs for minor differences.

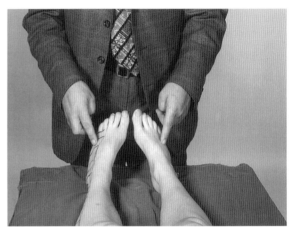

Figure 2.11   Clinical exam for sensory changes should test each dermatome in turn, comparing the two legs for minor differences.

dermatome and myotome in turn (Table 2.2) and the best way to detect minor change is to compare the two legs (Figs 2.10–2.12).

The common L5 and S1 signs are weakness of the ankle and toes, sensory loss in the foot, and a diminished ankle reflex (Table 2.2). You should concentrate on these unless symptoms suggest a higher lumbar root or a widespread neurologic disorder.

The exact pattern of leg pain and a brief examination for nerve irritation and compression signs should usually allow you to diagnose a nerve root problem. Referred leg pain is simply part of more severe, but still "ordinary" backache.

INVESTIGATIONS

When there are clinical red flags, the ESR and plain X-rays should form part of your routine assessment.

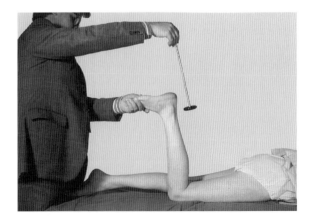

Figure 2.12   Examination for minor changes in the reflexes depends on the patient being relaxed.

You do not need them in every patient with recent onset of ordinary backache. You must be clear about the role and limitations of these tests. The ESR and plain X-rays are complementary. X-rays show anatomic detail and structural problems that may not affect the ESR. The ESR is sensitive to soft-tissue or systemic disease that may not affect bones. The ESR may also rise earlier while radiographic changes take time to develop.

The erythrocyte sedimentation rate

The ESR is old-fashioned and non-specific, but it is still a useful screening test for disease. It is simple and easy to perform and the result can be ready while the patient is having X-rays or seeing a therapist.

The limitation is that the ESR is quite crude, with many false-negatives and -positives, and so a normal ESR does not exclude disease. We must also use the ESR in a way that reduces the impact of false-positives. The upper limit of normal in the standard Westergren method is variously given as 15–25 mm in the first hour. In our series only one patient with serious spinal pathology fell between these limits, so in this context I feel it is better to use a limit of 25 mm. In our series, all the patients with a raised ESR due to serious spinal pathology also had clinical red flags. Twenty-seven patients with a raised ESR but no clinical red flags all turned out after investigation and follow-up to have no spinal pathology. So I suggest that you use the ESR selectively. If there are no clinical red flags, then do not do an ESR, because it would be more likely to mislead than to help triage. If there are clinical red flags, then perform the ESR while the patient is having X-rays. A raised ESR provides a useful check on your clinical triage and supports the need for further investigation. A normal ESR and normal X-rays mean that serious spinal pathology is less likely, but you must still judge on the basis of the clinical red flags whether this patient needs further referral or investigation.

Plain X-rays

The main value of plain X-rays is to show structural problems in the bones. The main limitation is that they do not show soft-tissue problems such as backache or a disk prolapse. X-rays are the first

investigation in trauma if there is any question of a possible fracture. Most serious spinal pathology affects the vertebral body and shows on X-rays as bone destruction. New bone formation is less common. However, these bone changes are non-specific. The pattern of radiographic change may suggest a diagnosis, but this is unreliable. X-rays cannot diagnose histology or bacteriology and it is wiser not to attempt specific diagnosis from X-rays. Bone destruction must also have advanced beyond a certain point before it will show on X-ray. Routine spinal X-rays do not detect osteoporosis until there is 30% loss of the bone mass. A lateral X-ray of the lumbar spine will only detect a focal lesion when at least 50% of the cancellous bone is destroyed, and there must be even greater destruction for it to show on the anteroposterior view. So X-rays can only detect pathology after it has been present for a certain time or reached a certain stage. The most virulent disk infection may not show any radiographic change for several weeks. Metastases may take many months to show on X-ray. *A normal X-ray does not rule out spinal pathology.*

Nachemson claims that if there are no red flags on careful clinical assessment then X-rays only detect significant spinal pathology once in 2500 patients. The caveat is "on careful clinical assessment." Spinal X-rays cannot compensate for inadequate clinical assessment.

There are now guidelines on the use of plain lumbar X-rays (Ch. 15), but efforts to reduce the number of unnecessary X-rays have had limited success (Jarvik 2001). X-rays of the lumbar spine still account for 5% of all radiographic exams in UK National Health Service hospitals (Kendrick et al 2001). Several recent studies may help to explain this. Kerry et al (2000) did a randomized controlled trial (RCT) of routine X-ray for patients with back pain in UK primary care. Early X-ray did not improve physical outcomes, or the number of repeat consultations or specialist referrals. The authors claimed X-ray improved psychological well-being over the next 12 months, but that was based on a single question that reached borderline significance. Routine X-rays led to higher irradiation and costs, for no clear benefit. Kendrick et al (2001) did another RCT in UK primary care. Patients who got X-rays reported *more* pain and poorer general health status at 3 months. Selim et al (2000) found that US patients with more severe pain and disability were more likely to be X-rayed, which is as expected. However, repeated X-rays were associated with more distress and poorer mental health rather than any physical indications. They suggested that repeat lumbar X-rays in particular are overused, and often inappropriate. Espeland et al (2001) found that Norwegian patients' views on the value of lumbar X-rays depended on several factors (Table 2.3). Inappropriate referrals were associated with stronger beliefs about the importance and usefulness of X-rays. They suggested other and better strategies to address patients' concerns (Table 2.3).

For all these reasons, routine X-rays have little value or place in ordinary backache. We should only order X-rays when there are clinical indications and when they are likely to produce useful further information.

MRI

Over the last two decades there have been great advances in sophisticated imaging. Computed tomography (CT) and magnetic resonance imaging (MRI) now provide wonderful information about the anatomy of spinal pathology and neurologic compression, which is what they were designed for. For the patient who needs investigation of possible spinal pathology or who needs surgery, MRI is the investigation of choice. (Even if I sometimes wonder if we may have lost sight of the old-fashioned bone scan.)

But we must be equally clear about the limitations of imaging. X-rays do not tell us much about ordinary backache (with the possible exception of pain provocation techniques). MRI images are much more impressive but still tell us little, if anything, about backache. Most of the findings bear little relationship to clinical symptoms and are equally common in patients with back pain and normal asymptomatic people. Most degenerative changes are a normal age-related process. We now realize back pain is usually due to conditions that cannot be diagnosed on imaging and most images do not help routine management of ordinary backache (Jarvik & Deyo 2000).

Table 2.3 Patients' concerns, lumbar X-rays, and reassurance

Issue of importance to patients	Suggested strategies
Severe, worsening, and worrisome symptoms	Clearer indications for X-ray, which may need to be narrowed
Advice from doctors	Doctors should follow guidelines on indications for lumbar X-rays. They should elicit and discuss issues of importance to the patient. They may then negotiate with patients to influence their expectations of X-rays
Need for emotional support from doctor	Consider the patient's concerns and how this need might be better met in other ways
Need for certainty and reassurance	Reassurance may be given by careful clinical history and exam, and by information and advice tailored to the individual patient. Do not rely on X-rays for reassurance (they are often counterproductive)
Need for explanation of symptoms and diagnosis	X-rays rarely provide this in ordinary backache! Explore patients' own views of what is wrong and what other explanations they may have received. Provide simple, accurate explanations
Belief that X-rays are more reliable than clinical exam	Explain that a careful clinical history and exam can usually exclude serious disease and are actually more reliable than X-rays
Expectation that X-rays will lead to treatment, referral, compensation, etc.	Explain the limitations of X-rays for diagnosis and treatment of ordinary backache. X-rays should only be used for clinical X-rays and not as the basis for receiving care or compensation

Adapted from Espeland et al (2001).

These investigations were not designed for diagnostic triage. Imaging has become more and more sensitive, but the more sensitive the investigation, the higher the number of false-positive findings in normal people (Table 2.4). These are very inefficient screening tools.

The role of investigations

As a clinician, I would argue strongly that diagnostic triage should be based on clinical assessment. There is a growing tendency to rely on imaging, but that is no substitute for a focused clinical history and physical exam. Deyo (1995) offers a very good introduction to understanding the accuracy of diagnostic tests.

Some doctors argue that we can use such tests to reassure patients, but I believe that is a false argument. Overall, the trials suggest that X-rays do *not* reassure patients and reduce distress. Rather, the decision to order an X-ray may cause worry that the doctor thinks there may be something serious. Even a normal test result may not outweigh that anxiety (McDonald et al 1996). And any minor radiologic "abnormalities" may be disastrous. The trouble is that modern high-quality images are seductive and almost irresistible. The greatest risk is that minor changes, and even false-positive findings, may then drive clinical management. We fall into the trap of treating images instead of patients. Beware of shadows on the wall! The more subtle danger is that imaging becomes a lazy substitute for a careful clinical history and exam, and proper clinical decision-making. There is growing concern about the amount of radiation from plain X-rays. A standard set of three lumbosacral views gives 120 times the radiation dose of a chest X-ray. These investigations are also expensive and use health care money that could be spent in better ways for the patient with ordinary backache.

Diagnostic triage is a clinical decision, based on clinical assessment. Investigations should be based on clear indications, and used when the likely benefits outweigh the risks and costs. When there is real doubt that might influence management, then of course you should use investigations to supplement the decision. But you must be clear what information you are looking for and select the investigation that will answer your question. You must match the investigation results to the clinical findings and always remain aware of the role and limitations of each investigation. The best image is no substitute for a proper clinical assessment and diagnostic triage will always be a clinical decision.

THE MAJOR CLINICAL PROBLEM

Diagnostic triage takes much longer to explain than to carry out in practice. Start from the main presenting symptoms. Clinical history and physical exam focus on the key items of information to answer the diagnostic questions. This should lead automatically to triage into one of three major clinical problems (Figs 2.1 and 2.13). Each of these clinical problems has different prognosis, investigations, and treatment. Thus triage sets the scene for management and final outcome.

One of the most common fears of all health professionals working with back pain is that we will miss the patient with serious pathology. This is understandable, particularly in primary care where such pathology is rare. However, we are all so aware of the danger that with the present approach and reasonable care the risk is very low. We must get triage into perspective. Most back pain is benign and non-specific and all the serious problems put together are probably less than 5%. In the case of serious spinal pathology, it is better to err on the

Table 2.4 The false-positive rate of radiographic investigations in normal asymptomatic people. The more sensitive the test, the higher the false-positive rate

	Degenerative and other abnormalities (%)	Disk prolapse (%)
Plain radiographs	0–90	–
Oil myelography	20	4
Water-soluble myelography	25	10
CT scan	10–35	10–20
MRI scan	35–90	20–35

When there is a range, it shows the increase with age.
CT, computed tomography; MRI, magnetic resonance imaging.
See also Jarvik & Deyo (2000), Nachemson & Vingard (2000).

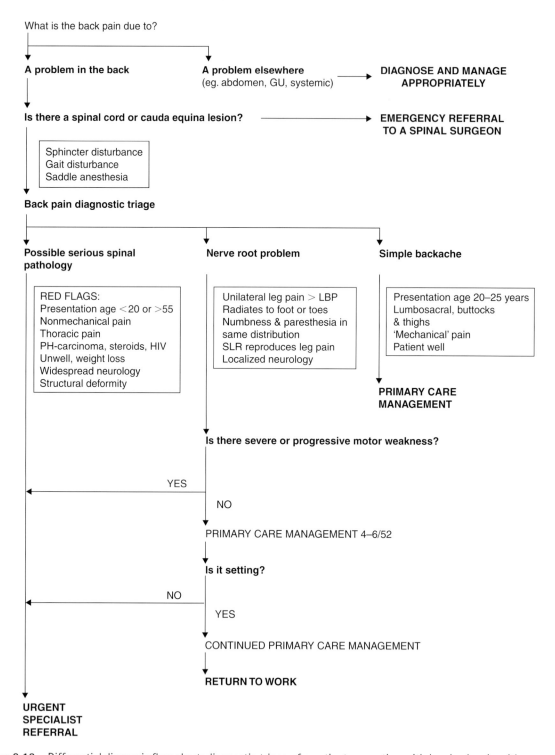

What is the back pain due to?

A problem in the back

A problem elsewhere
(eg. abdomen, GU, systemic) → DIAGNOSE AND MANAGE
APPROPRIATELY

Is there a spinal cord or cauda equina lesion? → EMERGENCY REFERRAL
TO A SPINAL SURGEON

Sphincter disturbance
Gait disturbance
Saddle anesthesia

Back pain diagnostic triage

Possible serious spinal pathology

Nerve root problem

Simple backache

RED FLAGS:
Presentation age <20 or >55
Nonmechanical pain
Thoracic pain
PH-carcinoma, steroids, HIV
Unwell, weight loss
Widespread neurology
Structural deformity

Unilateral leg pain > LBP
Radiates to foot or toes
Numbness & paresthesia in same distribution
SLR reproduces leg pain
Localized neurology

Presentation age 20–25 years
Lumbosacral, buttocks & thighs
'Mechanical' pain
Patient well

PRIMARY CARE
MANAGEMENT

Is there severe or progressive motor weakness?

YES

NO

PRIMARY CARE MANAGEMENT 4–6/52

Is it setting?

NO

YES

CONTINUED PRIMARY CARE MANAGEMENT

RETURN TO WORK

URGENT
SPECIALIST
REFERRAL

Figure 2.13   Differential diagnosis flow chart: diagnostic triage of a patient presenting with low back pain with or without sciatica. GU, genitourinary; PH, previous history; HIV, human immunodeficiency virus; LBP, low back pain; SLR, straight leg raising. After CSAG (1994), with permission.

side of caution and investigate further when there is any doubt. In the case of nerve root pain, however, overdiagnosis is likely to be more harmful than underdiagnosis. The most common mistake in practice is to overdiagnose nerve root problems, and here the sins of commission are worse than those of omission. It may be helpful to take a legal perspective: how much real evidence do you have of a nerve root problem and how would that evidence stand up in a court of law? Stop and think before you rush into action.

I must offer one caveat. This approach is logical and has a strong clinical basis. I have found it highly successful in my clinical practice over many years, and to the best of my knowledge I have rarely missed anything serious. Practicing all that time in one tightly knit and stable community we all

heard about our mistakes! All my fellows have found it equally successful. Family doctors have welcomed the triage approach in clinical guidelines. But as van den Hoogen et al (1995) and Little et al (1996) point out, there is limited empiric evidence on its effectiveness in primary care. This approach was developed in hospital practice, where patients are already preselected. The basic problem and the approach are the same in primary care, but clinical presentations and decision-making may be subtly different. We need more primary care studies on the accuracy of diagnostic triage and referral.

Despite that caveat, triage is fundamental: ordinary backache, nerve root pain, or possible serious spinal pathology. The rest of this book is about the complex and fascinating problem of "simple" backache.

References

Abraham I, Killackey-Jones B, Deyo R A 2002 Controversies in internal medicine. (Specific -v- non-specific diagnosis in low back pain.) Archives of Internal Medicine 162: 1442–1448

AHCPR 1994 Clinical practice guideline number 14. Acute low back problems in adults. Agency for Health Care Policy and Research, US Department of Health and Human Services, Rockville, MD

Binkley J, Finch E, Hall J, Black T, Gowland C 1993 Diagnostic classification of patients with low back pain: report on a survey of physical therapy experts. Physical Therapy 73: 138–155

Bogduk N 1999 Draft clinical practice guidelines for the management of acute low back pain. Prepared on behalf of the Australasian Faculty of Musculoskeletal Medicine for the National Musculoskeletal Medicine Initiative

Bogduk N, Govind J 1999 Medical management of acute lumbar radicular pain: an evidence-based approach. Newcastle Bone and Joint Institute, Newcastle, New South Wales

CSAG 1994 Clinical Standards Advisory Group report on back pain. HMSO, London

Delitto A, Cibulka M T, Erhard R E et al 1993 Evidence for use of an extension–mobilization category in acute low back syndrome: a prescriptive validation pilot study. Physical Therapy 73: 216

Deville W L J M, van der Windt D A W M, Dzafeeragic A, Bezemer P D, Bouter L M 2000 The test of Lasegue: systematic review of the accuracy in diagnosing herniated discs. Spine 25: 1140–1147

Deyo R A 1995 Understanding the accuracy of diagnostic tests. In: Weinstein J N, Ryderik B L, Sonntag K H (eds) Essentials of the spine. Raven, New York, pp 55–69

Deyo R A, Rainville J, Kent D L 1992 What can the history and physical examination tell us about low back pain? Journal of the American Medical Association 268: 760–765

Edgar M A, Park W M 1974 Induced pain patterns on passive straight leg raising in lower lumbar disc protrusion. Journal of Bone and Joint Surgery 56B: 658–667

Espeland A, Baerheim A, Abrektsen G, Korsbrekke K, Larsen J L 2001 Patients' views on importance and usefulness of plain radiography for low back pain. Spine 26: 1356–1363

Jarvik J G 2001 Editorial: Don't duck the evidence. Spine 26: 1306–1307

Jarvik J G, Deyo R A 2000 Imaging of lumbar intervertebral disk degeneration and ageing, excluding disk herniation. Radiological Clinics of North America 38: 1255–1266

Kellgren J H 1939 On the distribution of pain arising from deep somatic structures with charts of segmental pain areas. Clinical Science 4: 35–46

Kendrick D, Fielding K, Bentley E et al 2001 Radiography of the lumbar spine in primary care patients with low back pain: randomised controlled trial. British Medical Journal 322: 400–405

Kerry S, Hilton S, Patel S, Dundas D, Rink E, Lord J 2000 Routine referral for radiography of patients presenting with low back pain: is patients' outcome influenced by GPs' referral for plain radiography? Health Technology Assessment 4: no. 20. Available online at: www.ncchta.org

Little P, Smith L, Cantrell T, Chapman J, Langridge J, Pickering R 1996 General practitioners' management of acute back pain: a survey of reported practice compared with clinical guidelines. British Medical Journal 312: 485–488

McDonald I G, Daly J, Jelink V M, Panetta F, Gutman J M 1996 Opening Pandora's box: the unpredictability of reassurance by a normal test result. British Medical Journal 313: 329–332

Merskey H, Bogduk N (eds) 1994 Classification of chronic pain. Descriptions of chronic pain syndromes and definition of pain terms, 2nd edn. International Association for the Study of Pain (IASP) Press, Seattle

Moffroid M T, Haugh L D, Henry S M, Short B 1994 Distinguishable groups of musculoskeletal low back pain patients and asymptomatic control subjects based on physical measures of the NIOSH low back atlas. Spine 19: 1350–1358

Nachemson A, Vingard E 2000 Assessment of patients with neck and back pain: a best-evidence synthesis. In: Nachemson A, Jonsson E (eds) Neck and back pain: the scientific evidence of causes, diagnosis and treatment. Lippincott Williams & Wilkins: Philadephia, pp. 189–235

RCGP 1996, 1999 Clinical guidelines for the management of acute low back pain. Royal College of General Practitioners, London

Selim A J, Fincke G, Ren X S, Deyo R A, Lee A, Skinner K, Kazis L 2000 Patient characteristics and patterns of use for lumbar spine radiographs. Spine 25: 2440–2444

Spitzer W O, Leblanc F E, Dupuis M et al 1987 Scientific approach to the assessment and management of activity-related spinal disorders. A monograph for physicians. Report of the Quebec Task Force on spinal disorders. Spine 12 (7S) s1–s59

van den Hoogen H M M, Koes B W, van Eijk J T H M, Bouter L M 1995 On the accuracy of history, physical examination and erythrocyte sedimentation rate in diagnosing low-back pain in general practice. A criteria-based review of the literature. Spine 20: 318–327

von Korff M, Moore J C 2001 Stepped care for back pain: activating approaches for primary care. Annals of Internal Medicine 134: 911–917

Waddell G 1982 An approach to backache. British Journal of Hospital Medicine 23: 187–219

Chapter 3

Pain and disability

This book is about low back pain and disability. Before we go any further, we need to look more closely at pain and disability and the difference between them.

Pain and disability often go together. We talk about them as if they were one and the same, but that kind of sloppy thinking leads to much confusion. Pain and disability are not the same, and we must make a clear distinction between them in our thinking and in clinical practice. This is equally true of assessment and of management.

Pain is a symptom, not a clinical sign, or a diagnosis, or a disease. Disability is restricted activity. We cannot assess pain directly, but always depend on the patient's report of his or her experience. So the report of the symptom of pain depends on how the patient thinks and feels and how he or she communicates it. Assessment of disability also relies on patients' own reports of what they do or do not do, so again it is subjective and open to these same influences.

Failure to distinguish pain and disability has a major impact on management. Many patients, doctors, and therapists assume it is simply a question of pain causing disability and so if we treat the pain, disability will disappear. Too often, that just does not work. This is partly because our treatment for back pain is not very effective. More fundamentally, it is because there is not a simple 1:1 relationship between pain and disability.

I believe one of the roots of our current difficulty dealing with back pain is this assumption that pain and disability are the same. It is a basic mistake that has had far-reaching consequences. Pain and disability are obviously related to each other, but they are quite different aspects of the illness. Having back pain and being disabled by it are not the same. Clinical experience shows that back pain does not always lead to disability, and that the amount of disability is not always proportionate to the severity of pain. We often see patients who manage to lead surprisingly normal lives despite serious spinal pathology or severe pain. Yet ordinary backache may totally and permanently disable other patients, even when they have little objective pathology. Closer scientific study confirms that the relationship between pain and disability is weaker than we might think.

- Pain is a symptom.
- Disability is restricted activity.
- Clinical assessment relies on the patient's *report* of pain and disability.

PAIN

Pain is the main presenting symptom in 99% of patients with back trouble. Pain is the most common symptom in health care, but despite this it is one of the least understood. Lewis was one of the modern pioneers of the study of pain, yet he freely admitted the problem in the opening sentences of his classic book (Lewis 1942):

> Reflection tells me that I am so far from being able satisfactorily to define pain, of which I here write, that the attempt could serve no useful purpose. Pain, like similar subjective things, is known to us by experience and described by illustration. The usage of the term in this book will be clear enough to anyone who reads its pages. To build up a definition in words or to substitute some phrase would carry neither the reader nor myself farther. But in using the undefined word it is necessary to take care that it is never allowed to confuse phenomena that may be distinct. When there is such possibility, the bare word pain is not enough; it needs and will be given qualification.

Over 60 years on, we should still heed Lewis's warning! Descartes (1596–1650), the leading

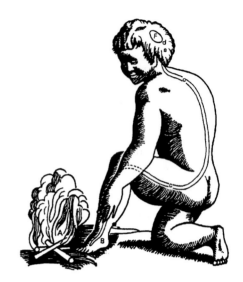

Figure 3.1   The traditional Cartesian model of specific pain pathways.

If for example fire (A) comes near the foot (B), the minute particles of this fire, which as you know have a great velocity, have the power to set in motion the spot of the skin of the foot which they touch, and by this means pulling upon the delicate thread (c–c) which is attached to the spot of the skin, they open up at the same instant the pore (d–e) against which the delicate thread ends, just as by pulling at one end of a rope one makes to strike at the same instant a bell which hangs on the other end (Descartes 1664, as translated by Foster 1901).

European philosopher after the Renaissance, has had a major impact on western thinking about pain for more than three centuries. What is commonly known as the Cartesian model is a very mechanistic view of pain as a signal of tissue damage (Fig. 3.1).

> A pain, an ache, a discomfort – these are the common complaints of those who seek the doctor's help. Pain issues a warning with kindly intent. She calls to action and, pointing the way, brooks no delay. And thus the ancient cycle is served, from pain to cause, to treatment to cure (Penfield 1969).

In most routine practice, doctors and therapists still consider pain in this way – "pain-as-a-signal." But thoughtful clinicians have always known this does not explain many clinical observations of pain. Different patients with similar injuries seem to experience very different amounts and kinds of pain, and they react in very different ways. When pain becomes chronic, it sometimes seems to become dissociated from any original tissue damage and almost develops an identity of its own. This simple approach to pain may work for acute injury, but it has been much less successful for many chronic pains.

Over the past 30 years we have begun to face up to the clinical reality that pain is more complex. From the time of Aristotle, philosophers have distinguished pain from the five senses and classed it as one of the "passions of the soul." Pain has some elements in common with touch, taste, smell, vision, and hearing. However, Wall (1988) pointed out that we cannot define or identify pain independently of the person who experiences it. We can measure sound waves and the electrical activity in the auditory nerve or cortex, and these correspond to what the listener hears. We have no such objective measure for pain. We can only know that someone is in pain by his or her statements or actions. We may try to measure noxious stimuli, electrical activity in nerves, or brain activity on functional magnetic resonance imaging (MRI), but that tells us little about the individual's experience, much less his or her suffering. Wall suggests that pain functions more as a basic human drive, like hunger or thirst, leading to highly predictable responses. Pain always produces some response in the person experiencing it. It usually also produces some response from those around the individual.

Loeser (1980) described four aspects or dimensions of pain (Fig. 3.2):

1. *Nociception* refers to mechanical or other stimuli that could cause tissue damage. These stimuli act on peripheral pain receptors to produce activity in nerve fibers.

2. *Pain* is the perception of the sensation of pain. This has two important implications. First, we must perceive nociception before it is pain. Second, it is possible to perceive pain even when no tissue damage is occurring.

3. *Suffering* is the unpleasant emotional response generated in higher nervous centers by pain and other emotional situations. Suffering is not unique to pain, but also occurs with grief, stress, anxiety, or depression. Indeed, we often use the

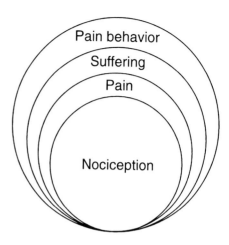

Figure 3.2   Loeser's conceptual model of the dimensions of chronic pain. (From Loeser 1980, with permission.)

language of pain to describe our suffering in these situations. But pain and suffering are different. We can have pain without suffering and suffering without pain.

4. *Pain behavior* includes all acts and conduct that we commonly understand to suggest the presence of pain. Pain behaviors include talking, moaning, facial expressions, and limping, taking painkillers, seeking health care, and stopping work. Note the phrase "which we commonly understand": pain behavior is a form of communication. This does not necessarily mean it is conscious or intended. Most pain behavior is unconscious.

Pain and disability often involve all of these aspects of pain. Treatment of pain-as-a-signal fails to address these other dimensions of pain, which is why it is often unsuccessful.

Loeser's (1980) model begins to give us a better picture of clinical pain, but has a fundamental problem. It uses the word pain in two very different ways: we have the single element of pain-as-a-signal, but we also have pain as the whole experience, in all its complexity. On second thoughts, perhaps this is an accurate reflection of our dilemma. We often confuse pain-as-a-signal with the whole clinical syndrome of pain.

Health care places great emphasis on pain, and most doctors and therapists spend much of their working life treating pain. Engel (1959) suggested that "the relief of pain is the primary social role of the physician." Some idealists still hanker after the unrealistic goal that medicine should provide relief for all pain. The International Pain Foundation states flatly that "no one should have to live with pain" (Liebeskind & Melzack 1987). They then go even further: "By any reasonable code, freedom from pain should be a basic human right, limited only by our knowledge to achieve it." Many philosophers and theologians through history would dispute this as a narrow medical perspective on life. Of course we must improve our management of clinical pain, but we will never abolish all pain and it is supreme medical arrogance even to try.

The same muddled thinking appears in clinical practice. Some workers suggest that the patient's report of pain is the only symptom that matters. That is naive. It presents pain either as a simple physical symptom or so complex that we cannot even attempt to understand it except at the most pragmatic level. I believe that we must understand pain better if we are going to improve our management of back trouble, but we must also deal with clinical reality.

The neurophysiology of pain

Stimulation of a nociceptor produces impulses in peripheral nerves that enter the dorsal column of the spinal cord. Traditional physiology then described specific pain pathways in the spinal cord, leading to the sensory cortex. We might imagine it as a kind of giant telephone exchange. Pressing a peripheral button would ring a bell in the corresponding area of the cortex and bring the stimulus to conscious attention as pain. This oversimplification may seem attractive but it is inaccurate.

Modern neurophysiology provides a more complex but much better basis for understanding clinical pain. There are three fundamental ideas. First, pain signals do not pass unaltered into the central nervous system (CNS), but are filtered, selected, and modulated at every level. Second, pain is not a purely physical sensation that passes all the way up to consciousness and only then produces secondary emotional effects. Emotions are hardwired. The neurophysiology of pain and emotions are closely linked throughout the higher levels of

the CNS. Sensory and emotional events occur simultaneously and influence each other. Third, pain does not depend only on conscious reaction to produce changed behavior. Rather, sensory and motor elements are also closely linked at every level of the CNS, so that pain behavior is an integral part of the pain experience.

Melzack & Wall's (1965) gate control theory of pain crystallized these ideas. Their graphic concept of a pain "gate" made it easy to understand and popularized the theory (Fig. 3.3). Stimulation of nociceptors produces impulses in peripheral nerves that enter the dorsal column of the spinal cord. Melzack & Wall suggested that the dorsal horn then acts as a gate control mechanism. Sensory information arrives in both large and small afferent fibers. Immediate, sharp pain is transmitted by large myelinated A fibers, and slow, diffuse, or aching pain by small unmyelinated C fibers. The balance of activity in different afferent fibers may stimulate or inhibit the next cells in the dorsal horn and so open or close the gate for transmission

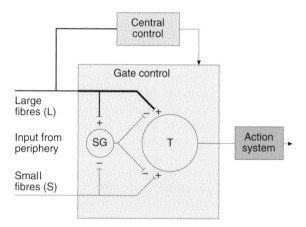

Figure 3.3 Gate control theory I (GCT–I). L, the large diameter fibers. S, the small diameter fibers. The fibers project to the substantia gelatinosa (SG) and first central transmission (T) cells. The inhibitory effect exerted by the SG on the afferent fiber terminals is increased by activity in L fibers and decreased by activity in S fibers. The central control trigger is represented by a line running from the large fiber system to the central control mechanisms; these mechanisms, in turn, project back to the gate control system. The T cells project to the action system (+, excitation, −, inhibition.) From Melzack & Wall 1965, p. 971, reproduced with permission.

of impulses higher up the nervous system. Thresholds to excitation depend on pre-existing levels of activity within the spinal cord. Higher CNS activity can also influence the gate, both by descending nerve impulses (Ren & Dubner 2002) and by the release of analgesic chemicals such as endorphins.

But filtering at the first synapse in the dorsal horn is only the start of a continuous process of selection and modulation of information. It was previously thought that different parts of the CNS might serve different aspects of the pain experience. For example, the spinothalamic tract might process information about the location and sensory qualities of the pain. The brainstem, reticular formation, and limbic system might be more concerned with the emotional or affective qualities of the pain. Fast dorsal column pathways and central control mechanisms at a cortical level might evaluate the sensory information, and relate it to other sensory information and past experience. That might then produce feedback to influence how all the other parts of the system deal with the incoming information. Now, we think instead that it all works as a complex, integrated, neural network or neuromatrix (Melzack 1999). It is genetically determined, but modified by earlier learning. It allows multiple stress, endocrine, autonomic and immune system inputs, and mental functions, as well as the traditional sensory inputs, to interact and modulate pain. Recent studies with functional brain imaging confirm that many parts of the brain are active in pain states (Casey & Bushnell 2000). We are coming back to the holistic view that pain is a response of the whole human brain (Devor 2001).

There is also a close link between afferent and efferent activity at all levels in the nervous system. Segmental reflexes can produce reflex muscle spasm or autonomic activity. Multisegmental efferents from the spinal cord and medulla may produce coordinated motor withdrawal responses. Higher CNS motor activity forms the basis of all pain behavior.

Since 1965, there have been many attacks on the neurophysiologic detail of the gate control theory, but there is now general agreement on the main events (Melzack 1996, Wall 1996). Pain signals do not pass unaltered to the cerebral cortex, but are always and constantly modulated within the CNS before they reach consciousness. Pain, emotions, and pain behavior are all integral parts of the pain experience. The spinal cord and the brain are best seen as a neural matrix rather than as pain tracts. The CNS is not like some enormous telephone exchange, but more like a complex computer network that responds actively to incoming signals.

These concepts provide a physiologic basis for many clinical observations:

- Fundamental to all understanding of pain, they explain how the pain and suffering that we experience may diverge greatly from peripheral nociception.

- Other afferent inputs and neural activity in other parts of the CNS can greatly modify pain signals. This may explain the effects of counterirritation, acupuncture, and transcutaneous electrical nerve stimulation (TENS).

- Pain transmission may be modulated by endorphins. These are chemical substances in the cerebrospinal fluid that act as analgesics like opiates. Certain cells in the CNS produce these and a number of similar substances. The concentration rises in the cerebrospinal fluid after exercise.

- The complex neurophysiology of pain explains why surgical division of a nerve or pain tract is unlikely to give long-term relief of pain. Pain soon recurs and associated sensory disturbance may make it even more unpleasant. This kind of ablative surgery is rarely, if ever, indicated for back pain.

There may also be neurophysiologic changes in chronic pain. The CNS is not a set of rigid electrical circuits, but is plastic in nature. We are all familiar with axon injury and regrowth, but there is little evidence of structural nerve damage in most cases of ordinary backache. Rather, chronic pain may involve more functional changes in the nervous system (Devor 1996, Doubell et al 1999, Ren & Dubner 2002). Tissue damage or inflammation can cause peripheral sensitization of peripheral nociceptors, so that normal stimuli produce pain. Sensory neurones can become hyperexcitable and cause neuropathic pain. Central sensitization may occur in the spinal cord and higher levels of the CNS. But, crucially, in many normal people the

CNS seems to adapt to continued pain and reduce its sensitivity. Chemical and morphologic changes in the dorsal horn of the spinal cord *may either raise or lower* receptor thresholds. Summation or habituation may occur in the spinal cord. There may be changes in the electrical and chemical activity of the spinal cord and the brain itself. Neural networks and their function can change and may be altered by neural activity itself over time. There is experimental evidence for all of these events. These changes may be lasting, which could explain how pain may persist after the original stimulus has stopped. They could also account for spread, so that pain seems to affect a wider area. Many pain lectures give the impression that these neurophysiologic changes are irreversible, but that is untrue, as shown by the relief of chronic pain after joint replacement.

Yet even the best neurophysiology cannot fully explain human pain. Neurophysiology is about the CNS, even the brain, but it is not the mind. Neurophysiology can only explain the physiologic mechanisms, the bodily substrate, or electrochemical correlates of mental events. Clinical pain is a complex and subtle experience in a thinking, feeling human being. To understand the pain experience fully we must also look at emotions, psychology, and human behavior. We might draw an analogy with grand prix racing. Of course we depend on the internal combustion engine and the chemistry of high-octane fuel to compete, but we need much more than that if we are to win the race.

Neurophysiology and psychology are not alternatives: they go together. Pain is not only filtered and modulated through the nervous system. Pain is also filtered and modulated though the individual's genetic make-up, previous experience, and learning. And through current physiological status, emotional state, and sociocultural environment (Turk 2002). Sensitization may be both neurophysiologic and psychological (Eriksen & Ursin 2002). The major advance of modern neurophysiology is to offer an explanation for how physiologic *and* psychological events interact to influence afferent input and the pain we feel, our suffering and pain behavior (Villemure & Bushnell 2002).

At this point it is worth revisiting Descartes. Earlier, we looked at the Cartesian model, which is a very mechanistic and biologic view of pain. It reflects Descartes' earlier writing and his distinction between the physical substance of the body and the non-physical aspects of thought and mind. It is the famous mind–body dichotomy. But Descartes was a philosopher, whose concern was with the soul and the meaning of life. He was not a scientist. His biology reflected knowledge in the 17th century, and no one uses him as a scientific authority. So why did 19th- and 20th-century medicine adopt that model so enthusiastically? Perhaps that tells us more about "modern" medicine with its focus on disease and physical treatment than it tells us about Descartes. Philosophically, Descartes took a much more holistic approach. Philosophers since Socrates have stressed the importance of mind and Descartes agreed. "I think, therefore I am." Descartes spent the last decade of his life insisting on the interdependence of body and mind to form a complete human being (Cottingham 2000). He described feelings of pain as a prime example of "confused perceptions" that must not be referred to the body alone or the mind alone. Pain arises from "the close and intimate union of the mind with the body" (Cottingham 1993).

Pat Wall devoted his life to neurophysiology, yet Devor (2001) suggested that Wall's last message was that pain is a function of the complex human organism and we must not lose sight of the mind. In the final analysis, neurophysiology and philosophy agree!

Definition of pain

Let us return to clinical pain and try to integrate these clinical and neurophysiologic ideas (Anand & Craig 1996).

Pain is a complex sensory and emotional experience. It is much more than just a signal of tissue damage:

- Pain signals do not pass unaltered to the cerebral cortex. They are always and constantly modulated within the CNS before they reach consciousness.
- The sensation of pain, emotions, and pain behavior are all integral parts of the pain experience.

> • The CNS is plastic in nature, and there may be neurophysiologic changes over time with the development of chronic pain.

We all know what pain is from our own experience, but defining it in words is surprisingly difficult. Most people start with examples of what causes pain rather than describing pain itself. Even when we get beyond that stage, it is difficult to define pain precisely and comprehensively. From a clinical perspective, I believe the best definition of pain is still that from the International Association for the Study of Pain (Merskey 1979):

> An unpleasant sensory and emotional experience associated with actual or potential tissue damage, or described in terms of such damage.

This is a profound statement that was the outcome of much thought and debate. Read it several times. Stop and think it through. It has many clinical implications:

• Stimulation of peripheral receptors and activity in neural pathways is not pain. Pain is always a mental state, even if we most often associate pain with such physiologic events. We experience, assess and act upon pain at a conscious level. A dentist once examined Bertrand Russell and asked: "Where does that hurt?" "In my mind, of course. Where else could it hurt?" replied the philosopher.

• This definition avoids tying pain to the stimulus. All pain is real to those who suffer. It feels just the same to them, whether or not we can identify tissue damage. If they regard their experience as pain and if they report it as pain, then we should accept it as pain. Attempts to separate mental and physical pain, organic and non-organic, betray a fundamental misunderstanding. They do not help to understand the clinical problem and will destroy our relationship with the patient. We should simply accept the pain is real to the patient and direct our efforts to understanding the clinical problem.

• The definition lays equal weight on the sensory and emotional aspects of pain. Pain is unquestionably a sensation about a part of the body but it is also unpleasant and therefore always an emotional experience.

• Pain is a subjective and personal experience. The way in which each of us deals with and expresses our pain varies. It depends on our experience of pain in general and this pain in particular. It also depends on our current mental and emotional state.

• The definition allows for actual events, anticipation of possible future events, and the patient's interpretation of the pain. Anticipation and fear of pain may be as potent as pain itself.

• Because pain is so subjective, it is difficult to communicate across the barriers of language. The *way patients report the pain* will always be influenced by how they think and feel and by their communication ability and style. There is a major gap in communication about pain between patients and health professionals.

Acute and chronic pain

Doctors traditionally classify low back pain as acute or chronic. Acute pain is usually defined as being less than 6 weeks' duration. Many patients have recurrent attacks, but these often continue to be like acute pain. In the past, the definition of chronic pain was more than 6 months, which stressed its intractable nature. But 6 months is probably too late to begin thinking about and dealing with chronic pain, and many workers now classify chronic pain as being of more than 3 months' duration. In terms of clinical progress and the risk of chronic pain and disability, 6 weeks may actually be a better cut-off. The key distinction is not the duration of the pain, but the persistence of chronic pain beyond expected recovery times and the intractable nature of chronic pain.

There are marked clinical differences between acute and chronic pain, which too many doctors and therapists ignore at their patients' peril. Loeser once exclaimed that "acute and chronic pain have nothing in common but the four letter word pain." Acute and experimental pains usually have a simple relation to nociception and tissue damage. There may be some anxiety about the meaning and future effects of acute pain, but that is easy to understand

and is not usually a major problem. Acute pain and disability are usually in proportion to the physical findings. The natural tendency of most acute pain is to recover, and physical treatment is relatively effective. Management *should* be easy.

The clinical presentation of chronic pain is very different. Chronic pain and disability often seem to become dissociated from the original physical problem. There may indeed be very little evidence of any remaining tissue damage or nociception. Instead, chronic pain and disability seem to become self-sustaining. They are also intractable to treatment. Continued attempts to treat tissue damage do not relieve symptoms, but may actually reinforce pain and perpetuate the problem. Clinical patterns of chronic pain become complex and varied. Management is far from easy, and indeed is one of the most difficult challenges of health care.

Sternbach (1974, 1977) was one of the first to explore the differences between acute and chronic pain. He compared acute pain to the sympathetic reaction of "fight or flight." There is release of epinephrine (adrenaline); heart rate, blood pressure, and blood flow increase; breathing becomes faster; palms sweat; pupils dilate. Acute pain has biologic meaning and value as a warning of tissue damage. But these changes are also characteristic of anxiety states. Sternbach argued that acute pain and anxiety are closely linked. Treatment of acute pain tries to deal with the cause, but it should also deal with anxiety, as this can help to reduce pain. We can reduce anxiety by *repeated* explanations and reassurances.

With the passage of time these autonomic responses habituate and disappear, and a pattern of "vegetative changes" now emerges. Patients often develop sleep and appetite disturbance, loss of libido, and irritability. There is gradual withdrawal from social activities, and feelings of helplessness and hopelessness. Chronic pain loses its biologic meaning and purpose, and becomes counterproductive. These changes are also characteristic of depression. Sternbach believed that chronic pain is almost always accompanied by some degree of depression. We can best treat depression by rehabilitation with increasing activity, retraining and giving reasons to be hopeful.

These observations let us begin to see the problem of chronic pain, but we should not overstate the distinction between acute and chronic pain. There is no absolute cut-off in time – acute pain merges into chronic pain. Only a very small proportion of back patients develop chronic intractable pain, and the rate and the manner at which this happens may vary greatly.

We will consider many of these issues in greater depth throughout this book. Suffice to say, at this point, that we cannot understand or treat chronic back pain like the acute pain of tissue damage. We may treat acute back pain with simple physical measures and reassurance and expect early recovery. But chronic back pain persists, and is almost by definition a failure to recover properly or to respond to treatment. So we cannot treat it simply by continuing the management that has already failed. We must now deal with the whole pain syndrome.

Assessment of pain

Assessment of pain is a routine and basic part of clinical practice (Turk & Melzack 2001). Yet once we accept the complexity of pain, it should be no surprise that assessment is difficult and often inadequate.

Assessment of pain

- anatomic distribution
- time course
- severity
- quality.

For all the reasons we have discussed, only the patient can really assess his or her pain. Clinical assessment is only an attempt to put the patient's report into medical terms. It always remains the patient's report of his or her own symptoms, and so is open to subjective influences. However, the report of pain is not as straightforward as it may seem. It varies with the level of distress. It may be colored by previous encounters with health professionals, and cultural influences on consulting behavior. Previous failed treatment may have a profound effect on the report of pain, as may expectations about further treatment. These are not only of theoretic importance, but have a direct effect on how patients respond when asked about their pain. Doctors and therapists who are not aware of these issues may easily misinterpret the patient's report of pain. That is why we must always look at pain in the context of the whole clinical picture, and not base diagnosis and management on the report of pain alone.

Anatomic distribution

We generally define low back pain as being between the lowest ribs and the inferior gluteal folds. The simplest and most reliable classification is from the Quebec Task Force (Spitzer et al 1987):

- low back pain alone
- low back pain with radiating pain into the thigh but not below the knee
- nerve root pain, with or without neurologic deficit.

Many workers feel this is too simple, but it is one of the few classifications of back pain on which different specialists and therapists can agree. It reflects the diagnostic triage in Chapter 2 and is a very practical working classification.

Selim et al (1998) tested this in practice. They found a clear clinical gradient across four groups:

- group 1 – back pain alone
- group 2 – back pain with radiating leg pain above the knee
- group 3 – back pain with leg pain below the knee
- group 4 – back pain with leg pain below the knee and a positive straight leg raising test.

Intensity of pain, level of disability, and analgesic consumption all increased from groups 1 to 4. Group 4 patients were more likely to have MRI scan and surgery. Loisel et al (2002) showed that the initial Quebec grade predicted pain, functional status, and return to work at 1-year follow up.

Time pattern – acute, subacute or chronic

The basic clinical classification is (Spitzer et al 1987):

- acute: less than 6 weeks
- subacute: 6–12 weeks
- chronic: more than 3 months of continuous pain.

This classification rests on the assumption that patients start with an episode of acute pain that either recovers after a varying period of time, or fails to get better and continues indefinitely. But when we look at the epidemiology (Ch. 5), we will see that is not an accurate picture. One of the main characteristics of back pain is that it often runs a fluctuating or recurring course. An isolated acute attack with no previous history and complete relief of pain after x weeks is unusual. Most people have some previous history and many have some persisting or recurring symptoms. Each attack, or episode of health care, may occur against a background of recurrent attacks or persisting minor symptoms. Even chronic pain usually fluctuates in intensity. The most important feature of chronic pain, perhaps, is not its duration but its impact on the patient's life and its intractable nature.

So back pain is often neither acute nor chronic in the traditional sense of these terms, and the duration of each episode or time to remission may not give a true picture of its outcome. von Korff et al (1993) suggested it might be better to assess either the total days in pain over a period of time, or the characteristic severity of the episodes. For example, in one study they classified low back pain as:

- occasional – pain present on less than 30 days in the past 6 months
- frequent – pain present on more than 50% of days for the past 6 months.

Measuring pain

The real difficulty comes when we try to measure the intensity of low back pain (Jensen et al 1986, Jensen & McFarland 1993). Despite the emphasis on pain for the diagnosis of underlying pathology, our training and practice pay little attention to the assessment of pain itself. We usually rely on clinical impression or observer judgments of pain, but these correlate poorly with the patient's own report of pain. They are unreliable and prone to observer bias. Bartfield et al (1997) found that doctors used their own impression of pain intensity to influence management, but these only correlated 0.40 with the patient's own rating.

Pain can be assessed on a scale, by the words patients use to describe it, or by drawings. Some form of scale is the most widely used and probably the best method for both clinical practice and research (Figs 3.4 and 3.5). It is simple to give and

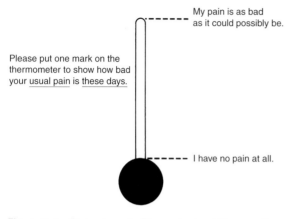

My pain is as bad as it could possibly be.

Please put one mark on the thermometer to show how bad your <u>usual pain</u> is <u>these days</u>.

I have no pain at all.

Figure 3.4 The pain scale. The scale should be exactly 100 mm long and the level marked by the patient is scored as a percentage. Some patients find it easier to mark this on a thermometer scale, but you must make sure they do not mistake this for an anatomic diagram of the back! (From Waddell 1987, with permission.)

to score, and most patients find it easy to use. The scale is exactly 100 mm long. Ask the patient to put a mark on the scale and then measure that mark in millimeters to give a score from 0 to 100%. A diagram of a thermometer may help patients who do not understand the concept of a scale, but make sure they do not mistake it for a diagram of the spine (Fig. 3.4).

The difficulty is how to interpret what the score means. It is not an objective measure of pain and does not match any physiologic or pathologic change. It is still the patient's report of pain, and reflects all the influences we have discussed. It is not clear to what extent the pain scale measures pain or distress, as the two are closely linked. It may be idiosyncratic (Williams et al 2000). So we must not overinterpret the pain score, but accept it simply as a measure of how bad this patient reports his or her pain to be. The pain scale is most useful to

McGill pain questionnaire
Please tick those adjectives that describe your pain, as mild, moderate or severe.

	None	Mild	Moderate	Severe
Throbbing				
Shooting				
Stabbing				
Sharp				
Cramping				
Gnawing				
Hot – burning				
Aching				
Heavy				
Tender				
Splitting				
Tiring – exhausting				
Sickening				
Fearful				
Punishing – cruel				

Visual analog scale

No pain ├────────────────────────────────┤ Worst possible pain

Present pain intensity
0 – no pain
1 – mild
2 – discomforting
3 – distressing
4 – horrible
5 – excruciating

Scoring
Adjectives 1 – 11 are "sensory" and adjectives 12 – 15 are "emotional".
Score each adjective: none = 0, mild = 1, moderate = 2, severe = 3.
Add the sensory and emotional scores separately.
The visual analog scale and present pain intensity scale are also included to provide overall pain intensity scores. The visual analog scale is exactly 100 mm long and the score is measured by ruler.

Figure 3.5 The short form of the McGill Pain Questionnaire. From Melzack R, The short-form McGill Pain Questionnaire, Pain 30; 191–197, 1987, with kind permission from Elsevier Science, NL, Sara Burgerhartstraat 25, 1055 KV, Amsterdam, the Netherlands.

follow a patient's progress over time, rather than to compare different patients.

We have little epidemiologic data about the severity of back pain. Table 3.1 presents US data from *The Nuprin Pain Report* (Taylor & Curran 1985) and Table 3.2 UK data from the Consumers' Association survey (1985). These illustrate the problem of how to interpret the pain scale. They simply tell us how these people scored their pain. Does this really tell us more about back pain in the US or in the UK? H Raspe et al (unpublished communication) found considerable variation in pain reports in different countries. Perhaps surprisingly, the UK and West Germany seemed to be the two extremes of a European range between low back "toughness" and "catastrophizing."

The adjectives that patients use to describe their pain can assess the quality of the pain in a very crude way. The most widely used method is the McGill Pain Questionnaire (Melzack 1975) and there is a shorter version that is more practical for routine use (Melzack 1987) (Fig. 3.5). The adjectives are divided broadly into those that describe the sensory qualities and those that describe the emotional qualities of the pain (Table 3.3).

A pain drawing may provide information about the anatomic distribution of the pain and a very crude estimate of the amount of pain. However, it really provides a different kind of information that we will consider later in Chapter 10.

DISABILITY

I have tried to emphasize that pain and disability are not the same (Table 3.4). This is so fundamental and important that I will repeat it without apology.

Definition

Disability is restricted activity. The standard definition is by the World Health Organization (WHO

Table 3.1 Duration and severity of back pain in American adults

Duration (days in year)		Percentage of adults
1–5		22
6–10		7
11–30		12
31–100		6
101 or more		9

Severity	Scale (1–10)	Percentage of those with back pain
Slight	1–3	16
Moderate	4–6	44
Severe	7–9	23
Unbearable	10	14

Data from Taylor & Curran (1985).

Table 3.2 Severity of back pain in British adults

Severity of back pain on a scale of 0–10	Percentage of those who in the last 12 months reported back pain
0 (minimal)	1
0–1	2
1–2	7
2–3	10
3–4	14
4–5	17
5–6	12
6–7	9
7–8	8
8–9	6
9–10	5
10 (intolerable)	8

Data from the Consumers' Association (1985).

Table 3.3 Sensory and emotional adjectives for pain

Sensory	Emotional
Throbbing	Tiring
Shooting	Exhausting
Stabbing	Sickening
Sharp	Fearful
Cramping	Punishing
Gnawing	Cruel
Hot and burning	
Aching	
Heavy	
Tender	
Splitting	

From the McGill Pain Questionnaire.

Table 3.4 Low back disability among those with back pain for at least 2 weeks

Self–rated pain	Percentage who reduced activities	Mean days work loss per annum	Mean days in bed per annum
Mild	40	11	4
Moderate	54	18	7
Severe	55	34	13

Data from Deyo & Tsui-Wu (1987).

1980): "Any restriction or lack (resulting from an impairment) of ability to perform an activity in the manner or within the range considered normal for a human being." To that we might add: compared to a healthy person of the same age and sex. The fifth edition of the *Guides to the Evaluation of Permanent Impairment* (American Medical Association (AMA) 2000) gives a similar definition. Disability is "an alteration of an individual's capacity to meet personal, social or occupational demands because of an impairment." The new *International Classification of Functioning, Disability and Health* (ICF) changes the emphasis to *activity* and *activity limitation* (WHO 2000). ICF defines activity as "something a person does, ranging from very basic elementary or simple to complex." Activity limitation is "a difficulty in the performance, accomplishment, or completion of an activity. Difficulties in performing activities occur when there is a qualitative or quantitative alteration in the way in which activities are carried out. Difficulty encompasses all the ways in which the doing of the activity may be affected." Across the different wording, the core of all the definitions is that disability is restricted activity.

Administrative definitions for the purpose of compensation focus on incapacity for work. For example, the US Social Security Administration (2001) requires "inability to engage in any substantially gainful activity." But incapacity for work is only one aspect of disability. Unfortunately, every official body seems to feel the need to produce its own terms and definitions for disability, which may cause confusion. You must obviously learn and use the official terms where you work.

We may agree that disability is restricted activity: but the how and why often lead to false assumptions. It often assumes that disability is the direct physical consequence of pain, and that continued pain automatically means incapacity for work. And it implies that disability is a health problem, that can only be resolved by treatment of the pain. That simple model is how most doctors, therapists, and patients think about pain and disability.

Pain $\longrightarrow$ Disablity $\longrightarrow$ Incapacity for work

Unfortunately, this is too simplistic. Pain and disability and (in)capacity for work are all subjective issues. Pain is a symptom, not a diagnosis nor a disease. Some patients have pain but little disability. Others have disability that seems to be out of proportion to their pain. Some continue working despite severe pain. Others stop work with little apparent justification. A physical disorder in the back may give *both* pain and disability but the relationship between them depends on many influences as well as the presence of pain.

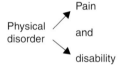

The new Chapter 18 on pain in the AMA *Guides* (AMA 2000) uses the concept of "pain-related activity restrictions." "I have severe back pain. I can't walk more than 50 yards. I avoid lifting. I obviously can't work because I have this pain. And, anyway, I've lost my job." But what is the distinction or the relation between pain and disability? Disability is restricted activity, and all that we can assess is what this patient does or does not do. That is not necessarily what the patient is *able* or *unable* to do. In practice we assess performance, not capability. This person does not bend or walk more than 50 yards and attributes these limitations to back pain. They are restricted bending, walking, and working, and therefore that is their disability. Or, to be more precise, that is their report of their disability.

Clinical assessment of disability

We have already seen the problems of measuring pain, and to some extent we face the same problems

---

Assessment of disability

- activities of daily living
- questionnaires
- physical performance measures
- work loss
- capacity for work.

---

3. standing – standing in one place generally limited to less than 30 minutes at a time before needing to move around
4. walking – walking generally limited to less than 30 minutes or 1–2 miles at a time before needing to rest
5. traveling – traveling in a car or bus generally limited to less than 30 minutes at a time before needing to stop and have a break
6. social life – regularly miss or curtail social activities and normal social mobility (not sports, which are a very different level of disability)
7. sleeping – sleep regularly disturbed by pain, i.e., two or three times per week
8. sex life – reduced frequency of sexual activity because of pain
9. dressing – help regularly required with footwear (tights, socks, or shoelaces).

Simple yes or no answers about each of these activities give a basic disability score out of nine that is sufficient for clinical purposes. This may seem crude, but the scale is robust and useful in clinical practice. Despite, or because of, its simplicity, it compares well with more elaborate disability questionnaires (Beurskens et al 1995). If you wish, you can build a complete disability evaluation on the basic scale. You can explore the exact limit in each of the nine basic activities and how they affect the patient's work, home, and leisure activities. You obtain and record this as "medical" information, but always remember it is the patient's own subjective report of disability.

with disability. Once again we depend largely on the patient's own report, which is subject to the same influences. Despite that, we can define and assess disability better than pain. Measures of disability are more reliable and give a more valid account of what we are trying to measure. This is perhaps because reports of disability simply require description of concrete activities, while reports of pain depend on complex evaluation of subjective experiences. Many research groups around the world agree that the best way to assess low back disability is on activities of daily living. This gives a direct measure of basic activity. Back pain may affect many daily activities, such as bending and lifting, sitting, standing, walking, traveling, social life, sleeping, sex, and dressing. A few simple questions can give an accurate picture of the impact of back pain on the patient's life.

When asking about disability, you must focus on limited activity rather than pain. Your questions should be clear and precise. "Are you actually restricted in that activity?" rather than "Is that activity painful?" "Does your back limit how much you do?" "Do you now require help with that activity?" Any restriction must be from the onset of back pain and because of back pain. You should note the common or usual effect, not occasional effects or special efforts. Our studies (Waddell & Main 1984) have shown that the clinical interview can give a reliable assessment of disability in activities of daily living. We found the following limits are most useful for low back pain:

1. bending and lifting – help required or avoid heavy lifting (30–40 pounds, a heavy suitcase, or a 3- to 4-year-old child)
2. sitting – sitting in an ordinary chair generally limited to less than 30 minutes at a time before needing to get up and move around

Disability questionnaires

Patients can give the same information on a questionnaire. These are suitable for routine clinical use, but also give high-quality information for research. They are more consistent and reliable than interviews because they present the questions in exactly the same way to every patient, every time.

There are many questionnaires that all give comparable, though slightly different, measures of low back disability. There is no doubt that the two most widely used and standard measures are the Oswestry (Fairbank et al 1980) and the Roland questionnaires (Roland & Morris 1983). Both have been carefully developed, and have stood the test of time (Fairbank & Pysent 2000, Roland & Fairbank

Box 3.1   The Roland disability questionnaire (from Roland & Fairbank 2000)

When your back hurts, you may find it difficult to do some things you normally do.

This list contains some sentences that people have used to describe themselves when they have back pain. When you read them, you may find that some stand out because they describe you *today*. As you read the list, think of yourself *today*. When you read a sentence that describes you today, put a tick against it. If the sentence does not describe you, then leave the space blank and go to the next one. Remember, only tick the sentence if you are sure it describes you today.

1. I stay at home most of the time because of my back.
2. I change position frequently to try and get my back comfortable.
3. I walk more slowly than usual because of my back.
4. Because of my back I am not doing any of the jobs that I usually do around the house.
5. Because of my back, I use a handrail to get upstairs.
6. Because of my back, I lie down to rest more often.
7. Because of my back, I have to hold on to something to get out of an easy chair.
8. Because of my back, I try to get other people to do things for me.
9. I get dressed more slowly than usual because of my back.
10. I only stand for short periods of time because of my back.
11. Because of my back, I try not to bend or kneel down.
12. I find it difficult to get out of a chair because of my back.
13. My back is painful almost all the time.
14. I find it difficult to turn over in bed because of my back.
15. My appetite is not very good because of my back pain.
16. I have trouble putting on my socks (or stockings) because of the pain in my back.
17. I only walk short distances because of my back.
18. I sleep less well on my back.
19. Because of my back pain, I get dressed with help from someone else.
20. I sit down for most of the day because of my back.
21. I avoid heavy jobs around the house because of my back.
22. Because of my back pain, I am more irritable and bad-tempered with people than usual.
23. Because of my back, I go upstairs more slowly than usually.
24. I stay in bed most of the time because of my back.

2000). They also have the advantage that they have now been used in many published studies, which provide a basis for comparison.

The Roland disability questionnaire (Box 3.1) is simple, quick, and easy to use. It is sensitive to change (Beaton 2000), and gives the best measure of early and acute disability and recovery. Its main disadvantage is that it is less able to measure very severe levels of chronic disability. I believe the Roland disability questionnaire is the best available at present, for most clinical use and research on back pain in primary care.

The Oswestry disability questionnaire is slightly more complicated to fill in and score, but that is not a problem in practice. It is less sensitive to low levels of disability, but is better able to measure severe disability. It has been used more and is probably more suitable for surgical studies.

Classification of chronic pain and disability

Chronic low back pain is not the same as chronic pain-related disability. So it may be better to classify pain and functional outcomes over time.

von Korff et al (1992) developed a simple method of grading the severity of chronic back pain and disability. They originally designed this for population studies and tested it on 2389 American

Table 3.5 Factors influencing the diagnosis of *chronic* low back pain

Clear physical or mechanical symptoms and signs	85%
Psychosocial problems	85%
Long course of treatment (not just symptoms)	73%
Work-related problems	52%

Adapted form Cedraschi et al (1999).

patients. They used pain intensity, disability, duration, and persistency to give a simple grading into:

- grade I: low disability – low intensity
- grade II: low disability – high intensity
- grade III: high disability – moderately limiting
- grade IV: high disability – severely limiting.

Cassidy et al (1997) studied 1133 adults in the general population in Canada. Seventy-two percent reported some back symptoms during the past 6 months: 48.2% had grade I; 12.4% grade II; 7.2% grade III; and 4.7% grade IV. Smith et al (1997) also found it a useful, reliable, and valid measure in UK patients.

This takes us back to our classification of acute, recurrent, and chronic pain. The importance of chronic pain is not simply the duration of the pain but also its impact on the patient's life. von Korff's classification reflects the severity and impact of chronic pain and the importance of both pain and disability (McGorry et al 2000).

Cedraschi et al (1999) looked at how doctors and therapists used the term "chronic" in practice. They did *not* use it strictly by duration. Instead, they based it mainly on the impact on the patient's physical function and psychological well-being and on treatment (Table 3.5). They really used "chronic" to describe problem patients or their situation.

Physical performance measures

Clinical assessment of disability, whether by interview or questionnaire, is limited by its dependence on the patient's self-report. In principle, we should be able to get a more objective measure by independent observation of actual performance.

Functional capacity evaluation (FCE) does exactly that (Blankenship 1986, Hart et al 1993, Yeomans & Liebenson 1996). FCE measures whole-body ability and limitations such as cardiovascular fitness, lifting capacity, and fitness for work. It puts patients through a standard protocol of physical tasks while a trained observer records their performance and limitations. It is simple, safe, low-tech, and gives reliable results. It contains tests and checks that try to tell if the patient is cooperating fully and giving maximum effort. The report is in a standard format, and contains normal population values for comparison. It can be used to describe clinical progress and outcomes, to prescribe rehabilitation needs and goals, and for vocational assessment.

Unfortunately, FCE also has limitations, which is probably why it has never been very popular in Europe. Full FCE is complex, needs a specialist, takes several hours, and is costly. Although it is standardized and much better than clinical impression, it is not as wholly objective as some of its users claim. There are many competing systems of FCE. Reducing clinical observations to numbers may give a false impression of accuracy. FCE is also misnamed. It is not an evaluation of capacity but of performance, so it still depends on effort. I also have doubts about some of the methods used in FCE to assess effort and symptom magnification, which will become clearer in later chapters.

Simpler clinical test batteries can also directly observe the patient's capacity to perform everyday activities in a controlled setting. Harding et al (1994) developed such a battery for severely disabled patients with various chronic pain problems. Box 3.2 shows a simplified version they now use in routine clinical practice. They found the tests reliable and sensitive to change after a pain management program. Simmonds' group developed a similar but more comprehensive battery for patients with low back pain (Simmonds et al 1998, Novy et al 2002, Simmonds 2002). They again found it to be simple and easy to use, acceptable to patients, and reliable. On analysis, the tests fell into two groups. The larger and more powerful group assesses speed and coordination. The smaller assesses endurance, strength, and balance. Individual performance tests showed moderate

---

Box 3.2   A simple physical performance measure (VR Harding, personal communication)

The test area should be quiet and free of passing people. Put up warning signs for staff and other patients when tests are taking place. The patient should not need to walk a long distance to reach the test area or between the different tests. Ask the patient to wear comfortable shoes and loose clothing.

- *Five minutes of walking.* The distance walked up and down between marks 20 m apart in 5 min. Choose a quiet, empty corridor with a non-slip surface or hard carpet. There should be walls or doors on either side that can be used if necessary for support, but not handrails. Patients should not use walking aids but can use the walls for support or can sit down for a rest. Inform patients of the time at the end of each lap or every minute if they are slower (mean, 185 m).

- *One minute of stair climbing.* Climbing up and down a straight flight of standard stairs with one handrail and an opposite wall within easy reach. Have a chair available for resting if the patient needs it. Count the number of steps up and down, e.g., 20 up + 15 down = 35 steps (mean, 48 steps).

- *One minute of stand-ups.* The number of times the patient can stand up from a chair in 1 min. Use a firm, upright chair with a padded seat and back rest but no arm rests. The seat height should be about 45 cm, or 18 inches. There should not be any wall or other furniture within reach that the patient could use for support (mean, 11 stand-ups).

- *Standardization of test instructions.* The tester should have written instructions. The tester must respond neutrally at all times and maintain a test atmosphere. Do not give patients any advice or encouragement during the tests as feedback influences their performance. Only give information on the time to help patients to pace themselves if they are able. Tell patients this is a test of current performance. It is a measure of how much they can manage, bearing in mind the journey home after their assessment. These instructions are designed to prevent anxiety and overexertion.

Note: These values are for chronic pain patients. Other patient groups may be fitter and show different values.

---

correlation with self-reported disability ($r = 0.4$–0.6) but variable correlation with pain intensity.

Several studies in back pain have used the *shuttle walk test* alone (Box 3.3). This is again a general measure of fitness or disability (Singh et al 1992). Fogg & Taylor (1997) found the shuttle walk test to be simple, reliable, and a sensitive measure of response to treatment for back pain.

Such assessments of physical performance can give a more objective measure to supplement and compare with the patient's self-report of disability. But they cannot overcome the basic limitation that we can only observe what the patient does. This does not tell us what he or she is *able* to do or *should be able* to do. As an oversimplification, capacity may be limited by physiology, but performance is limited by psychology. What the patient does or does not do will always depend on effort and motivation. Even the most "objective"

Box 3.3   The shuttle walk test

The patient walks up and down a 10 m course, round two cones inset 0.5 m from either end to avoid the need for abrupt changes in direction. On the first test the patient has to walk 30 m in 1 min. The speed of walking is increased by 10 m each minute, so that in the 12th minute the patient has to walk 140 m. The end of the test is either when the patient decides to stop due to fatigue or back symptoms, or when the observer finds the patient has not met the target speed. The observer then simply counts the total number of meters the patient has managed to walk up to that point.

assessment is not of actual capacity but only of performance.

Incapacity for work

Health care concentrates on symptoms. The most important outcome, however, is not any clinical measure of pain or disability, but how the problem affects the patient's life. The single most crucial impact of low back pain is on ability to work, which pervades all else. For working patients, sickness absence, loss of earnings, and loss of their job have the greatest potential ill effects on them and their families. Sickness absence is also the most important measure of the social impact of back pain for employers, the economy, and social costs. This is the reason for political interest in back pain. For all these reasons, incapacity for work is the most important measure of low back disability.

Sickness absence does have limitations as a measure of disability and of health care outcomes. (In)capacity for work is only weakly related to clinical measures of pain or disability. It only applies to people who are working, and not to the young, the elderly, housewives, or the unemployed. Sickness absence only measures more severe disability and only one aspect of disability due to back pain. It misses lesser degrees of disability and finer aspects of work such as limited duties, lower productivity, loss of overtime, and loss of promotion. The greatest problem is that sickness absence and return to work depend on other influences as well as pain and disability – and many of these influences have nothing to do with illness or health care. They include the demands and conditions of the person's job, ability to modify the job, and job satisfaction. Broader issues include job availability, local economic conditions, other sources of income, compensation, and retirement.

We can measure sickness absence easily and accurately. We can check sickness records. Sickness absence, sick certification, and social security benefits, however, are not the same. Most people with more than a few days off work get some form of medical sick certification. Payment of benefits, however, depends on entitlement. As a result, many people may lose time from work yet not be entitled to benefits and therefore are not included in official statistics. On the other hand, patients may get sick certificates and benefits without work loss, e.g., if they are unemployed.

Despite these limitations, there is growing agreement that incapacity for work is the single most important social measure of low back disability and health care (Spitzer et al 1987, Fordyce 1995). That does not mean that pain is unimportant, or that work is the sole purpose of life. What it means is that we must consider both pain and its impact on the patient's life.

CONCLUSION

Pain, disability, and (in)capacity for work are linked, but the relationship between them is complex and influenced by many factors. We must make a clear distinction between pain and disability, and assess each separately. We may ask patients to keep a pain diary of pain intensity, use of medication, and sleep and activity patterns over a week, and this may give some insight into how pain and disability are related. Understanding the other influences that link low back pain and disability will take us a long way to understanding the clinical problem and our present epidemic.

References

AMA 2000 Guides to the evaluation of permanent impairment, 5th edn. American Medical Association, Chicago

Anand K J S, Craig K D 1996 New perspectives on the definition of pain. Pain 67: 3–6

Bartfield J M, Salluzzo R F, Raccio-Robak N, Funk D L, Verdile V P 1997 Physician and patient factors influencing the treatment of low back pain. Pain 73: 209–211

Beaton D E 2000 Understanding the relevance of measured change through studies of responsiveness. Spine 25: 3192–3199

Beurskens A J, de Vet H C, Koke A J, van der Heijden G J, Knipschild P G 1995 Measuring the functional status of patients with low back pain: assessment of the quality of four disease-specific questionnaires. Spine 20: 1017–1028

Blankenship S K 1986 Functional capacity evaluation: the procedure manual. American Therapeutics, Macon, GA

Casey K L, Bushnell M C 2000 Pain imaging. Progress in pain research and management, vol. 18. IASP Press, Seattle

Cassidy J D, Carroll L, Cote P, Senthilselvan A 1997 The prevalence of graded chronic low back pain severity and its effect on general health: a population based study. Presented to the International Society for the Study of the Lumbar Spine, Singapore

Cedrasschi C, Robert J, Georg D, Perrin E, Fischer W, Vischer T L 1999 Is chronic non-specific low back pain chronic? Definitions of a problem and problems of a definition. British Journal of General Practice 49: 358–362

Consumers' Association 1985 Back pain survey. Consumers' Association, London

Cottingham J 1993 A Descartes dictionary. Blackwell, Oxford

Cottingham J 2000 Descartes' philosophy of mind. In Monk R, Raphael F (eds) The great philosophers. Phoenix, London, pp 93–134

Descartes R 1664 L'homme (translated by Foster M). Cambridge University Press, New York

Devor M 1996 Pain mechanisms and pain syndromes. In: Campbell J N (ed.) Pain – an updated review. International Association for the Study of Pain refresher course. IASP Press, Seattle, pp 103–112

Devor M 2001 Obituary: Patrick David Wall 1925–2001. Pain 94: 125–129

Deyo R A, Tsui-Wu Y-J 1987 Functional disability due to back pain. Arthritis and Rheumatism 30: 1247–1253

Doubell T P, Mannion R J, Woolf C J 1999 The dorsal horn: state-dependent sensory processing, plasticity and the generation of pain. In: Wall P D, Melzack R (eds) Textbook of pain, 4th edn. Churchill Livingstone, Edinburgh, pp 165–181

Engel G L 1959 Psychogenic pain and the pain prone patient. American Journal of Medicine 26: 899–918

Eriksen H R, Ursin H 2002 Sensitization and subjective health complaints. Scandinavian Journal of Psychology 43: 189–196

Fairbank J C T, Pysent P 2000 The Oswestry disability index. Spine 25: 2940–2953

Fairbank J C T, Mbaot J C, Davies J B, O'Brien J P 1980 The Oswestry low back pain disability questionnaire. Physiotherapy 66: 271–273

Fogg A J B, Taylor A E 1997 The usefulness of the shuttle walk test in a population of low back pain patients. Presented to the 24th Annual Meeting of the International Society for the Study of the Lumbar Spine, Singapore

Fordyce W E 1995 Back pain in the workplace: management of disability in non-specific conditions. IASP Press, Seattle, pp 1–75

Foster M 1901 Lectures on the history of physiology during the sixteenth, seventeenth and eighteenth centuries. Cambridge University Press, Cambridge (translated from Descartes R 1664 L'homme)

Harding V R, Williams A C, Richardson P H et al 1994 The development of a battery of measures for assessing physical functioning of chronic pain patients. Pain 58: 367–375

Hart D L, Isernhagen S J, Matheson L N 1993 Guidelines for functional capacity evaluation of people with medical conditions. Journal of Orthopedic and Sports Physical Therapy 18: 682–686

Jensen M P, McFarland C A 1993 Increasing the reliability and validity of pain intensity measurement in chronic pain patients. Pain 55: 195–203

Jensen M P, Karoly P, Braver S 1986 The measurement of clinical pain intensity: a comparison of six methods. Pain 27: 117–126

Lewis T 1942 Pain. Macmillan, New York

Liebeskind J C, Melzack R 1987 The International Pain Foundation: meeting a need for education in pain management (editorial). Pain 30: 1–2

Loeser J D 1980 Perspectives on pain. In: Turner P (ed.) Clinical pharmacy and therapeutics. Macmillan, London, pp 313–316

Loisel P, Vachon B, Lemaire J et al 2002. Discriminative and predictive validity assessment of the Quebec Task Force classification. Spine 27: 851–857

McGorry R W, Webster B S, Snook S H, Hsiang S M 2000 The relation between pain intensity, disability and the episodic nature of chronic and recurrent low back pain. Spine 25: 834–841

Melzack R 1975 The McGill pain questionnaire; major properties and scoring methods. Pain 1: 277–299

Melzack R 1987 The short-form McGill pain questionnaire. Pain 30: 191–197

Melzack R 1996 Gate control theory: on the evolution of pain concepts. Pain Forum 5: 128–138

Melzack R 1999 From the gate to the neuromatrix. Pain 6(suppl.): S121–S126

Melzack R, Wall P D 1965 Pain mechanisms: a new theory. Science 150: 971–979

Merskey R 1979 Pain terms: a list with definitions and notes on usage. Pain 6: 249–252

Novy D M, Simmonds N J, Lee C E 2002 Physical performance tasks: what are the underlying constructs? Archives of Physical Medicine and Rehabilitation 83: 44–47

Penfield W 1969 Foreword. In: White J, Sweet W H (eds) Pain and the neurosurgeon. CC Thomas, Springfield, Illinois

Ren K, Dubner R 2002 Descending modulation in persistent pain: an update. Pain 100: 1–6

Roland M, Fairbank J 2000 The Roland–Morris disability questionnaire and the Oswestry disability questionnaire. Spine 25: 3115–3124

Roland M, Morris R 1983 A study of the natural history of back pain. Part I: development of a reliable and sensitive measure of disability in low back pain. Spine 8: 141–144

Selim A J, Ren S R, Fincke G et al 1998 The importance of radiating leg pain in assessing health outcomes among patients with low back pain: results from the Veterans Health Study. Spine 23: 470–474

Simmonds M J 2002 The effect of pain and illness on movement: assessment methods and their meanings. In: Giamberardino M A (ed.) Pain 2002 – an updated review: refresher course syllabus. IASP Press, Seattle, pp 179–187

Simmonds M J, Olson S L, Jones S et al 1998 Psychometric characteristics and clinical usefulness of physical performance tests in patients with low back pain. Spine 23: 2412–2421

Singh S J, Morgan M D L, Scott S, Walters D, Hardman A E 1992 Development of a shuttle walking test of disability in patients with chronic airways obstruction. Thorax 47: 1019–1024

Smith B H, Penny K I, Purves A M et al 1997 The chronic pain grade questionnaire; validation and reliability in postal research. Pain 71: 141–147

Social Security Administration 2001 Social Security handbook. US Government Printing Office, Washington, DC

Spitzer W O, Leblanc F E, Dupuis M et al 1987 Scientific approach to the assessment and management of activity-related spinal disorders. A monograph for physicians. Report of the Quebec Task Force on spinal disorders. Spine 12(7S): s1–s59

Sternbach R A 1974 Pain patients: traits and treatment. Academic Press, New York

Sternbach R A 1977 Psychologic aspects of chronic pain. Clinical Orthopaedics and Related Research 129: 150–155

Taylor H, Curran N M 1985 The Nuprin pain report. Louis Harris, New York, pp 1–233

Turk D C 2002 Remember the distinction between malignant and benign pain? Well, forget it (editorial). Clinical Journal of Pain 18: 75–76

Turk D C, Melzack R (eds) 2001 Handbook of pain assessment, 2nd edn. Guilford Press, New York

Villemure C, Bushnell M C 2002 Cognitive modulation of pain: how do attention and emotion influence pain processing? Pain 95: 195–199

von Korff M, Ormel J, Keefe F, Dworkin S F 1992 Grading the severity of chronic pain. Pain 50: 133–149

von Korff M, Deyo R A, Cherkin D, Barlow W 1993 Back pain in primary care: outcomes at one year. Spine 18: 855–862

Waddell G 1987 Clinical assessment of lumbar impairment. Clinical Orthopaedics and Related Research 221: 110–120

Waddell G, Main C J 1984 Assessment of severity in low back disorders. Spine 9: 204–208

Wall P D 1988 The John J Bonica distinguished lecture: stability and instability of central pain mechanisms. In: Dubner R, Gebhart G, Bond M (eds) Proceedings of the Vth world congress on pain. Elsevier, Amsterdam, pp 13–24

Wall P D 1996 Comments after 30 years of the gate control theory. Pain Forum 5: 12–22

WHO 1980 International classification of impairments, disabilities and handicaps. World Health Organization, Geneva

WHO 2000 International classification of functioning, disability and health (ICF). World Health Organization, Geneva

Williams A, Davies H T O, Chadury Y 2000 Simple pain rating scales hide complex idiosyncratic meanings. Pain 85: 457–463

Yeomans S G, Liebenson C 1996 Quantitative functional capacity evaluation: the missing link to outcomes assessment. Topics in Clinical Chiropractic 3: 32–43

Chapter 4

Back pain through history

Gordon Waddell   David B. Allan

Back pain is not new. Human beings have had back pain through recorded history, and probably long before. So what has changed? How did back pain become such a problem? Let us try to put our present epidemic into historic perspective (Allan & Waddell 1989).

UNDERSTANDING AND MANAGEMENT OF BACK PAIN

The symptom of pain in the back is the common link between the ordinary backache that most people have at some time in their life, a number of serious spinal diseases, and low back disability. We should try to keep these different perspectives in mind as we look at the history of back pain.

The oldest surviving text about back pain is the Edwin Smith papyrus from about 1500 BC (Fig. 4.1). It is a series of 48 case histories, the last of which is an acute back strain (Breasted 1930):

> Examination. If thou examinest a man having a sprain in a vertebra of his spinal column, thou shouldst say to him: extend now thy two legs and contract them both again. When he extends them both he contracts them both immediately because of the pain he causes in a vertebra of the spinal column in which he suffers.
>
> Diagnosis. Thou shouldst say to him: One having a sprain in the vertebra of his spinal column. An ailment I shall treat.
>
> Treatment. Thou shouldst place him prostrate on his back; thou shouldst make for him …

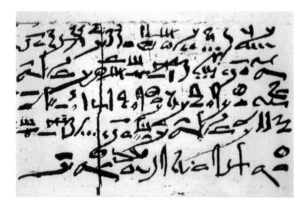

Figure 4.1   The oldest surviving description of back pain. The Edwin Smith papyrus (c. 1500 BC). From Breasted (1930), with permission.

At this tantalizing point the unknown Egyptian scribe died and the papyrus lay in his tomb for almost 3500 years. This is an early 20th-century translation that reflects thinking at that time, but the accuracy of the clinical description only adds to our frustration. We do not know what the ancient Egyptians thought about back pain or how they treated it. The ambiguity of the last sentence is particularly frustrating when we look at the recent debate about rest or staying active. From the contemporary evidence, however, it is unlikely this was a prescription of rest. It is more likely to have been the start of some form of local application or manual therapy.

The *Corpus Hippocraticus* (c. 400 BC) was the collected writings of the Greek library at Cos and Cnidus. It included reports of spinal deformities and fractures, and described pain in the back in that context. Back pain itself received little attention.

The writings of Galen (c. 150 AD) and his disciples dominated medicine for the next 1200 years. Galen thought that disease was due to disturbed "humors" and treatment was empiric. Back pain was a symptom of many illnesses but also one of the "fleeting" pains affecting joints and muscles. Treatment was symptomatic with spas, soothing local applications, and counterirritants. Galen was the original source of the oft-repeated saying that "The physician is but nature's assistant."

When the Graeco-Roman empire fell, exiled Christians took medical learning to Persia. The Arab world preserved that knowledge and reintroduced it to Europe after the Dark Ages, but Islamic laws largely limited them to the preservation of the ancient writings. Medical thought almost ceased during the Dark Ages as patient care moved into the hands of the church. Monks saved the ancient writings but only in degenerate forms. Back pain was a matter for folk medicine. The Welsh "shot of the elf" and the German "witch's shot" reflected beliefs that pain was due to external influences.

Modern western medicine began with the European Renaissance. The scientific method used careful observation to unlock nature's secrets by the power of human reason rather than by religious revelation. Studies of anatomy, physiology, and pathology laid the foundation. Paracelsus (1493–1541) rebelled against the ancient writings and began clinical freedom by treating each patient on the basis of his own observation and diagnosis. Sydenham (1624–1689) made a clear distinction between illness and underlying disease and introduced our present concept of clinical syndromes. They should be "reduced to certain and determinate kinds with the same exactness as we see it done by botanic writers in the treatises of plants." Diagnosis depends on "certain distinguishing signs, which Nature has particularly affixed to every species." Sydenham classified back pain or lumbago with the rheumatic diseases. The word rheumatism came from the Greek *rheuma*, a watery discharge or evil humor that flowed from the brain to cause pain in the joints or other parts of the body.

Modern use of the term rheumatism started in the 17th century. At that time it included what we now recognize as many musculoskeletal disorders ranging from acute rheumatic fever to arthritis. The only common feature was pain in the joints or muscles. Doctors at that time thought that rheumatism was due to cold and damp. They did not relate it to trauma. Gradually, different workers identified a number of diseases within this group. Sydenham, who himself suffered from gout, distinguished gout from acute rheumatism and described lumbago as a third form of rheumatism.

By 1800, physicians began to look for the cause of back pain. They suggested that it was due to a buildup of rheumatic phlegm in the muscles, so they used both local and systemic treatment to remove the phlegm. Scudamore (1816) published the first systematic treatise on chronic rheumatism. He blamed inflammation of the white fibrous tissue of the body "unaccompanied by fever but aggravated by motion." The inflammation was attributed to cold and damp. Through the 19th century, treatment of back pain was by general measures against rheumatism such as relief of constipation, counterirritants, blistering, and cupping. The theory was to remove the rheumatic exudi from the affected area, and surgeons removed septic foci in the teeth, toenails, and bowel.

Two key ideas in the 19th century laid the foundations for our modern approach to back pain: that it comes from the spine and that it is due to trauma. In 1828 a physician called Brown in Glasgow Royal Infirmary published a paper on *spinal irritation* (Fig. 4.2). Brown suggested for the first time that the vertebral column and the nervous system could be the source of back pain. He also described local spinal tenderness. The concept of spinal irritation swept the US and Europe, and held sway for nearly 30 years. For a time, nervous "irritability" got a kind of false legitimacy because it was compared with inflammation. However, inflammation was a local condition with objective features; irritation was only a hypothesis based on distant, subjective complaints. The concept of spinal irritation had a profound influence. Neither Brown nor his followers ever demonstrated its pathology and the diagnosis gradually fell into disrepute. But spinal irritation introduced the idea that the spine is the source of back pain; and the idea that a painful spine must somehow be irritable lingers in our thinking to this day.

It is difficult for us to believe that all through history neither doctors nor patients thought that back pain was due to injury. This idea only came in the latter half of the 19th century. The industrial revolution, and particularly the building of the railways, led to a spate of serious injuries. Violent trauma could cause spinal fractures and paralysis, so perhaps less serious injuries to the spine might be the cause of lumbago. There might be cumulative or repetitive trauma. Some people even thought the speed and nature of railway travel could damage human health.

Erichsen (1866) described what he called *railway spine* (Fig. 4.3; Keller & Chappell 1996). He suggested that severe jarring or shaking of the spine and nervous system could disturb spinal cord

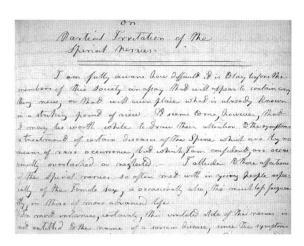

Figure 4.2 Spinal irritation. The copperplate minutes of Brown's original presentation to the Glasgow Medical Society in January 1923. With thanks to the Royal College of Physicians and Surgeons of Glasgow.

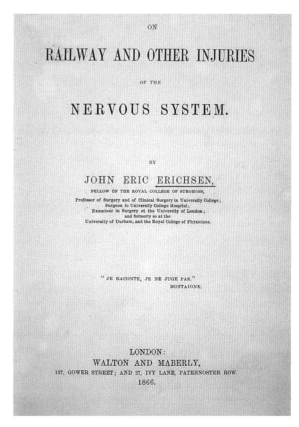

Figure 4.3 Erichsen's classic description of railway spine. With thanks to the Royal College of Physicians and Surgeons of Glasgow.

function, and compared it to disturbed mental function after concussion of the brain. It might be a form of molecular derangement, so was impossible to demonstrate. Alternatively, there might be an insidious and even more ominous disorder. A slight blow to the spine could lead to meningitis or myelitis with back pain, motor or sensory disturbance in the arms or legs, and mental symptoms of confusion and lassitude. Railway spine was a syndrome of subjective weakness and disability. As you might expect, no one ever confirmed its pathology and this diagnosis also eventually fell into disrepute. Railway spine, like spinal irritation, was a key act in this story that we will see again. Suffice to say that, for the first time, it linked back pain to trauma. Most health professionals and patients still regard back pain as an injury.

Sciatica

The word sciatica has been in use from Greek times, and is derived from "ischias" or pain around, or coming from, the hip and thigh. It was only with modern ideas of pathology that it came to mean pain in the distribution of the sciatic nerve.

Hippocrates (460–370 BC) noted that "ischiatic" pain mainly affected men aged 40–60 years. In younger men it usually lasted 40 days. Contrary to modern ideas, radiation of pain to the foot had a good prognosis but pain that stayed in the hip was dreaded. (This was probably tuberculosis or other serious disease of the hip joint.) Areteus (150 AD) first distinguished nervous and arthritic "schiatica." He blamed nervous sciatica on an excess of cold and suggested that the remedy was local heat – spas, soothing ointments, counterirritants, and cautery.

Hippocrates first mentioned cautery and it appears throughout the ancient writings (Fig. 4.4). "Dung cautery" was in use by 100 AD and probably came from Arabic use of goat's dung. Albucasis (1100 AD) described local and wrist cautery for sciatica and drew a number of the instruments.

Domenico Cotugno (1765) wrote the first book on sciatica (Boni et al 1994). He combined new knowledge of anatomy and pathology with clinical observation. He separated nervous and arthritic sciatica and divided nervous sciatica into anterior and posterior types. He knew that the condition could be continuous or intermittent. He noted that sometimes

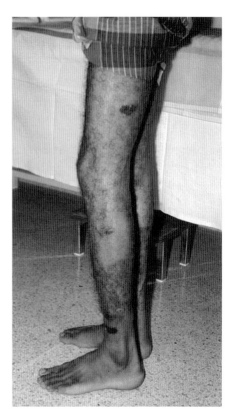

Figure 4.4 Cautery with a red hot iron is still in use in parts of the world today. See the S1 distribution.

the continuous became intermittent but never the other way around. Apart from a comment by Hippocrates that most attacks recover in 40 days, this was one of the first observations on the natural history of recovery. Cotugno thought that sciatica was due to an excess of fluid surrounding the nerve, which is perhaps not surprising as he was first to describe the dura and the cerebrospinal fluid. His treatment was to remove the excess fluid by cupping, blistering, and aquapuncture (sic), which put needles into the nerve itself to draw off the excess fluid. For many years sciatica was known as Cotugno's disease.

In the 19th century, sciatica was again thought to be a kind of rheumatism. Inflammation of the sciatic nerve might be primary or secondary. Primary causes included gout, rheumatism, syphilis, neuromata, poisons, trauma, and cold. Secondary causes included pelvic tumors, a distended rectum and bone disease, especially hip joint disease. This shows the new emphasis on identifiable pathology, but still no one understood sciatica itself. Fuller (1852) concluded that "the history of sciatica is, it must be confessed, the record of pathologic ignorance and therapeutic failure."

Orthopedic principles

Modern medical treatment for back pain is closely linked to the emergence of the specialty of orthopedics.

Early orthopedics was mainly about childhood deformities, and orthopedics first took an interest in sciatica because of sciatic scoliosis. From these roots, orthopedics expanded in the second half of the 19th century to include all musculoskeletal problems. Interest in spinal deformities spread to sciatica and back pain, and focused on the spine. Previously, back pain and sciatica were regarded as separate diseases. From now on, they were linked in the spine. Ever since, failure to distinguish our ideas and treatment of back pain and sciatica has caused much confusion, which continues to this day.

There was no precedent for the scale of casualties in World War I. For the first time, medical concern with trauma matched previous concern with disease. It also brought the treatment of fractures within the scope of orthopedics. Between the two world wars orthopedic surgeons struggled to gain control of fractures and trauma and so expand their professional practice. As back pain was an injury, it automatically fell within the growing province of orthopedics.

The discovery of X-rays opened up a whole new perspective. For the first time it was possible to visualize the spine during life. Soon, every incidental radiographic finding became an explanation for back pain and sciatica. Different authors blamed lumbosacral anomalies, facet joint degeneration, and sacroiliac disease. The 1920s and early 1930s saw operations to correct these anomalies by sacroiliac fusion, lumbosacral fusion, transversectomy, and facetectomy. The problem of back pain remained intractable.

In the UK, the father of modern orthopedics was Hugh Owen Thomas, who was a qualified medical practitioner from Liverpool (Fig. 4.5). He came from a long line of Welsh bonesetters but worked with his father for less than a year before separating from him. There was an inevitable conflict of

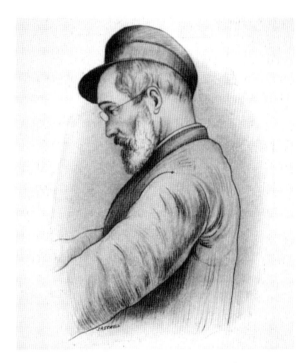

Figure 4.5   Hugh Owen Thomas (1834–1891), the father of English-speaking orthopedics. From a sketch made about 1884 (Keith 1919), with thanks to the Royal College of Physicians and Surgeons of Glasgow.

interest between the new orthopedic doctors and lay bonesetters. Thomas (1874) incorporated many of the bonesetters' manipulative skills into orthopedic treatment of fractures and dislocations, but rejected many of the bonesetters' principles. In particular, he would have nothing to do with manipulation for musculoskeletal symptoms. Instead, Thomas proposed rest as one of the main orthopedic principles for the treatment of fractures, tuberculosis, and joint infection, which was actually quite reasonable in the days before antibiotics and modern surgery. Therapeutic rest must be "enforced, uninterrupted and prolonged." Orthopedics achieved this by bracing, by bed rest, and later by surgical fusion.

Bonesetters, like their descendants the osteopaths and chiropractors, held to the competing principle of mobilization. Their patients continued their daily lives and normal activities. Medicine moved back pain into a medical context. Back pain was now a disease and the sufferer became a patient. Medical treatment often made the patient stop normal activities and actually prescribed disability.

Rest

Seriously ill people always went to "the sick bed," but that was a consequence of disease and not a treatment. Sydenham (1734) kept arthritic or rheumatic patients mobile: "For keeping bed constantly promotes and augments the disease."

John Hunter (1794) first proposed rest as a treatment, in a treatise on wounds and the new pathologic idea of inflammation:

> The first and great requisite for the restoration of injured parts is rest, as it allows that action, which is necessary for repairing injured parts, to go on without interruption, and as the injuries excite more action than is required, rest becomes still more necessary.

Hunter only devoted two pages to rest, but the theme was implicit in his whole book and had enormous influence.

Hilton popularized the idea in *Rest and Pain*, a course of lectures to the Royal College of Surgeons in 1860–1862 (Hilton 1887). He considered the influence of mechanical and physiologic rest in the treatment of accidents and surgical diseases, and the diagnostic value of pain. He proposed rest as a curative agent or natural therapeutics in surgical practice. His argument ranged from biblical quotations to contemporary ideas about cardiac, liver, renal, pulmonary, and brain disease. The divine gift or solace for mankind is rest from his labors. Sleep at night has a restorative function and is essential for the growth of plants and children. Psychiatric disease is linked to physical and mental exhaustion. More prosaically, after Hunter, he claimed that rest is the natural treatment for the inflammation of injury and wounds. Hilton's main contribution was to link rest to pain. Pain is the prime agent "suggesting the necessity and indeed compelling to seek rest." Hilton laid out this thesis in 14 introductory pages, while the rest of his book is a dated and uninteresting set of lectures on surgical conditions.

Hunter and Hilton were surgeons dealing with surgical disease, yet their ideas had an impact across the whole of medicine.

Injury ➞ Inflammation ➞ Rest ➞ Healing
(irritability) + pain

These were powerful and influential ideas, aided and abetted by the seductive title *Rest and Pain*.

Over the next century, physicians used rest to treat a wide range of conditions, from myocardial infarction to normal childbirth.

The rationale of rest for back pain and sciatica started from the 19th-century idea that they were due to injury. This caused traumatic inflammation so rest was essential for healing, or else chronic pain would develop. This was closely linked to the lingering idea that the spine and the nervous system were "irritable." Movement and physical activity may increase pain, and so must be harmful. Above all, the patient must avoid repeated injuries, for these would aggravate inflammation, prevent healing, and lead to chronic pain. This thinking was later updated in terms of the disk. The ruptured disk is clearly an injury and the disk "comes out." Disk pressure is lowest when lying down, so bed rest will somehow let the disk "go back." Unfortunately, none of these ideas had much pathologic validity. So it should come as no surprise that there was never any scientific evidence to support the dogma of bed rest for back pain. Such minor details have never held back medical enthusiasts.

As sciatica and later back pain came under the care of orthopedics, they got orthopedic treatment. Like all professionals, when we do not know what to do, we do what we are trained to do. So, when orthopedic doctors did not know how to treat back pain and sciatica, they prescribed their standard treatment of rest (Thomas 1874). Thus began "modern" treatment for back pain.

By 1900, a standard orthopedic text recommended 2–6 weeks' bed rest for acute back pain. Gradually, and especially after World War II, orthopedics became the leading specialty dealing with spinal disorders and rest became standard teaching and routine management. Up to the 1990s, one British textbook stated unequivocally: "The principle is to provide rest for the lumbar spine … [either] by a plaster jacket or bed rest. … Rest for the spine must be continued for six to twelve weeks according to progress." This was not finally updated till the 1995 edition. Another blithely continued till 1997: "REST: With an acute attack the patient should be kept in bed, with hips and knees slightly flexed and 10 kg traction to the pelvis … for two weeks." By implication this was in hospital (Fig. 4.6).

However, that teaching did not go unchallenged. The French school of orthopedics, from

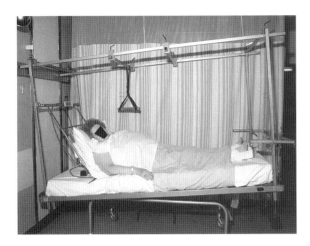

Figure 4.6   Hospital bed rest on traction in 1984.

Nicholas André in the early 18th century, promoted mobilization. One of the earliest English orthopedic texts on back pain was a lecture by Johnson (1881), who advised against bed rest. Indeed, he saw that bed rest might cause back pain!

> When the nutrition of the muscles has been impaired by long inaction, the results of confining to bed by illness or mechanical injury … pains in the back and limbs often follow the first attempts at exercise during convalescence. And these pains usually continue with more or less severity until by degrees the muscles regain their normal state of nutrition and vigour.

Asher (1947) waxed lyrical:

> It is my intention to justify placing beds and graves in the same category and to increase the amount of dread with which beds are usually regarded … There is hardly any part of the body which is immune to its dangers.

Cyriax (1969) was his usual forthright self:

> Recumbency admits failure and should be the doctor's last thought, not his first.

But these were voices in the orthopedic wilderness. The principle of therapeutic rest became the dominant medical treatment for back pain.

The dynasty of the disk

Vesalius (1543) described the intervertebral disk, but that was of purely anatomic interest. In the 19th century there were a number of postmortem reports of major trauma and disk damage causing paraplegia. Luschka (1858) first described two cases of prolapsed intervertebral disk with a connection from the nucleus pulposus through the posterior longitudinal ligament to the protrusion. Later Schmorl (1929) and Andrae (1929) made postmortem studies of large series of spines and described both posterior disk protrusions and protrusions into the vertebral bodies (Schmorl's nodes). They considered that most were asymptomatic in life! However, although pathologists saw these disk lesions, no one related them to the clinical symptom of sciatica.

Despite these reports, clinicians remained unaware of the disk. Middleton & Teacher (1911) then reported a case of fatal paraplegia from a central disk prolapse. They related it to the "sprains and racks of the back" and did a crude experiment to produce a disk prolapse. Goldthwait (1911) described a case of paresis after manipulation of the back for a "displaced sacroiliac joint." Harvey Cushing carried out a laminectomy and found nothing apart from "narrowing of the canal" at the lumbosacral junction. In an anguished search for the cause of this iatrogenic disaster, Goldthwait and Cushing considered compression of the nerve at the lumbosacral joint. They suggested the disk might be the cause of "many cases of lumbago, sciatica and paraplegia." Dandy (1929) gave the first complete account of disk surgery, a description of two cases with beautiful illustrations. They had paraplegia, myelographic evidence of complete block, a presumptive diagnosis of spinal cord tumor, and histologic proof of a sequestrated disk. Both cases recovered. Dandy probably deserves the real credit for the first description of disk prolapse. However, he only described the rare cauda equina syndrome and failed to recognize that disk prolapse was the common cause of sciatica. And so he missed his place in surgical history.

Mixter & Barr (1934) discovered "the ruptured disk" as the cause of sciatica. Mixter was a prominent neurosurgeon and Barr a young orthopedic surgeon. Barr had a patient with recurrent sciatica after a skiing accident. He had "several months in absolute recumbency on a Bradford frame" but his neurologic symptoms failed to improve. Barr thought he might have a spinal tumor and referred him to Mixter. A myelogram did not show a block

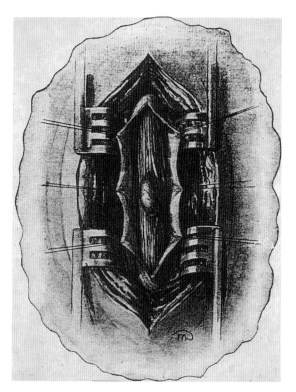

Figure 4.7 Surgery for "the ruptured disk." From Mixter & Barr (1934), with permission.

and so was reported normal. Despite that, Mixter went ahead with laminectomy and the operative diagnosis and pathology report were of enchondroma. Barr was not convinced and wondered if this might not be similar to Schmorl's pathologic description of posterior disk protrusion. Mixter & Barr then reviewed the histology of previous cases and compared them with normal disks, having to make special sections as no one had looked at the disk before. Of 16 surgical specimens of "enchondromas," they found that 10 were normal disk cartilage. Mixter & Barr then began to look for patients, and on December 19, 1932 operated on the first patient with a preoperative diagnosis of disk prolapse (Fig. 4.7). Their classic paper (Mixter & Barr 1934) gave the first complete clinical, pathologic, and surgical description of disk prolapse as the cause of sciatica. It also showed that surgical treatment was possible.

Mixter & Ayer (1935) wrote a much more radical paper the following year. This was very influential, although few authors quote it now. It added several

key ideas to the concept of disk prolapse. It suggested that disk rupture might cause back pain, even when there were no objective neurologic signs. It started modern myelography by describing the use of large quantities of dye and indentation of the dye column rather than a complete block. Even at that early stage, they admitted the results of disk surgery were less than ideal. Surgery cured leg pain in all but one case, but "some patients complain subsequently of lame back." Most important was their idea that the lesion was traumatic, although only 14 of their 23 cases reported even minor injuries. Disk lesions were now injuries to the spine, which the authors admitted "opens up an interesting problem in industrial medicine." This paper was the real start of the dynasty of the disk.

Disk rupture brought together the 19th-century ideas that back pain was an injury, an injury to the spine, and a mechanical problem that should be treated according to orthopedic principles. If all else failed, it could be fixed by surgery. Disk rupture made this into a marketable package. For the next 50 years the disk dominated medical thinking about back pain.

The first surgeons made the diagnosis of disk prolapse on hard neurologic signs. Their successors soon relied on symptoms alone, partly because of the risks and costs of early myelography. These moves away from the early strict criteria unleashed on an unsuspecting public a wave of surgical enthusiasm held back only by World War II. Key (1945) caused a furore at a meeting of the Southern Surgical Association in 1945 by claiming that "intervertebral disk lesions are the most common cause of low back pain with or without sciatica." Even the published discussion was heated. Magnuson retorted this was no more logical than saying that "all kittens born in an oven are biscuits!"

From the 1950s there was an explosion of disk surgery, closely related to the growth of orthopedics and neurosurgery. Indeed, it was claimed at one time that the average US neurosurgeon made half his income from disk surgery. But the rapid growth of disk surgery soon exposed its limitations. Even the enthusiasts admitted it was difficult to assess the results: "The question of liability, compensation and insurance loom large on the horizon and add complications compounded to an already knotty problem" (Love & Walsh 1938). By 1970, one authority on spinal surgery admitted that "no oper-ation in any field of surgery leaves in its wake more human wreckage than surgery on the lumbar spine" (De Palma & Rothman 1970). Surgeons gradually came to realize that disk surgery only helps the few patients with a surgically treatable lesion and that success depends on careful selection.

Undaunted, orthopedic surgeons extended the concept of "disk lesions." If sciatica is caused by disk prolapse, then back pain might be caused by disk degeneration. They ignored the normal age-related nature of these X-ray changes and their poor rela-tion to symptoms. They used biomechanical studies to support the hypothesis, despite the lack of clinical correlation. Once again, they could blame the disk for most back pain. The answer was spinal fusion, and this re-established the role of surgery in back pain. It also reinforced the influence of ortho-pedics in the management of ordinary backache. This approach has gravely distorted health care for the 99% of people with back trouble who do not have a surgical condition. It caused us to see back pain as a mechanical or structural problem, and therefore patients expect to be "fixed." Just as when they take their car to a mechanic, it is the doc-tor or therapist's responsibility to fix their backs. By the time they discover there is no such magic cure for back pain, they are trapped. They no longer have ordinary backache, but have become patients with a serious back injury or irreversible degenera-tion. This has led to unrealistic expectations and has diverted resources from attacking the real problem of back pain.

Disk surgery has survived the test of time for more than half a century because 80–90% of care-fully selected patients get good relief of sciatica. Sadly, this approach did not solve the problem of ordinary backache.

A HOLISTIC APPROACH

Since the ancient Greeks, most philosophers and many doctors have stressed the relationship between body and mind. It is fundamental to human existence and to medicine. Plato encapsu-lated this in the fourth century BC:

> So neither ought you to attempt to cure the body without the soul ... for part can never be well unless the whole is well.

In 100 AD, Rufus of Ephesus saw the need for a complete clinical assessment:

> And I place the interrogation of the patient first, since in this way you can learn how far his mind is healthy or otherwise; also his physical strengths and weaknesses, and get some idea of the part affected.

Stahl (1660–1734), writing at the time of the Renaissance, felt that the new physical sciences were not enough in themselves to explain human behavior. He was one in a long line of doctors since Hippocrates who took this view. His work has a surprisingly modern ring:

- the essential unity of the organism
- the personal element in liability to illness
- the part played by mental factors in mental and physical disease
- emotional life is important in treating patients and is independent of reason.

Sadly, the mechanistic approach of orthodox medicine soon swamped such holistic ideas. In the mind–body dichotomy, medicine dealt with the body, and pain was a simple signal of disease. Haller (1707–1777) founded modern physiology, so illness became a matter of disordered physiol-ogy. Pasteur (1822–1895) showed that infections are caused by microbes, and paved the way for modern treatment with antibiotics. The German pathologist Virchow (1858) proposed the concept of cellular pathology, which led to the disease model of human illness:

- Recognize patterns of symptoms and signs – history and examination
- Infer underlying pathology – diagnosis
- Apply physical therapy to that pathology – treatment
- Expect the illness to recover – cure.

The business of orthodox medicine was physical disease. We have already seen how the disease model changed medical thinking about back pain. Haller's concept of nerve excitability or irritability led to Brown's spinal irritation and Charcot's *grande hystérie*. So began our modern approach to the spine. But by concentrating entirely on physi-cal disease it also introduced a bias that has con-tinued to the present day. Brown (1828) described the syndrome of spinal irritation in young women. They had spinal tenderness, pain in the left breast, and many vague bodily symptoms. But these patients were unaware of their spinal tenderness until medical examiners drew it to their attention! The beauty of the diagnosis was that there was nothing physically wrong with the spine. But the more dramatic the treatment, the more effective it was for psychosomatic symptoms: "The ensuing orgy of blistering, leeching and cupping of the spine probably represents the first (unwitting) use of placebo therapy in modern surgery" (Shorter 1992). During the 1820s an increasing number of young women presented with spinal complaints augmented by medical suggestion.

Railway spine is one of the most distressing episodes in the history of back pain (see above). Erichsen (1866) brought together the spate of railway accidents, the new compensation laws, and Brown's concept of spinal irritation (Fig. 4.8). He suggested that minor railway injuries to the spine could have long-term effects. Controversy raged over the nature and indeed the existence of railway spine for many years in both medical and legal circles. In Europe, Valleix (1841) suggested that many

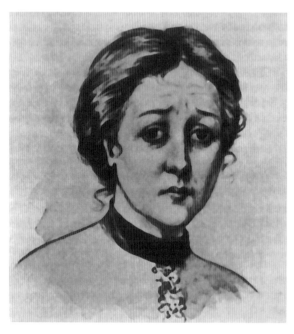

Figure 4.8 A railway spine victim. From Hamilton (1894), reproduced with permission from *Spine*.

of these symptoms were hysteric. In the USA, Page (1885) denounced railway spine as little more than traumatic lumbago, or a nervous disturbance with overtones of simulation or hysteria, combined with the deleterious effects of lawsuits. This view that the psychic shock of the accident produced "neurasthenia" gradually prevailed. "Exhaustion of the nervous system" or "disease of civilization related to industrialization" were in vogue by the end of the 19th century. At about the same time, the great French neurologist Charcot developed his theories of hysteria. Shortly before his death in 1896, Erichsen himself agreed that railway spine was probably a form of traumatic neurasthenia. As the diagnosis of railway spine fell into disrepute, so doctors, lawyers, and claimants shifted their attention to this new diagnosis. The condition spread from the railways to other work, road, and domestic accidents. With the acceptance of high-speed travel, better clinical examination, and the new X-rays, the diagnosis of railway spine faded. But Erichsen's railway spine caused a great deal of trouble before it was extinguished. And, like spinal irritation, some of its concepts endure to this day. Both medicolegal and lay circles came to accept that back pain is an injury and that minor trauma can lead to severe and permanent low back pain and disability.

The striking aspect of the stories of spinal irritation and railway spine is that vague clinical features gained such ready medical acceptance as physical diseases. This is not unique to back pain. Even today, many health professionals seem uncomfortable dealing with psychosomatic problems. They search desperately for a purely physical or neurophysiologic explanation, however unlikely, for the vaguest symptoms.

Medicine's struggle with these problems coincided with the growth of psychology and psychiatry. Heinroth first coined the term "psychosomatic" in 1818. He did not imply a psychological cause but simply wanted to describe the mutual interaction between psychological and physical events. It is now nearly a century since Freud reaffirmed the importance of psychological factors in medicine. He showed how doctors could assess psychoneurotic symptoms and gain insight into emotional processes. Meyer, one of the founders of American psychiatry, recognized that psychological factors affect the course and outcome of every illness, physical as well as mental.

People have always had psychosomatic or stress-related symptoms, but the form they take varies depending on what each culture accepts as legitimate. Complaints must be acceptable to the patient's family, health professionals, and society. What is acceptable changes over time and the history of psychosomatic disorders is of "ever-changing steps in a pas-de-deux between doctor and patient" (Shorter 1992). Up to the 18th century, psychosomatic symptoms were largely related to folk beliefs about external influences on health. In the 19th century, medical ideas focused on the nervous system and irritability. Psychosomatic symptoms changed to hysteric paralysis, then neurasthenia and traumatic neurosis. As medical ideas changed in the 20th century, so did psychosomatic systems. Now we focus on pain and fatigue. They are not only symptoms, but have become accepted as syndromes. People are also now much more aware of their health. From 1928 to 1931, a survey of US adults reported 82 episodes of illness per 100 people per annum. By 1982, that had risen to 212 episodes. People are now much more likely to regard themselves as "ill" and to seek health care, despite vast advances in nutrition, health care, and public health. At the same time medicine has lost much of its authority, and patients develop their own fixed beliefs about disease.

MANUAL THERAPY

The value of massage to soothe pain has been known since the fifth century (Schiotz & Cyriax 1975). It is still a common lay remedy today (Fig. 4.9).

Manual therapy is use of the hands to mobilize, adjust, manipulate, apply traction, massage, stimulate, or otherwise influence joints and muscles. In back pain, the basic idea is to *influence* spinal motion and so relieve pain and dysfunction. It may also produce change in neurophysiologic function and reduce muscle spasm. However, we still do not have a clear understanding of *how* manipulation works (McClune et al 1997).

Manual therapy includes manipulation and mobilization. Manipulation is generally defined as the application of a high-velocity, low-amplitude thrust to the spinal joint, slightly beyond its passive

range of motion. Mobilization is the application of force within the passive range of the joint, without a thrust. However, different therapists use the term "manipulation" loosely to describe a wide range of procedures. There are striking similarities in the techniques developed by different health professions, yet it is surprising how unaware the various practitioners seem to be of these similarities.

Ancient medical texts, from Hippocrates and Galen to Paré in the 16th century, describe manipulation. These were powerful spinal manipulations usually combined with traction and were probably for fractures and dislocations, or deformities of the spine (Fig. 4.10).

Spinal manipulation for back pain appears in folk medicine over many centuries from places as far apart as Norway, Mexico, and the Pacific Islands. The most common form was "trampling" for lumbago. For several hundred years, professional bone-setters or "sprain rubbers" also developed manual

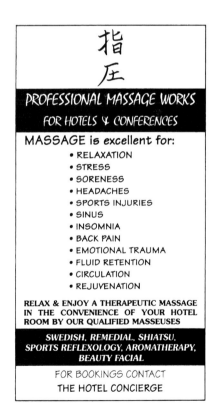

Figure 4.9   Massage is still in widespread use. An advert in an international hotel, 1997.

Figure 4.10 Most old medical descriptions of manipulation from the time of Hippocrates to the 17th century were probably for fracture-dislocation or deformity. From Sculteti (1662), with thanks to Glasgow University library.

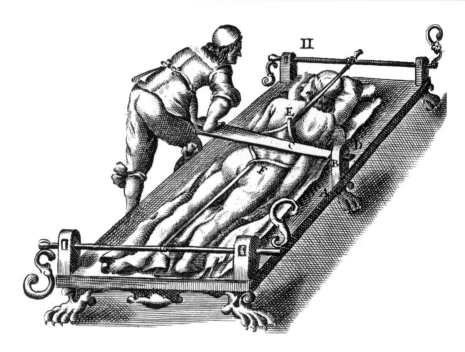

skills in manipulation. This was usually a family business handed down from one generation to the next by apprenticeship. St Bartholomew's Hospital in London had bonesetters on its staff in the 17th century, and one was even knighted.

They were called bonesetters because they attributed the pain to "a little bone lying out of place." Manipulation *reset* the bone to relieve the pain. The relationship between orthodox medicine and bonesetters varied from respect and cooperation to outright hostility. Paget gave a lecture to medical students in St Bartholomew's Hospital in 1866 on "cases that bonesetters cure." "Few of you are likely to practice without having a bonesetter as an enemy …" He cautioned against "the mischief that they do," but also admitted that "it sometimes does some good," with lumbago as an example. "Learn then to imitate what is good and avoid what is bad in the practice of bonesetting." The success of bonesetters was partly due to their practical skill and experience, but also to medical ignorance and neglect of common musculoskeletal symptoms. (Oh, how little has changed today!)

Although orthopedics took over the manipulation of spinal fractures and dislocations, orthodox medicine in the 19th century rejected manual therapy for symptomatic relief. This reflected its focus on identifiable pathology and "science." As

medicine struggled for professional status, it was happy to leave such hands-on therapy to others. In the UK, the Medical Act of 1858 registered medical practitioners and made it unethical to refer patients to unregistered practitioners. The result was to leave a vacuum, to be occupied by alternative health care, for people with spinal pain for whom orthodox medicine had little interest or help.

In the US, osteopathy and chiropractic developed to meet this need.

Osteopathy

On June 22, 1874, Dr Andrew T Still "flung to the breeze the banner of osteopathy" (Fig. 4.11). Still was an old school physician in Kansas and Missouri. He had little formal medical education but learned his trade by apprenticeship, as was normal practice for the time. He received an MD from the Kansas City Medical School, and practiced as a physician for a few years. Still lost three of his children in an epidemic of meningitis, and orthodox medicine could not save them. His brother was also a morphine addict through medical treatment. Still then started a campaign against orthodox medicine and "the indiscriminate use of drugs." He sought a better alternative, so he combined ancient principles of holistic medicine with the bonesetter's art, and

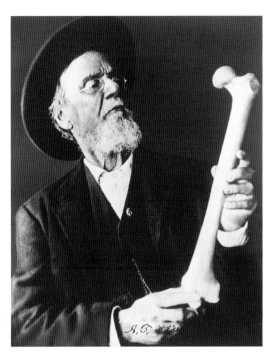

Figure 4.11   Dr Andrew T Still (1828–1917), the founder of osteopathic medicine. Courtesy of the British School of Osteopathy, with thanks.

based osteopathy on two main principles (Still 1899):

1. The body has within itself the power to combat disease. Hippocrates recognized that "it is our natures that are the physicians of our diseases. We must not meddle with nor hinder Nature's attempt towards recovery. First, do no harm."

2. The human framework is a machine, subject to the same mechanical principles and disturbed function as a steam engine. The cause of disease is "dislocated" bones, abnormal ligaments, and contracted muscles – especially in the back – that cause pressure on blood vessels and nerves, and also lead to ischemia and necrosis, in part due to a disturbance of the life force traveling along nerves. This dislocation was the original "osteopathic lesion."

Manipulation did not in itself cure the problem. Rather, it allowed the body to heal the osteopathic lesion. The structure–function concept was of an intimate bond between the framework and the workings of the human body. Still combined his

holistic approach to health and the healing power of nature with a practical approach to mechanical factors in health and disease. This provided a philosophy for manipulative therapy. But osteopathic medicine is more than just manipulation. It is a whole system of diagnosis, assessment, therapy, and prophylaxis. It is "a therapeutic system based on the belief that the body, in normal structural relationship and with adequate nutrition, is capable of mounting its own defences against most pathologic conditions" (DiGiovanna & Schiowitz 1991). Even if used primarily to treat symptoms, it also aims to help restore the individual to a more nearly ideal physiologic state of well-being.

DiGiovanna & Schiowitz (1991) gave a succinct modern summary of osteopathic principles:

- Osteopathic physicians … are primarily interested in the achievement of normal body mechanics as central to good health.
- The neuromusculoskeletal system is salient to the full expression of life.
- Structure governs function.
- The heart of osteopathy is the recognition of the body's ability to heal itself, with some external help, of most pathologic conditions.

Martinke (1991) and Seffinger (1997) presented the same ideas in a slightly different way:

- The body is a unit. It does not function as a collection of separate parts but is an integrated unit. The person is a single entity of body and mind.
- Structure and function are reciprocally interrelated.
- The body is capable of self-regulation, self-healing, and health maintenance.
- Rational treatment is based upon an understanding of the basic principles of body unity, self-regulation and the interrelationship of structure and function.

Chiropractic

D D Palmer (Fig. 4.12) carried out the first chiropractic treatment in Iowa on September 18, 1895. Palmer was a magnetic healer, who knew the early medical literature well and the methods of the bonesetters. He was probably also acquainted with osteopathic techniques in neighboring Missouri. There

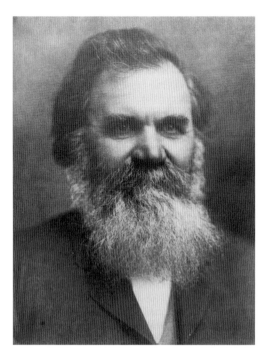

Figure 4.12   D D Palmer (1845–1913), the founder of chiropractic. Courtesy of Palmer College of Chiropractic Archives, David D Palmer Health Sciences Library.

are many similarities between chiropractic and osteopathy, though they have always had distinct professional identities and philosophies.

Chiropractic dealt with *subluxations* – reduced mobility and slight malposition of a vertebral segment. It laid more emphasis on the resulting pressure on nerves and ignored the flow of blood or body fluid. Palmer (1910) also placed more stress on the method of manipulation or *adjustment*:

> I do claim ... to be the first to replace displaced vertebrae by using the spinous or transverse processes as levers whereby to rack displaced vertebrae into normal position, and from this basic fact, to create a science, which is destined to revolutionize the theory and practice of the healing art...

Chiropractic also had, and still has, a strong philosophic base (Coulter 1999). Palmer founded chiropractic on the twin pillars of science and vitalism, with strong emphasis on the mind–body relationship (Box 4.2). The mechanical side was the manipulation of subluxations. Vitalism gave an equally strong metaphysical and spiritual side. Palmer saw

---

Box 4.1   Modern chiropractic (Chapman–Smith 2000)

Chiropractic is a health care discipline that emphasizes the inherent recuperative power of the body to heal itself without the use of drugs or surgery. The *practice of chiropractic* focuses on the relationship between structure (primarily the spine) and function (as coordinated by the nervous system) and how that relationship affects the preservation and restoration of health. In addition, doctors of chiropractic recognize the value and responsibility of working in cooperation with other health care practitioners when in the best interests of the patient.

- Chiropractors are first-contact physicians who possess the diagnostic skills to differentiate health conditions that are amenable to their management from those conditions that require referral or co-management
- Chiropractors provide conservative management of neuromusculoskeletal disorders and related functional manifestations including, but not limited to, back pain, neck pain, and headaches
- Chiropractors are expert providers of spinal and other therapeutic manipulation/adjustments. They utilize a variety of manual, mechanical, and electrical therapeutic modalities. Chiropractors also provide patient evaluations and instructions regarding disease prevention and health promotion through proper nutrition, exercise, and lifestyle modification, among others

---

this as a life force, expressed in the individual as innate intelligence that controls and coordinates bodily activity and influences health and illness. It is the fundamental ability of the body to heal itself. Vitalism is holistic and naturopathic. Holism integrates body, mind, and spirit. It considers that health depends on obeying certain natural laws and on lifestyle, and that deviation can lead to illness. The innate intelligence gives purpose, balance, and direction to all biologic function. The naturopathic approach is the opposite of orthodox or allopathic

Box 4.2   A humanistic philosophy (Coulter 1999)

- Naturalism   – the body is built on nature's order
                – look to nature for the cure
- Vitalism   – the healing power of nature
                – recognize the patient's own capacity for self-healing
- Holism   – mind, body, and spirit
                – focus care on the whole patient, in the context of his or her life
- Therapeutic   – "first, do no harm"
  conservatism – the least care is the best care
- Humanistic   – inalienable human rights to dignity and care
                – recognize and respect the patient's point of view
- Egalitarian   – share responsibility for care with the patient

medicine. The allopathic approach considers that disease is due to an external cause overcoming the body's resistance, e.g., germs cause infection. Orthodox medicine's answer is to counter the external cause, e.g., with antibiotics. The naturopathic approach considers that illness is largely due to the person's lowered resistance, e.g., only a few of those exposed to germs become infected. So the answer is to strengthen the person, rather than attack the external cause. Healing depends on mobilizing the innate recuperative powers within the patient.

The emphasis of chiropractic is on natural remedies. It restores musculoskeletal integrity and neurophysiologic function. It stresses a proper diet, lifestyle, and a healthy environment. It uses conservative, safe treatments and avoids drugs and surgery. It helps the patient to understand that his or her illness is the result of the body's failure to maintain a healthy state. Manipulation may stimulate healing, but the patient also has to change and return to more healthy living. It is a patient-centered, hands-on approach that depends on good communication between doctor and patient. Touch and physical contact between doctor and patient help to mobilize this internal healing power. It is

wellness-oriented rather than sickness-oriented, and is concerned with the person who is ill rather than the illness that the person has.

Rereading these two sections, I may have given the impression that chiropractic is more holistic than osteopathic medicine. That is not the case. Both have strong holistic roots, and, today, both emphasize a biopsychosocial approach. However, there are widely differing views in both professions. At one extreme are those practitioners who see themselves as musculoskeletal specialists. At the other extreme are those with an almost evangelic faith in the benefits of their treatment for the human condition. There is also some variation between views in the US and the UK.

There is a danger, of course, that if this philosophy is carried to extremes it may become dogma. We must balance the holistic and the mechanistic approaches. "First do no harm" (Hippocrates), but at the same time remember that "it ill behoves the skilled physician to mumble charms over ills that crave the knife" (Sophocles). Modern osteopathic medicine and chiropractic have a holistic approach but incorporate and use knowledge from the mechanistic, scientific approach.

Practice, of course, tends to leave philosophy some way behind. Many osteopaths and chiropractors, like many orthodox doctors and therapists, simply get on with treating the patient's physical symptoms.

The reaction of orthodox medicine

We must see the origins of osteopathy and chiropractic in the context of their time (Northup 1966). In the late 19th century, Kansas, Missouri, and Iowa were still the American frontier. This was an age of heroic medicine. The primitive state of medical science meant that some of the new invasive treatments for disease did as much harm as good, leading to public outrage and a search for safer alternatives. The medical reform movement in the US stressed the need for personal responsibility for health, lifestyle recommendations, and professional alternatives to orthodox medicine. Osteopathy and chiropractic sought to preserve some of the ancient principles that orthodox medicine seemed to be abandoning. This was the Bible belt, and the medical reform movement had strong evangelic overtones. That philosophic base has helped to sustain the professional identity of osteopathic medicine and chiropractic to this day.

This background also helps us to understand the reaction of orthodox medicine. Osteopathy and chiropractic were direct competitors at a time when orthodox medicine was struggling to establish its own professional status. They vehemently accused orthodox medicine of abandoning ancient medical principles. It is little wonder that orthodox medicine met the new health professions with outright hostility and persecution. From 1896 to as late as 1949, hundreds of chiropractors went to jail in the US for giving "unlawful treatment" and for the unlawful practice of medicine. Litigation between chiropractic and the American Medical Association was not finally settled till 1987 (Chapman-Smith 2000). Despite that, osteopathic medicine and chiropractic survived, supported by patients who continued to choose them in preference to orthodox medicine.

They also developed professional education, the equal of orthodox medicine, with virtually no external funding. Andrew Still founded the American School of Osteopathy in 1892 and D D Palmer founded the first school of chiropractic in 1896. During the 20th century, osteopathic training in the US gradually became very like medical training, though with more emphasis on musculoskeletal disorders and manual therapy. By 1968 the American Medical Association finally withdrew its opposition and proposed eventual amalgamation of orthodox and osteopathic medicine. By the 1980s osteopathic medicine was fully recognized in every state. A DO is now equivalent to an MD. Osteopathic physicians are once again part of mainstream medicine and they practice in every medical specialty. Chiropractic stayed completely independent and recognition as a health profession was slower. There are now 15 colleges of osteopathy and 16 colleges of chiropractic in the US. Progress in Europe has been slower. The British School of Osteopathy opened in 1917, but the Anglo-European College of Chiropractic did not open until 1965. In the UK, Acts of Parliament to register and regulate osteopaths and chiropractors were not passed until 1993 and 1994. Even today, most osteopaths and chiropractors practice independently from orthodox medicine.

There are now about 70 000 chiropractors in the US, 6000 in Canada, 1500 in the UK, and about 90 000 internationally (Chapman-Smith 2000, www.chiropracticreport.com). The number of practicing osteopaths is harder to estimate because in the US they are now integrated into mainstream medicine.

Manual medicine

Orthodox medicine has been slow to concede that it can learn anything from osteopathy and chiropractic. Early enthusiastic claims that spinal manipulation could cure distant diseases ranging from diabetes to goiter laid osteopathy and chiropractic open to medical ridicule. There is still a major problem of communication and misunderstanding. For example, subluxation means very different things to a chiropractor and an orthopedic surgeon. Patients still frequently misinterpret osteopathic and chiropractic explanations of segmental dysfunction as "disks out" which orthodox physicians deny.

But orthodox medicine never wholly abandoned manual therapy. In the 19th century physicians stopped doing manipulation themselves, but were still interested in physical therapies. Magnetism, electrotherapy, and hydrotherapy were all in vogue. In Europe this was the age of the spa, where new wealth and ease of travel let middle-class women congregate to indulge in these therapies.

In the mid 20th century, there was also re-emergence of an orthodox specialty of "manual medicine." Cyriax (1969) in England led the fight to restore the place of manipulation in the treatment of musculoskeletal disorders. He strongly rejected osteopathic and chiropractic theories and philosophies as quackery. Instead, he tried to reintegrate manipulation as a purely physical modality. However, there are still few physicians who have learned these skills, and musculoskeletal medicine has remained a tiny specialty. Orthodox medicine has largely delegated manual therapy to physiotherapists.

Physical therapy

Physiotherapy in the UK, Europe, and in the rest of the English-speaking world is the same thing as physical therapy in the US.

"Physiotherapy is a health care profession that emphasizes the use of physical approaches in the prevention and treatment of disease and disability" (CSP 1991). The *Standards of Physiotherapy Practice* (CSP 1993) expand this:

> Physiotherapy is a health care profession with an emphasis on analysis of movement based on the structure and function of the body and the use of physical approaches to the promotion of health, and the prevention, treatment and management of disease and disability … The aim is to identify and diagnose the specific components of movement or function responsible for the patient's physical problems.

This "is based on an assessment of movement and function" and also "takes account of the patient's current psychological, cultural and social factors."

In 1894, a group of British nurses started the Society of Trained Masseuses for women practicing massage or "medical rubbing" (Wickstead 1948). Their original aim was "to make massage a safe, clean and honorable profession for British women." At first, the society and its examinations were entirely about massage. By 1920, it got a Royal Charter "to promote a curriculum and standard of qualification for the persons engaged in the practice of massage, medical gymnastics, electrotherapies and kindred methods of treatment." In 1994, a writer in the centennial issue of *Physiotherapy* commented:

> While not wishing to enter into the debate about their use, misuse or disuse in every day practice, suffice to comment that they remain, in one form or another, the basis of practice today.

Physiotherapists have also always used manual therapy. Since the 1970s, in the face of growing competition from chiropractic and osteopathy, they have taken even greater interest in mobilization and manipulation. Therapists in Australia and New Zealand have played a leading part.

Physical therapy in the US started officially during World War I (Murphy 1995). The Surgeon General of the US army saw the need for a core of young women to assist the "reconstruction" of maimed and disabled soldiers (Fig. 4.13). They were led by Mary MacMillan, who qualified in physical education and then did postgraduate physiotherapy and orthopedic studies in England. By the end of the war there were 1200 reconstruction aides with

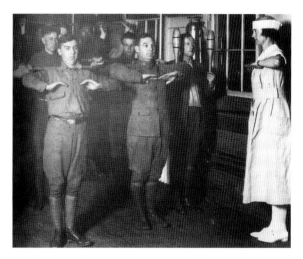

Figure 4.13   A rehabilitation class in a reconstruction center in 1919. Reprinted with permission of the American Physical Therapy Association from Murphy W. Healing the generations: A history of physical therapy and the American Physical Therapy Association. Alexandria, VA: American Physical Therapy Association 1995.

valuable clinical experience. They also had the respect and support of orthodox medicine, and in 1921 they set up the American Physical Therapy Association (APTA).

There have always been close links between US and UK physiotherapy. However, from the start, physical therapy in the US had a stronger emphasis on exercise and rehabilitation. This reflected the different background of its early leaders, and its whole *raison d'être* for rehabilitation of the injured. Its work with polio and then in World War II, the Korean war, and the Vietnam war reinforced the focus on neuromuscular and musculoskeletal disabilities.

The APTA (1997) *Guide to Physical Therapist Practice* put this first. Physical therapy is about "the preservation, development and restoration of maximum physical function." It is "the examination, evaluation, treatment and prevention of neuromuscular, musculoskeletal, cardiovascular and pulmonary disorders that produce movement impairments, disabilities and functional limitations." This includes:

- examining patients with impairments, functional limitations, and disability or other health-related conditions in order to determine a diagnosis, prognosis, and intervention

- alleviating impairments and functional limitations by designing, implementing, and modifying therapeutic interventions that include, but are not limited to, the following (note the order):
  - therapeutic exercise (including aerobic conditioning)
  - functional training in self-care and home management (including activities of daily living)
  - functional training in community or work reintegration activities
  - manual therapy techniques (including mobilization and manipulation)
  - prescription, fabrication, and application of assistive, adaptive, supportive, and protective devices and equipment
  - physical agents and mechanical modalities
  - electrotherapeutic modalities
  - patient-related instruction
- preventing injury, impairments, functional limitations, and disabilities, including the promotion and maintenance of fitness, health, and quality of life.

This continued an ancient Greek tradition of physical culture and remedial exercises, and drew on the Swedish movements of the early 19th century. In the UK, also, experience in two world wars, and close links with orthopedics, increased the emphasis on remedial exercises and re-education. This changing role led to a change of name to the Chartered Society of Physiotherapy (CSP), with passionate debate. Some therapists felt that to reduce the role of massage was to forfeit the birthright of the profession. However, the change of name did acknowledge the increasing role of "restoration of function by active work on the part of the patient." That dilemma is still not fully resolved on either side of the Atlantic. A more critical writer in the centennial edition of *Physiotherapy* still had reservations in 1994:

> Most current treatments are really only dealing with symptoms and giving short-lived relief. They are usually received by a passive patient, from a therapist who very much *gives* a treatment.

Physiotherapy has always been closely allied to orthodox medicine. At the end of the 19th century, like the nursing profession from which it arose, it was subservient. The CSP's first rule of professional conduct stated: "no massage to be undertaken except under medical direction." Not until the 1970s did UK doctors stop prescribing the modalities and course of physiotherapy treatment. The current rules of the CSP date from 1987, following a major revision in collaboration with the British Medical Association: "Chartered physiotherapists shall communicate and co-operate with registered medical practitioners in the diagnosis, treatment and management of patients." It still assumed that patients would make first contact with a physician but did accept that the therapist was now properly involved in clinical assessment and diagnosis. By 1993, the *Standards of Physiotherapy Practice* were much more confident (CSP 1993): "Physiotherapists, where appropriate, are members of the multi-disciplinary team caring for the patient." However, "this role does not restrict chartered physiotherapists who so wish from accepting the responsibility of independent professional practice."

There has been a similar but faster trend in the US. The American Medical Association accredited schools of physical therapy until 1980, when the APTA finally took over. Academic standards have steadily risen. Four-year bachelor degrees had become standard by the early 1950s. During the 1960s and 1970s there was a rapid expansion of research activities and increasing numbers of physical therapists gained PhDs. Sahrmann (1998) described the trend over the past 40 years: "the transition from a technical field with individuals skilled in the application of physical modalities to a profession with knowledge of the movement function of the body."

THE HISTORY OF LOW BACK DISABILITY

There is little mention of low back disability in ancient times, although, in fairness, medical writing did not show much interest in any form of disability. Seriously ill people who took to the sick bed usually did not survive long. Chronic disability depends on some form of social support. Some cripples became beggars, but that was always a precarious existence. Early codes of compensation dealt with serious bodily mutilation, and did not mention a minor problem like back pain. It seems very unlikely that back pain was accepted as a reason for chronic disability in the harsh conditions of earlier times. Chronic low back disability was simply not possible for most ordinary people.

Ramazzini (1705) gave the first report of work-related back pain in *A Treatise on the Diseases of Tradesmen*. He found that servants at court who stood for long periods and weavers because of the violent action of their looms were liable to "pains in the loyns." Fowler (1795) noted that "the lumbago is a very common disease among laboring farmers from their frequent exposure to cold and hardships." However, these were solitary reports and did not mention disability.

Modern concepts of disability, compensation, and social security date from the industrial revolution. The spate of accidents and injuries led to growing acceptance of society's responsibility to care for "the wounded soldiers of industry" (Fig. 4.14). Over many decades this led to financial support or compensation for all who are sick or disabled and unfit for work.

The first report of low back disability was on the railways. A *Lancet* commission (1862) on "The influence of railway travel on the public health" found that railway workers had more sickness than seamen, miners, or laborers. Lumbago was one of the most common causes. As we have seen, railway spine became an increasing problem between 1860 and 1880, and introduced the concept of back injury. By the 1880s and 1890s, the first reports of long-term low back disability were in the context of compensation.

New laws led to a spate of legal and medical activity. Many injuries were severe and fully justified compensation, but there was soon a problem of many claims for trivial injuries. Some of these claimants had subjective symptoms without much objective evidence of injury and "sprains and strains" of the back were soon a leading example. The limitations of medical examination made the problem worse: "Lawyers and judges appear to have a pretty generally formed opinion that a doctor's statement concerning disability of the lower back is largely a matter of guesswork" (Wentworth 1916). As legislation extended the scope of compensation, so the scale of the problem grew. By 1915, "pain in the back as a result of injury is the most frequent affection for which compensation is demanded from the casualty company." King (1915) summed up the dilemma neatly: "Lumbago is a condition of most frequent occurrence. The laborer however seldom suffers from the pain of lumbago but is a frequent victim of pain in the back due to injury." He did not imply that the worker was always lying.

> It is easy to trace the mental process of a patient who, after a hard previous day's work, honestly concludes that the lumbago of today had its origin in the employment of yesterday. Such an individual is scarcely a malingerer, but rather the victim of a false conception, the more deep rooted often because of tactless disputes at previous examinations (Conn 1922).

There was growing interest in low back pain and disability in an industrial context during the first two decades of the 20th century. The medical answer was better diagnosis, better treatment, and the detection of malingering. The industrial answer was better selection of employees and better working practices. The US Draft Board in the First World War agreed. Many conscripts were rejected because of "static problems" that they thought might lead to back pain. Despite this, many recruits broke down with back pain during training. The alarmed authorities set up special training battalions and the results were striking. They quickly made 80% of these "derelicts" fit for service.

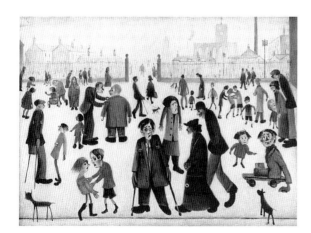

Figure 4.14 The "wounded soldiers of industry." *The Cripples* by L S Lowry, courtesy of City of Salford Museums and Art Gallery.

Table 4.1 The historic parallels between low back pain, sciatica, disability, and compensation

Date	Backache	Sciatica	Disability	Illness behavior	Compensation
2000 1500	1500 Edwin Smith papyrus – case presentation				≈1750 Code of Hammurabi
1000 500		≈400 Hippocrates – clinical description		Hippocrates	≈800 ius Taliones Military pensions Roman law
BC 100 0 AD 100					
150	150 Galen – symptom of disease – "fleeting pains" of joints and muscles	≈150 Aretaeus – nervous – arthritic			
200					
500					
1000				Arabian medicine – isolated case presentations	
1500	1681 Sydenham – rheumatism	1765 Contugno – modern clinical entity	1705 Ramazzini – occupational back pain		
1800	1828 Brown – spinal irritation			1816 Heberden 1828 Spinal irritation	1836 First personal injury case in English High Court 1846 Fatal Accident Act
1850	1866/ Erichsen – railway spine 1874 Thomas – orthopedic surgery, therapeutic rest		1866 Railway spine	1866 Railway spine 1880 Freud – psychologic medicine	1880 Employers' Liability Act 1897 Workmen's Compensation Act – compulsory insurance
1900		1934 Mixter & Barr – disk rupture – disk surgery	1900–1920 Industrial back pain 1930 First population morbidity statistics Post World War II epidemic of low back disability Chronic pain syndrome	1910 Medicolegal assessment	1911 National Health Insurance Act – state insurance for injury and sickness 1948 National Health Service and comprehensive social security
1950	Degenerate disk disease Chronic pain syndrome			1960 Mechanic-illness behavior	

They suggested that back pain might be "a fitness problem" rather than a medical problem.

Early epidemiology was about mortality, infectious disease, and child health. Not until 1921 did the UK Ministry of Health commission a report on rheumatic diseases. This found that 16% of all disabilities were due to rheumatism, and more than half of these were due to lumbago, muscular pain, and undefined rheumatism.

The Department of Health for Scotland gathered some of the first morbidity data in the world during the 1930s. They made a national survey of people who had been sick-listed continuously for 12 months. Rheumatism caused 12.6% of all chronic disability, and three-quarters of these cases were lumbago, muscular and undefined rheumatism. Rheumatism was now a more common cause of long-term disability than tuberculosis, even though tuberculosis was still rife. Only mental diseases were more common (21.4%). They made the important point that rheumatic disability was mainly found in younger adults. They also found that chronic disability due to rheumatism was growing faster than any other form of disability.

There were similar changes in low back disability in the British Army between the two world wars. Lumbago caused 0.23% of "medical admissions" in 1914–1918, and 1.07% in 1939–1945. (This military term is closer to sick certification than hospitalization.) This increase in back pain contrasted with sciatica, which caused 0.2% of medical admissions in both wars. In World War I, back pain was still usually diagnosed as either "fibrositis" or other rheumatic conditions. By World War II, it was more likely to be a "strain." The outcome also changed. In World War I, 50% returned to duty within 2 weeks, but in World War II the average period off duty was 2 months and "the men are often reconciled to being a chronic case." By World War II, "fibrositis" and mild referred sciatica pain had ousted dyspepsia, diarrhea, and headache as the chief cause of withdrawal from army duties.

There is one fascinating footnote. The above history of low back disability is almost entirely about men. There was very little mention of low back disability in women. In this respect, women lagged behind men for many years, which may reflect the different social roles of men and women, particularly in work. Only recently have trends of sexual equality allowed women to have low back disability as well. Table 4.1 summarizes the history of low back pain and disability.

TIME FOR A REVOLUTION

By the last decade of the 20th century the scene was set for a revolution in the management of back pain. Many divergent strands were coming together. Traditional and increasingly high-tech medicine had been very successful at dealing with many serious spinal diseases. It was ineffective for ordinary backache and had not halted the growing epidemic of low back disability. Many specialist doctors and therapists might still be happy and confident "doing their thing" but many family doctors, patients, and policy makers were dissatisfied. There was increasing evidence against traditional treatment by rest and for a more active approach. There was gradual recognition and acceptance that, after all, osteopathy and chiropractic might have something to offer. There was growing demand for a more holistic approach.

Summary

- Human beings have had back pain all through history. There is no historic evidence it has changed
- What has changed is how we understand and manage the symptom of pain in the back. Three key ideas in the 19th century laid the foundation for traditional 20th-century management:
  - back pain comes from the spine and involves the nervous system
  - it is due to injury
  - the back is irritable and should be treated by rest
- The discovery of the disk brought these ideas together and made them into a marketable package. After World War II, orthopedics came to dominate medical thinking and the treatment of back pain and sciatica
- Osteopathy and chiropractic have always had a very different approach to back pain
- By the end of the 20th century the time was ripe for a revolution in back care

References

Allan & Waddell (1989) provide a more comprehensive bibliography to the historic literature

Allan D B, Waddell G 1989 An historical perspective on low back pain and disability. Acta Orthopaedica Scandinavica (suppl. 234) 60: 1–23

Andrae A 1929 Ueber Knorpelknotchen am hinteren Ende der Wirbelbandscheiben im Bereich des Spinalkanals. Beiträge zur pathologischer Anatomie und zur allgemeines Pathologie 82: 464–474

APTA 1997 Guide to physical therapist practice: a description of patient management, 2nd edn., vol. I. American Physical Therapy Association, Alexandria, VA

Asher R A J 1947 The dangers of going to bed. British Medical Journal 967–968

Boni T, Benini A, Dvorak J 1994 Historical perspectives: Domenico Felice Antonio Cotugno. Spine 19: 1767–1770

Breasted J H 1930 The Edwin Smith papyrus: published in facsimile and heiroglyphic transliteration with translation and commentary in two volumes. University of Chicago Press, Chicago

Brown T 1828 On irritation of the spinal nerves. Glasgow Medical Journal 1: 131–160

Chapman-Smith D A 2000 The chiropractic profession. Its education, practice, research and future directions. NCMIC Group, West Des Moines, Iowa

Conn H R 1922 The acute painful back among industrial employees alleging compensable injury. Journal of the American Medical Association 79: 1210–1212

Cotugno D 1765 De ischiade nervosa commentarius. Neapoli apud frat Simonios (a treatise on the nervous sciatica or nervous hip gout). English translation 1775. Wilkie, London

Coulter I D 1999 Chiropractic: a philosophy for alternative health care. Butterworth-Heinemann, Oxford

CSP 1991 Curriculum of study. Chartered Society of Physiotherapists, London

CSP 1993 Standards of physiotherapy practice. Chartered Society of Physiotherapists, London

Cyriax J 1969 Textbook of orthopaedic medicine. Williams & Wilkins, Baltimore

Dandy W E 1929 Loose cartilage from intervertebral discs simulating tumour of the spinal cord. Archives of Surgery 19: 660–672

De Palma A F, Rothman R H 1970 The intervertebral disc. W B Saunders, Philadelphia

DiGiovanna E L, Schiowitz S (eds) 1991 An osteopathic approach to diagnosis and treatment. Lippincott, Philadelphia

Erichsen J E 1866 On railway and other injuries of the nervous system. Six lectures on certain obscure injuries of the nervous system commonly met with as a result of shock to the body received in collisions in railways. Walton & Maberly, London

Fowler T 1795 Medical reports of the effects of blood letting, sudorifics and blistering in the cure of acute and chronic rheumatism. Johnstone, London

Fuller H W 1852 On rheumatism, rheumatic gout and sciatica: the pathology, symptoms and treatment. Churchill, London

Goldthwait J E 1911 The lumbosacral articulation. An explanation of many cases of "lumbago", "sciatica" and paraplegia. Boston Medical and Surgical Journal 164: 365–372

Hamilton A M 1894 Railway and other accidents. William Wood, New York, pp 15–44

Hilton J 1887 Rest and pain. In: Jacobson W H A (ed.) A course of lectures at the Royal College of Surgeons of England, 4th edn. Bell & Sons, London

Hunter J 1794 A treatise on the blood, inflammation and gun-shot wounds. Nicol, London

Johnson G 1881 A lecture on backache and the diagnosis of its various causes with hints on treatment. British Medical Journal 1: 221–224

Keith A 1919 Menders of the maimed. Oxford Medical Publications, London

Keller T, Chappell T 1996 Historical perspective: the rise and fall of Erichsen's disease (railway spine). Spine 21: 1597–1601

Key J A 1945 Intervertebral disk lesions are the most common cause of back pain with or without sciatica. Annals of Surgery 121: 534–544

King H D 1915 Injuries of the back from a medical legal standpoint. Texas State Journal of Medicine 11: 442–445

Lancet commission 1862 The influence of railway travelling on public health. Lancet 1: 15–19, 48–53, 79–84

Love J G, Walsh M N 1938 Protruded intervertebral disks: report of one hundred cases in which operation was performed. Journal of the American Medical Association 111: 396–400

Luschka H 1858 Die Halbgelenke des menschlichen Korpers. G Reimer, Berlin

Martinke D J 1991 The philosophy of osteopathic medicine. In: DiGiovanna E L, Schiowitz S (eds) An osteopathic approach to diagnosis and treatment. Lippincott, Philadelphia, pp 3–6

McClune T, Clarke R, Walker C, Burton K 1997 Osteopathic management of mechanical low back pain. In: Giles L G F, Singer K P (eds) Clinical anatomy and management of low back pain. Butterworth-Heinemann, Oxford, pp 358–368

Middleton G S, Teacher J H 1911 Injury of the spinal cord due to rupture of an intervertebral disk due to muscular effort. Glasgow Medical Journal 76: 1–6

Mixter W J, Ayer J B 1935 Herniation or rupture of the intervertebral disk into the spinal canal. New England Journal of Medicine 213: 385–395

Mixter W J, Barr J S 1934 Rupture of the intervertebral disk with involvement of the spinal canal. New England Journal of Medicine 211: 210–215

Murphy W 1995 Healing the generations: a history of physical therapy and the American Physical Therapy Association. American Physical Therapy Association, Alexandria, VA

Northup G W 1966 Osteopathic medicine: an American reformation. American Osteopathic Association, Chicago

Page H W 1885 Injuries of the spine and spinal cord. Churchill, London

Palmer D D 1910 The science, art and philosophy of chiropractic. Portland Printing House, Oregon

Paracelsus (Bombastus A B Hohenheim – Aureolus Philipus Theorastus) 1493–1541 Samtliche Wenke Harausg (14 vols). von K Sudhoff und W Mathiessen (1922–1923), Munchen, Berlin, Barth und Oldenburg

Ramazzini B 1705 A treatise on the diseases of tradesmen. Bell, London

Sahrmann SA 1998 Moving precisely? Or taking the path of least resistance? Physical Therapy 78: 1208–1218

Schiotz E H, Cyriax J 1975 Manipulation past and present. Heinemann, London

Schmorl G 1929 Ueber Knorpel knoten an der Hinterflache der Wirbelbandschieben. Fortschritte ander Geb.der Rontgenstrahlen 40: 629–634

Scudamore C 1816 A treatise on the nature and cure of gout and rheumatism. Longmans, London

Sculteti I 1662 Armamentarium chirurgicum. Amstellodami

Seffinger M A 1997 Development of osteopathic philosophy. In: Ward R C (ed.) Foundations of osteopathic medicine. Williams & Wilkins, Baltimore, pp 3–12

Shorter E 1992 From paralysis to fatigue: a history of psychosomatic illness in the modern era. Free Press, New York

Still A T 1899 Philosophy of osteopathy. A T Still, Kirksville, MO

Sydenham T 1734 The whole works of that excellent physician Dr Thomas Sydenham (translated by John Pechey), 10th edn. W Feales, London

Thomas H O 1874 Contributions to medicine and surgery. Lewis, London

Valleix F L I 1841 Traité des neuralgies ou affections douloureuses des nerfs. J B Baillière, Paris

Vesalius A 1543 De humani corporis fabrica. Basileae ex off Ioannis Oporini

Virchow R 1858 Die cellular Pathologie in ihrer Begrundurg auf physiologische und pathologische. A Hirschwald, Berlin

Wentworth E T 1916 Systematic diagnosis in backache. Journal of Bone and Joint Surgery 8: 137–170

Wickstead J H 1948 The growth of a profession. Being the history of the Chartered Society of Physiotherapy 1894–1945. Edward Arnold, London

Chapter 5

The epidemiology of back pain

What is the impact of back pain today? There is no doubt it is a common problem, however we judge it. We may look at back pain as a symptom in the general population, as disability, as a reason for health care, or in terms of short- and long-term work loss. By any of these measures, back pain is a major problem. But do we really have an epidemic of low back pain? As we saw in Chapter 3, we must consider pain and disability separately. First, we will look at the occurrence of back pain today. Then we will look at the present scale of low back disability. Finally, we will try to see whether back pain and disability are changing.

DEFINING THE PROBLEM

To understand the epidemiology of back pain, we must first consider what we are trying to measure and how we measure it. Most surveys define *low back pain* between the costal margins and the gluteal folds. Some surveys include a diagram (Fig. 5.1).

We should also remind ourselves about common epidemiologic terms:

- *Prevalence* is the percentage of people in a known population who have the symptom during a particular period of time.
- *Point prevalence* is the percentage who have pain now, on the day of interview.
- *One-month* or *1-year prevalence* is the percentage who have pain at some time during that period.
- *Lifetime prevalence* is the percentage who can remember pain at some time in their life, whether or not they have it now.

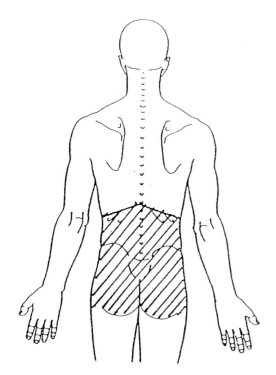

Figure 5.1   The diagram of low back pain used in all recent British surveys. From Papageorgiou et al (1995) with permission.

● *Incidence* is the percentage of a known population who develop new problems within a given time. It is commonly applied to those who report injuries or present for health care.

There is a problem defining low back *pain*. Do we include any low back symptoms, no matter how mild or how brief their duration? How do we draw a line between symptoms, ache, and pain? Many surveys ask about pain that lasts for a certain time, e.g., for a day or more. Is the pain severe enough to stay off work? but then we are talking about disability or incapacity for work rather than pain. Is the pain severe enough to seek health care? We must distinguish back pain, associated disability, and health care for back pain. We have already seen that pain and disability are not the same. Surveys show that the rates of low back pain, of back disability, and of health care use for back pain are very different. About 40% of people say they have had back pain in the past month: but only a third of these report any restriction and less than a tenth report time off work or health care.

There is another major limitation to the information we can get. Most people with back pain have few objective physical findings and we depend on their own report of pain and disability. As we have already seen, this is open to all the errors of subjective bias. Psychological, social, work-related, and legal issues may influence perceptions of symptoms and how they are reported. There is a problem of recall bias: the longer the time we ask about, the more unreliable the answers. If we try to overcome this by asking about a shorter period, such as 1 month or 1 year, subjects with more severe trouble may "slide" earlier events into their answer. We can get data about work loss, health care use, sick certification, and sickness benefits from various records, but these usually give lower rates than self-reports of these events from population surveys.

There may also be bias from the sample we study. Most epidemiologic studies of back pain are from North America and Europe. Many of the earlier surveys looked at particular groups of patients or workers, who were selected in different ways and are probably not typical of the general population. Many surveys are not directly comparable. For example, at one time various authors claimed that back pain was less common in the US than in Europe. They quoted Deyo & Tsui-Wu (1987) for a 1-year prevalence of 10.3% and a lifetime prevalence of 13.8% in the US, compared with 40–60% in Europe. But that did not compare like with like. Many of the early American surveys looked at "significant" back pain. Deyo & Tsui-Wu used the Second National Health and Nutrition Examination Survey (NHANES II), which only included back pain that lasted "most days for at least two weeks." Another early US survey only counted back pain that caused days in bed or led to health care. These were clearly only the more severe cases. Those US studies that ask more open questions about back pain get very similar results to Europe (Lawrence et al 1998).

The South Manchester Study

The best evidence on the epidemiology of back pain is from large, longitudinal surveys of the general population. Let me describe the South Manchester Study because it is a good example, and may help us to understand such surveys. It appears frequently in

Table 5.1   Reviews of the epidemiology of back pain

Review	Topic	Literature reviewed	Number of studies included
Leboeuf-Yde & Lauritsen (1995)	Review of Nordic studies to assess trends in the prevalence of low back pain	1954–1992	26
Volinn (1997)	The prevalence of low back pain in the rest of the world, including low- and middle-income countries	1980–1995	8 general population studies 9 occupational groups
Lawrence et al (1998)	Estimates of the prevalence of arthritis and selected musculoskeletal disorders in the US	Up to 1992	10 US data sets and surveys
Loney & Stratford (1999)	Methodologic review of the literature on the prevalence of low back pain	1981–1998	Only 13 studies considered methodologically acceptable
Bressler et al (1999)	Prevalence of low back pain in the elderly (>65 years)	1966–1997	12
Nachemson et al 2000	Various aspects of the epidemiology of neck and low back pain	1966–1997	15 selected studies on low back pain 21 on neck pain
Walker 2000	Review of world literature (all languages) to assess the population prevalence of low back pain in adults	1966–1998	56

the next three chapters. This was a prospective, community survey to investigate patterns and predictors of back pain and health care use. Data were collected through 1992–1993 and preliminary results were available by 1994 (Croft et al 1994) but the final parts of the analysis were not published till 1999. The study looked at 7699 adults aged 18–75 years who were registered with two family practices. One was in a large housing project with high social deprivation and unemployment. The other was in a well-established residential area with a broad social mix. An initial postal survey in March 1992 got a 59% response – 4500 subjects (Papageorgiou et al 1995). Health care use over the next 12 months was studied from medical records. Those who were free of back pain at baseline had a repeat postal questionnaire 12 months later, with a 60% response – 1540 subjects (Papageorgiou et al 1996). A total of 1412 who were free of back pain and employed at baseline had more detailed assessment of work-related psychosocial factors and distress, to find predictors of back pain over the next 12 months (Croft et al 1995, Macfarlane et al 1997, Papageorgiou

et al 1997). A group of 490 patients who consulted their general practitioner were followed for 12 months to see what happened to them (Croft et al 1998) and to find predictors of recovery or chronic back trouble (Macfarlane et al 1999, Thomas et al 1999). Croft et al (1997) provided an overview of the study and considered some of the conceptual issues it raised. You can see the practical difficulty even finding this large amount of data, published under different lead authors in different places over 5 years.

There are now well over 100 epidemiologic studies. Fortunately, we also have several good reviews (Table 5.1).

THE FREQUENCY OF BACK PAIN

Most people probably get some back symptoms at some time in their lives, but by no means all these symptoms are a health problem. Some authors describe those who present for health care as "the tip of an iceberg" and imply there is a hidden

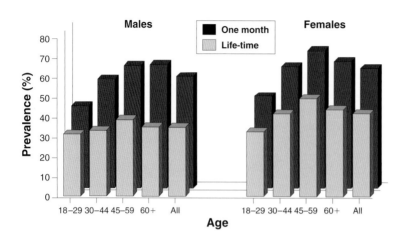

Figure 5.2   Age distribution of 1-month and lifetime prevalence of back pain lasting more than 24 h in British adults. From Papageorgiou et al 1995, with permission.

reservoir of disease awaiting treatment. That is a poor analogy. Rather, this is an island of health care amidst a sea of everyday bodily symptoms.

Many international studies show that 12–33% of people report some back symptoms on the day of interview; 19–43% report back pain in the last month; 27–65% in the last year; and 59–84% at some time in their lives (Walker 2000). The exact figures seem to depend on the wording of the questions rather than any differences between the people in each study.

The *Nuprin Pain Report* (Taylor & Curran 1985) found that back pain was the second most common pain in the US after headache. Fifty-six percent said they had at least 1 day of back pain in the previous year; 34% had pain for 6 days or more; and 14% had pain for more than 30 days in the year. Most back pain was mild and short-lived and had very little effect on daily life, but recurrences were common.

A recent CBS News Poll (2003) gave similar results, though it was small and gave little separate data for back pain. Fifty-three percent said they had back or neck pain often or sometimes; 12% said they had been diagnosed by a doctor to have some form of chronic pain.

Von Korff et al (1988) found that 41% of American adults aged 26–44 years had back pain in the previous 6 months. Most people had occasional short attacks of pain over a long period. Their pain was usually mild or moderate and did not limit activities. However, about a quarter of those with any back pain said they had it on more than half the days and that it caused some limitation of their activities.

Table 5.2   Total duration of pain during the previous year as a percentage of those reporting back pain

Duration of pain	Male (%)	Female (%)
<1 week	19	13
1–4 weeks	38	28
1–3 months	15	18
3–12 months	10	16
Complete year	17	22

From Mason (1994), with permission from the Office of National Statistics.

British surveys give similar figures. Mason (1994) found a point prevalence of 14%. The South Manchester Study found a 1-month prevalence of 39% (Papageorgiou et al 1995). Both Walsh et al (1992) and Mason (1994) found a 1-year prevalence of 36–37%. Both Walsh et al (1992) and Papageorgiou et al (1995) found a lifetime prevalence of 58%. The similarities between the results are striking, despite the differences in the surveys. Figure 5.2 shows the distribution of back pain in British adults. Walsh et al (1992) had similar results.

Mason (1994) asked how long people had back pain during the previous year (Table 5.2). Nearly half the people with back pain said that it had lasted less than 4 weeks in the year. However, for 19% it lasted the whole year, suggesting that about 6–7% of all adults have back problems more or less constantly.

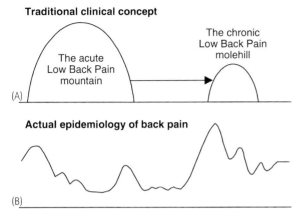

Traditional clinical concept

The acute Low Back Pain mountain

The chronic Low Back Pain molehill

(A)

Actual epidemiology of back pain

(B)

Figure 5.3 The time-course of back pain. (A) The assumed clinical course of acute low back pain. (B) The real course of low back pain. From Croft et al (1997), with permission.

UK General Household Surveys show that back problems are one of the most common causes of "chronic sickness." About 3–4% of the population aged 16–44 years and 5–7% of those aged 45–64 report back problems as a "chronic sickness." Back trouble is the most common cause of chronic sickness in both men and women under the age of 45 and one of the most common between age 45–65. Only in women aged over 45 and men aged over 65 do arthritis and rheumatism become more common than back trouble. Other bone and joint problems also become more common in both sexes over the age of 65.

Time–course

We saw in Chapter 3 that the traditional clinical classification of back pain is:

- acute – current attack less than 6 weeks
- subacute – current attack 6 weeks to 3 months
- chronic – current attack more than 3 months.

This may be convenient for clinical purposes, but population surveys show it is not a true picture. Back pain is often a recurrent or fluctuating problem (Fig. 5.3). Croft et al (1997) suggested that the most important epidemiologic concept is the pattern of back pain over long periods of the individual's life. They based this on four observations:

1. 60–80% of people get back pain at some time in their lives.

2. Most acute clinical attacks settle rapidly, but residual symptoms and recurrences are common.
3. 35–40% of people report low back pain lasting 24 hours or more each month and 15–30% of people have some low back symptoms each day.
4. The strongest predictor of a further episode of low back pain is a history of previous episodes.

Croft et al (1998) summed it all up neatly. "Low back pain should be viewed as a chronic problem with an untidy pattern of grumbling symptoms and periods of relative freedom from pain and disability interspersed with acute episodes, exacerbations, and recurrences." They suggested we should summarize the back pain experience by total days of pain over a year.

The South Manchester Study also looked at patterns of prevalence and incidence of new episodes over a 1-year period (Papageorgiou et al 1996, Thomas et al 1999). At the start of the year, the adult population fits into three groups (Fig. 5.4):

- group 1 – those who have been free of back pain for the previous 12 months (62%)
- group 2 – those who have had intermittent or less disabling low back pain during the previous 12 months (32%)
- group 3 – those who have had long-standing or serious disabling low back pain during the previous 12 months (6%).

Over the course of the following year, about one-third of people in group 1 will develop a new episode of low back pain. So the 1-year incidence of new episodes among previously painfree adults is 19%. However, few of them are really experiencing their first ever episode of back pain. [Because of the difficulty in defining "new" episodes, different studies give widely varying figures for incidence. Hillman et al (1996) found an annual incidence of first onset of back pain of only 4.7%.] Almost half of group 2 will have further episodes during the following year. We often assume that severe and chronic back pain will continue indefinitely, but that is not true. One-third of those in group 3 will improve and have less severe problems during the following year. However, they will be replaced by a comparable number of people from groups 1 and 2 who develop more severe problems during the year. These figures all balance out and the size of

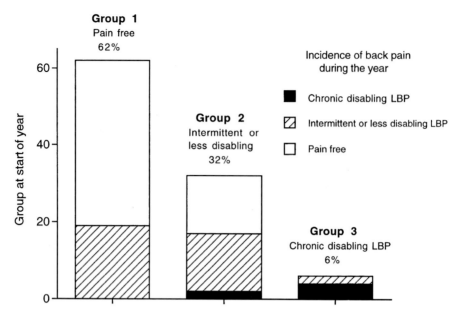

Figure 5.4   The incidence of low back pain (LBP) episodes in the adult population during the course of a year. Based on ideas and data from Croft et al (1997).

each group remains the same. The incidence of new episodes is balanced by the number of people who improve. So the annual prevalence stays at about 38%, and the pool of chronic disabling back pain stays at about 6% of the adult population. Individuals move between the different groups.

Nerve root pain

Few population surveys use strict criteria for nerve root pain. A number of reports give a lifetime prevalence of leg pain of 14–40%, but they do not distinguish true nerve root pain from the more common referred leg pain. Deyo et al (1992) in the US estimated the lifetime prevalence of "surgically important disk herniation" to be about 2%. Lawrence (1977) in the UK found the prevalence of "sciatica suggesting a herniated lumbar disc" to be 3.1% in men and 1.3% in women. Neither of these studies gave their diagnostic criteria. Heliovaara et al (1987) in Finland reported the only large population survey with proper clinical criteria of nerve root pain. The lifetime prevalence of back pain was 77% in men and 74% in women over the age of 30 years. Thirty-five percent of men and 45% of women had some associated leg pain. With strict diagnostic criteria, however, the lifetime prevalence of true

nerve root pain was only 5.3% in men and 3.7% in women.

Comorbidity

Back pain is the third most common bodily symptom, after headache and tiredness. So it is not surprising that people with back pain often report other symptoms. *The Nuprin Pain Report* (Taylor & Curran 1985) found that 90% of those with frequent back pain had multiple pains, though half of them said that back pain was the "most troublesome". Bergenudd (1989) found that back pain was the most common musculoskeletal complaint in 55-year-old men and women in Sweden, but it was often associated with other pains (Table 5.3). Clinical and epidemiologic studies show that up to 60% of people with low back pain also report some neck symptoms. Makela (1993) found that many chronic musculoskeletal pains go together. The strongest association was between back pain, neck pain, and osteoarthritis of the hips and knees, though inflammatory joint disease was quite separate.

The South Manchester Study showed the close association between the presence of other pains and the likelihood of developing new back pain (Table 5.4).

Table 5.3   Association of back pain and other pains

	Men (%)	Women (%)
Back pain	28	30
Shoulder pain	13	15
Knee pain	8	13
Hip pain	4	4
But of those with back pain		
Back pain alone	50	
Back pain and shoulder pain	25	
Back pain and knee pain	15	
Back pain and hip pain	10	

Based on data from Bergenudd (1989).

Table 5.4   Back pain as part of general pain complaints

No back pain at baseline Number of other pains at baseline	Percentage who develop new back pain in next 12 months (%)
0	23.6
1 area	38.7
2 areas	37.8
3 areas	40.5

From the South Manchester Study (P Croft, personal communication).

Men and women who attend their family doctor with back pain also attend more frequently with other complaints. Porter & Hibbert (1986) found that 17% of men who consult their family doctor with back pain also consult about neck pain at some time. Patients who consult with back pain and neck pain, but not sciatica, are also more likely to consult with stress and mental disorders. Or, at least, they may be more likely to get a diagnosis of stress and mental disorders.

In the US (Yelin 1997) and the UK (Erens & Ghate 1993), between one-third and one-half of social security claimants have more than one long-term health problem. Of Americans awarded social security disability pensions in 1996 for back pain, 40% also had neck pain and 25% also had a mental health diagnosis.

We can see that from an epidemiologic perspective, back pain is not a discrete clinical problem. It is often associated with other pains, comorbidities, psychological and stress-related symptoms, and work-related or other social problems. From a social security perspective, back pain has many features in common with other musculoskeletal complaints, and with mental health and stress-related conditions.

LOW BACK DISABILITY

The most important consequence of back pain is its impact on people's lives. It may affect general health and well-being, activities of daily living, and work.

Remember that all surveys give people's own report of their disability. This is entirely subjective and most surveys only ask about disability in the most general terms. There is no objective evidence or pathologic check on these figures.

The Nuprin Pain Report (Taylor & Curran 1985) found that 14% of adult Americans said that back pain interfered with their routine activities, work, or sleep for one or more days in the year. The CBS News Poll (2003) found that 14% of those with any form of pain said that it often interfered with their daily life. (Though again, note this poll did not give separate data for back pain.) Andersson (1999) found that back problems were the most common cause of activity limitation in people below the age of 45 and the fourth most common in those aged 45–64. Seven percent of adults reported a disability due to their back or due to both their back and other joint problems. On average, this limited their activities for about 23 days each year. These various figures suggest that 7–14% of adults in the US have some restriction due to back pain for a least 1 day each year, i.e., about 15–30 million people. Just over 1% of Americans are permanently disabled by back pain, and another 1% are temporarily disabled by back pain at any one time. That is about 4 million people.

There are several detailed surveys of low back disability in the UK. Mason (1994) found that 11% of adults said that back pain had restricted their activities during the last 4 weeks. Almost all those aged 16–24 years only had restrictions for a few days. However, there was then surprisingly little

Table 5.5 One-year and lifetime prevalence of back pain, disability and time off work

Prevalence (%)	Age (years)				
	20–29	30–39	40–49	50–59	Total
Male					
Back pain					
1 year	35.4	37.1	38.2	40.5	37.6
Lifetime	52.0	60.4	64.2	70.5	61.3
Disability score >8/16					
1 year	4.1	5.8	6.6	5.3	5.4
Lifetime	8.2	12.6	20.8	23.1	15.9
Time off work					
1 year	9.5	13.5	9.4	9.5	10.6
Lifetime	22.4	31.3	38.2	46.2	34.1
Female					
Back pain					
1 year	27.0	33.6	43.7	35.7	34.8
Lifetime	45.2	53.8	62.3	63.7	55.8
Disability score >8/16					
1 year	2.1	4.7	5.7	5.6	4.5
Lifetime	7.7	13.1	16.4	15.8	13.1
Time off work					
1 year	6.1	5.1	9.8	6.5	6.8
Lifetime	16.9	18.4	29.8	29.8	23.3

From Walsh et al (1992) with permission from the BMJ Publishing Group.

difference between those age 25 and >65 years. About one-third had restrictions for 1–5 days and about one-third had them for the whole 4 weeks. The effect on their lifestyle varied, but mainly involved restriction of normal activities in the home and garden, and restriction of sporting activities or mobility.

Walsh et al (1992) is the only population survey that is directly comparable to clinical disability questionnaires. They assessed eight activities of daily living to give a total disability score from 0 to 16. Table 5.5 shows the 1-year and lifetime prevalence of low back disability by age and sex.

Work loss

Different reports give very variable rates of work loss associated with back pain (Table 5.6). Reported or compensated work loss may obviously vary under different social security or workers' compensation systems. However, it appears that sickness absence may also vary in different countries. These studies are from very different times, and when we look at trends we will see this may be important.

Watson et al (1998) gave the most detailed UK data from the island of Jersey. Jersey is unique, because all work loss of more than 1 day requires medical certification, and all sick pay is by the state, not the employer. Jersey records all individual sickness, incapacity, and accident benefits on a computer database. Benefits are paid at a fixed rate and are not related to wages lost. Unique among western countries, Jersey has no unemployment benefit. However, the true unemployment rate is less than 3%, so in economic terms there is virtually full employment. All of these differences mean the Jersey data may not be typical of the rest of the UK. Despite this, the findings were quite close to other UK estimates. In 1994, the 1-year incidence of new claims for back pain causing more than 1 day's work loss was 5.6%. Including those still off work from the previous year, the 1-year prevalence of work loss due to back pain was 6.3%.

About half the total days lost are by the 85% of people who are off work for short periods, most commonly for less than 7 days. The other half is by the 15% of people who are off work for more than 1 month. This is reflected in the social costs of back pain. It is widely known that 80–90% of the health care costs of back pain are for the 10% of patients with chronic low back pain and disability. The Jersey data showed that the same is true for social costs. In 1994, back pain accounted for 10.5% of all sickness absence in Jersey. Only 3% of those off work with back pain were off for more than 6 months, but they accounted for 33% of the benefits paid (Fig. 5.5).

It is surprisingly difficult to estimate total sickness absence associated with back pain. Quite apart from actual differences in sickness absence, each system collects different data and has different obstacles to getting an accurate picture. In most countries, employers hold data about individual sickness absence and there are no national statistics. Health care systems do not generally keep data on patients' work loss. Social security and compensation systems keep data about claims and the

Table 5.6 Population studies of work loss associated with back pain

Country	Study	Year	Database		Annual prevalence in adults
US	Guo et al (1995)	1988	US population survey	Self-reported work loss	11.8% (17.6% of workers)
	Murphy & Volinn (1999)	1995	US workers' compensation database	Claims for work-related low back pain	1.8%
UK	Walsh et al (1992)	Late 1980s	8 family practices	Self-reported work loss	Annual prevalence: men 9.5%, women 6.5% Lifetime prevalence by by age 50: men 40%, women 30%
	Mason (1994)	1993	Population survey	Self-reported work loss	2.4%
	Watson et al (1998)	1994	Social security data Jersey	Benefits paid 1 day or more	Incidence 5.6 Prevalence 6.3%
	Hillman et al (1996)	1995	Population survey Bradford	Self-reported work loss	6.4% (21.8% of workers with low back pain)
	Working Backs Scotland[a]	2001	Population surveys	Self-reported work loss	0.8%
Norway	Hagen & Thune (1998)	1995–1996	National social security database	Social security benefits for 2 weeks' sickness absence	Men 1.9% Women 2.7%
Sweden	Linton et al (1998)		Population survey 35–45-year-olds	At least 1 day of sickness absence	Official sick leave: 12.5% +"unofficial" absence: 10%
Switzerland	Santos-Eggimann et al (2000)	1992–1993	Population survey	Self-reported "reduction in professional activities"	Men 9.1% Women 6.9%

[a]Unpublished data.

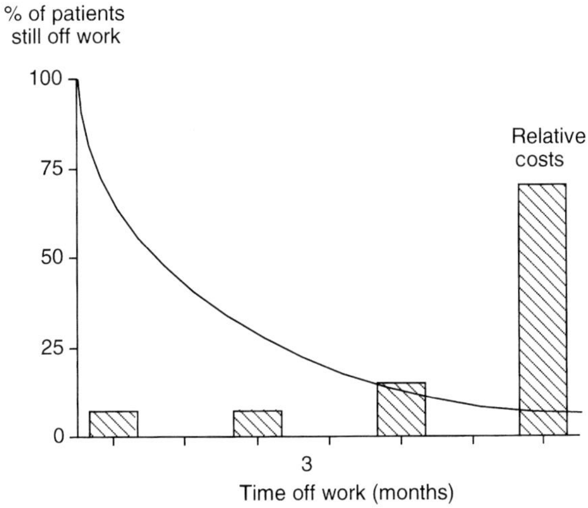

Figure 5.5 The large percentage of wage replacement costs accounted for by a small percentage of claimants. Based on data from Watson et al (1998).

payments they make, but that is not the same as sickness absence because it depends on entitlement to the particular benefit. For example, many US authors quote workers' compensation figures, but that is a selected part of the picture. Many UK authors misquote figures for social security benefits, but that is quite different from work loss. Most sickness absence from work in UK is covered by sick pay from the employer for up to 28 weeks. So a worker who is off work for up to 28 weeks with back pain may not receive any social security benefits or appear in official statistics. The social security system does not even know they exist. Conversely, over three-quarters of the people who receive incapacity benefits were not working anyway but were unemployed or on other social security benefits.

Guo et al (1995) provided the best estimate of work loss due to back pain in the US, using data on 30 074 workers from the National Health

Interview Survey. In 1988, about 22.4 million people, i.e., 17.6% of all US workers, lost 149 million working days due to back pain. This is the best available estimate, though it is difficult to cross-check, and is now more over 15 years out of date.

CSAG (1994) estimated there were about 52 million days of work loss due to back pain in UK in 1993, but that was a very rough estimate. It was based on a small sample, with a wide range of possible error. Recent unpublished data from Working Backs Scotland suggests the figure might be much lower. The Labour Force Survey estimated that about 360 000 people in the UK had 3.7 million days' sickness absence with work-related back pain in 1995 (Jones et al 1998). Adding all musculoskeletal conditions involving any back symptoms increased that to 5.3 million days. However, the Labour Force Survey was only about "work-related" back pain, with all the problems about how that is interpreted.

Work-related back injuries

Most reports show that back sprains and strains make up nearly one-third of all work-related injuries in the US. By the mid-1990s, there were about 1 million compensation claims for work-related back injuries each year. Murphy & Volinn (1999) estimated that in 1995, the latest year for which they had data, there were 1.8 back injury claims per 100 workers. Twenty-nine percent of these were compensable. They estimated annual US workers' compensation costs for back injuries were about $8.8 billion.

The Health and Safety Executive (HSE) records all work injuries in the UK. Thirty-six percent of all accidents are caused by manual handling and half of them are sprains and strains of the back, usually causing more than three days off work. A total of 32 083 back injuries were reported in 2000–2001 (HSE 2001). Only 1.8% of back injuries were "major injuries" severe enough to need hospital admission and only 2.1% of all major injuries were to the spine. Ninety-eight percent of back injuries were less serious "sprains or strains", but they accounted for 24% of all minor work injuries.

Minor back injuries lead to longer time off work, and to higher health and compensation costs than other minor injuries (Table 5.7).

Table 5.7 The relative severity of back and other sprains and strains

	Back sprains and strains	Other sprains and strains
Days off work	38	23
Days of medical treatment	21	8
Total costs (1984 US$)	$308	$167

Based on data from various US workers' compensation sources.

Table 5.8 Common conditions receiving incapacity benefit in UK

Simple musculoskeletal disorders osteoarthritis, sprains, simple back pain	19%
More serious musculoskeletal disorders rheumatoid arthritis, ankylosing spondylitis, serious back conditions	7%
"Soft" mental health problems anxiety, stress, neurosis	9%
Depression	14%
More serious mental illness psychoses, personality disorders, severe learning disabilities	3%
Cardiovascular disorders myocardial infarction, ischemic heart disease, angina, hypertension	10%
Drug- and alcohol-related disorders	1.5%

Based on data from the Department for Work and Pensions.

Sickness benefits

There are many sources of sick pay, workers' compensation, and social security benefits in the US and it is not possible to get total national figures.

There are much better data available in the UK, despite the limitations we have already seen. These are now really statistics of social security benefits paid for long-term back incapacity and they omit short-term sickness absence. Musculoskeletal and mental health disorders are now the most common causes of chronic incapacity in all western countries (Table 5.8).

Back pain now accounts for 13.5% of all incapacity benefits in the UK, which is about half of all

Table 5.9 UK incapacity benefits paid for back conditions 1999–2000

	Spells		Days	
	Males	Females	Males	Females
Ankylosing spondylitis and other inflammatory spondylopathies	20 000	8000	6 628 000	2 723 000
Spondylosis and allied disorders	29 000	19 000	8 825 000	6 212 000
Intervertebral disk disorders	18 000	10 000	5 742 000	3 408 000
Dorsalgia	177 000	103 000	47 594 000	29 839 000
Sprain and strain of neck	3000	2000	541 000	545 000
Sprain and strain of lumbar spine and pelvis	2000	1000	460 000	418 000
Sprain and strain of unspecified parts of back	4000	2000	443 000	404 000
Total back incapacities	254 000	148 000	70 554 000	43 566 000
All incapacities	1 899 000	1 125 000	526 747 000	314 960 000

Spells are the number of periods of sickness benefits.
Days are the total number of days benefit was paid.
All figures rounded to nearest thousand.
Based on statistics from the Department for Work and Pensions.

musculoskeletal incapacities. Table 5.9 shows the social security statistics for back pain for 1999–2000. Remember that these diagnoses reflect what doctors put on certificates, which may not be the same as actual pathology.

TRENDS OVER TIME

Pain

Palmer et al (2000) claimed that there was a dramatic increase in the prevalence of back pain in the UK between 1988 and 1998. However, there were problems to their study that cast doubt on this conclusion. It was based on a single question in two very different surveys. A second question showed no change in disability. Macfarlane et al (2000) looked at two more comparable surveys and found a slight *decrease* in prevalence between 1991 and 1998.

Most epidemiological studies for the past 40 years show a constant picture. Any differences seem to be due to the setting of the survey or the wording of the questions. Leboeuf-Yde & Lauritsen (1995) compared 26 Nordic studies from 1954 through 1992 and could not find any trend. Finland is the only country in the world that has used identical questions in annual surveys since 1978. Leino et al

(1994) reported that the prevalence of back pain stayed the same from 1978 to 1992. Preliminary analysis of further data up to 1997 suggests that, if anything, the prevalence may have fallen slightly (P Leino, personal communication).

There were three detailed and identical Omnibus surveys on back pain in the UK between 1993 and 1998 (Table 5.10). An unpublished Scottish survey in 2001 gave similar findings. These show no significant change in the prevalence of back pain or disability over the past decade.

Both the historic review and modern epidemiologic surveys agree. Back pain does not appear to have changed. Back pain is no more common, no different, and no more severe than it has always been. Nor is there any reason to expect any change in the biologic basis of ordinary backache.

Work-related back injuries

All earlier US workers' compensation studies showed a large increase in the number of back injury claims over several decades. The National Council for Compensation Insurance (NCCI) showed an 80% increase in all claims during the 1980s (NCCI 1992). There was a marked shift

Table 5.10   Prevalence of back pain in Britain 1993–2001

	March–June 1993	March–June 1996	March–June 1998	January–June 2001[a]
12-month prevalence	37%	40%	40%	39%
Restricted activities in previous 4 weeks[b]	30%	30%	33%	
Time off work in previous 4 weeks[c]	6%	5%	5%	2%
Medical sick certification in previous 4 weeks[c]		4%	2%	

[a]Scotland only. Slightly different questions.
[b]Of those with back pain.
[c]Of those with back pain and employed.
Based on data from the Omnibus surveys.

Table 5.11   Recent trends in US workers' compensation claims

Year	Back injury claims	Non–back injury claims	All claims
1988	148 917	818 077	966 994
1990	131 102	693 439	824 541
1992	106 961	504 245	611 206
1994	105 333	514 273	619 606
1996	88 766	513 059	601 825
% fall 1988–1996	40.4	37.3	37.8

Data supplied by B Webster, personal communication.

towards soft-tissue injuries such as sprains, strains, and low back claims. However, the *proportion* of all injuries to the low back only increased very slightly from 29.2 to 31.8% between 1981 and 1990. Backs simply followed the general workers' compensation trend.

That trend has reversed from about the late 1980s or early 1990s. US Bureau of Labor statistics (www.nasi.org/workcomp/1997-98Data) show that the number of all occupational injuries and illnesses with days off work fell steadily from 2.6 million in 1991 to 1.7 million in 1998. Table 5.11 shows data on back pain from one large workers' compensation provider that covers 10% of the privately insured labor force (Hashemi et al 1998,

Murphy & Volinn 1999). Between 1988 and 1996 there was a 37.8% fall in all claims and a 40.6% fall in back injury claims. Once again, backs seemed to follow the general workers' compensation trend. In addition, however, the average duration of back injury claims fell from 156 to 61 days. There was a particular fall in the number of long-duration, high-cost, back injury claims. The proportion of all workers' compensation claim costs accounted for by back injuries fell from 38.4% to 22.7%. Murphy & Volinn (1999) confirmed these findings on Washington State and US Bureau of Labor data.

O'Grady (2000) reported that workers' compensation claim rates in Canada peaked in 1986. Since then, they have fallen 40%.

The UK had a similar fall of 20% in all reported non-fatal work injuries between 1990–1991 and 2000–2001 (HSE 2001). Over that decade, back injuries fell 7.5% from 34 720 to 32 083.

We can only speculate about the causes of these recent trends. During this period, there was a growing emphasis on health and safety at work. US workers' compensation systems, insurers, and employers have made major efforts to control claims and costs. They introduced medical fee schedules, utilization review procedures, and managed care. There are schemes for disability management, modified work, and early return to work. The number of employers with back injury prevention and rehabilitation schemes rose to one-third by 1992. It is difficult to prove the impact of any of these interventions. More generally, this all took place during the economic boom of the 1990s and that may be the greatest influence on workers' compensation claims and costs.

Disability

Remember that we have little objective or clinical data on trends of low back disability over the years. All that we have are surveys of people's own reports of their perceptions of disability. And most of the data is in very general terms.

US National Health Interview Surveys ask about chronic back pain lasting more than 3 months and causing inability to work or go to school. These are people who regard themselves as "chronically and permanently disabled by back pain." This number increased from about 1 million in 1987 to 1.5 million in 1993. Preliminary analysis by E Volinn (personal communication) suggests that it then fell significantly between 1993 and 1996.

There is very little data on any trend in low back disability in the UK. Palmer et al (2000) asked about back pain that had made it impossible to put on socks, stockings, or tights. The prevalence was the same in two surveys in 1987–1988 and 1997–1998. However, we have already seen the limitations of that report.

We need to view these findings against a more general background. Many surveys in the US, UK, Europe, and Japan show that most self-reported symptoms and disability are gradually increasing over the years. That is despite improvement in most objective measures of health. The UK Labour Force Survey is a good example. The number of working-age people reporting any long-term health problem or disability increased gradually from about 10 to 14% between 1984 and 1998. That was partly due to an increase in the number of older workers and changes in the wording of the questions. But the survey team concluded it was mainly due to changing attitudes and increased awareness of disability rather than any real change in the level of disability (LFS 1998).

Social security benefits

Everyone must now be aware of the dramatic rise in social security benefits for back pain in all

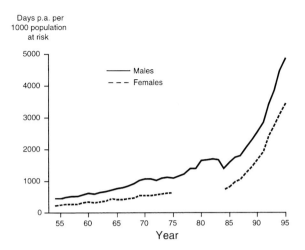

Figure 5.6 Male and female sickness and invalidity benefits for back incapacities in the UK, expressed as the rate per 1000 members of the eligible population. Based on statistics from the Department of Social Security.

western countries between the 1950s–1960s and the 1990s (Fig. 1.1). However, remember the limitations of the data. Over this period, repeated changes to the rules excluded many people from the statistics, so the real increase in chronic back disability was probably even greater. More important, this was not an epidemic of back pain. These are not trends of low back pain or back disability. They are not even statistics of sickness absence, though they are often misquoted as such. More specifically, they show an increase in sick certification and social security benefits paid for long-term incapacity attributed to some form of back trouble.

The UK has had the best social security statistics on back pain in the world over many years (Waddell et al 2002). The Department of Social Security (now the Department for Work and Pensions) has kept diagnostic statistics for disability and incapacity benefits since 1953–1954.

Figure 5.6 shows the rates for men and women separately. We saw in our review of the history of back pain that for many years low back disability was a male problem. By the 1990s, women were catching up, which probably reflects social trends toward gender equality. Figure 5.7 shows that back incapacities rose faster than any other conditions.

Figure 5.8 shows that the number of people going on to benefits each year remained more or

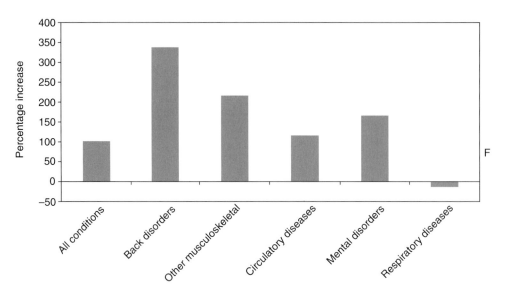

Figure 5.7   Between 1978–1979 and 1994–1995, sickness and invalidity benefits for back pain rose faster than for any other condition. Based on statistics from the Department of Social Security.

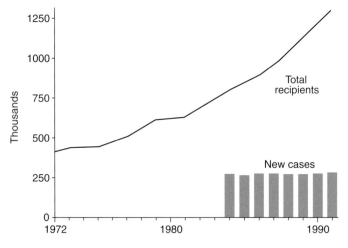

Figure 5.8   UK invalidity benefit trends in the 1990s. The number of new awards remained constant. However, more people stayed on benefit longer and fewer came off, so the number of recipients of continuing benefits rose.

less steady. The problem was that more people stayed on benefit longer, and fewer people came off benefit. So the total number of recipients on continuing benefit gradually rose. It was not that more people were becoming disabled by back pain. The problem was, despite all our medical advances and resources, we were less successful at getting people off benefits and back to work.

The latest UK statistics show that trend has reversed since 1994–1995. The number of days of benefit paid for back incapacities appears to have passed its peak (Fig. 5.9). Since 1994–1995, there has been a 42% fall in new awards for back pain (Fig. 5.10), compared with a 25% decrease for all conditions. The number of people on continuing benefits for back pain has fallen 13% (Fig. 5.11), while the number on benefits for all conditions remains unchanged.

Just over half the fall in new awards for back pain reflects all conditions and is probably due to

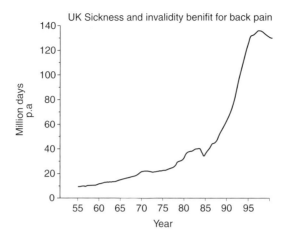

Figure 5.9   Current UK trend of incapacity benefit for back incapacities. Based on statistics from the Department for Work and Pensions.

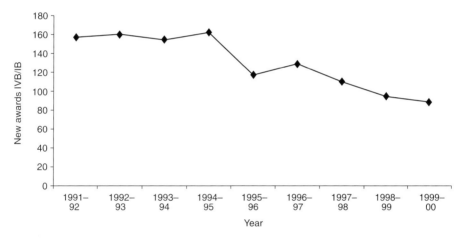

Figure 5.10   New awards of incapacity benefit for back pain in the UK. IVB, invalidity benefit, replaced by incapacity benefit (IB) from April 1995. Based on statistics from the Department for Work and Pensions.

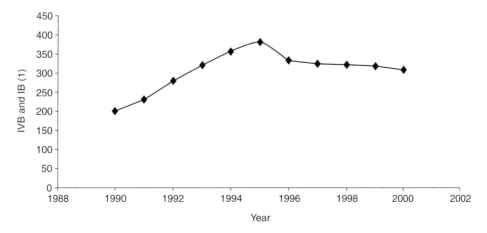

Figure 5.11   Number of recipients of continuing incapacity benefit for back pain in the UK. IVB, invalidity benefit, replaced by incapacity benefit (IB) from April 1995. Based on statistics from the Department for Work and Pensions.

Table 5.12   Low back disability in Sweden

Year	Percentage losing time off work with back pain	Average days lost per annum
1970	1	20
1975	3	22
1980	4	25
1987	8	36
1992	8	39

Based on data from the Swedish Council for Technology Assessment in Health Care.

changes in the social security system. Rather less than half is unique to back pain. It is unlikely that any single factor explains this, but rather the cumulative effect of many influences. It is possible the social security changes could have a differential effect on back pain, though we have no direct evidence of that. This trend coincides with more active clinical management of back pain. Changed medical thinking about back pain could also have a more indirect effect on social attitudes and practices. The real explanation, both of the earlier rise and the recent fall, may be enigmatic but fundamental cultural change. To put it simply, perhaps back pain is becoming a less fashionable reason for sick certification and social security benefits. Whatever, there is a very real shift in social behavior with back pain, which differs from other health conditions.

The main improvement has been in the number of people developing chronic back pain and incapacity, who claim and start benefits. That was the main target of health care and social security initiatives in the 1990s. The problem is that if people do develop chronic low back disability and lose their jobs, they then often remain on benefits long-term. So the number of people on continuing benefits for back pain is falling more slowly. The major challenge now is to find a better health care or rehabilitation answer for them.

Most other western countries have had comparable problems (Waddell et al 2002). For many years, Sweden seemed to be worst affected. There was a dramatic increase in the number of people staying off work with back pain, and in the

average time off, from the early 1970s to the early 1990s (Table 5.12). Nachemson even forecast that early in the new millennium there would not be enough people still working to pay for those retired with back pain! Since that time, there has been great political interest in back pain. Successive governments tightened the social security rules with reduced benefits, and then relaxed the rules and gave more generous benefits again. The number of people getting early retirement for back pain rose fivefold from the early 1970s to its peak in 1993. It then fell more than a third by 1997. Since then it has risen and is once again approaching the levels of the early 1990s (A Nachemson, personal communication). It is difficult to tell how much these Swedish statistics reflect changes in social attitudes, health care, or the sickness benefit system. They probably all acted together. Indeed, it may be difficult to change one without the others.

Because of the many sources of financial support for sickness in the US, it is difficult to get national figures. It is also unbelievably difficult to get data on back pain out of the Social Security Administra-tion (SSA), even under the Freedom of Information Act. It is like extracting hens' teeth! Many earlier authors quoted the 2000% rise in SSDI awards from 1957 through 1975. This is a true figure from the SSA, but it gives a very false impression. It refers to the single diagnosis of "displacement of the intervertebral disk." It reflects medical fashion for that particular diagnosis rather than the total impact of back pain. There was then a fall of 42% from 1977 through 1984 that few authors quote.

E Volinn (personal communication) finally succeeded in getting some more recent SSA data. Figure 5.12 shows the number of awards of SSDI and SSI benefits to adults of working age with "back disorders." Unfortunately, this information is still very incomplete. It is a single diagnostic code for "other and unspecified disorders of the back." We cannot get data on the other codes, particularly those for "intervertebral disk disorders" or "sprains and strains." So the present data are probably only about half the total number of awards for back conditions. And, as we saw with the earlier SSA data on disk displacement, we cannot tell if there has been a change in diagnostic

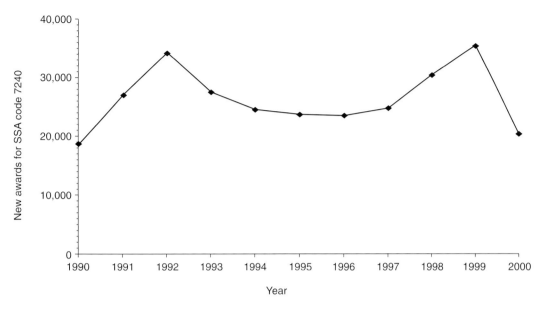

Figure 5.12   Initial awards of SSDI and SSI disability benefits for "back conditions" to adults of working age. (Data supplied by Social Security Administration: Volinn E, personal communication, August 2000).

practice. So, unless or until SSA produces better data, it is not possible to draw any conclusions about US social security trends for back incapacities.

CONCLUSION

This may surprise you. Despite popular belief, there never was an epidemic of back pain. Back pain has always been a common bodily symptom, but it is no more common today than it has always been. Rather, the evidence is of an epidemic of disability associated with ordinary backache. More specifically, all western countries had a dramatic increase in sick certification, social security benefits, and early retirement attributed to back pain between the 1950s–1960s and the early–mid-1990s.

You may notice that throughout this chapter I have carefully written about disability *attributed to* or *associated with* back pain rather than *due to* or *caused by* back pain. From a clinical point of view, we have already stressed that pain and disability are not the same. The epidemiology shows the same. The real change is not in pathology or even in clinical symptoms, but in patterns of sick

certification and social security benefits. This is very much a social phenomenon.

Up to the mid-1990s, the rising trend of back disability seemed irreversible. When writing the first edition of this book, there were the first tentative hints that the situation might be improving. The latest statistics show a dramatic shift in what is happening with back pain, at least in some settings in some countries.

Some clinicians object this is all just tinkering with the social security system and any improvement is cosmetic. It does not do anything about the real clinical problem. Even worse, they suggest any recent fall in the number of awards is because patients are being denied benefits. There is some truth in this view, but it goes to the heart of the current dilemma. Similar comment could apply equally to the rising trend up to 1995. We have already seen that we cannot understand or deal with these trends purely as a clinical or health care problem. There is no epidemic of spinal pathology, nor even of back pain. The dramatic increase in benefit claims and payments was for self-reported, non-specific, low back symptoms. It was supported by a change in the pattern of sick certification, without any clear pathologic basis. The more recent fall is equally a social change rather that any change in spinal pathology. If this really has been a social epidemic, then it is entirely proper to address it at least partly by social measures.

The epidemiology, like the clinical analysis, shows that we must distinguish low back pain from disability. We should make a clear distinction between the epidemiologic sea of those with low back symptoms and the small proportion who seek health care or receive sickness benefits. We must also consider low back disability and sickness benefits in their social context.

Summary

A back pain epidemic?

- There is no evidence of any change in low back pathology
- The prevalence of low back pain has not changed
- There was an exponential increase in chronic disability, medical certification, and social security benefits associated with nonspecific low back pain up to the mid-1990s
- At least in some countries and some systems, these trends appear to have reversed since the early–mid-1990s

References

Andersson G B J 1999 Epidemiological features of chronic low back pain. Lancet 354: 581–585

Bergenudd H 1989 Talent, occupation and locomotor discomfort. PhD Thesis, Malmo. Chapter 6 Occurrence and incidence of some common locomotor complaints in 55 year old men and women

Bressler H B, Keyes W J, Rochon P A, Badley E 1999 The prevalence of low back pain in the elderly: a systematic review of the literature. Spine 24: 1813–1819

CBS News Poll 2003 Ouch! We're a hurting group. Available online at: www.cbsnews.com/stories/2003/01/28/opinion/polls/main538259.shtml

Croft P, Joseph S, Cosgrove S et al 1994 Low back pain in the community and in hospitals. A report to the Clinical Standards Advisory Group of the Department of Health. Arthritis & Rheumatism Council, Epidemiology Research Unit, University of Manchester

Croft P R, Papageorgiou A C, Ferry S, Thomas E, Jayson M I V, Silman A J 1995 Psychological distress and low back pain: evidence from a prospective study in the general population. Spine 20: 2731–2737

Croft P, Papageorgiou A, McNally R 1997 Low back pain. In: Stevens A, Rafferty J (eds) Health care needs assessment, 2nd series. Radcliffe Medical Press, Oxford, pp 129–182

Croft P R, Macfarlane G F, Papageorgiou A C, Thomas E, Silman A J 1998 Outcome of low back pain in general practice: a prospective study. British Medical Journal 316: 1356–1359

CSAG 1994 Epidemiology review: the epidemiology and cost of back pain. Annex to the Clinical Standards Advisory Group *Report on back pain.* HMSO, London, pp 1–72

Deyo R A, Tsui-Wu Y-J 1987 Functional disability due to back pain. Arthritis and Rheumatism 30: 1247–1253

Deyo R A, Rainville J, Kent D L 1992 What can the history and physical examination tell us about low back pain? Journal of the American Medical Association 268: 760–765

Erens B, Ghate D 1993 Invalidity benefit: a longitudinal study of new recipients. Department of Social Security Research report no. 20. HMSO, London, pp 1–127

Guo H-R, Tanaka S, Cameron L L et al 1995 Back pain among workers in the United States: national estimates and workers at high risk. American Journal of Industrial Medicine 28: 591–602

Hagen K B, Thune O 1998 Work incapacity from low back pain in the general population. Spine 23: 2091–2095

Hashemi L, Webster B S, Clancy E A 1998 Trends in disability duration and cost of workers' compensation low back pain claims (1988–1996). Journal of Occupational and Environmental Medicine 40: 1110–1119

Heliovaara M, Impivaara O, Sievers K et al 1987 Lumbar disc syndrome in Finland. Journal of Epidemiology and Community Health 41: 251–258

Hillman M, Wright A, Rajaratman G, Tennant A, Chamberlain M A 1996 Prevalence of low back pain in the community: implications for service provision in Bradford, UK. Journal of Epidemiology and Community Health 50: 347–352

HSE 2001 Health and Safety Statistics 2000/01. Health and Safety Executive, London. Available online at: www.hse.gov.uk/statistics

Jones J R, Hodgson J T, Clegg T A, Elliott R C 1998 Self-reported work-related illness in 1995: results from a household survey. HSE Books. Her Majesty's Stationery Office, Norwich

Lawrence J S 1977 Rheumatism in populations. Heinemann, London

Lawrence R C, Helmick C G, Arnett F C, Deyo R A 1998 Estimates of the prevalence of arthritis and selected musculoskeletal disorders in the United States. Arthritis and Rheumatism 41: 778–799

Leboeuf-Yde C, Lauritsen J M 1995 The prevalence of low back pain in the literature: a structured review of 26

Nordic studies from 1954 to 1993. Spine 20: 2112–2118

Leino P L, Berg M A, Puschka P 1994 Is back pain increasing? Results from national surveys in Finland. Scandinavian Journal of Rheumatology 23: 269–276

LFS 1998 Disability data from the Labour Force Survey: comparing 1997–98 to the past. Labour Market Trends June 1998: 321–325

Linton S J, Hellsing A-L, Hallden K 1998 A population based study of spinal pain among 35–45 year old individuals. Spine 23: 1457–1463

Loney P L, Stratford P W 1999 The prevalence of low back pain in adults: a methodological review of the literature. Physical Therapy 79: 384–396

Macfarlane G F, Thomas E, Papageorgiou A C, Croft P R, Jayson M I V, Silman A J 1997 Employment and work activities as predictors of future low back pain. Spine 22: 1143–1149

Macfarlane G F, Thomas E, Croft P R, Papageorgiou A C, Jayson M I V, Silman A J 1999 Predictors of early improvement in low back pain amongst consulters to general practice: the influence of pre-morbid and episode-related factors. Pain 80: 113–119

Macfarlane G F, McBeth J, Garrow A, Silman A J 2000 Life is as much of a pain as it ever was. British Medical Journal 321: 897

Makela M 1993 Common musculoskeletal syndromes. Prevalence, risk indicators and disability in Finland. Publications of the Social Insurance Institution, Finland (ML 123)

Mason V 1994 The prevalence of back pain in Great Britain. Office of Population Censuses and Surveys, Social Survey Division (now Office of National Statistics). HMSO, London, pp 1–24

Murphy P L, Volinn E 1999 Is occupational low back pain on the rise? Spine 24: 691–697

Nachemson A, Waddell G, Norlund A I 2000 Epidemiology of neck and low back pain. In: Nachemson A, Jonsson E (eds) Neck and back pain: the scientific evidence of causes, diagnosis and treatment. Lippincott, Williams & Wilkins, Philadelphia, pp 165–187

NCCI 1992 Workers compensation back claim study. National Council on Compensation Insurance, Florida, pp 1–25

O'Grady J 2000 Joint health and safety committees: finding a balance. In: Sullivan T (ed.) Injury and the new world of work. University of British Columbia Press, Vancouver, pp 162–197

Palmer K T, Walsh K, Bendall H, Cooper C, Coggon D 2000 Back pain in Britain: comparison of two prevalence surveys at an interval of 10 years. British Medical Journal 320: 1577–1578

Papageorgiou A C, Croft P R, Ferry S, Jayson M I V, Silman A J 1995 Estimating the prevalence of low back pain in the general population. Evidence from the South Manchester back pain survey. Spine 20: 1889–1894

Papageorgiou A C, Croft P R, Thomas E, Ferry S, Jayson M I V, Silman A J 1996 Influence of previous pain experience on the episode incidence of low back pain: results from the South Manchester Back Pain Study. Pain 66: 181–185

Papageorgiou A C, Macfarlane G F, Thomas E, Croft P R, Jayson M I V, Silman A J 1997 Psychosocial factors in the workplace – do they predict new episodes of low back pain? Spine 22: 1137–1142

Porter R W, Hibbert C S 1986 Back pain and neck pain in four general practices. Clinical Biomechanics 1: 7–10

Santos-Eggimann B, Wietlisbach V, Rickenbach M, Paccaud F, Gutzwiller F 2000 One year prevalence of low back pain in two Swiss regions. Spine 25: 2473–2479

Taylor H, Curran N M 1985 The Nuprin pain report. Louis Harris, New York, pp 1–233

Thomas E, Silman A J, Croft P R, Papageorgiou A C, Jayson M I V, Macfarlane G J 1999 Predicting who develops chronic low back pain in primary care: a prospective study. British Medical Journal 318: 1662–1667

Volinn E 1997 The epidemiology of low back pain in the rest of the world: a review of surveys in low- and middle-income countries. Spine 22: 1747–1754

Von Korff M, Dworkin S F, Le Resche L A et al 1988 An epidemiologic comparison of pain complaints. Pain 32: 173–183

Waddell G, Aylward M, Sawney P 2002 Back pain, incapacity for work and social security benefits: an international literature review and analysis. Royal Society of Medicine, London

Walker B F 2000 The prevalence of low back pain: systematic review of the literature from 1966 to 1998. Journal of Spinal Disorders 13: 205–217

Walsh K, Cruddas M, Coggon D 1992 Low back pain in eight areas of Britain. Journal of Epidemiology and Community Health 46: 227–230

Watson P J, Main C J, Waddell G, Gales T F, Purcell-Jones G 1998 Medically certified work loss, recurrence and costs of wage compensation for back pain: a follow-up study of the working population of Jersey. British Journal of Rheumatology 37: 82–86

Yelin E 1997 The earnings, income, and assets of persons aged 51–61 with and without musculoskeletal conditions. Journal of Rheumatology 24: 2024–2030

Chapter 6

Risk factors for back pain

Kim Burton   Gordon Waddell

Who gets back pain? The simple answer, of course, is that most of us get back pain but there is obviously more to it than that. So, more specifically, are some people more at risk of serious back trouble or do some circumstances increase the risk?

There are hundreds of studies of risk factors in back pain, but fortunately we also now have good reviews (Table 6.1).

Table 6.1   Reviews of risk factors in back pain

Review	Topic
Burdorf & Sorock (1997)	Positive and negative evidence of risk factors for back disorders
NIOSH (1997)	Musculoskeletal disorders and workplace factors
National Research Council (1999)	Work-related musculoskeletal disorders: report, workshop summary, and workshop papers
Hoogendoorn et al (1999)	Physical load during work and leisure time as risk factors for back pain
Hoogendoorn et al (2000)	Psychosocial factors at work and private life as risk factors for back pain
Nachemson & Vingard (2000)	Individual influences on neck and low back pain
Linton (2000)	Psychological risk factors for neck and back pain
National Research Council & Institute of Medicine (2001)	Musculoskeletal disorders and the workplace: low back and upper extremities

---

Box 6.1   Potential risk factors for back pain

Individual
- Genetics
- Gender
- Age
- Body build: height, weight, leg length inequality
- Physical fitness
- Smoking
- Social class, education
- Emotional distress

Environmental
Physical
- Manual handling
- Heavy lifting
- Bending and twisting
- Repetitive movements
- Static work postures and sitting
- Driving and whole-body vibration
- Leisure activities and sports

Psychosocial aspects of work
- Job satisfaction
- Work "stress"
- High job demands and pace
- Poor job content: low decision latitude, low job control, and monotonous work
- Low social support
- Job "strain"

We can broadly divide potential risk factors for back pain into individual and environmental (Box 6.1). This does not imply a dichotomy. Rather, it suggests there are both individual susceptibilities and environmental stressors that may interact.

RISK FACTORS

Before we go any further we ought to be clear what we mean by "risk." Our first thought might be that a risk factor is something that causes back pain. So if we can remove or reduce that factor we might prevent some back pain. Sadly, risk is more complex than that and can have various implications.

As we saw in Chapter 5, most people get back pain at some time in their lives and it is commonly recurrent. Because back pain is a recurrent problem,

the most consistent and by far the strongest predictor of future back pain is the individual's previous history (Waddell & Burton 2000). So other risk factors are usually weaker, *additional* influences that simply modify the natural history.

Most of the early research was on physical risk factors for back injuries, particularly at work. The UK Health and Safety Executive (HSE 2000) distinguished "hazard" and "risk." A hazard is anything with the potential to cause harm; risk is the probability of someone actually coming to harm. Obviously, if there is no hazard, then there is no risk. However, even if there is a hazard the risk might be very low. Some hazards may have such serious consequences that we must try to eliminate them, even if the risk is very low. But at a practical level, the most cost-effective control strategies address hazards that carry a higher risk.

Many of the early studies of risk factors were cross-sectional in design. Strictly speaking, these only show statistical associations between possible risk factors and the prevalence of reported symptoms. Most were retrospective studies looking at small groups of workers and matched controls. The groups were often highly selected and not at all typical of the general population. Most studies depended on self-reports of work and of symptoms, which are often unreliable. In short, these early studies had many serious limitations.

Scientific study of risk factors and proof of cause and effect require prospective cohort studies. These measure risk factors in people who are initially free of symptoms and then study the incidence of new symptoms over time. Some factors turn out to be only risk markers that are associated with symptoms, but do not necessarily demonstrate cause and effect. For example, a cross-sectional study may show that workers in a certain job have more sickness absence due to back pain. This could be because that job causes back injuries. Or it may be the job aggravates pre-existing back symptoms. Or workers who have back pain for some other reason may have more difficulty doing that job. Or that workplace may have poor industrial relations, with high sickness absence rates, and workers who are more likely to stay off work when they have ordinary backache. True risk factors predict the development of future problems and also provide information about their etiology and causal mechanisms, e.g., certain physical demands of work. Still others may be "pantechnicon" variables, e.g., gender, which contain complex biologic, psychological, and social issues that require further analysis.

Proof of cause and effect requires strict criteria (Bombardier et al 1994, Rothman & Greenland 1998):

- strength of association: sometimes described as the "effect size." Weak effects may be statistically significant but are unlikely to be clinically important. For complex statistical reasons that we need not go into here, this usually requires an odds ratio (OR) or relative risk (RR) of >3–4.
- consistency in different studies
- biologic plausibility: does it fit our theoretic understanding? This may be difficult for a condition like non-specific back pain where we do not really understand the pathology!
- temporal sequence of exposure and effect: which can only be shown in a longitudinal study
- dose–response gradient: greater or cumulative exposure to the hazard increases the risk
- specificity: it is usually only possible to demonstrate this with an uncommon exposure and an uncommon condition, e.g., asbestos and mesothelioma. It is difficult to demonstrate with a common condition like back pain
- reversibility: stopping exposure to the hazard reduces the risk. Thus back pain that develops some time after stopping work is unlikely to be caused by that job.

We should also ask – risk of what? In this chapter we are mainly concerned with risk factors for the *onset* of back pain. These are closest to what we might think of as possible *causes* of back pain. Over the next seven chapters we will consider the wide range of factors that are linked to the various consequences of back pain: chronic pain and disability, sickness absence, and health care use. These are sometimes described as risk factors for these different outcomes. However, it seems to make more sense to think of them as *influences* on back pain after it has occurred.

Adams et al (2002) considered various risk factors for back trouble and possible relationships

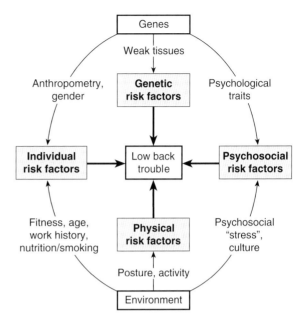

Figure 6.1   Risk factors for low back trouble and the relationship between them. Reproduced with permission from Adams et al (2002).

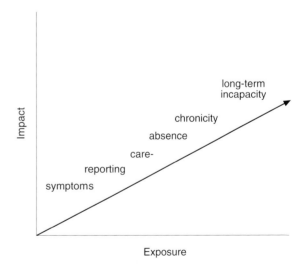

Figure 6.2   The dose–response gradient: increased exposure produces increased risk and impact.

between them (Fig. 6.1). Figure 6.2 expands on the possible consequences of back pain, and shows the dose–response gradient. This started from the concept that increasing or cumulative exposure leads to increased risk of the outcome, e.g., back pain. Today, it places more emphasis on increasing exposure leading to more serious consequences. Both may be true.

Before we look at individual risk factors, it is worth repeating that we must keep them in perspective. The high prevalence of back pain means that most risk factors can only have a modest *additional* effect. If 50% of people get back pain at some time anyway, then most risk factors might increase that to 60–70%. What then matters is the effect size and the clinical importance of the risk.

INDIVIDUAL RISK FACTORS

Genetics

Genetic factors play a role in certain spinal disorders, such as spondylolisthesis, scoliosis, and ankylosing spondylitis. A few clinical studies suggest there may sometimes be a familial or genetic predisposition to disk prolapse. However, all of that is of little relevance to ordinary backache.

We now have various twin studies that investigate genetic factors in back pain. The evidence seems clearer for degenerative changes than for symptoms, but we must remember that the correlation between them is low.

The classic Finnish twin study (Battie et al 1995) found that identical twins showed very similar magnetic resonance imaging (MRI) changes in their spines, despite different occupational histories (Fig. 6.3). This is often misquoted as showing that genetic factors determine degenerative changes in the spine. These findings are hardly surprising, as identical twins have the same body build and metabolism. But they also usually share their early lives. The main message of this study was that familial factors (which includes genetics, body build and make-up, and early environment) have more influence than occupation on the degeneration that occurs in everyone with age. The authors themselves point out that this kind of study cannot separate genetic, anthropometric, and metabolic factors from the effect of shared early environment and lifestyle (T Videman, personal communication). Moreover, this study still left a great deal of degenerative changes unexplained, particularly at the lower lumbar levels, which are most important clinically.

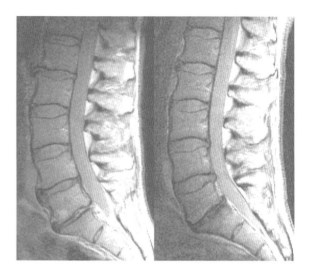

Figure 6.3 Occupational exposure has little impact on degenerative changes. These magnetic resonance imagings are from 50-year-old twins. One was a farmer who had always done heavy manual work. The other was a journalist. Can you tell which is which? You have a 50% chance of guessing correctly! Reproduced with permission from Battie & Videman (2003).

A study of British twins came to broadly similar conclusions (Sambrook et al 1999). Lumbar disk height, disk bulge, and osteophytes appeared to be highly heritable, but there was a confounding influence from shared environment.

Even more fascinating are preliminary studies of the human genome. A few genes have been identified that are related to disk degeneration – those for the vitamin D receptor (Videman et al 1995), for collagen type IX (Paassilta et al 2001), and for proteoglycans (Kawaguchi et al 1999). It has been suggested that the search for genes should be extended to pathologic, physiologic, and behavioral mechanisms. It is still early days, but studies of gene–environment interactions might lead eventually to a better understanding of risk factors and causal mechanisms. Gene studies might even lead to new treatments.

Twin studies of back symptoms give inconsistent results. MacGregor et al (1999) found a large genetic contribution to the prevalence of moderately severe back pain in females. Not surprisingly, however, this was only partly explained by any genetic influence on degenerative changes on MRI. In a study of pain thresholds, MacGregor et al

(1997) found that learned patterns of behavior within families were much more powerful than any genetic influence.

The Danish twin study (Hartvigsen et al 2003) could not detect any significant genetic influence on short- or long-term back pain. They concluded that physical workload might be more important that any genetic effect.

A much earlier twin study by Heikkila et al (1989) found that only about 10% of "sciatica" could be explained by constitutional similarity.

In summary, it appears that certain aspects of back pain may have a genetic or at least a constitutional or familial element. We still need to disentangle these elements. Most important, there is no evidence that genetic or constitutional factors determine who is going to become a back cripple.

Gender

Most large population surveys show a slightly higher prevalence of back pain in women. (For example, see Fig. 5.2.) However, we must interpret this against a background that women report a slightly higher level of most symptoms. This could be due as much to body awareness, pain perception, and willingness to report symptoms as to any physical difference in their backs. When it comes to actual studies of risk factors for back pain, gender consistently turns out to have a limited effect (Burdorf & Sorock 1997).

The evidence on low back disability is conflicting, with no clear pattern. The evidence on work loss is also conflicting. There are biomechanical reasons to suggest that women may be more at risk of increased loading during heavy lifting than men (Marras et al 2002). However, that is balanced by women generally having lighter jobs. Almost all workers' compensation figures show more work-related back injuries and claims in men, although in some series women stay off work longer (Waddell et al 2002). However, these data only cover work-related back pain in selected groups of workers. Social security data may be more representative of the general population. This shows different patterns in different countries (Waddell et al 2002). In the UK, benefits paid for chronic back incapacity have always been higher in men than in women, although women do now seem to

be catching up (Fig. 5.6). This seems to be largely a matter of more women working and becoming entitled to benefits. In Sweden, sickness absence due to back pain is higher for women than for men. However, this difference is largely explained by sick leave during pregnancy. When that is excluded, there is no difference between men and women (Sydsjö et al 2003).

All of these findings may reflect their social settings rather than any biologic difference between men and women. Overall, there does not appear to be any major difference in low back disability between men and women.

Women seek slightly more health care for back pain, as for all health complaints (McCormick et al 1995, Vingard et al 2002: for example, see Table 19.4).

Sciatica does appear to be more common in men than in women (Heliovaara et al 1987). Clinical reports all show more men coming to spinal surgery, although this may also be due to different referral patterns and different selection for surgery in men and women.

There is one condition that is absolutely gender-specific: pregnancy. Many women have temporary back pain during the later stages of pregnancy, possibly related to altered posture and hormonal changes in soft tissues. However, this does not appear to have any lasting effect. Several early reports suggested that women with multiple pregnancies might continue to have more back pain. More careful studies do not seem to confirm this. Ostgaard et al (1996) suggested there might have been confusion between posterior pelvic pain and lumbosacral pain. The main problem in pregnancy may be pelvic pain, which usually settles after delivery. When they distinguished this, pregnancy did not appear to influence future back pain. As epidurals became more common during labor, there were many claims that they caused chronic low back pain. However, long-term follow-up of a randomized controlled trial of epidural pain relief in labor showed no significant difference in spinal movements, back pain, or disability (Howell et al 2002).

Age

Population surveys suggest that the age of first onset of back pain is spread fairly evenly from the

Summary

Back pain in men and women

- Women report a slightly higher prevalence of back pain, as is the case for most bodily symptoms
- Sciatica is more common in men
- There is conflicting evidence and probably little difference in low back disability
- Women seek slightly more health care for back pain, as is the case for most health conditions
- Back injuries at work, time off work, sickness benefits, and compensation claims may reflect different social and work patterns rather than any biologic difference between men and women

teens to the early 40s. It is uncommon to develop ordinary backache for the first time after the mid-50s.

During the 1990s, many studies from all developed countries showed that back symptoms are also common in adolescents and teenage children aged 11–18 years (Balague et al 1999, Nachemson & Vingard 2000). These symptoms do not usually present for health care, and adult surveys suggest that most people forget about them. So we only detected them when we asked specifically about them. Burton et al (1996a) made a prospective study of 216 adolescents from 11 through 15 years of age. Only 12% of 11-year-olds said they had ever had back pain, but by age 15 it rose to adult levels of 50%. That is an annual incidence of 15%. Their back pain was often recurrent but did not deteriorate with time. Most important, however, all studies agree that it rarely causes significant disability and few seek health care (Burton et al 1996a, Wedderkopp et al 2001, Watson et al 2002, 2003).

We should be cautious how we interpret these findings. They are based entirely on leading questions that, as every parent with kids of this age knows, do not always produce reliable results! Brattberg (1993, 1994) carried out a longitudinal study of 471 schoolchildren aged 10, 13, and 15 years in Sweden. In each year's survey, about 26% of children said they had back pain, but only 9% of the children reported back pain in both surveys in 1989 and 1991. King & Coles (1992) found marked variation between different European countries, ranging from 3% for girls aged 15 in Finland to 22% in Belgium. However, Hakala et al (2002) found that the prevalence in Finland increased dramatically by the late 1990s. This all suggests that there may be a major cultural element in these findings.

It might seem plausible to suggest that the search for causes of back pain should start with children and adolescents, and that preventive measures should start at that time. But we should be careful. Balague et al (1999) reviewed risk factors for back pain in children and found serious weaknesses in the scientific evidence. They found moderate evidence that competitive sports activities are associated with increased back pain in adolescents. They found some evidence that a family history of back pain, increased height, smoking, high levels of physical activity, and depression and emotional stress are also associated with reported symptoms. But many of these are behavioral phenomena that may easily be confounded with psychosocial influences on self-report. Watson et al (2002, 2003) made one of the few studies that looked at both physical and psychosocial risk factors in children. They could not identify any mechanical risk factors, but found a stronger association with emotional difficulties and psychological problems.

There is little or no evidence that any of these adolescent risk markers have any direct biologic effect. Nevertheless, the search for a physical cause has led to a media frenzy over backpacks. There are no prospective studies looking at this issue, but there are studies that help to put it into perspective. One study in Italy found that children felt their backpacks were heavy, uncomfortable, and caused back pain. However, reports of back pain were not related to the weight of the backpack, but to the time spent carrying and subjective feelings of fatigue (Negrini & Carabalona 2002). Another study in the US looked at backpack injuries coming to emergency departments (Wiersema et al 2003). Only 11% of injuries in children involved the lower back, of which 59% involved carrying a backpack. However, most injuries were caused by tripping over a backpack or being hit by one!

Burton et al (1996a) suggested that we should consider most adolescent back trouble to be a normal life experience and not attach undue significance to it. Most important, there is no convincing evidence that back pain in adolescence is a risk factor for serious low back trouble in adult life. The history of adult back pain should teach us the danger of overmedicalizing back pain in children. The real risk would be if overenthusiastic intervention should turn a minor childhood symptom into a self-fulfilling medical disaster in adult life.

Schoene (2002) gave a very balanced discussion on what this means for clinical management (Box 6.2).

Most population surveys show that the prevalence of back pain increases with age up to about 45–50 and then levels off or falls slightly (Burdorf & Sorock 1997). However, such surveys usually focus on people of working age. Bressler et al (1999) reviewed 12 studies that gave separate data about back pain in people aged 65+ years. Methodologic weaknesses and small sample sizes gave wide variation in the estimates. Nevertheless, some studies again showed that the prevalence of symptoms fell slightly with age. Edmond & Felson (2000) studied a large cohort of 1037 Americans aged 68–100 years. The 1-year prevalence remained about 50% in those aged 68–80 and 81–100 years. It was slightly higher in women, particularly in the thoracic region. If older people did get back pain, however, it was likely to be more persistent. Twenty-two percent said they had back pain "most days."

Self-reported disability tends to increase with age (Table 6.2). We have already seen that Walsh et al (1992) provide the best population data on back disability (Table 5.4). They again found that disability increased up to age 40–49 years. Social security statistics in all countries show that sickness absence and long-term disability benefits rise dramatically some time after 50–55 years of age (Waddell et al 2002). This reflects all conditions. All chronic disability becomes much more common in the elderly, but we have little data for back pain. Edmond & Felson (2000) found that geriatric patients with poor general health who were confined to their homes had a particularly high prevalence of back pain and stiffness.

So, is age a risk factor in back pain? The answer is yes and no – it depends: on whether we are talking about symptoms or disability or health care. Clinically, there are similarities and differences between back pain in adolescents, adults of working age, and the elderly.

Body build

There are many clinical myths about back pain being related to body build. Doctors and therapists can't resist blaming obesity, or being tall, or leg length inequality.

Box 6.2   A clinical framework for thinking about back pain in adolescence

(a) During adolescence and teenage years the prevalence of back pain increases to adult levels. Most adolescent back pain is not due to any significant medical condition and does not present for health care

(b) When adolescent back pain does present clinically, a small but important proportion will be due to serious underlying pathology (which is why it is a "red flag"). In each case, you should consider if and when further investigation is required to exclude this

(c) But, remember (a) and keep (b) in proportion

Table 6.2   Self-reported restricted activities in the past 4 weeks due to back pain (as a percentage of those with back pain)

Age (years)	Men (%)	Women (%)
16–24	11	21
25–34	20	29
35–44	25	27
45–54	23	37
55–64	32	41
65+	36	39

Based on data from Mason (1994), with permission from the Office of National Statistics.

Contrary to popular belief, most studies show that body weight, and even obesity, does not make much difference. Leboeuf-Yde (2000a) reviewed 65 studies, of which only a third showed any significant association between body weight and symptoms. Even then it was weak. She concluded that there is no clear evidence that weight actually causes back pain. There is also no clinical evidence that weight loss is an effective treatment for back pain.

Reviews by Burdorf & Sorock (1997) and Nachemson & Vingard (2000) showed no consistent relation between height and back pain.

Doctors and therapists often get excited about unequal leg length, but the literature again does not show any consistent relationship (Nachemson & Vingard 2000).

In summary, contrary to individual cross-sectional reports, the evidence suggests that none of these aspects of body build is a significant risk factor for back pain or its consequences.

Physical fitness

There has been much interest in the possible role of physical fitness in back pain. Clinical evidence shows that patients with chronic back pain are less fit, but this could be effect rather than cause. The more specific idea that physically fit people get less back trouble rests mainly on a single, classic study. Cady et al (1979) found that physically fit firefighters got fewer back injuries than those who were less fit. However, that was a very select population in an unusual, high-risk situation. This study has never really been replicated. Reviews by Andersson (1997) and Nachemson & Vingard (2000) did not find convincing evidence that the level of general (cardiovascular) fitness is a risk factor for future back pain.

There are many health advantages to being physically fit. It is possible that physical fitness/strength may help to reduce the likelihood of new episodes of back pain in certain jobs. However it seems likely that fitness is more relevant if and when back pain does occur. There are theoretic reasons and some clinical evidence to suggest that fit patients make a more rapid recovery from acute back pain and are less likely to develop chronic pain and disability.

Smoking

Many studies describe smoking as a risk factor for various aspects of low back trouble. Battie et al (1991) and Goldberg et al (2000) reviewed theories about smoking. Smoking may cause chronic cough, which might influence disk prolapse and sciatica, although there is no direct evidence on this. Smoking reduces bone mineral content, so might cause osteoporosis and microfractures. It impairs fibrinolysis and promotes scar formation. It causes changes in disk nutrition. Battie et al (1991) found more degenerative changes on MRI in the disks of smokers compared with their non-smoking identical twins. Smoking could also have more indirect effects. There may be a relation between smoking, physical fitness, and body weight. Smoking is linked to how people report pain and is actually related more strongly to pain in the limbs than to pain in the neck or back. Smokers have lower physical and mental health status, and show more depressive symptoms (Vogt et al 2002). Smoking varies with social class, education, and occupation. So smoking may simply be a risk marker for a complex set of demographic, psychosocial, and lifestyle factors.

Two reviews of 47 studies show that the relation between smoking and back pain is weak and inconsistent (Leboeuf-Yde 1999, Goldberg et al 2000). Leboeuf-Yde (1999) concluded that smoking is only a weak risk marker of back pain and not a cause. There is also no evidence that stopping smoking is an effective treatment. This really shows the danger of overinterpreting some of these studies!

Several early studies questioned the possible role of alcohol. Do not worry! We are delighted to say that a review by Leboeuf-Yde (2000b) showed that alcohol is not a risk factor for back pain.

Social class

There are many social influences on back pain and disability. As a very crude starting point, we might look at social class. Most British surveys use a classification based on occupation:

  I: professional groups such as doctors, lawyers, and scientists
 II: intermediate groups such as teachers, nurses, and self-employed shopkeepers

III: skilled occupations

    IIINM: skilled non-manual, such as clerical workers

    IIIM: skilled manual, such as tradesmen

IV: partly skilled, such as process workers in industry or transport workers

 V: unskilled, such as laborers and cleaners.

This classification is really twofold. It is partly occupational, with a divide between manual and non-manual. That may be why studies of social class usually show more significant findings in men than in women. It is also partly socioeconomic, and serves as a marker for all facets of social disadvantage, such as education, housing, (un)employment, and income. That applies equally to men and women.

Walsh et al (1992) provided most detail on the relation between back pain and social class (Table 6.3). In men, the prevalences of back pain, disability, and work loss all rose between social classes I–II and IV–V. In women, the only correlation was with long-term disability. Croft & Rigby (1994) tried to disentangle the socioeconomic influences. In men, the only correlation seemed to be with unskilled manual labor. Women showed a correlation with the lowest income category and less formal education: in them it seemed to be a question of social disadvantage.

There is a stronger association between social class and the consequences of back pain (Waddell &

Waddell 2000). People in manual work are more likely to blame their back pain on work. They lose more time from work and stay off longer. People in social classes IV–V are more likely to lie down to rest and seek more health care.

Education

Dionne et al (2001) reviewed 64 studies of education as a risk factor. Most studies showed an association between lower education level and a higher prevalence of back pain, though the strength of the effect was weak. There was a stronger association with disabling back pain. There did not appear to be any association with outcome of treatment.

The problem is that it is difficult to disentangle education from other aspects of social class. In a very careful analysis, Makela (1993) concluded that education was simply an indirect measure of heavy work, work stress, and work injury. In an equally careful study, Deyo & Tsui-Wui (1987) found that education did have an independent effect. Dione et al (1995) made a longitudinal study of education and back-related disability in adults. Like most previous studies, they found that people with less than 13 years' schooling had more disability. More interesting was what happened over the next 2 years. Disability tended to improve, particularly in those with more education, but did not improve as much in those with less education. Dione et al (1995) considered possible mechanisms, and suggested that occupational and psychological factors were more important than health care access or use. Straaton et al (1996) also found that higher education level was associated with better rehabilitation outcome.

In summary, lower social class is probably a weak risk factor for back pain. There is a stronger association with resulting disability. The relationship to social class is fairly consistent in men but less clear in women. The problem is what this means. Social class appears to be another pantechnicon variable, which is a crude measure of a host of social, educational, occupational, economic, lifestyle, and psychosocial issues, any of which could affect the consequences of back pain. It is partly a matter of heavy manual work, particularly in men. It is probably also a matter of social disadvantage in both men and women, although

Table 6.3 Prevalence of back pain related to social class

		Men		Women	
Social Class		I–II	IV–V	I–II	IV–V
Back pain	1 year	23%	42%	No trend	
	Lifetime	51%	65%	No trend	
Low back disability	1 year	2.9%	8.1%	1.9%	6.2%
	Lifetime	No trend		No trend	
Work loss due to back pain	1 year	5.6%	13.9%	No trend	
	Lifetime	22.3%	38.5%	No trend	

From Walsh et al (1992), with permission.

we do not know exactly which aspects of this disadvantage are important or how they affect back pain.

Perhaps these are more important *social influences* on what happens to people after they develop back pain, rather than risk factors. We will consider this in more detail in Chapter 13.

Summary

The influence of social class on back pain
- Social class reflects occupation, particularly manual vs non-manual, and social disadvantage
- The prevalence of back pain may be slightly greater in those from a lower social class
- There is a clear and marked increase in work loss due to back pain with lower social class
- It is not clear what aspects of work, social disadvantage, lifestyle, or attitudes and behavior influence this

Emotional distress

Patients with back pain often show emotional distress, but it is usually a secondary consequence of their pain and disability. Here, we are considering the converse: is pre-existing distress a risk factor for developing back pain?

Let us look briefly at a couple of studies that tried to disentangle cause and effect.

Mannion et al (1996) studied 403 female nurses and health workers aged 18–40 who had no previous history of "serious" low back pain, by which they meant no medical attention or work loss. Thirty-five percent did have some previous back pain that did not require medical attention or work loss. At the start of the study, they found that those with more distress were more likely to report previous back pain. They also had lower experimental pain tolerance. Over 18 months' follow-up, 40% reported some low back pain but this was not associated with any rise in levels of distress. Twenty percent reported serious back pain and sought health care or took time off work. This latter group showed slightly increased levels of distress. Initial physical assessment did not predict those who

would develop any back pain or serious back pain. Workload also had little effect, whether judged by the job description or by the workers' own perception of their jobs. The best predictor was psychological distress, but the effect was weak and explained less than 3% of future back pain.

Burton et al (1996b) studied policemen in England and Northern Ireland, with different exposures to physical stressors (wearing heavy body armor and vehicular vibration). They also collected data on back pain history and psychosocial factors. Physical loading on the spine led to earlier first-onset back pain with a dose–response relationship. However, continued exposure to physical stress did not lead to chronic problems. Chronic pain and work loss seemed instead to depend mainly on psychosocial factors.

Linton (2000) reviewed this area. Most prospective studies show that various measures of distress are a risk factor for new onset of back pain. However, the effect is weak. Estimates vary, but it seems that psychological factors only increase the risk by about 5–10%. This does *not* mean that "5–10% of episodes are caused by a psychological disturbance." It is more likely that psychological issues play a variable but generally minor role in many people. We should also remember that the outcome in most of these studies was *self-reported* back pain or injury. And the effect of distress on back pain is weaker than the effect on other musculoskeletal injuries, cardiovascular disability, and depression (Manninen et al 1995). So it may be that distress simply makes people more likely to report symptoms. There is no good evidence linking individual psychology to the development of physical pathology in the spine. As you would expect, Manninen et al (1995) found that mental stress only predicted non-specific low back pain, and not spinal pathology such as disk prolapse and stenosis.

In summary, emotional distress does appear to be a risk factor for the incidence of new back pain in symptom-free people. However, the effect size is weak. This does not prove that back pain is caused by psychological factors or is "psychogenic". It seems more likely that psychological factors influence how people react to or report a bodily symptom like back pain. They also influence sickness absence and seeking health care. Once again, we will see in Chapter 11 that distress plays a much more important role in what happens after people develop back pain.

ENVIRONMENTAL RISK FACTORS: PHYSICAL

We sometimes assume that physical demands on the back must be risk factors for back pain, but that is not always true. Different physical activities may either load or unload the spine, and loading may be either good or bad for the spine. Physical activities may also be good or bad for us, quite apart from any direct effect they might have on the spine.

We might argue that standing and walking are the most natural human activities, creating a standard loading on the spine. Prolonged standing and walking are not risk factors for back pain (Hoogendoorn et al 1999). Indeed, natural selection would seem to make that unlikely. If standing upright had caused early hominids to develop (disabling) back pain, the experiment would have failed, and *Homo sapiens* would not have evolved!

Other physical activities fall into two broad categories: those that increase or decrease spinal loading compared with walking. Biomechanical measurements confirm that strenuous activities such as bending, lifting, and manual handling increase the load on the spine. Lying down has the greatest unloading effect. But some activities do not have quite the expected effect. Early biomechanical studies suggested that sitting increased disk pressure (Nachemson & Morris 1964). However, this was an isolated measurement in a single disk, with possible technical limitations. It is now possible to make more sophisticated measurements of different loads on different tissues and in different positions, e.g., on the disks, facet joints, ligaments, and different muscles (Adams et al 2002). These suggest that sitting, in any type of chair, may actually unload the spine relative to standing (Althoff et al 1992). Even some apparently strenuous tasks, such as working with the arms overhead, can lead to relative unloading (Burton et al 1994). Thus, normal physical activities at work and leisure expose our spines to both loading and relative unloading.

It is also wrong to suppose that all spinal loading is harmful. Quite the contrary, some loading is essential for spinal health. The same mechanical

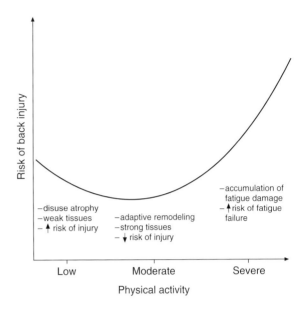

Figure 6.4 Proposed U-shaped relation between mechanical loading and risk of back injury. From Adams et al (2002), with permission.

loading that can deform and damage spinal tissues also stimulates growth and repair. Adaptive remodeling strengthens bone, collagen, and muscle. Risk may then be more a matter of certain patterns or levels of loading that exceed the capacity for repair (Adams et al 2002). The different rates at which spinal tissues are able to adapt to increased mechanical demands could mean that poorly vascularized tissues such as disks and ligaments might be more vulnerable. This may be important when levels of physical activity are suddenly increased, e.g., starting a new job or in sport.

It has been suggested that there might be a U-shaped risk between spinal loading and back pain (Fig. 6.4). This was originally an attempt to explain contradictory findings that both heavy physical work and light activities such as sitting were associated with back pain. There is some biomechanical face-validity to this as a model for back injury. There is a theoretic argument that it reflects the capacity of spinal tissues to adapt to loading and the balance between repair and damage. The concept is even philosophically attractive, of "moderation in all things" with virtuous roots as far back as Aristotle! However, some of these early findings no longer appear valid. Overall, the current epidemiologic evidence on risk factors for back pain is not entirely supportive of U-shaped risk. Nevertheless, the value of this model is to reinforce the idea that loading is not always harmful and some loading is essential for health.

Physical demands of work

The most important question is whether occupational loading leads to mechanical overload damage to the spine. In vitro experiments certainly show that certain levels of loading (both sudden loads and cyclical loading) can produce mechanical disruption of vertebrae, end plates, and disks. But does that level of loading occur in life and is there any evidence of damage in vivo?

Brinckmann et al (1998) made one of the most careful studies. They made precise measurements of spinal X-rays from 355 workers who had been exposed to extreme physical demands and 737 unexposed controls. They showed that very heavy lifting and handling, particularly in miners working in confined underground conditions, led to reduced disk height. Substantial exposure to whole-body vibration on unsprung seats had the same effect. However, these X-rays were from historic archives. The jobs and the physical demands far exceeded what would be permitted in any North American or European country today. Ergonomic improvements and current regulations mean that today's jobs rarely involve the kind of physical demands likely to cause any such lasting damage. This was most starkly demonstrated in Brinckmann et al's study by the contrast between the effect of vibration on operators with unsprung seats and the lack of effect on those with damped seats.

The study was not designed to assess the relation between overload damage and symptoms, but some data happened to be available. One cohort with overload damage did not have any higher prevalence of back pain. Another cohort with a high prevalence of back pain did not show overload damage. So even mechanical overload damage did not necessarily result in symptoms.

Even if modern work does not cause any structural damage, it is still important to ask whether it is a risk factor for back pain. Since the classic study by Magora (1970), there have been hundreds of studies on the relation between physical demands

of work and back pain. There are also many good reviews (Burdorf & Sorock 1997, Bigos et al 1996, Hoogendoorn et al 1999, Videman & Battie 1999, Waddell & Burton 2000, Adams et al 2002).

Videman & Battie (1999) reviewed the influence of occupation on lumbar degeneration. This is perhaps the most authoritative statement from leading world experts. They concluded that there is evidence that occupational exposure can influence disk degeneration. However, this is a weak effect that explains a very small portion of the degeneration found in the adult population. Further, the lack of a clear dose–response relationship casts doubt on any strong causal link. Contrary to popular belief, occupational loading does not appear to play a dominant role in disk degeneration.

The UK Occupational Health Guidelines (Carter & Birrell 2000, Waddell & Burton 2000) tried to summarize the evidence on the complex relationships between physical demands of work and back pain.

1. Most adults (60–80%) experience LBP at some time, and it is often persistent or recurrent. It is one of the most common reasons for seeking health care, and it is now one of the commonest health reasons given for work loss.

2. There is strong epidemiological evidence that physical demands of work (manual materials handling, lifting, bending, twisting, and whole body vibration) can be associated with increased reports of back symptoms, aggravation of symptoms and "injuries".

3. There is limited and contradictory evidence that the length of exposure to physical stressors at work (cumulative risk) increases reports of back symptoms or of persistent symptoms.

4. There is strong evidence that physical demands of work (manual materials handling, lifting, bending, twisting, and whole body vibration) are a risk factor for the incidence (onset) of LBP, but overall it appears that the size of the effect is less than that of other individual, non-occupational and unidentified factors.
[Note: evidence statements 2 and 4 are not incompatible. Whilst the epidemiological evidence shows that low back symptoms are commonly linked to physical demands of work, that does not necessarily

mean that LBP is *caused* by work. Although there is strong scientific evidence that physical demands of work can cause individual attacks of LBP, overall that only accounts for a modest proportion of all LBP occurring in workers.]

5. There is moderate scientific evidence that physical demands of work play only a minor role in the development of disc degeneration.

6. There is strong epidemiological and clinical evidence that care seeking and disability due to LBP depend more on complex individual and work-related psychosocial factors than on clinical features or physical demands of work.

Manual handling

Manual materials handling involves various combinations of lifting, moving, carrying, and handling physical loads. It is difficult to separate manual handling per se from generally heavy manual jobs. An important subgroup involves patient handling by nurses and other health workers. Patients are hardly "materials", but the principles are the same!

There is strong and consistent evidence that workers in jobs involving manual handling report more back pain (Burdorf & Sorock 1997, Hoogendoorn et al 1999). The effect size is weak–moderate (RR or OR ranging from about 1.5 to 3). The UK Labour Force Surveys of the 1990s consistently showed that manual workers report all musculoskeletal complaints more than non-manual workers. They also had more persistent symptoms 3 years after stopping work and attributed them to work (Jones et al 1998).

There is limited and inconsistent evidence on manual handling as a risk factor for disk prolapse or sciatica.

Most workers' compensation data suggest that men with heavy manual jobs report more back injuries at work. The data are less clear for women. Nurses and certain other groups of health workers report more back pain and injuries, but they are a special group.

Almost all data sets show that workers with heavy manual jobs lose more time from work with back pain. Some, but not all, studies show that workers with heavy manual jobs have more spells

off work with back pain. Others show that, when they are off, they return to work more slowly (Fig. 7.3). There is wide variation in long-term disability and early retirement rates in different jobs but, surprisingly, this does not correlate well with the physical demands of work. However, these data do not tell us whether or not heavy work is the cause of more disabling back pain. It could equally be effect. It may simply be more difficult to do a heavy job when you have back pain, whatever its cause.

In summary, workers in heavy manual jobs do get more back trouble, but we must be careful how we interpret this.

Lifting

Ideally, we would like to identify which physical activities in heavy manual work might cause back trouble. From biomechanical studies, lifting, bending, and twisting are most likely to damage the spine. These are also the activities that have been studied most in the workplace.

Industrial accident and workers' compensation statistics certainly show that back injuries are reported more commonly in jobs that involve:

- heavy lifting
- lifting objects which are bulky or must be held away from the body
- lifting from the floor
- frequent lifting.

The more general role of lifting as a risk factor for back pain is less clear. It is difficult to separate any specific effect of lifting from manual handling and heavy physical work in general. The reviews by Burdorf & Sorock (1997) and Hoogendoorn et al (1999) were unable to reach any definite answer. Perhaps we should simply accept that, in principle, frequent heavy lifting carries about the same risk as manual handling.

It might seem possible that handling unexpectedly heavy or asymmetric loads would carry a higher risk of injury. In fact, a recent biomechanical study found no evidence to support this (van der Burg et al 2000). It seems the neuromuscular apparatus is robust enough to cope.

The lack of clear epidemiologic evidence means that lifting and handling guidelines and regulations are based on theory and consensus. In theory, ability to lift and the risk of injury will vary with individual strength. Heavy lifting that exceeds the person's ability may carry greater risk. However, it is difficult to set safe limits. In addition to the weight, we must also consider the frequency and rate of lifting, the level of the lift, and the position of the body. The distance between the load and the body greatly increases the forces on the back. Lifting standards set by the US National Institute for Occupational Safety and Health (Waters et al 1993) or the UK Health and Safety Executive's guidance (HSE 1992) are simply based on experience and consensus.

Despite popular clinical belief, there is limited epidemiologic evidence on lifting as a risk factor for disk prolapse or sciatica.

There is little separate information on pushing and pulling, although heavy manual jobs often involve these activities as well. In one careful prospective study, Hoozemans et al (2002) found a limited relation between pulling and pushing and low back complaints.

Bending and twisting

There is strong biomechanical evidence that lifting combined with bending and twisting has the potential to injure spinal structures. The risk of disk prolapse is especially high with combined loading and twisting. Twisting alone, without lifting, probably does not carry much risk. This is probably because of the anatomic limitations to vertebral rotation.

Burdorf & Sorock (1997) found 10 studies giving strong and consistent evidence that frequent bending and twisting is a risk factor for back pain. The effect size is weak–moderate (RR or OR ranging from about 1.3 to 2.8).

Repetitive strain

Repetitive strain injury is currently fashionable, particularly in a medicolegal context. It usually affects the upper limb, although the pathology and the diagnosis itself are hotly disputed. Several legal claims about occupational back pain have explored the same concept.

It is certainly possible to produce fatigue failure due to repetitive strain in the laboratory. There are,

however, major differences between such experiments and clinical back pain. Most of the biomechanical studies are on bones and disks, which are probably not the source of most work-related back pain. There are some hypotheses about how this might apply to soft tissues but little experimental data. The many thousands of rapid cycles required to produce failure are quite different from the pattern of repeated everyday movements in work. In vitro experiments also fail to allow for biologic adaptation and healing in response to repeated strain.

There is little clinical evidence to support the idea of repetitive strain injury to the back. Most claimants have already done the same tasks over long periods without symptoms. There is nothing new or changed in their job when back pain develops. The symptoms are subjective and are the same as common, ordinary backache. No one has defined any specific clinical syndrome or objective pathology with repetitive strain injury. When back pain is present, such repetitive activities may aggravate symptoms, but yet again this is not proof of cause and effect. Burdorf & Sorock (1997) could only find three studies of repetitive work, and two out of three found no association.

In summary, repetitive strain injury seems to be more of a medicolegal concept than a clinical or pathologic reality.

Static work postures and sitting

Several early cross-sectional studies suggested that there was an association between sitting and back pain. This was linked to biomechanical theories about raised disk pressure, but we have already seen these findings were suspect. Moreover, this is static loading and any pressure is very low compared with that required to cause experimental damage. We have already discussed the more sophisticated U-shaped model of risk. Despite these theories, there is no actual biomechanical evidence that sitting damages the spine.

Hartvigsen et al (2000) reviewed 35 epidemiologic studies on sitting. Only eight had a satisfactory experimental design. Only one showed any significant relation between prolonged sitting at work and low back pain. Seven out of eight showed no effect. They concluded that the extensive evidence now available does not support the popular belief that sitting is a risk factor for back pain.

Seating has fluctuated greatly over the centuries in different cultures, from upright to slouched positions (Pynt et al 2002). There is no evidence that any type of seat or sitting position makes any difference to the risk of back pain. The current epidemiologic evidence demolishes debate about the best form of seating and the "ideal" seated posture. Biomechanical arguments for or against different positions now seem pretty irrelevant! So choice of seat is entirely a matter of subjective comfort.

In summary, sitting is *not* a risk factor for back pain. Prolonged sitting in one position may aggravate back pain that is already present, whatever its cause. Experience suggests that it is reasonable advice to change position and get up and move about regularly. But all of that is more a matter of coping with back pain rather than anything to do with risk or cause.

Driving and exposure to whole–body vibration

Driving is different from ordinary sitting, because it involves exposure to whole-body vibration. The dominant frequency of vibration in many vehicles is 4–6 Hz, which is also the resonant frequency of the spine (Pope et al 1991). Most of the biomechanical evidence is about whole-body vibration, but most of the epidemiologic evidence is about driving. However, driving exposes us to more than just vibration (Heliovaara 1999). It involves static and sometimes awkward postures with variable lumbar support. It requires use of the legs with imposed loads on the spine. Perhaps most important, there is exposure to transmitted shocks from the road, jolting, and various accelerations. Unfortunately, the epidemiologic evidence cannot distinguish the possible risks of driving and of whole-body vibration.

Kjellberg et al (1994) and Wickstrom et al (1994) made an extensive review of the health effects of whole-body vibration. They concluded that there was extensive evidence of an association with low back pain. However, at that time there was insufficient evidence to establish the exposure–response relationship.

The Finnish twin study (Battié et al 2002) found no association between lifetime driving exposure and disk degeneration. Videman et al (2000) took a more extreme example. They looked at top rally drivers who were regularly subjected to severe whole-body vibration and compared them with normal controls. This was a small study, but they did not find any MRI evidence of increased degenerative changes.

Lings & Leboeuf-Yde (2000) reviewed the more recent epidemiologic evidence. They concluded that there is strong evidence that driving is a risk factor for back pain and limited evidence for disk prolapse. However, there is only weak evidence on a dose–response relationship. The effect size is moderate: Burdorf & Sorock (1997) found RR or OR generally ranging from about 1.5 to 3.9. Lings & Leboeuf-Yde (2000) concluded that there is good reason to reduce exposure to whole-body vibration to the lowest practical level. Modern, damped, vehicle seats probably achieve this. There is little evidence of harm occurring on such modern seats. Perhaps being deliberately provocative, they suggested this is no longer an important problem.

Leisure activities and sports

Hoogendoorn et al (1999) reviewed 17 studies of sports and physical activity during leisure time. The results were inconsistent. There is no clear evidence that most sports activity or total physical activity during leisure time are risk factors for back pain. Most important, leisure activities such as swimming, walking, running, cycling, golf, or physical exercise do not appear to carry any risk. Overall, the prevalence of back pain is no higher in those who are physically active or take part in general athletic activities. On the contrary, as we saw earlier, improved physical and mental health and physical fitness are likely to be beneficial.

There is limited evidence that certain strenuous sports such as weightlifting and gymnastics may carry an increased risk of disk degeneration and vertebral damage (Sward et al 1990, 1991; Videman et al 1995). Some high-level and competitive sports may also be associated with an increased prevalence of back pain. That link could, however, involve both physical and psychosocial factors.

In summary, apart from certain high-level and competitive sports, most leisure and normal sporting activities seem likely to do more good than harm. Indeed, the clinical evidence shows that exercise and sports activities are the best treatment for back pain!

ENVIRONMENTAL RISK FACTORS: PSYCHOSOCIAL ASPECTS OF WORK

Work obviously imposes physical demands on workers, but it also imposes psychosocial demands.

During the 1990s, there was a lot of interest in job satisfaction and its possible influence on back pain. The classic Boeing Study (Bigos et al 1991) found that "hardly ever" enjoying the job was one of the few predictors of reporting a back injury over the next 4 years. However, it was actually a very weak predictor. The only reason it got so much attention was because so many of the findings of the Boeing Study were negative. There are now a large number of studies of job satisfaction and reported back pain, injury claims, seeking health care, and sick listing with back pain (Burdorf & Sorock 1997, Hoogendoorn et al 2000).

Over the past 20 years, there has been a great deal of research into more detailed psychosocial aspects of work:

- work "stress"
- high job demands and pace
- poor job content: low decision latitude, low job control, and monotonous work
- low social support from fellow workers or supervisors
- job "strain."

High job demands and conflict at work produce stress. Poor control over work and poor social support make it harder to cope with stress. This led to the "demand–control" theory that the level of job "strain" depends on the balance between high demands vs low control and support (Karasek 1979, Karasek & Theorell 1990). These concepts were originally developed for cardiovascular disease, but have since been applied to musculoskeletal disorders.

There are now at least 70 studies on psychosocial aspects of work and spinal pain, many of them from Scandinavia. Fortunately, there are also good reviews (Burdorf & Sorock 1997, Davis & Heaney 2000, Hoogendoorn et al 2000, Linton 2001).

Most of the studies in this area are cross-sectional, with all their limitations. Hoogendoorn et al (2000) could only find 11 cohort and two case–control studies. Davis & Heaney (2000) reviewed the methodologic problems in this field. "Psychosocial aspects of work" are by definition subjective. So individual *perceptions* or psychosocial reactions to the job are what matter, rather than any more "objective" measures of social or organizational characteristics of the job. There is a particular problem with potential confounding. We rely on self-report of both the risk factor and the outcome. Few studies allow for the physical demands of work. As we have already seen, we must be cautious how we interpret such complex associations.

Summary of evidence

The following is a brief summary of the evidence on each of these psychosocial aspects of work as risk factors for the onset of back pain. We will deal with their *influence* on sickness absence and the development of chronic incapacity separately in Chapter 13.

Job satisfaction

There is strong and consistent evidence that job satisfaction is a risk factor for reported back pain (Burdorf & Sorock 1997, Davis & Heaney 2000, Hoogendoorn et al 2000). The effect size is weak (RR or OR generally ranging from about 1.4 to 2.4). Part of the problem may be attempting to measure such a complex psychosocial issue by simple questions.

Job "stress"

Stress is now fashionable and the subject of intense professional, occupational, and legal debate. This is not the place to enter the fray that surrounds this area and we will limit ourselves to the evidence on stress as a risk factor for back pain.

There is actually limited epidemiologic evidence that job "stress" is a risk factor for reported back pain (Burdorf & Sorock 1997, Davis & Heaney 2000). The effect size is weak (RR or OR of the order of 1.3–2.1). Part of the problem may be attempting to measure such a complex psychosocial issue by simple questions.

High mental demands

There is inconsistent evidence on high mental demands and work pace. Some studies report positive findings, but as many fail to show a significant association. Burdorf & Sorock (1997), Davis & Heaney (2000) and Hoogendoorn et al (2000) all concluded that it is not possible to demonstrate that job demands are a risk factor for back pain.

As already noted, however, there is a practical difficulty defining and measuring "job demands" and "work stress."

Poor job content: low decision latitude, low job control, and monotonous work

There is inconsistent evidence on decision latitude, job control, and monotonous work. Different reviews reach different conclusions. Even if there is any effect, it appears to be weak. Hoogendoorn et al (2000) and Davis & Heaney (2000) concluded that there is insufficient evidence on poor job content as a risk factor for back pain.

Low social support

There is strong and generally consistent evidence that low social support from fellow workers and supervisors is a risk factor for reported back pain. The effect size is weak (RR or OR generally ranging from about 1.3 to 1.9).

Job "strain"

There is insufficient evidence to support the demand–control theory in back pain or musculoskeletal disorders.

Altogether, it is surprising that psychosocial aspects of work seem to have such a weak effect. Perhaps it is because we have quite crude methods of measuring what are really complex psychosocial issues. Perhaps it is because most studies and reviews look at each aspect individually.

Bartys et al (2001) showed that there might be a cumulative effect (Table 6.4). Individual and work-related psychosocial issues appear to interact, which is exactly what you would expect. Preliminary results from their prospective study are also encouraging. Such interactions appear to be a promising area for further research.

Table 6.4   Proportion of workers reporting back pain who had sickness absence in the past 12 months: the cumulative effect of psychosocial factors

Individual risk factors	Psychosocial aspects of work		
	None (%)	One (%)	Two or more (%)
No distress	2.5	3.5	7.8
Distress	4.0	5.8	9.8

Associations based on cross-sectional analysis.
Based on data from Bartys et al (2001).

Interactions between physical and psychosocial demands of work

Even more fascinating are possible interactions between physical demands and psychosocial aspects of work. A few years ago, there was an argument about which were more important risk factors in back pain, but that was naive. Both may play a role. So the real question is whether and how they might have an additive or interactive effect.

Davis & Heaney (2000) provided one of the most thoughtful reviews of these complex relationships (Fig. 6.5). They suggested three potential links. First, physical demands and psychosocial factors could each contribute independently to the onset or consequences of back pain. These might also have an additive effect. Second, psychosocial factors may modulate the relation between physical demands and back pain. For example, poor psychosocial conditions might reduce ability to cope with physical demands that would otherwise be tolerated. Third, physical demands and psychosocial aspects may co-vary. Many jobs involve both greater physical demands and poorer psychosocial conditions. Until recently, few studies investigated both physical demands and psychosocial aspects, which raises the possibility of confounding. Most studies of psychosocial aspects did not adjust for physical demands.

Biomechanical risk factors might cause back pain through excessive loading or repetitive loading. Psychosocial aspects of work were originally thought of as "stressors." There are various theories about the possible biologic effects of stress, but there is no convincing evidence that stress is a direct *cause* of physical pathology in the back. However,

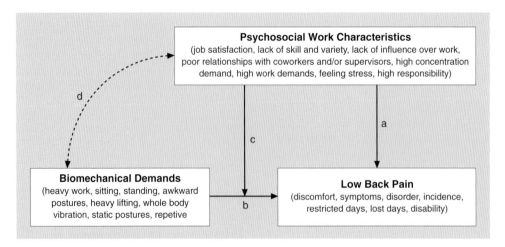

Figure 6.5 Possible relationships between biomechanical and psychosocial risk factors and occupational back pain. Reproduced with permission from Davis & Heaney (2000).

psychosocial factors might have more indirect effects on the biomechanics of the back. First, psychosocial factors could influence spinal loading by changes in muscles, forces exerted, and trunk movement. We will consider these *psychophysiologic* mechanisms in more detail in Chapter 9. Suffice to say at this point that they could involve changes in muscle tension, muscle activity, and patterns of movement. Second, these muscle changes or the neurohormonal changes that occur with stress could influence metabolic activity in various tissues of the back. Third, psychosocial factors could influence the neurophysiology of pain in various ways. Finally, psychosocial factors might influence the *reporting* of low back pain.

There are several tantalizing studies (Devereux et al 1999, Hoogendoorn et al 2002), but at present there is limited evidence for any of these mechanisms. This is clearly an area where much more research is needed. Whether or not these mechanisms turn out to be important for the initial *cause* of back pain, they have major implications for how we manage back pain at work.

CONCLUSIONS

Table 6.5 summarizes the epidemiologic evidence on risk factors for back pain. What does this information about risk factors mean in practice?

Approaches to prevention and control

Occupational back pain is an enormous problem, and the ideal answer would be to prevent it. Biomechanic and ergonomic approaches aim to reduce back injuries by controlling physical hazards and potential risk factors. This primary prevention may be an unrealistic goal (Burton 1997).

Reviews by van Poppel et al (1997) and Linton & van Tulder (2001) could not find good evidence on the effectiveness of primary prevention. Historically, this approach seems to have helped control more extreme physical demands and risks of work in previous generations. But there is little evidence that modern work is damaging to the back. So it is not surprising that there is also little evidence that this approach is effective in reducing the incidence of back trouble. And as back pain is so common, perhaps the goal of primary prevention is unrealistic.

Recent clinical developments also raise questions about that approach to risk. On the one hand, we try to prevent back trouble by reducing physical risk factors. On the other hand, modern treatment and rehabilitation aim to increase physical activity levels and challenge the musculoskeletal system.

This leads to a different approach to risk. We must continue to reduce more extreme hazards that might lead to damage. But controlling the physical demands of modern work is probably more a matter

Table 6.5 Summary of the evidence on risk factors for back pain

Risk factor	Strength of evidence	Effect size
Individual risk factors		
Previous history of back pain	Strong	Large – the overwhelming risk factor
Genetic/familial	Moderate/ strong?	Variable
Gender	Strong	Variable
Age	Strong	Variable
Body build: height, weight, leg length inequality	Strong	No effect
Physical fitness	Moderate	No effect
Smoking	Inconsistent	Small
Social class, education	Strong (men)	Variable
Emotional distress	Strong	Small
Environmental risk factors: physical		
Manual handling/ lifting	Strong	Moderate (variable)
Bending and twisting	Strong	Small– moderate
Repetitive movements	Inconsistent	Unproven
Static work postures and sitting	Strong	No effect
Driving and whole- body vibration	Strong	Moderate– small[a]
Leisure activities and sports	Moderate	Most have no effect
Environmental risk factors: psychosocial aspects of work		
Job satisfaction	Strong	Small
Work "stress"	Limited	Small
High job demands and pace	Inconsistent	No effect
Poor job content	Inconsistent	No effect
Low social support	Strong	Small
Job "strain"	Inconsistent	Unproven

[a]Probably small on modern damped seats.

of comfort and enabling workers with back pain to cope (whatever the cause of their pain; Hadler 1997). This is secondary prevention – reducing the consequences of back pain, even if we cannot prevent it in the first place. As back pain is almost universal, and its natural history is to recur, this may be more realistic.

Physical demands of work remain important: manual handling, lifting, bending and twisting, and exposure to vibration. Ergonomics still has a role here. Ergonomics aims to improve the "fit" between people, the things they use, and the way they use them. Information about human abilities, attributes, and limitations is also used to improve the design of equipment and tasks. The goal is to maximize comfort and safety for workers, by preventing excessive fatigue, discomfort, or stress. Occupational health often uses the same approach to enable workers to remain at work, return to work when they have back pain, and reduce recurrences.

We must also recognize the importance of psychosocial as well as physical demands of work. Physical risk factors may be most important for the initial onset of back pain. But psychosocial issues are probably even more important for its impact and consequences, for management, and for chronic pain and disability. Addressing psychosocial aspects of work and providing support may be just as important as modifying the physical demands.

What should we tell patients?

The review of individual risk factors suggests that most of us are going to get back pain at some time in our lives. It does not make much difference whether we are male or female, young or old, tall and thin, or small and fat. There is not a lot we can do about these personal characteristics in any event, but we do not need to worry about them. We may all be fated to have some back pain, but there is nothing in our genes that dictates it will inevitably lead to chronic pain and disability.

This has implications for what we tell patients. Too often, we tell them that they have back pain because they are too tall, too fat, the wrong build, or their legs are of unequal lengths. This is nonsense, and it is a dangerous message because it implies their back pain is inevitable and there is nothing that they or we can do about it.

It is good general health advice to stop smoking, avoid excess weight, and be physically fit. This will probably make little difference to the chances of getting back pain, but we will see later that it may help to deal with it better.

Advice about work is a critical part of managing back pain, and that advice depends on whether work is a risk. Sadly, too much advice is based on old myths that current evidence shows are wrong. Many patients and health professionals are firmly convinced that heavy manual work must somehow cause back injury or degenerative changes. So further exposure might cause further damage and hinder recovery or lead to chronic pain and disability. Strong scientific evidence now explodes these myths.

Back pain is certainly work-related to the extent that people of working age commonly get back pain and it impacts on their work. Physical demands at work are clearly *associated* with occupational back pain. Extreme loading may cause lasting damage, but that is rare in modern work. Occupational exposure can affect disk degeneration, but the effect is weak. Physical demands of work may provoke episodes of back pain, but that only accounts for a small portion of such a common bodily symptom. Work may aggravate back pain, whatever its cause. And back pain may make it more difficult to meet certain physical demands. The influence of cumulative exposure remains uncertain, but it seems not to be related to persistent back trouble. Altogether, there is little convincing evidence that work is physically harmful to the back. On the contrary, as we will see in later chapters, work is generally good for people with back pain.

All too often, doctors and therapists tell patients that their back pain is due to their job. So they advise them to take time off work, change to lighter work, give up their job, and even to retire early. This review shows that there is very little evidence to support such advice. It is usually not possible to say with any certainty that a patient's back pain is due to his or her job, or that the job is bad for his or her back. Too often, we give such advice glibly without adequate thought for the impact on our patients and their families. Try to imagine if someone casually told you to give up your job, for no very good reason – except they "thought" it might be good for you. How would that affect you? Education, knowledge, and insight would probably allow you to discount such advice. Your patients may not be so lucky – they may trust you.

It is too important a matter to make these decisions lightly on such flimsy evidence. It is rarely justified to advise patients to stay off work, change their job, or give up work completely because of ordinary backache. Advice such as that can easily become self-fulfilling.

References

Adams M A, Bogduk N, Burton K, Dolan P 2002 The biomechanics of back pain. Churchill Livingstone, Edinburgh

Althoff I, Brinckmann P, Frobin W, Sandover J, Burton K 1992 An improved method of stature measurement for quantitative determination of spinal loading: Application to sitting postures and whole body vibration. Spine 17: 682–693

Andersson G B J 1997 The epidemiology of spinal disorders. In: Frymoyer J W (ed.) The adult spine: principles and practice, 2nd edn. Lippincott-Raven, Philadelphia, pp 93–141

Balague F, Troussier B, Salminen J J 1999 Non-specific low back pain in children and adolescents: risk factors. European Spine Journal 8: 429–438

Bartys S, Tillotson M, Burton K et al 2001 Are occupational psychosocial factors related to back pain and sickness absence? In: Hanson M (ed.) Contemporary ergonomics 2001. Taylor & Francis, London, pp 23–28

Battie M C, Videman T 2003 Genetic transmission of common spinal disorders. In: Herkowitz H (ed.) The lumbar spine, 3rd edn. Lippincott, Williams & Wilkins, Philadelphia (in press)

Battie M C, Videman T, Gill K et al 1991 Smoking and lumbar intervertebral disc degeneration: an MRI study of identical twins. Spine 16: 1015–1021

Battie M C, Videman T, Gibbons L E, Fisher L D, Manninen H, Gill K 1995 Determinants of lumbar disc degeneration. A study relating lifetime exposures and MRI findings in identical twins. Spine 20: 2601–2612

Battie M C, Videman T, Gibbons L E et al 2002 Occupational driving and lumbar disc degeneration: a case–control study. Lancet 360: 1369–1374

Bigos S J, Battie M C, Spengler D M et al 1991 A prospective study of work perceptions and psychological factors affecting the report of back injury. Spine 16: 1–6

Bigos S J, Holland J, Webster M et al 1996 Prevention and risks of reporting occupational back problems: a methodological literature analysis. American Academy of Orthopedic Surgeons Report. AAOS, Rosemount, Illinois

Bombardier C, Kerr M S, Shannon H S, Frank J W 1994 A guide to interpreting epidemiologic studies on the etiology of back pain. Spine 19 (18S): 2047S–2056S

Brattberg G 1993 Back pain and headache in Swedish school children: a longitudinal study. Quality of Life Research 3: 157–162

Brattberg G 1994 The incidence of back pain and headache among Swedish school children. Quality of Life Research 3: S27–S31

Bressler H B, Keyes W J, Rochon P A, Bradley E 1999 The prevalence of low back pain in the elderly: a systematic review of the literature. Spine 24: 1813–1819

Brinckmann P, Frobin W, Biggemann M, Tillotson M, Burton K 1998 Quantification of overload injuries to thoracolumbar vertebrae and discs in persons exposed to heavy physical exertions or vibration at the work-place. Part II. Occurrence and magnitude of overload injury in exposed cohorts. Clinical Biomechanics 13 (suppl. 2): S(2)1–S(2)36.

Burdorf A, Sorock G 1997 Positive and negative evidence of risk factors for back disorders. Scandinavian Journal of Work and Environmental Health 23: 243–256

Burton A K 1997 Back injury and work loss: biomechanical and psychosocial influences. Spine 22: 2575–2580

Burton A K, Tillotson K M, Boocock M G 1994 Estimation of spinal loads in overhead work. Ergonomics 37: 1311–1322

Burton A K, Clarke R D, McClune T D, Tillotson K M 1996a The natural history of low back pain in adolescents. Spine 21: 2323–2328

Burton A K, Tillotson K M, Symonds T L, Burke C, Mathewson T 1996b Occupational risk factors for first-onset and subsequent course of low back trouble. A study of serving police officers. Spine 21: 2612–2620

Cady L, Bischoff D, O'Connel E 1979 Strength and fitness and subsequent back injuries in firefighters. Journal of Occupational Medicine 21: 269–272

Carter J T, Birrell L N (eds) 2000 Occupational health guidelines for the management of low back pain at work – principal recommendations. Faculty of Occupational Medicine, London. Available online at: www.facoccmed.ac.uk

Croft P R, Rigby A S 1994 Socioeconomic influences on back problems in the community in Britain. Journal of Epidemiology and Community Health 48: 166–170

Davis K G, Heaney C A 2000 The relationship between psychosocial work characteristics and low back pain: underlying methodological issues. Clinical Biomechanics 15: 389–406

Devereux J J, Buckle P W, Vlachonikolis I G 1999 Interactions between physical and psychosocial risk factors at work increase the risk of back disorders; an epidemiological approach. Occupational and Environmental Medicine 56: 343–353

Deyo R A, Tsui-Wu Y-J 1987 Functional disability due to back pain. Arthritis and Rheumatism 30: 1247–1253

Dione C, Koepsell T D, Von Korff M, Deyo R A, Barlow W E, Checkoway H 1995 Formal education and back-related disability: in search of an explanation. Spine 20: 2721–2730

Dionne C E, Von Korff M, Koepsell T D, Deyo R A, Barlow W E, Checkoway H 2001 Formal education and back pain: a review. Journal of Epidemiology and Community Health 55: 455–468

Edmond S L, Felson D T 2000 Prevalence of back symptoms in elders. Journal of Rheumatology 27: 220–225

Goldberg M S, Scott S C, Mayo N 2000 A review of the association between cigarette smoking and the development of nonspecific back pain and related outcomes. Spine 25: 995–1014

Hadler N M 1997 Back pain in the workplace. What you lift or how you lift matters far less than whether you lift or when. Spine 22: 935–940

Hakala P, Rimpela A, Salminen J J, Virtanen S, Rimpela M 2002 Back, neck and shoulder pain in Finnish adolescents: national cross-sectional surveys. British Medical Journal 325: 743–745

Hartvigsen J, Leboeuf-Yde C, Lings S, Corder E H 2000 Is sitting while at work associated with low back pain? A systematic, critical literature review. Scandinavian Journal of Public Health 28: 230–239

Hartvigsen J, Kyvik K O, Leboeuf-Yde C, Lings S, Bakketeig L 2003 Ambiguous relation between physical workload and low back pain: a twin control study. Occupational and Environmental Medicine 60: 109–114

Heikkila J K, Koskenvuo M, Heiovaara M et al 1989 Genetic and environmental factors in sciatica. Evidence from a nationwide panel of 9365 adult twin pairs. Annals of Medicine 21: 393–398

Heliovaara M 1999 Editorial: Work load and back pain. Scandinavian Journal of Work and Environmental Health 25: 385–386

Heliovaara M, Impivaara O, Sievers K et al 1987 Lumbar disc syndrome in Finland. Journal of Epidemiology and Community Health 41: 251–258

Hoogendoorn W E, van Poppel M N M, Bongers P M, Koes B W, Bouter L M 1999 Physical load during work and leisure time as risk factors for back pain. Scandinavian Journal of Work and Environmental Health 25: 387–403

Hoogendoorn W E, van Poppel M N M, Bongers P M, Koes B W, Bouter L M 2000 Systematic review of psychosocial factors at work and private life as risk factors for back pain. Spine 25: 2114–2125

Hoogendoorn W E, Bongers P M, de Vet H C W, Ariëns G A M, van Mechelen W, Bouter L M 2002 High physical work load and low job satisfaction increase the risk of sickness absence due to low back pain: results of a prospective cohort study. Occupational and Environmental Medicine 59: 323–328

Hoozemans M J M, van der Beek A J, Frings-Dresen M H W, van der Woude L H V, van Dijk F J H 2002 Low-back and shoulder complaints among workers with pushing and pulling tasks. Scandinavian Journal of Work and Environmental Health 28: 293–303.

Howell C J, Dean T, Lucking L, Dziedzic K, Jones P W, Johanson R B 2002 Randomised study of long term outcome after epidural versus non-epidural analgesia during labour. British Medical Journal 325: 357–360

HSE 1992 Manual handling: guidance on regulations. Manual handling operations regulations 1992. HMSO, London

HSE 2000 Management of health and safety at work: management of health and safety at work regulations 1999 – approved code of practice and guidance (L21). HSE Books, Norwich

Jones J R, Hodgson J T, Clegg T A, Elliott R C 1998 Self-reported work-related illness in 1995: results from a household survey. HSE Books, Her Majesty's Stationery Office Norwich

Karasek R A 1979 Job demands, job decision latitude and mental strain: implications for job redesign. Administrative Science Quarterly 24: 285–308

Karasek R A, Theorell T 1990 Healthy work. Basic Books, New York

Kawaguchi Y, Osada R, Kanamori M et al 1999 Association between an aggrecan gene polymorphism and lumbar disc degeneration. Spine 24: 2456–2460

King A, Coles B 1992 The health of Canada's youth: views and behaviours of 11-, 13- and 15-year olds from 11 countries. Health and Welfare Canada, Ottowa: (data quoted in Waddell et al 2002, p. 3)

Kjellberg A, Wickstrom B O, Landstrom U 1994 Injuries and other adverse effects of occupational exposure to whole-body vibration. Arb Halsa 41

Leboeuf-Yde C 1999 Smoking and low back pain: a systematic literature review of 41 journal articles reporting 47 epidemiologic studies. Spine 24: 1463–1470

Leboeuf-Yde C 2000a Body weight and low back pain: a systematic literature review of 56 journal articles reporting on 65 epidemiologic studies. Spine 25: 226–237

Leboeuf-Yde C 2000b Alcohol and low back pain: a systematic literature review. Journal of Manipulative and Physiological Therapeutics 23: 343–346

Lings S, Leboeuf-Yde C 2000 Whole body vibration and low back pain: a systematic, critical review of the epidemiological literature 1992–1999. Archives of Occupational and Environmental Health 73: 290–297

Linton S J 2000 A review of psychological risk factors in back and neck pain. Spine 25: 1148–1156

Linton S J 2001 Occupational psychological factors increase the risk for back pain: a systematic review. Journal of Occupational Rehabilitation 11: 53–66

Linton S J, van Tulder M W 2001 Preventive interventions for back and neck pain problems: what is the evidence? Spine 26: 778–787

MacGregor A J, Griffiths G O, Baker J, Spector T D 1997 Determinants of pressure pain threshold in adult twins: evidence that shared environmental influences predominate. Pain 73: 253–257

MacGregor A J, Andrew T, Snieder H, Sambrook P, Spector T D 1999 A genetic model for lower back pain: a population-based MRI study of twins. Arthritis and Rheumatism 49: 5146 (abstract)

Magora A 1970 Investigation of the relation between low back pain and occupation. Industrial Medicine 39: 28–37, 504–510; 41: 5–9

Makela M 1993 Common musculoskeletal syndromes. Prevalence, risk indicators and disability in Finland. ML 23. Publications of the Social Insurance Institution, Finland

Manninen P, Riihimaki H, Heliovaara M, Makela P 1995 Mental distress and disability due to low back and other musculoskeletal disorders – a ten year follow up. Presented to the 22nd annual meeting of the International Society for the Study of the Lumbar Spine, Helsinki

Mannion A F, Dolan P, Adams M A 1996 Psychological questionnaires: do 'abnormal' scores precede or follow first-time low back pain? Spine 21: 2603–2611

Marras W S, Davis K G, Jorgensen M 2002 Spine loading as a function of gender. Spine 27: 2514–2520

McCormick A, Fleming D, Charlton J 1995 Morbidity statistics from general practice. Fourth national study 1991–1992. Office of Population Censuses and Surveys Series MB5 no. 3. HMSO, London, pp 1–366

Nachemson A, Morris J M 1964 In vivo measurement of intradiscal pressure. Journal of Bone and Joint Surgery 46A: 1077–1092

Nachemson A, Vingard E 2000 Influences of individual factors and smoking on neck and low back pain. In: Nachemson A, Jonsson E (eds) Neck and back pain: the scientific evidence of causes, diagnosis and treatment. Lippincott Williams & Wilkins, Philadelphia, pp 97–126

National Research Council 1999 Work-related musculoskeletal disorders: report, workshop summary and workshop papers. National Academy Press, Washington, DC. Available online at www.nap.edu

National Research Council & Institute of Medicine 2001 Musculoskeletal disorders and the workplace. National Academy Press, Washington, DC

Negrini S, Carabalona R 2002 Backpacks on! Schoolchildren's perceptions of load, associations with back pain and factors determining the load. Spine 27: 187–195

NIOSH 1997 Musculoskeletal disorders and workplace factors. A critical review of epidemiologic evidence for work-related musculoskeletal disorders of the neck, upper-extremity, and low back. NIOSH, Cincinnati

Ostgaard H C, Roos-Hansson E, Zetherstrom G 1996 Regression of back and posterior pelvic pain after pregnancy. Spine 21: 2777–2780

Paassilta P, Lohiniva J, Göring H H H et al 2001 Identification of a novel common genetic risk factor for lumbar disc disease. Journal of the American Medical Association 285: 1843–1849.

Pope M H, Wilder D G, Krag M H 1991 Biomechanics of the lumbar spine: A. Basic principles. In: Frymoyer J W (ed.) The adult spine: principles and practice. Raven Press, New York, pp 1487–1501

Pynt J, Higgs J, Mackey M 2002 Milestones in the evolution of lumbar spinal postural health in seating. Spine 27: 2180–2189

Rothman K J, Greenland S 1998 Causation and causal inference. In: Rothman KJ, Greenland S (eds) Modern epidemiology. Lippincott-Raven, Philadelphia, pp 7–28

Sambrook P N, MacGregor A J, Spector T D 1999 Genetic influences on cervical and lumbar disc degeneration: a magnetic resonance imaging study in twins. Arthritis and Rheumatism 42: 366–372.

Schoene M 2002 Back pain in children and adolescents: is medicine clinging to an outmoded view? The Back Letter 17(3): 25, 32–34.

Straaton K V, Maisiak R, Wrigley J M, White M B, Johnson P 1996 Barriers to return to work among persons unemployed due to arthritis and musculoskeletal disorders. Arthritis and Rheumatism 39: 101–109

Sward L, Hellstrom M, Jacobsen B et al 1990 Back pain and radiologic changes in the thoraco-lumbar spine of athletes. Spine 15: 124–129

Sward L, Hellstrom M, Jacobsson B, Nyman R, Peterson L 1991 Disc degeneration and associated abnormalities of the spine in elite gymnasts. Spine 16: 437–443

Sydsjö A, Alexanderson K, Dastserri M, Sydsjö G 2003 Gender differences in sick leave related to back pain diagnoses: influence of pregnancy. Spine 28: 385–389.

van der Burg J C E, van Dieen J H, Toussaint H M 2000 Lifting an unexpectedly heavy object: the effects on low-back loading and balance loss. Clinical Biomechanics 15: 469–477

van Poppel M N M, Koes B W, Smid T et al 1997 A systematic review of controlled clinical trials on the prevention of back pain in industry. Occupational and Environmental Medicine 54: 841–847

Videman T, Battie M C 1999 Spine update: the influence of occupation on lumbar degeneration. Spine 24: 1164–1168

Videman T, Sarna S, Battié M C et al 1995 The long-term effects of physical loading and exercise lifestyles on back-related symptoms, disability, and spinal pathology among men. Spine 20: 699–709

Videman T, Simonen R, Usenius J-P, Osterman K, Battie MC. 2000 The long-term effects of rally driving on spinal pathology. Clinical Biomechanics 15: 83–86

Vingard E, Mortimer M, Wiktorin C et al 2002 Seeking care for low back pain in the general population. Spine 27: 2159–2165

Vogt M T, Hanscom B, Lauerman W C, Kang J D 2002 Influence of smoking on the health status of spinal patients: the National Spine Network Database. Spine 27: 313–319

Waddell G, Burton A K 2000 Occupational health guidelines for the management of low back pain at work – evidence review. Faculty of Occupational Medicine, London. Available online at: www.facoccmed.ac.uk

Waddell G, Waddell H 2000 Social influences on neck and back pain and disability. In: Nachemson A, Jonsson E (eds) Neck and back pain: the scientific evidence of causes, diagnosis and treatment. Lippincott, Williams & Wilkins, Philadelphia, pp 13–55

Waddell G, Aylward M, Sawney P 2002 Back pain, incapacity for work and social security benefits: an international literature review and analysis. Royal Society of Medicine Press, London

Walsh K, Cruddas M, Coggon D 1992 Low back pain in eight areas of Britain. Journal of Epidemiology and Community Health 46: 227–230

Waters T R, Putz-Anderson V, Garg A, Fine L J 1993 Revised NIOSH equation for the design and evaluation of manual lifting tasks. Ergonomics 36: 749–776

Watson K D, Papageorgiou A C, Jones G T et al 2002 Low back pain in schoolchildren: occurrence and characteristics. Pain 97: 87–92

Watson K D, Papageorgiou A C, Jones G T et al 2003 Low back pain in school children: the role of mechanical and psychosocial factors. Pain (in press)

Wedderkopp N, Leboeuf-Yde C, Andersen L B, Froberg K, Hansen H S 2001 Back pain reporting pattern in a Danish population-based sample of children and adolescents. Spine 26: 1879–1883

Wickstrom B O, Kjellberg A, Landstrom U 1994 Health effects of long-term occupational exposure to whole-body vibration: a review. International Journal of Industrial Ergonomics 14: 273–292

Wiersema B M, Wall E J, Foad S L 2003 Acute backpack injuries in children. *Pediatrics* 111: 163–166

Chapter **7**

The clinical course of back pain

CHAPTER CONTENTS

Let us now return to the clinical picture. The last chapter was about predicting who gets back pain. This chapter is about what happens to them if they get it:

- What is the usual clinical course of non-specific low back pain?
- How does it start?
- How does it progress and recover?
- How do chronic pain and disability develop?
- Can we predict which patients will do well and who is at risk of developing chronic pain and disability?

THE ONSET OF BACK PAIN

We asked more than 500 British patients how their back pain started (Fig. 7.1). There was little difference between patients who saw their family doctor and those who came to a routine hospital clinic, or between men and women.

About 60% said their first attack began suddenly and the others said the pain came on gradually. Of those whose pain began suddenly, almost two-thirds said it was "an accident." The other third said the pain began spontaneously and they could not think of any precipitating event. For most people, however, the "accident" was an everyday activity such as bending or lifting. They had done the same thing many times before and had done nothing different on this occasion. At most, it was what some authors describe as "overexertion."

Fewer of these patients could identify the cause of their present attack, despite it being more recent.

Figure 7.1   Onset of back pain in a personal series of 500 patients.

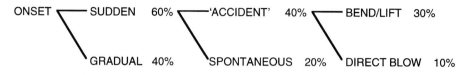

ONSET ⟨ SUDDEN 60% ⟨ 'ACCIDENT' 40% ⟨ BEND/LIFT 30%

GRADUAL 40%   SPONTANEOUS 20%   DIRECT BLOW 10%

Table 7.1   Onset of work-related backache and sciatica

Type of onset	Percentage of patients
Spontaneous	51
Sudden, during normal activity	
Lifting and handling	14
Other	3
Accidental event leading to injury	
Slips and falls	12
Handling	9
Blow on the back	4
Other	7

Based on data from Lloyd & Troup (1983).

Table 7.2   Factors people think are related to the onset of back pain

Factors related to start of back pain	Percentage of those with back pain	
	Men	Women
Accident/injury at work	21	9
Type of work done	35	18
Accident/injury at home	6	9
Accident/injury playing sport	16	5
Accident/injury elsewhere	5	9
Doing housework/garden	11	18
Pregnancy or childbirth	–	18
Arthritis and rheumatism	13	17
Other reasons	31	35

Based on data from Mason (1994), with permission from the Office of National Statistics.

That is surprising. Usually, patients can give more detail of recent events and are less sure about their earlier medical history. Also, only about one-third could say what usually caused recurrent attacks. Two-thirds felt their attacks came on spontaneously or unpredictably. This inability to identify the cause of present and recurrent attacks casts doubt on their certainty about the first attack.

Troup and his colleagues made one of the early studies of back pain in an occupational health setting (Troup et al 1981, Lloyd & Troup 1983). They saw nearly 1000 workers when they returned to work after an episode of back pain. In half, the current attack was spontaneous with no question of any kind of injury. In a sixth, the pain began unexpectedly at work with normal activity, most often lifting or handling. One-third described what Troup et al accepted was a true accidental event leading to injury (Table 7.1). Remember, however, this was a selected series of workers with work-related back pain.

Population studies show a different picture. *The Nuprin Pain Report* (Taylor & Curran 1985) found that 27% of Americans with back pain thought it was due to an injury. In the UK, Mason (1994) also looked at factors that people thought were related to the onset of their back pain (Table 7.2). The most common single factor they mentioned was work, either a work-related injury or simply the nature of their work. However, the reasons varied with sex and age. Two-fifths of men aged 18–34 said sports injuries. Over a third of women of that age said pregnancy or childbirth. A fifth of women over 35 blamed housework. A quarter of men and a third of women over 55 mentioned arthritis or rheumatism. A third of people gave a host of other reasons. Many gave more than one reason. Obviously, the factors people blame must vary at different stages of their lives!

The UK Labour Force Survey showed the importance of the context in which we ask these questions (Jones et al 1998). Back pain was by far the most common "illness, disability or other physical problem caused or made worse by work." This household survey estimated that 510 000 people had work-related back trouble in the UK in 1995. Another 130 000 with a musculoskeletal condition said it also affected their back. Thirty percent of men and 18% of women with back pain attributed it to their job. The most common job demands they blamed were manual handling in 66% and posture in 37%. The only remotely comparable work-related problem was "stress, depression and anxiety" in 252 000 people.

An earlier Labour Force Survey recognized that many people overestimate the role of work in musculoskeletal problems. So Jones et al (1998) looked more closely at "non-specific back pain and strain." They estimated 21% had some kind of "work accident": in 43% work was "the main cause," in 22% it was "a contributory cause" and 13% had "a symptomatic link only." However, they started with a strong presumption about back pain being work-related, and based these figures on workers' own perceptions and self-report. This was not objective data. Only 7% of these incidents were actually reported to the Health and Safety Executive as "work accidents" (Ch. 5).

There were a number of other inconsistencies. There was no clear association with heavier work. Symptoms did become more common with longer duration of employment. However, they were even more common among people who were not working at the time of the survey and increased with increasing time since last worked. And even when symptoms did not begin till after stopping work, people were still as likely to attribute them to their previous work! These questions are reinforced by a study of blue-collar workers in Sweden (Lindstrom et al 1994). Sixty percent of those with back pain attributed it to work. However, neither the physical demands of work nor calculated loads predicted duration of sick leave or return to work.

A study of nearly 8000 people who attended the Canadian Back Institute may help to explain some of these contradictory findings (Hall et al 1998). Two-thirds of people who were responsible for their own health care expenses and had no litigation said they did not know what caused their back pain. In contrast, 91% of people with compensation or litigation blamed it on some kind of work event. Whether their job was light or heavy made little difference: what mattered was the social context of their pain. However, that same social framework also influenced what they did. They could only get into the workers' compensation system if they had

some kind of accident, so there was some automatic selection.

We must recognize that these are simply patients' attempts to explain their pain. The answers tell us more about how people think about back pain than about what really causes it. Most of the answers seem to reflect the normal activities of the different groups when they happen to have back pain. They tell us little about the physical cause or pathology of back pain. The truth is that we have very little information about what causes or even triggers back pain. Most episodes of back pain probably start spontaneously or while doing an everyday activity that we have done many times before. But we should not discount these beliefs altogether. We will see later (Ch. 12) that even if what people believe about their back pain and its causes is inaccurate, these perceptions may affect what they do.

THE COURSE OF A CLINICAL EPISODE

Remember the epidemiology. Most people have back symptoms at some time in their lives, and about 40% have back pain each year and each month. Back pain is a recurrent and fluctuating symptom and we must view any clinical episode against that background.

Clinical teaching used to be that 75–90% of acute attacks of low back pain recover within about 4–6 weeks. This figure is quite consistent in clinical series over the past 40 years. Vernon (1991) looked closely at a small group of chiropractic patients. He found 25% improvement in pain, disability, and lumbar flexion in 7–10 days; 50% improvement took 2–3 weeks; 75% improvement varied from 4–6 weeks; and 100% improvement took 6–9 weeks or more. Disability and lumbar movement lagged behind improvement in pain. This is a typical picture of a clinical episode, but it is a limited, health care perspective.

In contrast, Lloyd & Troup (1983) found that 70% of people still had residual symptoms when they returned to work. Also, when we view back pain as a recurrent problem, the outcome of a clinical episode appears less favorable. Perhaps we should say more cautiously that up to 90% of acute attacks that present for health care settle sufficient to stop health care and return to work within 6 weeks.

Table 7.3 Prospective studies of low back pain in primary care

Country	Studies
US	Von Korff et al 1993, Von Korff & Saunders 1996 Carey et al 1995, Carey et al 2000
UK	Klenerman et al 1995 Burton et al 1995 The South Manchester Study (Papageorgiou et al 1996, Croft et al 1998, Thomas et al 1999)
France	Coste et al 1994
Belgium	Szpalski et al 1995
The Netherlands	van Tulder et al 1996, van den Hoogen et al 1997
Denmark	Schiottz-Christensen et al 1999

Table 7.4 Recurrent back pain 1–4 years after initial presentation for osteopathic treatment

Recurrent back pain between years 1 and 4	Initial presentation		
	Acute	Subacute	Chronic
No further attacks	29%	20%	5%
1–5 further attacks	57%	35%	15%
Many attacks (>5)	10%	33%	40%
Never got better	4%	12%	40%

K Burton, personal communication.

Clearly, we need to look more carefully at what happens over a longer period of time. We now have a wonderful set of large, prospective studies of low back pain in primary care (Table 7.3). Hestbaek et al (2003) recently reviewed a total of 36 studies, with widely varying results. Wasiak et al (2003) reviewed some of the problems of how we measure recurrences, but I do not want to go into that here. Let me simply highlight some key clinical messages from a few of the best studies.

The South Manchester Study looked at the claim that 90% of episodes of back pain resolve within a month. It followed 463 patients who consulted their family doctor with back pain. Sixty-nine percent presented with a new attack, and 20% with an acute exacerbation of a more chronic or persistent complaint. For 8%, the consultation was simply part of a continuing problem. Fifty-nine percent only consulted once, and 90% stopped consulting within 3 months, which fits traditional teaching. However, when they interviewed these patients they found a very different picture. At 3 months, only 21% said they had no pain or disability. At 12 months, only 25% had complete relief of pain and disability. So, 90% of acute episodes do "settle" in the sense that symptoms improve, and patients stop consulting and return to work. But only a minority "fully recovered" in the sense of being completely symptom-free.

Klenerman et al (1995) studied a more select group of 123 British patients who saw their family doctor within the first week of a new episode. They looked at patterns of pain, disability, and work loss when they presented and 2 and 12 months later. At follow-up, 21% patients had no pain, 72% continued to have intermittent pain, and 7% had constant pain. These three types of patients showed very different progress over the year. In patients with no pain or intermittent pain at follow-up, their pain, disability, and work loss had all improved by 2 months. Those with no pain showed further improvement in disability and had no further work loss between 2 and 12 months. Those with intermittent pain continued to have comparable levels of pain, disability, and work loss between 2 and 12 months. Patients with constant pain showed a slight improvement in pain by 2 months, but their pain then got worse again by 12 months. They did not show any improvement in disability or work loss over the whole 12-month period.

Burton et al (1995) showed a similar pattern in osteopathic practice (Table 7.4).

von Korff et al (1993) studied 1128 American patients presenting to a large health maintenance organization. These were different patients from Klenerman et al's, because only 17% had back pain of recent onset and a first ever attack within the past 6 months. One year later, 70–80% said they still had some back pain in the past month. However, von Korff et al distinguished patients with only occasional back pain (<30 days in the previous 6 months) from those with frequent pain (>90 days in the previous 6 months). Patients who had only occasional pain when first seen usually continued to have only occasional pain at 1 year. Those who presented with frequent pain usually continued to have frequent pain. About 90% of patients who presented with low-intensity, non-disabling back pain had a similar good outcome at 1 year. For patients with severe pain and severe disability at first presentation, the outcome depended on their previous history. If they had previously only had occasional pain, they had a two-thirds chance of a good outcome at 1 year. But if they had previously had frequent pain, they only had a one-third chance of a good outcome.

von Korff et al (1993) and von Korff & Saunders (1996) summed up the likely course of an acute episode presenting for health care:

- *Short-term outcomes*: most primary care patients who seek treatment for back pain will improve considerably over the first 4 weeks, but only 30% will be painfree. At 1 month, one-third will continue to experience back pain of at least moderate intensity, while 20–25% will still have substantial activity limitations.

- *Long-term outcomes*: at 1 year, 70–80% will still report some recurrent back symptoms, and one-third will continue to have intermittent or persistent pain of at least moderate intensity. About 15–20% will have a poor functional outcome.

Carey et al (1995, 2000) perhaps put this into perspective. They found that 31% of patients who consulted with acute back pain still had minor levels of functional disability at 6 months. Despite that, 95% were able to return to their usual activities of daily living. It was really only the few who still had functionally disabling pain at 3 months who then had a poor long-term prognosis.

Back pain is a recurrent problem, so it is not surprising that the best predictor of future progress is the previous history. However, the longer the time since the last attack, the lower the chance of recurrence (Table 7.5). So there is some suggestion that recurrences do diminish over several years.

von Korff et al (1993) considered how we might explain this to patients who ask what the future holds (Box 7.1).

It is worth reminding ourselves of Croft's summary of the epidemiology (Croft et al 1998). "Low back pain should be viewed as a chronic problem

Table 7.5   The likelihood of further attacks diminishes with the time since the last attack

Time since last attack	Likelihood of further attack(s) in the next year (%)
Less than 1 week	76
1–4 weeks	63
1–12 months	52
1–5 years	43
More than 5 years	28

Based on data from Biering-Sorensen (1983).

Box 7.1   Information for patients

- We can reassure them honestly that their pain is likely to improve
- Most people either stay at work or can return to work quickly, even if they still have some pain
- Back pain often recurs. Attacks may settle over several years, but back pain sometimes becomes chronic. However, even chronic back pain does not inevitably continue forever, and about one-third of people improve spontaneously each year
- It may also help to tell them that most people with back pain do manage to continue most activities and to work despite their pain

At a population level
- Most acute exacerbations settle in days or a few weeks without work loss or health care
- Most people return to work in days or a few weeks, with or without health care
- Most episodes requiring health care settle sufficiently to allow return to work within a matter of weeks
- However, that is often against a background of continuing or recurring symptoms (not necessarily requiring health care) over long periods of our lives

---

with an untidy pattern of grumbling symptoms and periods of relative freedom from pain and disability interspersed with acute episodes, exacerbations, and recurrences." Clinical management of a particular episode must be seen against that background. The paradox is that from a pathologic point of view most minor low back injuries *should* recover quite quickly, but the clinical *reality* is that many attacks do not. Or at least they do not under traditional management, because most of these reports are about patients who sought health care. That may once again raise questions about our current management of back pain.

RETURN TO WORK

How long do people stay off work with back pain and how fast do they return to work? Burdorf et al (2002) reviewed the literature on the natural course of sickness absence associated with low back pain. They found 10 high-quality studies from the past 25 years. On average, of workers who lost any time off work, 39% returned to work by 1 week, 67% by 2 weeks, 80% by 1 month, 91% by 3 months, 95% by 6 months, and 99% by 1 year (Fig. 7.2). Return to work in the different series varied most in the first few weeks and converged on 98–99% by 1 year.

However, in particular settings the long-term outcome may be much more variable (Hestbaek et al 2003). Coste et al (1994) found that 90% of patients who presented to their family doctor within 3 days of onset had complete recovery of pain and disability within 2 weeks. On the other hand, some recent workers' compensation and social security data suggest that as many as 5–10% of claimants go on to long-term incapacity (Reid et al 1997, Waddell et al 2002). In fairness, these may be selected groups of people at low or high risk. It also depends on initial work status. Disability trends certainly suggest that the number going on to chronic disability increased greatly in most western countries through the 1980s–1990s.

Let us look at a few of the factors that seem to influence rate of return to work.

As you might expect, progress is slower with nerve root pain than with back pain alone. Vroomen et al (2002) estimated that about one-third of patients with nerve root pain will "recover" in 2 weeks and about three-quarters by 3 months. However, many have residual, long-term symptoms. Mahmud et al (2000) found that workers' compensation patients who had back pain alone were off work for an average of 17 days. Those who

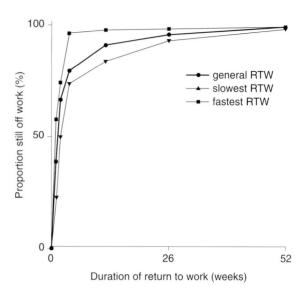

Figure 7.2 Return to work (RTW) after an acute episode of back pain. Based on data from Burdorf et al (2002).

also had leg pain were off for 48 days. Andersson et al (1983) found that about 10% of those with low back pain were still off work at 3 months, compared with about 25% of those with "sciatica."

Watson et al (1998) showed that return to work is faster in a first episode of work loss and slower in repeat episodes. Most important, they found that only 1% were still off work after 1 year in a first episode, compared with 4.5% in a repeat episode.

Nordin et al (2002) found that workers who have comorbidities return to work more slowly than those with back pain alone. After 6 months, about twice as many remained off work long-term.

Andersson et al (1983) found that blue-collar workers with back pain return to work more slowly than white-collar workers (Fig. 7.3). Perhaps surprisingly, however, they found that the same proportion did manage to get back to heavy physical work.

The social setting and the compensation system seem to be very important (Waddell et al 2002, 2003). Figure 7.4 compares the general population of Jersey, UK with two Canadian workers' compensation series in British Columbia and Ontario. This is not just an effect of work-related injury and compensation, because the Jersey data in this graph also include claims about back injuries at work. Nor is it simply a changing pattern over the

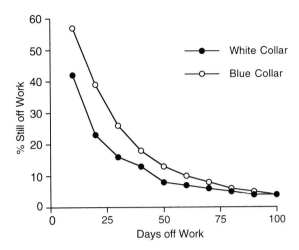

Figure 7.3   Workers with heavy manual jobs return to work more slowly after an attack of back pain. Based on data from Andersson et al (1983).

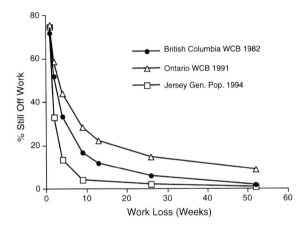

Figure 7.4   Return to work after a back injury at work. Based on workers' compensation data from British Columbia (Hrudey, personal communication), Ontario (Frank, personal communication), and Jersey (Watson et al 1998). WCB, workers' compensation board.

years. If we look more closely at what happens during the first month, there are even more fascinating differences (Fig. 7.5). The initial plateau in the Jersey data probably reflects the fact that no sickness benefit is paid for the first day. It seems that if people claim benefits at all, they are then likely to stay off for a working week. The rate of return to work and the number going on to chronic disability seem to vary with different socioeconomic circumstances.

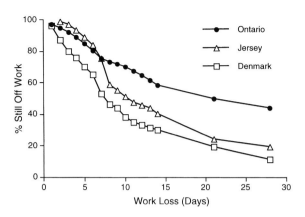

Figure 7.5   Return to work in different settings in the 1990s. Based on data from Ontario Workers' Compensation Board (Frank, personal communication), Jersey (Watson et al 1998) and Denmark (Hansen, personal communication).

So return to work is generally slower in the following situations:

- if the patient has nerve root pain or specific spinal pathology
- if it is a recurrent attack (compared with a first attack)
- if the patient has poor general health or comorbidities
- in manual workers and those of lower social class
- in different socioeconomic settings
- the longer the patient is off work.

We have already hinted that there are limitations to this rather artificial view of return to work after a single episode. von Korff et al (1993) showed that up to 40% of patients may still be taking at least odd days off work at 1 year. Just as it is more meaningful to consider the number of days of back pain over 12 months, so it may be better to look at total days of work loss in a year. Baldwin et al (1996), Johnson et al (1998), and Krause et al (1999) looked at longer-term patterns of work disability in US workers' compensation data. They found that the initial period of sickness absence seriously underestimated total work disability. Over 60% of workers had further periods of work loss, which could add 50–300% to total days off over several years. About a third made one or more unsuccessful attempts before successful return to work. A small proportion eventually went on to early retirement, often after repeated periods of sickness absence. So first return to work, like clinical discharge, may simply mark the end of this episode. It is often not the end of the story. What matters is *sustained* return to work, and we must always look at longer-term patterns.

Sustained return to work is no simple matter. It depends on complex interactions between worker, injury, health care, and employer characteristics and responses. Different factors influence short-term outcomes, which in turn influence long-term outcomes. There may be different influences on initial sickness absence and return to work, reinjury, further sickness absence, and early retirement (Pransky et al 2002).

Probability of return to work

We can look at this graph of return to work in another way. For any given time off work, we can use the data in Figure 7.2 to calculate the probability of returning to work (Fig. 7.6). McGill (1968) first pointed out that the longer anyone is off work with back pain, the lower the chance he or she will return to work. More recent large data sets confirm this (Krause et al 1999). It is equally true today and it is fundamental to management. This may seem obvious, but many health professionals caring for back pain still seem oblivious to the disastrous impact of prolonged time off work.

Most people recover from an acute attack and return to work quite rapidly, so the initial prognosis is very good. However, we should not be too sanguine. Depending on the particular health care and benefits system, the day someone stops work with back pain they have a 1–10% chance of still being off work a year later. And this prognosis soon deteriorates (Table 7.6). Once they are off work for 4–6 weeks, they have a 20% risk of long-term disability. Once they are off work for 6 months, they have only a 50% chance of ever returning to their previous job. Once they have been off work for 1–2 years or have lost their job, *which may be earlier*, then they are unlikely to work again in the foreseeable future. The further patients slide down that slippery slope, the harder it is for them to escape. *And this is almost irrespective of the physical condition of their back or any health care they then receive.*

Both recovery from the acute attack and the development of chronic pain and disability are processes that take place over time. Health professionals are certainly aware of patients' clinical progress. However, this epidemiologic view stresses that the passage of time, *in itself*, changes the patient's whole situation. This is so simple and so obvious that we often dismiss it as a truism, to our patients' peril.

Frank et al (1996, 1998) pointed out another implication. The factors that influence recovery vary over time, and the course and duration of illness itself may play a role in the process. As time passes we must consider other factors that may not have been important, or even present, at onset but only develop over time. These not only include physical changes in the patient's back. They also include patients' reaction to "failure to recover as

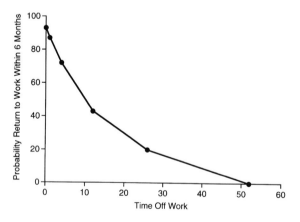

Figure 7.6 The probability of returning to work within the next 6 months with "usual care." Based on Canadian workers' compensation data. (JW Frank, personal communication.)

Table 7.6 Probability of return to work as a function of time off work

Time off work	Odds of still being off work 1 year later (%)
Day 1	1–10
1 month	20
6 month	>50
2 years (or lose job, which may be much earlier)	Up to 100

expected," the health care they receive, and changes in their work situation. Those factors at onset that predict chronic pain and disability may differ from those at 3–4 weeks, or at 3 months. The influence of some factors may reduce over time, while other factors may become more important. For example, the type and circumstances of injury and severity of symptoms may be useful predictors of recovery in the early stages, but their effects diminish over the first few months. Conversely, the patient's psychological reaction to failure to recover as expected only develops with the passage of time.

There may also be a threshold effect. The assumption that this whole sequence of events starts from the *initial injury* is simplistic and is not true for many patients. Many have a background of recurrent or chronic problems that sets the scene for their current episode. So it may be more appropriate to consider this as a sort of equilibrium. Stopping work may sometimes be more of a threshold when the patient is no longer able to tolerate more pain. This may be brought to a head by a more acute exacerbation of pain. But it may simply be that they are worn down by months of symptoms and are no longer able to cope. Or they may be overwhelmed by changed circumstances, or demands at work or at home may have increased. Or unrelated factors may influence the decision to go off sick.

Return to work may involve tilting the equilibrium to cross the threshold in the opposite direction. The change from working to being off sick is a dramatic social threshold. A person's whole social situation is very different when he or she goes off sick. This is not only in such obvious ways as financial effects or how he or she spends the day. It also involves change in the employer's attitudes to the worker and the patient's attitudes to work. Return to work then depends partly on the physical state of the patient's back and his or her pain. But it also depends on whether those factors in the worker's life and his or her feelings that encourage return to work outweigh those that make it easier to stay off.

THE DEVELOPMENT OF CHRONIC PAIN AND DISABILITY

Let us relate this to clinical progress. After we rule out serious pathology, there are basically two kinds of patients with non-specific low back pain. Most patients who present with an acute attack get better quite rapidly, no matter what we do. They need little more than analgesics, reassurance, and advice. We can rely on nature to cure them, and our job is only to assist and make sure we do not obstruct that process. The other 10–20% are at risk of developing chronic pain and disability. Once that occurs they present complex clinical and occupational problems for which we have no easy answer.

Frank et al (1996, 1998) proposed a three-phase model of work-related disability (Fig. 7.7): acute, subacute, and chronic. The acute phase lasts from stopping work through about 3–4 weeks. The subacute phase lasts from 3–4 weeks through about 12 weeks off work. The chronic phase is beyond about 3 months. The slope of the curve is quite different in these three phases, which reflects the *rate* of recovery and return to work.

During the acute stage, the curve is steep because most patients are recovering quite quickly. This is consistent with the natural history of back pain as a benign and self-limiting condition. For most patients in this phase the prognosis is good, irrespective of health care. Treatment at this stage may provide relief of symptoms, but has little or no effect on getting patients back to work. Instead, there is a danger that overinvestigation or overtreatment might be counterproductive and actually become an obstacle to recovery. So clinical management should provide simple symptomatic relief, with advice and support to maintain or return to ordinary activities as early as possible.

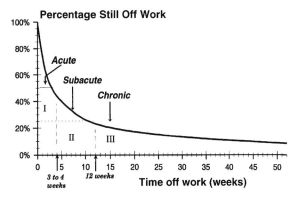

Figure 7.7   Three stages in the development of chronic disability. Reproduced with permission from Frank et al (1996).

By 3–4 weeks most patients have returned to work, even if they still have symptoms. For those who are still off work, the whole situation now changes fundamentally. The graph becomes less steep and this reflects the changing clinical problem. This is when everyone becomes worried about failure to recover as initially expected. The rate of return to work becomes slower and the risk of chronic disability rises. Those who are still off work in the subacute phase now have a 10–20% risk of long-term incapacity. By this phase, we can no longer rely on natural history alone. This is when we want to intervene more actively to control pain and help patients restore activity levels. This is the phase when treatment is likely to be most effective. It is when it becomes most efficient to deliver maximum resources.

By about 3 months the graph levels off. Any patient who is still off work is now "chronic," with all the implications of that. Ordinary backache has become the source of major suffering and disability. These patients become trapped in a vicious circle of pain, disability, and failed treatment. It impacts on their whole lives, their family, and their work. This 10–15% minority has a disproportionate impact on health care use and social costs to society. Treatment is more difficult and has a lower success rate. Successful rehabilitation is difficult and becomes even less likely with time. It is those who have disabling pain and are still off work at 2–3 months who then go on to become chronic pain patients.

Philips & Grant (1991a, b) made one of the earliest longitudinal studies of acute back pain, and questioned the traditional distinction between acute and chronic pain. By the end of the first week, 44% of their patients were already improving and 31% were getting worse. Most patients still expected to recover gradually over a period of 3 or 4 weeks. They were mildly frustrated and anxious about their pain, but they did not have clinical anxiety or depression. The main effect of acute pain was to reduce exercise tolerance. There was less impact on their housework, social activities, and family relationships. Most chronic pain patients were broadly similar. The main differences were that they reported much greater impact of pain on their lives and had lower expectations of recovery.

At 6 months, 40% of patients reported continuing pain. If we define chronic pain purely by duration, then they had chronic pain. Half of them described their pain as moderate or severe. However, most of them gradually adjusted and returned to their usual activities despite continuing pain. Very few went on to chronic intractable pain and disability. Most of the emotional changes developed within the first 3 months and then remained quite stable. In contrast, their pain and disability continued to improve up to 6 months.

Philips & Grant's study included few real "chronic pain patients." It probably tells us more about how most normal people deal with continuing pain than about the few who become problem pain patients. Hadjistavropoulos & Craig (1994) compared patients with acute back pain and a group of chronic back pain sufferers. They also found that most acute and chronic patients are actually quite similar. It is a small subgroup of patients who develop emotional and behavioral problems out of proportion to their physical problem; and some of these patients develop these changes at an early stage. It is this subgroup of patients who are different, rather than there being any difference between acute and chronic pain.

These studies raise doubts about the traditional division between acute and chronic pain. Acute pain merges into chronic pain, but although many people with back trouble continue to have pain, most of them adjust to it, and manage to return to most activities and a reasonably normal lifestyle. Chronic pain may not be something new or different that develops with time. Rather, we may understand chronic pain better as a failure of acute pain to resolve as it should. Chronic pain patients continue to present as if they still had an acute problem, rather than developing new reactions and behavior. Many of the changes may depend more on the severity and impact of pain and disability than on the duration of symptoms. Failure to restore normal function appears to be worse than chronic pain alone. The rate of development and severity of these changes also vary from patient to patient. Acute and chronic pain are not different in kind, but rather in effect. The major difference may be in the established nature of chronic pain, its impact on the patient's life and its intractable nature – and this may develop surprisingly early. If this is correct, we should look for factors that delay or prevent recovery, rather than factors that cause chronicity. We should also look at the influence of health care. It may be not just that chronic pain patients continue to present as if they had acute pain. It may be also that doctors and therapists treat them as if they still had acute pain.

However, this still does not explain *why* some people develop chronic pain and disability, while others recover. Clearly, different mechanisms must operate in different people. Clinical progress is not always smooth and uninterrupted, but may involve crises. There may be decision points and different paths that lead to widely divergent outcomes. (Of course, that does not mean that these are necessarily conscious decisions.) Frank et al (1996) looked at concepts of equilibrium and thresholds. Given the natural history of back pain, most people must cope and maintain some sort of equilibrium most of the time. But they may sometimes reach a crisis or breakpoint, and may slide or fall uncontrollably into a different situation (Fig. 7.8). It may then be much more difficult to return to their previous state. The most dramatic example is when they stop work. They then face a very different set of influences and obstacles to return to work, which requires recrossing the threshold in the opposite direction.

Krause & Ragland (1994) offered a social perspective on phases of occupational disability over time (Fig. 7.9). Phase 1 is the onset of symptoms before any health care or work loss. This has little social impact, although it may interfere with work performance to some extent. Phase 2 is the formal reporting of an injury or medical certification of the condition, which is the official, public registering of sickness. Phase 3 covers most acute episodes

of low back pain. The worker may rely on self-treatment, or seek medical care or alternative health care. Most acute attacks settle rapidly, sufficient to permit return to work with minor social, work, and economic impact.

Phase 4 is work disability for 1–7 weeks. Virtually all are receiving health care by this time. This is commonly regarded as the normal healing time or, perhaps more accurately, the normal recovery time. Treatment is most likely to be effective. Most western countries require medical certification, and some form of sick pay or sickness benefit begins. Krause & Ragland suggested this phase is the opportunity for timely health care and occupational interventions.

In phase 5, the worker is beginning to enter the chronic stage, with all its medical and social implications. Prognosis and expectations deteriorate. By phase 6, the chance of successful medical treatment falls and there is now a major rehabilitation challenge. Through phases 6–8 there is increasing social and economic impact on the worker and family, loss of employability, need for retraining or placement, and major social adaptation. Society must meet escalating health care costs and financial support, and there may be adversarial legal proceedings. Perspectives change. Instead of a medical condition with social implications, chronic back pain becomes a disability problem with medical elements.

Once again, disability is not static but dynamic. The disabling process evolves through distinct phases over time, and each phase involves a different set of social interactions. Capacity for work deteriorates and the difficulties of rehabilitation and return to work increase. Patients have to revise their expectations about getting well and returning to work. Their social status changes through each of these phases, at some points quite dramatically. The outcome of any intervention may be quite different in different phases, so the timing of intervention is critical.

Let me repeat: timing is vital to the clinical management of back pain. The clinical situation, return to work, the risk of long-term incapacity, and the intensity of intervention are all functions of time. Ideally, we want to identify as early as possible those who are at risk of developing chronic problems. In principle, prevention is better than cure for both the patient and for society. It is also easier

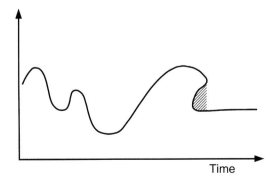

Figure 7.8 Clinical progress is not smooth and uninterrupted but involves crises and sudden shifts from one state to another. Based on catastrophe theory.

Figure 7.9 A social perspective on occupational disability due to low back pain. Different phases imply breakpoints and shifts from one social situation to another. From Krause & Ragland (1994), with permission.

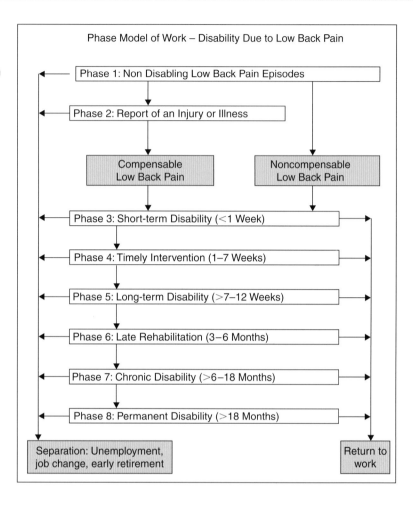

Phase Model of Work – Disability Due to Low Back Pain

Phase 1: Non Disabling Low Back Pain Episodes

Phase 2: Report of an Injury or Illness

Compensable Low Back Pain

Noncompensable Low Back Pain

Phase 3: Short-term Disability (<1 Week)

Phase 4: Timely Intervention (1–7 Weeks)

Phase 5: Long-term Disability (>7–12 Weeks)

Phase 6: Late Rehabilitation (3–6 Months)

Phase 7: Chronic Disability (>6–18 Months)

Phase 8: Permanent Disability (>18 Months)

Separation: Unemployment, job change, early retirement

Return to work

to prevent chronic pain and disability than to reverse it once it becomes intractable. If we could identify those patients at risk, we could direct more intensive health care and rehabilitation to them, and the sooner the better. This would direct treatment where it is needed and likely to do the most good. It would also be the most effective and cost-effective use of finite resources. At the other extreme, we may be able to identify some patients who are never going to return to work whatever we do. For them, we may need to look at more realistic goals and treatments.

IDENTIFYING PATIENTS AT RISK OF CHRONIC PAIN AND DISABILITY

Time, and particularly duration of time off work, is one of the best predictors of chronic disability

(Fig. 7.6). *Every* patient who has been off work more than about 12 weeks with back pain is at serious risk of long-term incapacity.

However, we do not want to wait several months till our patients are already well on the way to chronic incapacity. Rather, we want to identify those at risk as early as possible, ideally at the first consultation. This has become a kind of holy grail in back care.

So, the first and obvious purpose of screening is to identify patients at high risk of developing chronic pain and disability.

But the second and equally important purpose of screening is more detailed assessment of those patients who are at risk. Why and how are they likely to develop chronic pain and disability? What are the obstacles to them recovering and returning to work? What might we do to

Table 7.7   Reviews of predictors of chronic pain and disability

Review	Area covered
McIntosh et al (2000)	Low back pain prognosis – critical methodological issues
Pransky et al (2001)	Methodological and practical considerations
Burdorf et al (2002)	Natural course of sickness absence in low back pain
Frank et al (1996, 1998)	Secondary prevention of disability from occupational low back pain
Kendall et al (1997)	New Zealand Guide to "yellow flags" – psychosocial risk factors for chronic pain and disability
Turk (1997)	Demographic and psychosocial factors in the transition from acute to chronic pain (not only back pain)
Pincus et al (2002)	Psychological factors in the transition from acute to chronic pain and disability
Linton (2000a, b, 2002)	Psychological risk factors at all stages
Main et al (2000)	Yellow flags, conceptual issues
Burton & Main (2000)	
Truchon & Fillion (2000)	Biopsychosocial predictors of chronic disability
Turner et al (2000)	Predictors of chronic disability in injured workers
Shaw et al (2001)	Early prognosis for occupational disability
Waddell & Burton (2000)	Evidence review for UK occupational health guidelines for workers with back pain
Nordin (2001)	Return to work
Høgelund (2001)	Work incapacity and reintegration
Waddell et al (2002)	International social security literature
Crook et al (2002)	Determinants of occupational disability (This is probably the most comprehensive review of clinical and other predictors of chronic disability in low back pain)
Waddell et al (2003)	Screening tools for long-term incapacity

reduce the risk and to help them overcome those obstacles?

Screening depends on identifying risk factors. These may be any items of information that predict chronic pain and disability, but that does not necessarily imply cause and effect. Some may be demographic, e.g., age, and cannot be changed. Some may simply be early markers of chronic problems, e.g., depression. Some may actually tell us something about the mechanisms of developing chronic pain and disability or about obstacles to recovery, e.g., certain psychosocial or occupational factors. Others may be pantechnicon items that reflect more complex issues, e.g., gender or family status: these may need more detailed assessment. So predictors of chronic pain and disability are not necessarily the same as obstacles to recovery that we can address, and we may need to assess them separately.

Over the past decade, there have been many studies of screening and there is now an extensive literature. Fortunately, once again, we have good reviews (Table 7.7).

Historically and conceptually, there are two kinds of screening:

1. Administrative/actuarial screening: this forms the basis of the insurance industry. It is largely sociodemographic information, available in an administrative database.

2. Clinical and psychosocial screening: health care is more interested in how and why some patients develop chronic problems, and what can be done about it. This kind of data usually requires more detailed individual assessment by a health professional.

However, the distinction between these two types of screening is not absolute. They overlap. We may use them in combination or in sequence.

Table 7.8 summarizes some of the key predictors from this literature.

Table 7.8   Predictors of chronic pain and disability

Sociodemographic	Clinical and psychosocial predictors
Gender	Older age (>50–55 years)
Age	Previous history of back pain
Marital/family status (lone parent/young children, partner retired or disabled)	Nerve root pain
	Pain intensity/functional disability
Health condition (mental health conditions, musculoskeletal conditions, comorbitities)	Poor perception of general health
	Psychological distress/ depression
Occupation/education level	Fear avoidance
	Catastrophizing
Time since last worked	Pain behavior
Occupational status (no longer employed)	Job (dis)satisfaction
	Duration of sickness absence
Local unemployment rate	Occupational status (no longer employed)
	Expectations about return to work

From Waddell et al 2003, with permission from Royal Society of Medicine Press.

Clinical factors

Because back pain is a recurrent problem, we have already seen that the best predictor of future progress is the previous history:

- Where is this patient in the time-course of illness?
- How many previous episodes?
- How many days of pain in the past year?
- Previous medical consultations – number of doctors consulted; previous admissions to hospital; and most important of all, any previous low back surgery?
- Any loss of time from work? How often? How much? How long off work at present and how many days off in the past year?
- Any work-related back injuries and claims for compensation?

Similarly, observation of progress over time may be better than assessment at one point in time. The simplest and surest way of identifying those who are developing chronic pain and disability is the passage of time. But it is not good enough simply to "wait and see": it may then be too late to do anything about it. Our aim should be to spot what is happening as early as possible.

In the first edition of this book I reviewed the earlier clinical literature. Certainly, patients with a nerve root problem progress more slowly and are at higher risk of chronic pain and disability. Clinical findings are less helpful when it comes to the patient with ordinary backache. Here, the initial injury and clinical findings in the back are not useful guides to future progress or recovery. Several studies have found that persisting pain intensity at 3–6 weeks is one of the best predictors of pain and work status at 1 year, but others disagreed. Unfortunately, apart from the previous history of back pain, medical history and examination are poor guides to how a patient with ordinary backache is likely to progress.

Patients who report poor general health, general bodily symptoms, and "always feeling sick" are more likely to develop chronic low back disability. However, these symptoms appear to reflect general psychosomatic condition rather than severity of physical illness.

Box 7.2 gives an example of one of the best clinical screening questionnaires.

Box 7.2

The Vermont Disability Prediction Questionnaire. Templates permit easy scoring of each question as 0, 1, or 4 and all the scores are added together. The final score is the total score divided by the total possible score. If the answer to question 1 is "yes," the total possible score is 19. If the answer to question 1 is "no," the total possible score is 17. So a patient who answers question 1 as "yes," with a total score of 8, will have a final score of 8/19 = 0.42. Another patient who answers question 1 as "no," with a total score of 8, will have a final score of 8/17 = 0.47. The higher the score, the higher the risk of chronic disability. As a rough guide, a score of more than about 0.50 indicates a risk of disability, but you are probably better to develop your own cut-off for your patients and your needs. (From Hazard et al 1996, with permission.)

(Continued)

Box 7.2   (Continued)

For each of the following questions, please check the ONE
answer that best applies to you:

SCORING

| 0 | 4 | 1. | Have you ever had back problems before this injury? |

☐ Yes (Continue with Question 2)
☐ No (Stop to Question 5)

| 0 | 4 | 2. | How many times have you visited a medical doctor in the past for back problems? |

☐ Never
☐ 1 to 5 tiems
☐ 6 to 10 times
☐ 11 to 20 times
☐ More than 20 times

| 0 | 1 | 3. | How many times have you been hospitalized for low back pain? |

☐ Never
☐ One
☐ Two
☐ Three or more times

SCORING

| 4. | How many times have you had surgery for low back pain? | 0 | 4 |

☐ Never
☐ One
☐ Two
☐ Three or more times

5. Who or what do you think is to blame for your back problem?

☐ Work
☐ Yourself
☐ No one
☐ Something Else

| 6. | How many times have you been married? | 0 | 1 |

☐ Never
☐ One
☐ Two
☐ Three or more times

| 0 | 4 | 7. | On a scale of 0 to 10, how much pain in your back do you have RIGHT NOW? Think of 0 as meaning NO PAIN AT ALL and 10 as meaning the WORST PAIN POSSIBLE |

NOT PAIN AT ALL ☐0☐ ☐1☐ ☐2☐ ☐3☐ ☐4☐ ☐5☐ ☐6☐ ☐7☐ ☐8☐ ☐9☐ ☐10☐ WORST PAIN POSSIBLE

| 0 | 1 | 8. | On a scale of 0 to 10, how physically demanding is your present: job? Think of 0 as meaning NOT AT ALL DEMANDING and 10 as meaning VERY DEMANDING |

NOT AT ALL DEMANDING ☐0☐ ☐1☐ ☐2☐ ☐3☐ ☐4☐ ☐5☐ ☐6☐ ☐7☐ ☐8☐ ☐9☐ ☐10☐ VERY DEMANDING

| 0 | 4 | 9. | On a scale 0 to 10, how much trouble do you think you will haev sitting or standing long enough to do your job, six weeks from now. Think of 0 as meaning NO TROUBLE AT ALL SITTING OR STANDING, and 10 as meaning SO MUCH TROUBLE SITTING AND STANDING THAT YOU WON'T BE ABLE TO DO YOUR JOB AT ALL |

NO TROUBLE AT ALL ☐0☐ ☐1☐ ☐2☐ ☐3☐ ☐4☐ ☐5☐ ☐6☐ ☐7☐ ☐8☐ ☐9☐ ☐10☐ SO MUCH TROUBLE I WON'T BE ABLE TO DO MY JOB AT ALL

| 0 | 1 | 10. | On a scale of 0 to 10, how well do your co-workers? Think of 0 as meaning you DON'T GET ALONG WELL AT ALL and 10 as meaning you GET ALONG VERY WELL |

DON'T GET ALONG WELL AT ALL ☐0☐ ☐1☐ ☐2☐ ☐3☐ ☐4☐ ☐5☐ ☐6☐ ☐7☐ ☐8☐ ☐9☐ ☐10☐ GET ALONG VERY WELL

| 0 | 1 | 11. | On a scale of 0 to 10, how certain are you that will be working in six months? Think of 0 as meaning NOT AT ALL CERTAIN and 10 as meaning VERY CERTAIN |

NOT AT ALL CERTAIN ☐0☐ ☐1☐ ☐2☐ ☐3☐ ☐4☐ ☐5☐ ☐6☐ ☐7☐ ☐8☐ ☐9☐ ☐10☐ VERY CERTAIN

Total Score: _____

Psychosocial factors

There is now overwhelming evidence that psychosocial factors are important in the development of chronic pain and disability (Chs 10–12). Perhaps surprisingly, psychosocial factors appear to be better predictors of return to work than the physical condition of the back or the physical demands of the job. This is certainly true by 6–8 weeks, and possibly within the first 3 weeks. One of the strongest influences on return to work and work status at 6–12 months is patients' own perceptions of their pain. These include their beliefs about what has happened to their backs, beliefs that their back pain is work-related, and fear of reinjury if they return to work. This may be expressed most concisely in patients' own expectations about return to work. In this situation, patients are better at predicting what is going to happen to them (or what they are going to do) than doctors!

Kendall et al (1997) introduced the concept of "yellow flags" – psychosocial risk factors that identify patients at increased risk of developing chronic disability (Box 7.3). This was part of the New Zealand guide to the management of acute low back pain. Kendall, Linton, and Main are three clinical psychologists from New Zealand, Sweden, and the UK, who are international experts in pain management. Their main focus was clinical and psychological, though they also included occupational and compensation elements.

Boxes 7.4 and 7.5 give an example of one of the best psychosocial screening questionnaires (Linton & Halldén 1998, Boersma & Linton 2002).

Sociodemographic factors

The focus on psychological issues has perhaps diverted attention from the value of simple sociodemographic predictors. However, social security and workers' compensation studies show that sociodemographic factors can also predict long-term incapacity (Waddell et al 2003). Box 7.6 gives an example of a sociodemographic screening tool.

The accuracy of screening

We must be realistic about what we can expect from screening. Individual items (Table 7.8) are

---

Box 7.3   Yellow flags – psychosocial risk factors

Reproduced with permission from Working Backs Scotland, adapted from Kendall et al (1997)

When conducting an assessment, it may be useful to consider psychosocial "yellow flags" (beliefs and behaviors on the part of the patient which predict poor outcomes).

The following factors are important and consistently predict poor outcomes:
- Beliefs that back pain is harmful or potentially severely disabling
- Fear-avoidance behavior (avoiding a movement or activity due to misplaced anticipation of pain) and reduced activity levels
- Tendency to low mood and withdrawal from social interaction
- Expectation that passive treatments rather than active participation will help

Suggested questions to the worker with low back pain (to be phrased in your own style):
- Have you had time off work in the past with back pain?
- What do you understand is the cause of your back pain?
- What are you expecting will help you?
- How is your employer responding to your back pain? Your co-workers? Your family?
- What are you doing to cope with your back pain?
- Do you think you will return to work? When?

A worker may be considered to be at risk if:

- There is a cluster of a few very salient factors
- There is a group of several less important factors that combine cumulatively

The presence of risk factors should alert the clinician to the possibility of long-term problems and the need to prevent their development.

---

usually not very accurate predictors, but we can do better if we combine a number of items into a screening tool (e.g., Boxes 7.3, 7.4, 7.6). Even then, we must recognize the limitations of current screening tools for back pain. They may suggest that certain patients are at risk, but they are never 100% accurate and always make some errors.

Box 7.4   From Linton & Hallden 1998

Today's Date __/__/__

Name _____   ACC Claim Number _____

Address _____   Telephone (__) _____ (home)

_____   (__) _____ (work)

Job Title (occupation) _____   Date stopped work for this episode __/__/__

These questions and statements apply if you have aches or pains, such as back, shoulder or neck pain. Please read and answer each question carefully. Do not take too long to answer the questions. However, it is important that you answer every question. There is always a response for your particular situation.

1. What year were you born?   19__

2. Are you: ☐ male   ☐ female

3. Were you born in New Zealand? ☐ Yes   ☐ No

2X count ☐

4. Where do you have pain? Place a ✓ for all the appropriate sites.

☐ neck   ☐ shoulders   ☐ upper back   ☐ lower back   ☐ leg

5. How many days of work have you missed because of pain during the past 18 months? Tick (✓) one.

☐ 0 days [1]   ☐ 1–2 days [2]   ☐ 3–7 days [3]   ☐ 8–14 days [4]   ☐ 15–30 days [5]

☐ 1 month [6]   ☐ 2 months [7]   ☐ 3–6 months [8]   ☐ 6–12 months [9]   ☐ over 1 year [10]

☐

6. How long have you had your current pain problem? Tick (✓) one.

☐ 0–1 weeks [1]   ☐ 1–2 weeks [2]   ☐ 3–4 weeks [3]   ☐ 4–5 weeks [4]   ☐ 6–8 weeks [5]

☐ 9–11 weeks [6]   ☐ 3–6 months [7]   ☐ 6–9 months [8]   ☐ 9–12 months [9]   ☐ over 1 year [10]

☐

7. Is your work heavy or monotonous? Circle the best alternative.

    0   1   2   3   4   5   6   7   8   9   10
    Not at all   *Extremely*

☐

8. How would you rate the pain that you have had during the past week? Circle one.

    0   1   2   3   4   5   6   7   8   9   10
    No pain   *Pain as bad as it could be*

☐

9. In the past 3 months, on average, how bad was your pain? Circle one.

    0   1   2   3   4   5   6   7   8   9   10
    No pain   *Pain as bad as it could be*

☐

10. How often would you say that you have experienced pain episodes, on average, during the past 3 months? Circle one.

    0   1   2   3   4   5   6   7   8   9   10
    Never   *Always*

☐

11. Based on all the things you do to cope, or deal with your pain, on an average day, how much are you able to decrease it? Circle one.

    0   1   2   3   4   5   6   7   8   9   10
    Can't decrease it at all   *Can decrease it completely*

10–x ☐

12. How tense or anxious have you felt in the past week? Circle one.

    0   1   2   3   4   5   6   7   8   9   10
    Absolutely calm and relaxed   *As tense and anxious as I've ever felt*

☐

(Continued)

Figure 7.10 considers 100 patients who have been off work about 12 weeks, where 20% are going to develop chronic disability.

• Screening incorrectly predicts 24 individuals will develop chronic disability, but they actually return to work. These are false-positives. We might give these patients an intervention they did not need. They would have got better without it.

• Screening incorrectly predicts four individuals will return to work, but they actually develop

Box 7.4 (Continued)

13. How much have you been bothered by feeling depressed in the past week? Circle one.

    0   1   2   3   4   5   6   7   8   9   10
Not at all   *Extremely*

14. In your view, how large is the risk that your current pain may become persistent? Circle one.

    0   1   2   3   4   5   6   7   8   9   10
No risk   *Very large risk*

15. In your estimation, what are the chances that you will be working in 6 months? Circle one.

    0   1   2   3   4   5   6   7   8   9   10   10−x
No chance   *Very large chance*

16. If you take into consideration your work routines, management, salary, promotion possibilities and work mates, how satisfied are you with your job? Circle one.

    0   1   2   3   4   5   6   7   8   9   10   10−x
Not at all   *Completely*
satisfied   *satisfied*

Here are some of the things which other people have told us about their back pain. For each statement please circle one number from 0 to 10 to say how much physical activities, such as bending, lifting, walking or driving would affect your back.

17. Physical activity makes my pain worse.

    0   1   2   3   4   5   6   7   8   9   10
Completely   *Completely*
disagree   *agree*

18. An increase in pain is an indication that I should stop what I am doing until the pain decreases.

    0   1   2   3   4   5   6   7   8   9   10
Completely   *Completely*
disagree   *agree*

19. I should not do my normal work with my present pain.

    0   1   2   3   4   5   6   7   8   9   10
Completely   *Completely*
disagree   *agree*

Here is a list of 5 activities. Please circle the one number which best describes your current ability to participate in each of these activities.

20. I can do light work for an hour.

    0   1   2   3   4   5   6   7   8   9   10   10−x
Can't do it because   *Can do it without pain*
of pain problem   *being a problem*

21. I can walk for an hour.

    0   1   2   3   4   5   6   7   8   9   10   10−x
Can't do it because   *Can do it without pain*
of pain problem   *being a problem*

22. I can do ordinary household chores.

    0   1   2   3   4   5   6   7   8   9   10   10−x
Can't do it because   *Can do it without pain*
of pain problem   *being a problem*

23. I can go shopping.

    0   1   2   3   4   5   6   7   8   9   10   10−x
Can't do it because   *Can do it without pain*
of pain problem   *being a problem*

24. I can sleep at night.

    0   1   2   3   4   5   6   7   8   9   10   10−x
Can't do it because   *Can do it without pain*
of pain problem   *being a problem*   Sum

Box 7.5   Scoring instructions for the acute low back pain screening questionnaire (see Box 7.4; Linton & Hallden 1998)

- For Question 4, count the number of pain sites and multiply by 2
- For Questions 6, 7, 8, 9, 10, 12, 13, 14, 17, 18 and 19 the score is the number that has been ticked or circled
- For Questions 11, 15, 16, 20, 21, 22, 23, and 24 the score is 10 minus the number that has been ticked or circled
- Write the score in the shaded box beside each item – Questions 4 to 24
- Add them up, and write the sum in the box provided – this is the total score

Note: the scoring method is built into the questionnaire.

Interpretation of scores
Questionnaire scores greater than 105 indicate that the patient is "at risk".
This score produces:

- 75% correct identification of those not needing modification to ongoing management
- 86% correct identification of those who will have between 1 and 30 days of work
- 83% correct identification of those who will have more than 30 days off work

Box 7.6   Sociodemographic screening (from Waddell et al 2003, with permission from Royal Society of Medicine Press)

Sociodemographic risk factors
- Gender
- Age
- Marital/family status (lone parent/young children, partner retired/incapacitated)
- Health condition(s) (mental health disorders, musculoskeletal disorders, comorbidities)
- Occupation/education level
- Time since last worked
- Occupational status (still employed/not)
- Local unemployment rate (men < 50 years)

One additional question
When do you think you are likely to return to work?
1 month; 3 months; 6 months; 1 year; >1 year; probably never

Feedback
This in itself could form a potentially powerful intervention.
Client's estimate of return to work: realistic?/implications
Calculated risk of long-term incapacity
Agreement/divergence between these two estimates
On serial interview: estimates of return to work and risk of long-term incapacity improving or deteriorating

Follow-on questions
What do you think are the problems/obstacles to you returning to work?
How do you think these problems/obstacles might be overcome?
What might health professionals/employer/Department for Work and Pensions do to help overcome these problems/obstacles?
On serial interview: any progress?

chronic disability. These are false-negatives. These people need help but might not receive it.

We define the accuracy of a screening tool by its sensitivity and specificity.

- *Sensitivity*: the proportion of persons who do go on to chronic disability who are correctly predicted by screening. This is actual chronic disability minus the false-negatives. In this example, sensitivity = 16/20 = 80%.

- *Specificity*: the ability of screening to identify correctly those who will not go on to chronic disability. This is actual return to work minus the false-positives. In this example, specificity = 56/80 = 70%.

In practice, most screening tools for back pain have a sensitivity and specificity of about 70–80%, *at best*. That is better than chance, but we must not forget about the false-positives and false-negatives. Sociodemographic, clinical, and psychosocial

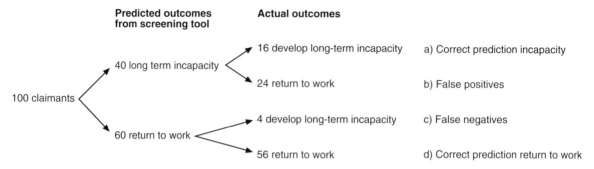

Figure 7.10   Predicted outcomes and actual outcomes from screening tool. From Waddell et al 2003, wiht permission.

screening tools all give more or less comparable accuracy. So there is a potential role for all types of screening, and we should not rely on one alone.

The other problem is that any screening tool is likely to be specific to the particular setting, patient group, and purpose. So you must be careful using a method or questionnaire from somewhere else. Ideally, you should test it out on your own patients. In routine practice, perhaps it is best simply to have a high index of suspicion. Be constantly aware of the insidious risk of chronic pain and disability. Understand the main risk factors. But, above all, strive to identify those patients at risk as early as possible.

CONCLUSION

On day 1, it is unfortunately not possible to identify which patient will go on to chronic pain and disability. The best guide is simply to look at the previous history and realize that some patients are not really at the start of their back pain story. The subacute stage, somewhere about 4–12 weeks, is the critical period. Back pain starts with a physical problem in the back, but by the subacute stage psychosocial factors progressively become more important in the development of chronic disability. That is when we should try to identify those at higher risk. That is when we should intervene and when intervention is most successful. By about 12 weeks, everyone who is still off work is at high risk of long-term incapacity and needs help. Now the emphasis of screening should shift to assessing why and how these patients are getting into trouble. What are the obstacles to their recovery and return to work? What can we do to help overcome these obstacles? There is now no more time to waste.

References

Andersson G B J, Svensson H-O, Oden A 1983 The intensity of work recovery in low back pain. Spine 8: 880–884

Baldwin M L, Johnson W G, Butler R J 1996 The error of using returns-to-work to measure the outcome of healthcare. American Journal of Industrial Medicine 29: 632–641

Biering-Sorensen F 1983 A prospective study of low back pain in the general public. 1 – Occurrence, recurrence and aetiology. Scandinavian Journal of Rehabilitation Medicine 15: 71–80

Boersma K, Linton S J 2002 Early assessment of psychological factors: the Orebro Screening Questionnaire for pain. In: Linton S J (ed.) New avenues for the prevention of chronic musculoskeletal pain and disability. Pain research and clinical management, vol. 12. Elsevier, Amsterdam, pp 203–213

Burdorf A, van Duijn M, Koes B 2002 The natural history of sickness absence due to low back pain and prognostic factors for return to work among occupational populations. (in preparation)

Burton A K, Main C J 2000 Obstacles to return to work from work-related musculoskeletal disorders. In: Karwowski W (ed.) International encyclopedia of ergonomics and human factors. Taylor & Francis, London, pp 1542–1544

Burton A K, Tillotson M, Main C J, Hollis S 1995 Psychosocial predictors of outcome in acute and subchronic low back trouble. Spine 20: 722–728

Carey T S, Evans A, Jackman A 1995 The outcomes and costs of care for acute low back pain among patients seen by primary care practitioners, chiropractors and orthopedic surgeons. New England Journal of Medicine 333: 913–917

Carey T S, Garrett J M, Jackman A M 2000 Beyond the good prognosis. Examination of an inception cohort of patients with chronic low back pain. Spine 25: 115–120

Coste J, Delecoeuillerie G, Lara A C, Le Parc J M, Paolaggi J B 1994 Clinical course and prognostic factors in acute low back pain: an inception cohort study in primary care practice. British Medical Journal 308: 577–580

Croft P R, Macfarlane G F, Papageorgiou A C, Thomas E, Silman A J 1998 Outcome of low back pain in general practice: a prospective study. British Medical Journal 316: 1356–1359

Crook J, Milner R, Schultz I, Stringer B 2002 Determinants of occupational disability following a low back injury: a critical review of the literature. Journal of Occupational Rehabilitiation 12: 277–295

Frank J W, Brooker A-S, DeMaio S E et al 1996 Disability resulting from occupational low back pain. Part II: What do we know about secondary prevention? A review of the scientific evidence on prevention after disability begins. Spine 21: 2918–2929

Frank L, Sinclair S, Hogg-Johnson S et al 1998 Preventing disability from work-related low-back pain. New evidence gives new hope – if we can just get all the players on side. Canadian Medical Association Journal 158: 1625–1631

Hadjistavropoulos H D, Craig K D 1994 Acute and chronic low back pain: cognitive, affective, and behavioral dimensions. Journal of Consulting and Clinical Psychology 62: 341–349

Hall H, McIntosh G, Wilson L, Melles T 1998 The spontaneous onset of back pain. Clinical Journal of Pain 14: 2

Hazard R G, Haugh L D, Reid S, Preble J B, MacDonald L 1996 Early prediction of chronic disability after occupational low back injury. Spine 21: 945–951

Hestbaek L, Leboeuf-Yde C, Manniche C 2003 Low back pain: what is the long-term course? A review of studies of general patient populations. European Spine Journal 11: 149–165

Høgelund J 2001 Work incapacity and reintegration: a literature review. In: Bloch F S, Prins R (eds) Who returns to work and why? A six country study on work incapacity and reintegration. Transaction Publishers, New Jersey, pp 27–54

Johnson W G, Baldwin M L, Butler R J 1998 Back pain and work disability: the need for a new paradigm. Industrial Relations 37: 9–34

Jones J R, Hodgson J T, Clegg T A, Elliott R C 1998 Self-reported work-related illness in 1995: results from a household survey. HSE Books, Her Majesty's Stationery Office, Norwich

Kendall N A S, Linton S J, Main C J 1997 Guide to assessing psychosocial yellow flags in acute low back pain. Accident Rehabilitation and Compensation Insurance Corporation and National Advisory Committee on Health and Disability, Wellington, NZ. Available online at: www.acc.org.nz

Klenerman L, Slade P D, Stanley I M et al 1995 The prediction of chronicity in patients with an acute attack of low back pain in a general practice setting. Spine 20: 478–484

Krause N, Ragland D R 1994 Occupational disability due to low back pain: a new interdisciplinary classification based on a phase model of disability. Spine 19: 1011–1020

Krause N, Dasinger L K, Deegan L J, Brand R J, Rudolph L 1999 Alternative approaches for measuring duration of work disability after low back injury based on administrative workers' compensation data. American Journal of Industrial Medicine 35: 604–618

Lindstrom I, Ohlund C, Nachemson A 1994 Validity of patient reporting and predictive value of industrial physical work demands. Spine 19: 888–893

Linton S J 2000a A review of psychological risk factors in back and neck pain. Spine 25: 1148–1156

Linton S J 2000b Psychological risk factors for neck and back pain. In: Nachemson A L, Jonsson E (eds) Neck and back pain: the scientific evidence of causes, diagnosis, and treatment. Lippincott Williams & Wilkins, Philadelphia, pp 57–78

Linton S J 2002 Psychological risk factors as "yellow flags" for back pain. In: Giamberardino M A (ed.) Pain 2002 – an updated review: refresher course syllabus. IASP Press, Seattle

Linton S J, Halldén K 1998 Can we screen for problematic back pain? A screening questionnaire for predicting outcome in acute and sub-acute back pain. Clinical Journal of Pain 14: 200–215

Lloyd D C E F, Troup J D G 1983 Recurrent back pain and its prediction. Journal of Social and Occupational Medicine 33: 66–74

Mahmud M A, Webster B S, Courtney T K, Matz S, Tacci J A, Christiani D C 2000 Clinical management and the duration of disability for work related low back pain. Journal of Occupational and Environmental Medicine 42: 1178–1187

Main C J, Spanswick C C, Watson P 2000 The nature of disability. In: Main C J, Spanswick C C (eds) Pain management: an interdisciplinary approach. Churchill Livingstone, Edinburgh, pp 89–106

Mason V 1994 The prevalence of back pain in Great Britain. Office of Population Censuses and Surveys Social Survey Division. HMSO, London

McGill C M 1968 Industrial back problems: a control program. Journal of Occupational Medicine 10: 174–178

McIntosh G, Frank J, Hogg-Johnson S, Hall H, Bombardier C 2000 Low back pain prognosis: structured review of the literature. Journal of Occupational Rehabilitation 10: 101–115

Nordin M 2001 International Society for the Study of the Lumbar Spine presidential address. Backs to work: some reflections. Spine 26: 851–856

Nordin M, Hiebert R, Pietrek M, Alexander M, Crane M 2002 The association of co-morbidity and outcome in episodes of non-specific low back pain in occupational populations. Journal of Occupational and Environmental Medicine 44: 677–684

Papageorgiou A C, Croft P R, Thomas E, Ferry S, Jayson M I V, Silman A J 1996 Influence of previous pain experience on the episode incidence of low back pain: results from the South Manchester Back Pain Study. Pain 66: 181–185

Philips H C, Grant L 1991a Acute back pain: a psychological analysis. Behavioural Research and Therapy 29: 429–434

Philips H C, Grant L 1991b The evolution of chronic back pain problems: a longitudinal study. Behavioural Research and Therapy 29: 435–441

Pincus T, Burton AK, Vogel S, Field A P 2002 A systematic review of psychological factors as predictors of chronicity/disability in prospective cohorts of low back pain. Spine 27: E109–E120

Pransky G, Shaw W, Fitzgerald T E 2001 Prognosis in acute occupational low back pain: methodologic and practical considerations. Human and Ecological Risk Assessment 7: 1811–1825

Pransky G, Benjamin K, Hill-Fotouhi C, Fletcher K E, Himmelstein J, Katz J N 2002 Work-related outcomes in occupational low back pain. A multidimensional analysis. Spine 27: 864–870

Reid S, Haugh L D, Hazard R G, Tripathi M 1997 Occupational low back pain: recovery curves and factor associated with disability. Journal of Occupational Rehabilitation 7: 1–14

Schiotz-Christensen B, Nielsen G L, Hansen V K, Schodt T, Sorensen H T 1999 Long-term prognosis of acute low back pain in patients seen in general practice: a 1-year prospective follow-up study. Family Practice 16: 223–232

Shaw W S, Pransky G, Fitzgerald T E 2001 Early prognosis for low back disability: intervention strategies for health care providers. Disability and Rehabilitation 23: 815–828

Szpalski M, Nordin M, Skovron M L, Melot C, Cukier D 1995 Health care utilization for low back pain in Belgium. Influence of sociocultural factors and health beliefs. Spine 20: 431–442

Taylor H, Curran N M 1985 The Nuprin pain report. Louis Harris, New York

Thomas E, Silman A J, Croft P R et al 1999 Predicting who develops chronic low back pain in primary care: a prospective study. British Medical Journal 318: 1662–1667

Troup J D G, Martin J W, Lloyd D C E F 1981 Back pain in industry: a prospective survey. Spine 6: 61–69

Truchon M, Fillion L 2000 Biopsychosocial determinants of chronic disability and low-back pain: a review. Journal of Occupational Rehabilitation 10: 117–142

Turk D C 1997 The role of demographic and psychosocial factors in transition from acute to chronic pain. In: Jensen T S, Turner J A, Wiesenfeld-Hallin Z (eds)

Proceedings of the 8th World Congress on Pain. Progress in pain research and management. IASP Press, Seattle, pp 185–213

Turner J A, Franklin G, Turk D C 2000 Predictors of chronic disability in injured workers: a systematic literature synthesis. American Journal of Industrial Medicine 38: 707–722

van den Hoogen H J M, Koes B W, Deville W, van Eijk J T M, Bouter L M 1997 The prognosis of low back pain in general practice. Spine 22: 1515–1521

van Tulder M W, Koes B W, Bouter L M (eds) 1996 Low back pain in primary care: effectiveness of diagnostic and therapeutic interventions. Institute for Research in Extramural Medicine, Amsterdam

Vernon H 1991 Chiropractic: a model incorporating the illness behaviour model in the management of low back pain patients. Journal of Manipulative and Physiological Therapy 14: 379–389

von Korff M, Saunders K 1996 The course of back pain in primary care. Spine 21: 2833–2839

von Korff M, Deyo R A, Cherkin D, Barlow W 1993 Back pain in primary care: outcomes at one year. Spine 18: 855–862

Vroomen P C A J, de Krom M C T F M, Knottnerus J A 2002 Predicting the outcome of sciatica at short-term follow-up. British Journal of General Practice 52: 119–223

Waddell G, Burton A K 2000 Occupational health guidelines for the management of low back pain at work – evidence review. Faculty of Occupational Medicine, London

Waddell G, Aylward M, Sawney P 2002 Back pain, incapacity for work and social security benefits: an international literature review and analysis. Royal Society of Medicine Press, London

Waddell G, Burton A K, Main C J 2003 Screening to identify people at risk of long-term incapacity for work: a conceptual and scientific review. Royal Society of Medicine Press, London

Wasiak R, Pransky G S, Webster B S 2003 Methodological challenges in studying recurrence of low back pain. Journal of Occupational Rehabilitation 13: 21–31

Watson P J, Main C J, Waddell G, Gales T F, Purcell-Jones G 1998 Medically certified work loss, recurrence and costs of wage compensation for back pain: a follow-up study of the working population of Jersey. British Journal of Rheumatology 37: 82–86

Chapter **8**

Physical impairment

In the last chapter we looked at the clinical course of back pain. As the next step towards trying to understand what is going on, let us now look at the clinical findings. We should start with actual physical observations, and try to avoid prejudging them against any theoretic ideas about pathology. So, what exactly are the objective findings in the backs of patients with back pain? What do they tell us about physical capacity or functional limitations? What does this tell us about low back disability?

This is not disability evaluation. I am well aware of the standard US methods of measuring impairment for workers' compensation and social security purposes. Descriptions are readily available (AMA 2000) and there is no need to repeat them here. I do not have the effrontery to propose a new personal rating system! Nor is this chapter about vocational assessment. Instead, I am simply trying to understand our clinical findings. What does physical assessment tell us about the problem?

ASSESSMENT OF SEVERITY

One of the most important measures of any illness is its severity, which helps to determine the impact on patients, the health care system, and society. Patients and their families are most concerned about severity of pain and its interference with their lives. The amount and type of treatment a patient receives depend on severity, particularly in a non-specific condition such as back pain. Fair and consistent rating of permanent impairment or incapacity for work is part of the legal basis for compensation and social support. For all these reasons, we need to assess the severity of low back trouble.

In most chronic disorders with clear pathology – such as osteoarthritis of the hip – assessment of severity is quite straightforward. Clinical assessment is reliable and valid, and different experts will agree. The patient's report of pain, disability, and (in)capacity for work is usually more or less in proportion to the diagnosis and the physical findings. But this is not the case in chronic back pain. Here, we often cannot diagnose any pathology. Clinical examination may not even be able to find any clear physical basis for the patient's continuing symptoms. It should be no surprise that we have difficulty assessing low back disability. Yet in view of the human and social impact of back pain, and despite the practical problems, we must try.

It is an instructive intellectual discipline to consider clinical assessment as evidence. How well would your findings and your interpretation of them stand up to cross-examination in a court of law? In health care, as in science or in law, we should be able to substantiate our findings.

Apply this test to diagnosis. Diagnosis of pathology is the usual basis for treatment and prognosis. Diagnosis gives a broad classification of the severity of an injury or disease. Diagnosis determines when rehabilitation is complete and what abnormality or loss we should consider permanent. At first sight, diagnosis looks like an important and useful measure of severity. In spinal fractures, this is true. There is an obvious range between a minor fracture of a transverse process and a severe T10–T11 fracture dislocation with paraplegia. Now try to apply this to non-specific low back pain. The first and insurmountable problem is that we cannot make any real diagnosis in most patients. We can diagnose injury to the bones or nerves of the spine and we can assess nerve root dysfunction, but none of that applies to ordinary backache. Clinical examination of the spine itself is not very helpful. X-rays tell us about fractures, but the common radiographic changes of degeneration tell us nothing about a patient's back pain. Even when we decide on some kind of diagnosis, different patients with the same diagnosis may have very different levels of pain and disability. So it is quite illogical to give every patient with a particular diagnosis the same rating. Unfortunately, diagnosis and X-rays provide little help in assessing the severity of back trouble.

Definitions

The medical model still forms the framework for how most health professionals and patients think about disability. It assumes a linear relationship between disease and disability, and works for clearcut physical pathology such as amputation or blindness.

Disease ⟶ Impairment ⟶ Disability ⟶ Incapacity for work

The *International Classification of Impairments, Disabilities and Handicaps* (World Health Organization (WHO) 1980) definitions were based on this medical model. The most recent, fifth edition of the American Medical Association (AMA) *Guides to the Evaluation of Permanent Impairment* (AMA 2000) still uses a similar approach. The key concepts are impairment and disability.

WHO (1980) defined impairment as "any loss or abnormality of anatomic, physiologic or psychological structure or function." The AMA *Guide* (AMA 2000) gives a similar definition. Impairment is "a loss, loss of use, or derangement of any body part, organ system or organ function." A more practical, clinical definition of *physical impairment* is "pathologic, anatomic or physiologic abnormality of structure or function leading to loss of normal bodily ability" (Waddell & Main 1984).

Compare this with the previous definitions for disability (Ch. 3). WHO (1980) defined disability as "any restriction or lack (resulting from an impairment) of ability to perform an activity in the manner or within the range considered normal for a human being." The AMA *Guide* (AMA 2000) gives a similar definition. Disability is "an alteration of an individual's capacity to meet personal, social or occupational demands because of an impairment."

Impairment and disability are two sides of the same coin, but we assess them on very different kinds of evidence. From the definition, we must assess impairment by objective observations. We must make a clear distinction between the health professional's assessment of impairment and the patient's report of pain and disability.

- pain $\Big\}$ subjective
- disability
- physical impairment – objective.

Most US jurisdictions insist on this distinction in the assessment of impairment and disability. Impairment is medically determined loss of structure or function of part of the body. But medical evidence on impairment is only one factor that the legal or compensation system takes into account in determining disability. They also consider the claimant's own evidence, circumstances and needs, and credibility. Consider a laborer and a concert pianist who each suffer amputation of their little finger. Medical assessment of impairment will be identical, but these two men have very different job demands and the consequences may be different. Social support and compensation place greatest value on incapacity for work, and a court may judge this very differently. The court may also allow for the patient's self-report of pain and suffering. Assessment of impairment is a professional responsibility. The final decision on disability rating and compensation is a legal or administrative responsibility. For more than a century, all parties have found this to be "a useful division of responsibility" (Drewry 1896, AMA 2000).

Let us consider physical impairment for a moment. The above definitions could cover two different kinds of impairment:

- pathologic or anatomic loss or abnormality of structure
- physiologic loss or limitation of function.

The US Social Security Administration (SSA) insists that impairment "can be shown by medically acceptable, clinical and laboratory diagnostic techniques" (SSA 2001). From this point of view, medical evaluation of impairment has always focused on tissue damage and structural impairment. However, in the context of back pain, physiologic loss of function may be just as important and could still meet the definition of impairment. The proviso is that we should be able to demonstrate any such loss of function objectively.

Again, compare back pain with other forms of physical impairment (Matheson et al 2000). We all agree about impairment in an amputee. Generally, we do not argue in court about the degree of impairment or disability. In cases of back pain, on the other hand, we cannot even agree on how to assess lumbar impairment, never mind agreeing on the result. Clinical assessment is often based on the examiner's impression, and different experts offer different opinions. Due to these problems, some research workers decry objective assessment of lumbar impairment. It certainly faces many problems and is not an absolute answer (Hadler 1999). However, some form of objective check on the patient's report of pain and disability is essential in logic, in clinical practice, and in law.

These criticisms mean that we must stop and rethink how we assess lumbar impairment. First, by definition, we must base it on objective physical characteristics. Second, we must use reliable clinical methods. Third, these clinical methods should provide a real and valid measure of the particular physical characteristic. Some clinical tests meet all these criteria, like nerve compression signs. Many routine methods of examination are not very reliable (Waddell et al 1982, McCombe et al 1989), e.g., posture, deformity, tenderness, palpation, and sacroiliac tests. So we must develop better techniques for routine clinical examination. We must also make sure that our tests are valid: that they really do measure what we intend to measure. The best example of this is lumbar flexion (Ch. 2). How well the fingers reach the toes tells us about total body movement, but if we want a valid measure of lumbar flexion we must look at the back.

We are trying to assess objective physical characteristics. This means that, as far as possible, we must discount subjective responses and behavior from our assessment. Many physical tests deliberately elicit pain, so the way individuals react will vary with their response to pain. This response may also vary due to conscious or unconscious exaggeration related to a claim for compensation. We must make a clear distinction between objective physical findings and behavior, and build cross-checks into our examination.

Finally, the aim of the exercise is to look for the objective physical basis of low back pain and disability. Lordosis is an example of a physical finding that is not helpful. Lordosis varies widely in normal people, and has little or nothing to do with low back pain or disability. So the degree of lordosis tells us nothing about impairment, and lordosis should not be part of how we assess impairment. We are looking for physical characteristics that *lead to loss of normal bodily ability*. That means they should correlate with low back disability and should distinguish patients with back pain from asymptomatic people.

METHODS OF RATING PHYSICAL IMPAIRMENT

Even if we agree on the principles of assessing lumbar impairment, it is difficult to put into practice. In the US, there has been constant effort to improve and standardize impairment ratings. The AMA *Guides to the Evaluation of Permanent Impairment* (AMA 2000) is now the standard for most musculoskeletal conditions. It is in its fifth edition and has been adopted as the official guide in 80% of states. It is also used in Canada and Australia. However, it has been attacked in court for having no scientific basis. It is a consensus document based on clinical experience and agreement about what is "reasonable" impairment. There is no scientific proof of the reliability or validity of the *Guides*, but they do give a more consistent rating than relying only on an expert's opinion. When it comes to back pain, however, the *Guides* are much less satisfactory. It may be worth reviewing the problems of various systems of rating lumbar impairment.

McBride

McBride (1936) made the first attempt to assess musculoskeletal impairment. He developed a comprehensive rating of quickness, coordination, strength, severity, endurance, safety, and physique (McBride 1963). These are all difficult to define, and this system depends on subjective judgments by the examiner. Many of McBride's concepts are clinically important, but his system does not give reliable ratings. It is almost impossible to apply to back pain and has never gained wide acceptance.

AMA and AAOS

More practical methods of rating lumbar impairment began about 40 years ago. Both the AMA (AMA 1958) and the American Academy of Orthopedic Surgeons (AAOS: AAOS 1962) produced guides to the evaluation of permanent impairment. Twenty years later, 60% of US surgeons used the AMA scale, 30% the AAOS scale, and only 5% the McBride system (Brand & Lehmann 1983). Today, the AMA *Guides* dominate the market. But the AMA and AAOS guides suffer similar problems. They work best in patients with objective bone or nerve damage.

We can demonstrate this with the most recent, fifth edition of the AMA *Guides* (AMA 2000). It does recognize the problems, so it suggests a two-stage evaluation of impairment.

In the first stage, you try the diagnosis-related estimates (DRE) model (Box 8.1). As the name says, this is a diagnostic approach, with the greatest weight on radiculopathy and neurologic findings, or X-ray findings. This is a very orthopedic approach to the spine, stressing tissue damage and structural impairment. Unfortunately, little of it is relevant to most patients with non-specific low back pain.

The AMA *Guides* recognize this, so they suggest that if (or, in the case of backache, when) this DRE model fails, you should use the range of motion (ROM) model instead. Goniometer measures of lumbar flexion, extension, and lateral flexion are entered into a table and converted to "percent whole-person impairment." Additional allowance is made for any neurologic deficit, though that again does not apply in backache. Obviously, the ROM impairment rating of backache depends more or less entirely on the range of spinal movement. We will discuss the interpretation and limitations of this later.

To confuse the issue further, the fifth edition of the AMA *Guides* now suggests a third alternative method of rating impairment. Some pain specialists feel that if a patient has chronic pain then a standard rating of objective physical impairment may not do them justice. (Or, perhaps more important, may not meet the legal requirements of the US workers' compensations and social security systems.) So a completely new Chapter 18 offers a method of rating "pain-related impairment." It does not actually define chronic pain, but deals with *chronic pain syndrome*. There is no explanation or logic for how the subjective symptom of pain meets the definition of objective impairment. And there is no scientific basis for the ratings under this system, which appear grossly inflated.

It is not surprising that questions have been raised about the reliability and validity of the AMA *Guides* for rating impairment in back pain (Nitschke et al 1999, Zuberbier et al 2001). Despite being the accepted standard, the fifth edition seems to pose more questions than it offers answers.

Waddell & Main (1984)

In the early 1980s, we made a first attempt to identify objective physical characteristics and to develop a clinical method of assessing lumbar impairment (Waddell & Main 1984). We looked at disability in 480 patients with various chronic low back problems. We used reliable methods of clinical examination and discounted behavioral reactions to examination. We then tried to find the physical characteristics that explained these patients' disability (Box 8.2). The problem was the very mixed group of physical characteristics, many of which only applied to patients with particular spinal pathologies. This reflected the patients in our hospital clinic. In this series, the findings were dominated by patients with serious spinal damage, nerve root problems, and previous surgery. Despite this, the study does provide some useful lessons. Only fractures, nerve compression signs, and previous surgery are true structural impairments, but none of these apply to the patient with non-specific low back pain. In practice, the patient's report of the anatomic and time pattern of pain had most influence on this score, but these do not meet the definition of physical impairment. The final problem was that we could not combine these characteristics statistically into a homogeneous scale. This study helped to show us the principles and the problems of assessing physical impairment in back pain, but it did not give us any answer.

NIOSH

The US National Institute for Occupational Safety and Health (NIOSH) also tackled this problem. Their approach was to put a great deal of effort into developing reliable methods of physical examination (Nelson & Nestor 1988). They used a literature review and an expert panel to find 105 clinical tests for back pain. They carried out extensive reliability studies in different centers. Their final "low back atlas" had 19 well-defined tests (NIOSH 1988), but unfortunately their only criterion was a very high level of reliability. This led to a rather bizarre group of tests. Six of the 19 tests were measures of pelvic tilt, and four were of lordosis. Yet pelvic tilt and lordosis have little or nothing to do with low back disability. The atlas did not include any form of palpation and the only movement was lateral flexion. It included a few measures of strength but they found them to be of doubtful reliability. That original set of tests may be reliable but they give a rather odd view of lumbar impairment.

Moffroid et al (1992) modified the NIOSH atlas slightly and confirmed its reliability. They then compared the tests in 115 patients with non-specific low back pain and 112 matched controls. About half the tests discriminated between the patients and asymptomatic people. The most powerful single test was pain on initiation of prone press-up. Box 8.3 presents the group of tests they found to provide the best discrimination.

Moffroid et al (1992, 1994) used the same data to try to separate four different symptom clusters. This was quite successful statistically, but clinically the clusters had a lot of overlap and it is difficult to see any clear clinical syndromes.

As far as I know, this NIOSH work has never gone any further.

Box 8.3   The National Institute of Occupational Safety and Health (NIOSH) atlas tests discriminating patients with back pain from normal people (after Moffroid et al 1992)

- Pain at initiation of press-up
- Lumbar mobility on forward bend
- Total range of hip rotation
- Whether the prone press-up test produces changes in the pattern of pain
- Pelvic tilt sitting
- Lower abdominal muscle strength

Other approaches

Several research groups in the 1980s tried to combine pain, physical impairment, and disability into a single scale (Lehmann et al 1983, Clark et al 1988, Greenough & Fraser 1992). The idea was to create an overall measure of severity for clinical, legal, and compensation purposes. This approach works for patients whose pain and disability are in proportion to the diagnosis and physical impairment. Often, however, that is not the case. This approach fails to address the common problem where the patient's report of pain and disability does not match the objective physical findings. The statistics reflect this. These different measures do not fit well into a single score, and the scales and the loading on each measure are arbitrary. The basic problem is that these combined scales fail to distinguish the distinct concepts of pain, disability, and physical impairment. The results have little clinical meaning.

Other groups tried to overcome this difficulty by using a panel of experts. This approach starts with a literature review, and then the experts select, based on their experience, the most useful tests for impairment. Statistical analysis of the experts' opinions puts a weight on each item to produce a scale. This does give a comprehensive scale that looks reasonable, as in the California Disability Rating Schedule (Clark et al 1988). Frymoyer & Cats-Baril (1987) also used this approach to predict chronic disability, and in their study it gave a useful starting point. However, the expert scale did not predict the outcome as accurately as the raw clinical data (see Box 7.2, Ch. 7). Moreover, I believe there is a basic flaw in this approach. No matter how sophisticated the methodology, it only gives a consensus of current clinical opinion. Statistical scoring of experts' votes is only an illusion of science. It cannot replace hard clinical data or a real understanding of the problem. In the past, such a committee would probably have *proved* that boiling tar was the best possible treatment for amputation stumps!

ASSESSMENT OF PHYSICAL IMPAIRMENT

There are problems associated with all of the methods described above, so we tried to develop a new method of assessing lumbar impairment, starting from basic principles (Waddell et al 1992). Our study had three aims:

1. to investigate physical impairment in patients with chronic low back pain
2. to develop a method of clinical evaluation suitable for routine use
3. to study the correlation between pain, disability, and physical impairment.

Our study was on patients with chronic low back pain, with or without referred leg pain. We excluded all patients with nerve root involvement, previous surgery, or structural problems like fractures and spondylolisthesis. This in effect excluded the permanent structural impairments that dominated our earlier study.

From the definition of physical impairment, we limited our assessment to objective findings on physical examination. We used reliable clinical tests and excluded behavioral responses. We studied 27 physical signs that might apply to ordinary backache, and did three pilot studies to develop reliable tests for 23 of the signs (Box 8.4). We had to exclude four tests because they were unreliable. We excluded a further nine tests because they were too behavioral in nature. Most of these were tests that reproduced pain and depended on how patients responded to pain.

We then looked at these 23 signs in 120 patients with chronic low back pain and 70 painfree, normal subjects. We wanted to find those signs that told us about physical impairment, so we went back to the definition. They should relate to back pain, so they should discriminate the patients from normal subjects. Physical findings are only an impairment if they cause disability, so they should also correlate with low back disability. Only the results will be considered here; the detailed statistics can be found in Waddell et al (1992).

We managed to produce a group of physical signs that combined into a scale of physical impairment (Table 8.1). This final scale could discriminate patients with back pain from normal people, and also correlated well with disability. Simple cut-offs made the scale simple and quick to use, with little loss of accuracy. This scale is suitable for routine use in patients with ordinary backache.

Box 8.4   Possible physical tests for lumbar impairment

- Lumbar lordosis and thoracic kyphosis
- Pelvic tilt and leg length
- Lumbar list
- Tenderness
  - lumbar
  - paravertebral
  - buttock
- Flexion
  - lumbar
  - pelvic
  - total
- Extension
- Lateral flexion
- Straight leg raising
- Passive knee flexion and pain[a]
- Passive hip flexion and pain[a]
- Hip flexion strength and pain[a]
- Hip abduction strength and pain[a]
- Prone extension
- Sit-up
- Bilateral active straight leg raising

[a]Reproduction of pain was subsequently excluded because it is too behavioral.

Table 8.1   Our final physical impairment scale

Physical test	Cut-off
Total flexion	<87°
Total extension	<18°
Average lateral flexion	<24°
Average straight leg raising	
Female	<71°
Male	<66°
Spinal tenderness	Positive
Bilateral active straight leg raising	<5 s
Sit-up	<5 s

Each scored 0/1 to give a total score out of 7.
From Waddell et al (1992), with permission.

Examination technique

Accurate assessment depends on careful and standard methods of examination. I am grateful to Duncan Troup for advice in refining this method.

Pre-examination procedure

The first step is to find the anatomic landmarks (Fig. 8.1). You will find it easiest to palpate these with the patient lying prone and relaxed. Make horizontal marks on the skin in the midline at S2 and T12–L1. The posterior superior iliac spines lie at the bottom of the posterior part of the iliac crest. They are just below and lateral to the dimples of Venus and correspond to S2. You can then find T12–L1 by counting up the spinous processes. Check that the iliac crests are at about the L4–L5 level. Then make further vertical marks in the midline over the spinous processes of T12 and T9.

Next, get the patient to perform warm-up exercises. They should flex and extend twice, rotate to the left and right twice, lateral flex to either side twice and then flex and extend once more. Therapists routinely use a warm-up before measuring any physical function, because it makes quite a difference to the results. A warm-up should now be standard before testing lumbar impairment.

You must then standardize the examination positions with care. We had considerable difficulty getting a consistent *erect* position, but reliable measures of movement depend on a standard starting point. It took a lot of trial and error to produce the following method. Have the patient stand in bare feet, with heels together, knees straight, and weight supported evenly on both legs. They should look straight ahead, with arms hanging at their sides. They should not hold themselves tense, but should relax without slumping. If a patient has severe muscle spasm, you should ask them to get as close to that position as they can hold comfortably for a few minutes. The *supine* position is with the patient lying flat on their back with their head on the couch without a pillow. They should relax with their arms by their sides, and extend their hips and knees as fully as possible without tension. The *prone* position is with the patient lying flat on their front on the couch without a pillow. They should relax with their arms by their sides.

The only equipment that you need is a ballpoint pen and some kind of inclinometer. We found an electronic inclinometer more convenient, but it is not essential.

Tests

You can perform the tests in any order you prefer. We found it simplest to arrange them in sequence in the erect, prone, and supine positions.

Flexion Measure flexion with the inclinometer (Fig. 8.2). Stand the patient in the erect position, and record at S2 (Fig. 8.2A) and then at T12–L1 (Fig. 8.2B). Hold the inclinometer on T12–L1, and ask the patient to reach down with the fingertips of both hands as far as possible towards their

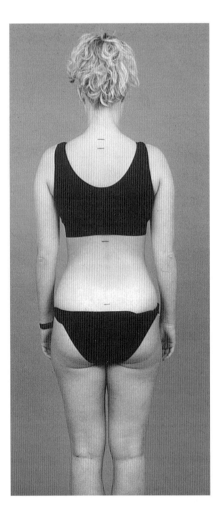

Figure 8.1 Reliable evaluation of physical impairment depends on a warm-up, a standard starting position, and careful marking of the anatomic landmarks.

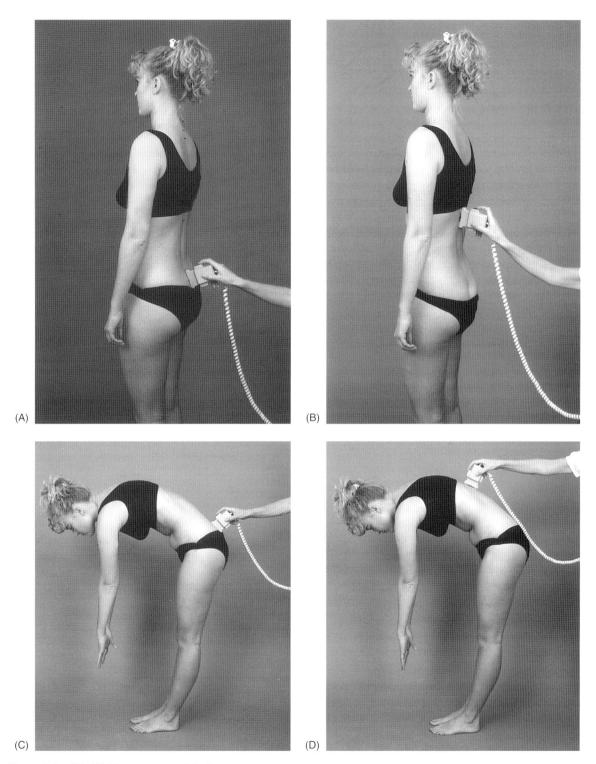

Figure 8.2   (A)–(D) Measurement of flexion.

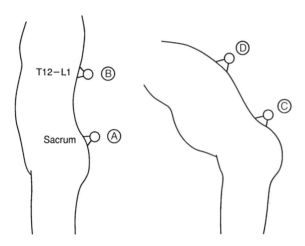

Figure 8.3   The inclinometer technique of measuring flexion: C−A = pelvic flexion; D−B = total flexion. The difference between them is lumbar flexion. In this diagram, pelvic flexion = 35°, total flexion = 60°, and therefore lumbar flexion = 25°.

toes. Check that the knees are straight. While the patient is fully flexed, make the third reading at T12–L1 (Fig. 8.2C). Tell the patient to hold that position and make the fourth reading at S2 (Fig. 8.2D). These four readings permit simple calculation of total flexion, pelvic flexion, and by subtraction, lumbar flexion (Fig. 8.3).

Extension   Measure extension at T12–L1 (Fig. 8.4). Take the first reading with the inclinometer while the patient is in the erect position. Then ask the patient to arch backwards as far as possible, looking up to the ceiling. Use one hand on the patient's shoulder as a support. This helps them to maintain their balance and gives them some feeling of security. Then take the second reading. Subtraction gives the measure of total extension.

Lateral flexion   To measure lateral flexion, use the longer bar on the inclinometer. While the patient is in the erect position, line up the bar between the spinous processes at T9 and T12 (Fig. 8.5). Take the first reading. Then ask the patient to lean straight over to the side as far as possible and to reach their fingers straight down the side of their thigh. Use one hand to support the patient's shoulder. Make sure that the patient does not flex forwards or twist round and that both feet remain flat on the floor. Measure lateral flexion to both sides.

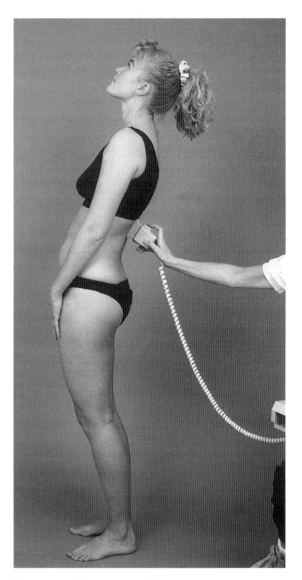

Figure 8.4   Measurement of extension.

Tenderness   Reliable testing for tenderness depends on particularly careful technique (Fig. 8.6). The patient should lie prone and you should make sure that they relax their muscles. Palpate the spine slowly without sudden pressure. Tenderness depends on eliciting pain, but do not hurt the patient unnecessarily. We will look at behavioral responses to examination in Chapter 10. It is enough at this point to note that widespread superficial or non-anatomic tenderness is behavioral. If these are present, you cannot examine for physical

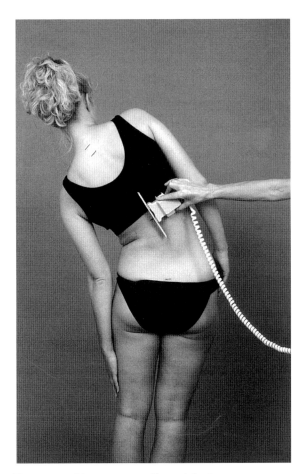

Figure 8.5 Measurement of lateral flexion.

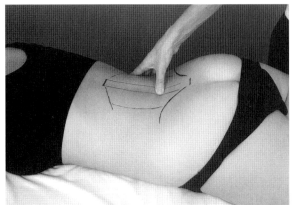

Figure 8.6 Lumbar spinal tenderness.

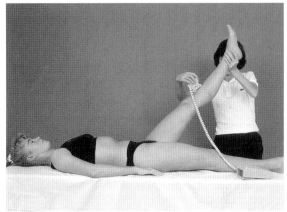

Figure 8.7 Straight leg raising.

tenderness. Look for local tenderness over the spinous processes and interspinous ligaments at each level from T12 to S2. Spinal tenderness is within half an inch (1 cm) of the midline. You should use exact wording: "Is that painful?" You should take *all* responses other than "no" to be positive, e.g., "only a little bit" should be taken to mean "yes". If the patient is doubtful or does not answer, then repeat the question: "Is that painful when I do that?"

Straight leg raising (SLR) Test SLR with the patient lying supine (Fig. 8.7). Make sure they stay relaxed and do not lift their head to watch what is happening. Hold their foot with one hand and make sure the hip is in neutral rotation. Use the other hand to hold the inclinometer on the tibia just below the tibial tubercle. Set the inclinometer

to zero. Then raise the leg passively, using your other hand to hold the inclinometer in place and also to hold the patient's knee fully extended. Raise the leg slowly to the highest SLR that the patient will tolerate, not just to the onset of pain. Record the highest reading in degrees. If SLR is limited, you should always check this while you distract the patient at a later stage (see Ch. 10). If distraction SLR is positive, then you should discount SLR on formal examination.

Bilateral active SLR This is a strength test, which should be carried out in the supine position (Fig. 8.8). Ask the patient to lift both legs together 6 inches (15 cm) off the couch and hold that position for 5 seconds. They should raise both heels and calves clear of the couch. You should not count aloud or give any verbal encouragement. Do not allow the patient to use their hands to lift their legs. Only if the patient manages to hold their legs clear for the full 5 seconds should you count the test as successful. If they fail to lift their legs clear of the couch, or lift them clear but lower them again in less than 5 seconds, that is a positive impairment.

Active sit–up Like bilateral active SLR, this is also a strength test, and should also be carried out in the supine position (Fig. 9.9). Ask the patient to bend their knees to 90° and to place the soles of both feet flat on the couch. Use one hand to hold down both feet. Then ask the patient to reach up with the fingertips of both hands to touch their knees. They should rest their fingers on their knees and not hold on. They should hold that position for 5 seconds. Again, you should not count aloud or give verbal encouragement. If the patient fails to reach the fingertips of both hands to their patellae, or does not hold the position for 5 seconds, that counts as a positive impairment.

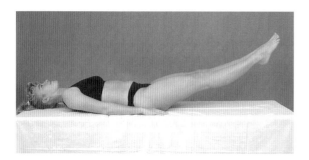

Figure 8.8   Bilateral active straight leg raising.

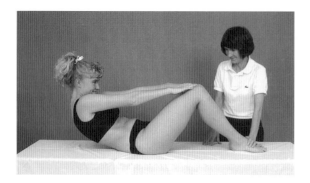

Figure 8.9   Active sit-up.

Interpretation of physical impairment

This is a comprehensive group of clinical tests for physical impairment in non-specific low back pain (Table 8.1). It includes spinal movement, SLR, spinal tenderness and strength tests. It has some similarities to the AMA *Guides* DRE and ROM models, and to Moffroid's scale. In our study, it discriminated patients with back pain from normal subjects and helped to explain low back disability. It provides an objective, clinical check on the patient's own report of disability.

To interpret this scale we must look again at the definition of impairment. This is a pragmatic method based entirely on clinical findings. It does not depend on pathologic or clinical diagnosis. Our previous study showed that the only permanent lumbar impairments were structural deformities, fractures, surgical scarring, and neurologic deficits. None of these apply to the patient with non-specific low back pain, and they do not appear in the present scale. This method provides an objective clinical evaluation, but it is not a measure of anatomic or structural impairment. Instead, all the tests in our scale are really measures of physical function. They are functional limitations associated with pain or disuse. More graphically, they are measures of "inability to do" because of pain. It is a matter of perspective whether we regard these findings as physiologic impairment as in the WHO definition or as clinical observations of performance. In any event, performance in these tests depends on how the patient reacts to pain and on the patient's effort, just as much as on the physical or physiologic disorder. We cannot interpret "inability to do" purely in terms of physical impairment. Inevitably, it is also a matter of performance.

One of our most surprising findings was that these patients with chronic low back pain did not have significant loss of lumbar flexion. Many studies suggest that lumbar flexion may be the most specific measure of true lumbar impairment. It is the most useful test of clinical severity and clinical progress in serious spinal pathology such as infection, and for disk prolapse and nerve root problems (Ch. 2). It is also the most useful measure of recovery from an acute attack of back pain. Direct measurement of lumbar flexion includes distraction and is hard to fake. It is the test that is least behavioral. For all these reasons, lumbar flexion may be the most valid single measure of true lumbar impairment.

Nevertheless, we found that lumbar flexion is more or less normal in patients with chronic low back pain. This may surprise many clinicians. One reason may be that we looked only at patients with ordinary backache. Most previous clinical studies, like our 1984 study, included patients with fractures, nerve root problems, or spinal surgery. Our normal subjects were also from the entire age range, whereas many previous studies used young and athletic normal controls.

However, we are not alone in our findings. Burton et al (1989) measured lumbar movement in nearly 1000 people aged 10–84 years. They compared those with no history of back pain, those with a previous history, and those with current pain. They found relatively minor differences in flexion in each group. Age and sex had a much greater effect. Esola et al (1996) found changes in the *pattern* of lumbar flexion, but no restriction in the range of flexion in adults with a history of back pain. Gronblad et al (1997) also looked at spinal mobility, pain, disability assessments, and physical performance tests in patients with chronic low back pain. They found very little relation between spinal mobility and any of these measures of severity. Marras et al (1999) could not quantify low back disorders using range of movement alone. They were able to discriminate patients from normal subjects, but only using complex measures of trunk motion, including velocity and acceleration. These findings question the nature of impairment in chronic low back pain. They are all consistent with physiologic change in the pattern of movement and reduced total body performance, rather than any structural impairment of the lumbar spine.

By the nature of these tests, they can only be measures of current impairment. In practice, we assess a patient at one point in time. We cannot know what was previously normal function for that individual; we can only compare our findings with the average for normal people. We can try to allow for age, sex, and build. Ultimately, however, these tests only tell us about the current state. This is an objective clinical evaluation of current functional limitation in patients with back pain.

We made every effort to separate our assessment of physical impairment from how patients respond to examination. Despite our efforts, we were only partly successful. All the tests in our scale still correlated to some extent with pain behavior. Our final scale was more closely related to the emotional than to the sensory scale of the McGill pain questionnaire. It correlated more with measures of illness behavior than with pain itself. By their very nature, performance in these tests will depend on how the individual reacts to pain, on motivation, and on effort, just as much as on the underlying physical or physiological disorder. All of these tests may also be open to exaggeration.

Summary

Objective clinical evaluation of physical impairment in ordinary backache:

- There is no clinical evidence of any permanent anatomic or structural impairment
- These findings are of current physiologic impairment or functional limitation associated with pain
- These clinical findings are a measure of performance, and depend on effort
- This physiologic impairment has the potential to recover

IMPAIRMENT AND DISABILITY

Back pain, impairment, and disability go together in clinical practice. The very definitions of impairment and disability relate them to each other. Impairment is that which causes disability; disability is that which results from impairment. But it is not a 1:1 relationship (Fig. 8.10). Many other studies have shown similar results. We often see patients with severe pain and disability, in whom we can find little impairment. Other people have severe pain or impairment, yet refuse to admit they have much disability. Disability must depend on other influences, as well as pain and impairment. Before we look at these other influences in the following chapters, we should stop and reflect further on impairment and disability (Fordyce 1995).

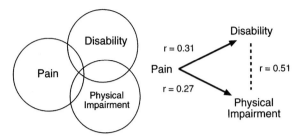

Figure 8.10 The relation between pain, disability, and impairment. *r* is the correlation coefficient, where 0 is no relation at all and 1 is complete identity. $r = 0.30$ is about 10% overlap in common, and $r = 0.50$ is about 25%.

We may assume that impairment and disability reflect loss of physical capacity, but we assess them on reduced activity. The fundamental limitation of clinical examination is that we cannot distinguish capacity and performance. Performance depends on anatomic and physiologic abilities, but also on psychological and social resources. Functional limitations on examination depend on how the patient reacts to pain, and on motivation and effort, just as much as on the underlying physical or physiologic disorder. Testing itself may cause pain and inhibit performance. As an oversimplification, capacity may be set by physiologic limits, but performance is set by psychological limits. Reduced performance may reflect actual loss of capacity, or the person may stop before they reach their physical limits, or their performance may be inhibited by pain, or they may not even attempt the activity because of expectations of pain. Fordyce (1995) defined disability as: "when the person prematurely terminates an activity, under-performs or declines to undertake it."

The limitation is that we cannot assess back pain: we can only assess the person with back pain. We cannot separate body and mind. Pain, suffering, and pain behavior all confound our assessment of impairment. Physical defects shape the person's beliefs and expectations about his or her situation. On the other hand, beliefs and expectations modify the impact of physical defects on function. Concepts of impairment and disability must allow for this dynamic interaction. We must not underestimate the extent to which psychosocial processes influence physical function, and vice versa.

Disability may imply the presence of illness, reduced capacity, restricted activity, or limited participation in life. But, conversely, impairment does not always cause disability. At first, minor dysfunction may not even cause any symptoms. If it gets worse, it may produce symptoms and become an illness, but that person may still not have any disability. People may draw on their resources and make greater effort to maintain activity. Even once they no longer have the physical capacity for a previous activity, they may modify their approach to do it a different way. If a patient cannot bend, he may squat to lift. He may split a load and make several smaller lifts. He may even buy a hoist. Only when no alternative remains, or when he gives up the effort, is he actually disabled.

Assessment at one point in time is inevitably limited, because impairment and disability are not static or passive. Both can vary with time, disuse, and rehabilitation. We have not found any physical basis for permanent disability in ordinary backache, and physiologic impairments at least have the potential to recover. Psychological, behavioral, and social impairments may all be remediable. Functional limitation may persist as long as pain lasts, and there is good clinical and epidemiologic evidence to suggest that the chances of successful rehabilitation of chronic pain reduce over time (Ch. 7). But, in principle, this kind of impairment always has the potential to improve. Various groups have proved this, even in chronic low back cripples (Cox et al 1988, Watson 2001).

In practice, we must judge disability within a broad clinical framework. We start with diagnosis or at least try to recognize symptom clusters. The principle remains that we must try to assess any functional limitations objectively, even accepting the practical limitations and the problems of interpretation. We must allow for effort and for the coexistence of physical and psychological dysfunction. Patients give us their account of symptoms and disability and the impact on their life and work. This may be in the context of a claim for compensation and we must try to discount exaggeration or observer bias. We must distinguish temporary and permanent disability. We must assess the potential for recovery and how much of current impairment is likely to be permanent. The final judgment of severity depends on the balance between the patient's report of pain and disability and the examiner's diagnosis and assessment of impairment. Together these give a comprehensive picture. When all are in proportion, we can combine them into an unequivocal assessment of severity. The objective clinical evidence then supports the patient's report of symptoms and disability. Sometimes, however, there may be a significant discrepancy between the patient's claim of pain, disability, and incapacity for work and our assessment of pathology and impairment. We must then try to discover the reasons why. To understand disability, we must look at the entire clinical picture in more detail.

Summary

Assessment of severity
- Diagnosis
- Patient report
  - pain
  - disability
- Professional assessment
  - physical impairment
  - functional capacity evaluation
- Judicial decision
  - (in)capacity for work
  - compensation

References

AAOS 1962 Manual for orthopedic surgeons in evaluating permanent physical impairment. American Academy of Orthopedic Surgeons, Chicago

AMA 1958 A guide to the evaluation of permanent impairment of the extremities and back. Journal of the American Medical Association 166(suppl.): 1–122

AMA 2000 Guides to the evaluation of permanent impairment, 5th edn. American Medical Association, Chicago

Brand R A, Lehmann T R 1983 Low-back impairment rating practices of orthopedic surgeons. Spine 8: 75–78

Burton A K, Tillotson K M, Troup J D G 1989 Variation in lumbar sagittal mobility with low back trouble. Spine 14: 584–590

Clark W L, Haldeman S, Johnson P et al 1988 Back impairment and disability determination. Another attempt at objective reliable rating. Spine 13: 332–341

Cox R, Keeley J, Barnes D, Gatchel R, Mayer T 1988 Effects of functional restoration treatment upon Waddell impairment/disability ratings in chronic low back pain patients. Presented to the 15th annual meeting of the International Society for the Study of the Lumbar Spine, Miami

Drewry W F 1896 Feigned insanity: report of three cases. Journal of the American Medical Association 27: 798–801

Esola M A, McClure P W, Fitzgerald G K, Siegler S 1996 Analysis of lumbar spine and hip motion during forward bending in subjects with and without a history of low back pain. Spine 21: 71–78

Fordyce W E (ed.) 1995 Back pain in the workplace: management of disability in non-specific conditions. International Association for the Study of Pain (IASP) Press, Seattle, pp 1–75

Frymoyer J W, Cats-Baril W 1987 Predictors of low back disability. Clinical Orthopaedics and Related Research 221: 89–98

Greenough C G, Fraser R D 1992 The assessment of outcome in patients with low back pain. Spine 17: 36–41

Gronblad M, Hurri H, Kouri J-P 1997 Relationships between spinal mobility, physical performance tests, pain intensity and disability assessments in chronic low back pain patients. Scandinavian Journal of Rehabilitation Medicine 29: 17–24

Hadler N M 1999 Occupational musculoskeletal disorders, 2nd edn. Lippincott/Williams & Wilkins, Philadelphia

Lehmann T, Brand R A, O'Gorman T W O 1983 A low back rating scale. Spine 8: 308–315

Marras W S, Ferguson S A, Gupta P et al 1999 The quantification of low back disorder using motion measures: methodology and validation. Spine 24: 2091–2100

Matheson L N, Gaudino E A, Mael F, Hesse B W 2000 Improving the validity of the impairment evaluation process: a proposed theoretic framework. Journal of Occupational Rehabilitation 10: 311–320

McBride E D 1936 Disability evaluation and principles of treatment of compensable injuries, 1st edn. Lippincott, Philadelphia

McBride E D 1963 Disability evaluation and principles of treatment of compensable injuries, 6th edn. Lippincott, Philadelphia

McCombe P F, Fairbank J C T, Cockersole B C, Pynsent P B 1989 Reproducibility of physical signs in low back pain. Spine 14: 908–918

Moffroid M T, Haugh L D, Hodous T 1992 Sensitivity and specificity of the NIOSH low back atlas. NIOSH report RFP 200-89-2917 (P). National Institute of Occupational Safety and Health, Morgantown, West Virginia

Moffroid M T, Haugh L D, Henry S M, Short B 1994 Distinguishable groups of musculoskeletal low back pain patients and asymptomatic control subjects based on physical measures of the NIOSH low back atlas. Spine 19: 1350–1358

Nelson R M, Nestor D E 1988 Standardized assessment of industrial low-back injuries: development of the NIOSH low-back atlas. Topics in Acute Care and Trauma Rehabilitation 2: 16–30

NIOSH 1988 National Institute for Occupational Safety and Health low back atlas. US Department of Health and Human Services, Morgantown, West Virginia

Nitschke J E, Nattrass C L, Disler P B, Chou M J, Ooi K T 1999 Reliability of the American Medical Association Guides' model for measuring spinal range of motion. Spine 24: 262–268

SSA 2001 Social security handbook. Social Security Administration. US Government Printing Office, Washington, DC

Waddell G, Main C J 1984 Assessment of severity in low back disorders. Spine 9: 204–208

Waddell G, Main C J, Morris E W et al 1982 Normality and reliability in the clinical assessment of backache. British Medical Journal 284: 1519–1523

Waddell G, Sommerville D, Henderson I, Newton M 1992 Objective clinical evaluation of physical impairment in chronic low back pain. Spine 17: 617–628

Watson P J 2001 From back pain to work. A collaborative initiative between the NDDI and the Department of Behavioural Medicine, Salford Royal Hospitals Trust. Final report to UK Department for Education and Employment

WHO 1980 International classification of impairments, disabilities and handicaps. World Health Organization, Geneva

Zuberbier O A, Hunt D G, Kozlowski A J et al 2001 Commentary on the American Medical Association Guides' lumbar impairment validity checks. Spine 26: 2735–2737

Chapter 9

The physical basis of back pain

So there is no doubt, let me state very clearly: back pain is a physical problem. Over the past 25 years, we have focused a lot (perhaps too much at times) on psychosocial issues. Psychosocial factors influence how patients respond to back pain and they are important in low back disability, but they do not cause the pain. Back pain is not a psychological problem. Back pain starts with a physical problem in the back.

So, what is the physical basis of non-specific low back pain? It is time to look at the basic science.

Most books about back pain start with chapters on the anatomy and pathology of the spine. Ian Macnab described this as a form of Brownian movement: it seems very busy, but is really mindless and serves no useful purpose. He then went ahead and started that way, anyway! You already know I resisted that temptation, deliberately. I firmly believe that we must start with the clinical problem, and only then look for the basic science that helps to explain our clinical observations. The danger of starting from anatomy, biomechanics, or pathology is that they set the agenda. We too easily become prisoners of theory and then select or twist the clinical facts to fit the theory. That is why I waited till now, after we have set the clinical and epidemiologic scene. And now I will take a very clinical perspective on the basic science.

Structure and function are intimately related, and we must consider them together.

CLINICAL CHARACTERISTICS

Back pain is a mechanical problem. It is mechanical in the sense that symptoms arise from the

Box 9.1   "Mechanical" low back pain

- Pain is usually cyclic
- Low back pain is often referred to the buttocks and thighs
- Morning stiffness or pain is common
- Start pain is common
- There is pain on forward flexion and often also on returning to the erect position
- Pain is often produced or aggravated by extension, lateral flexion, rotation, standing, walking, sitting, and exercise in general
- Pain usually becomes worse over the course of the day
- Pain is relieved by a change of position
- Pain is relieved by lying down, especially in the fetal position

Table 9.1   Effect of physical activities on back pain in 200 osteopathic patients

	Aggravates (%)	Relieves (%)
Sitting	30	23
Walking	22	12
Movement	17	16
Lying	9	35

From Dr K Burton, with thanks.

Table 9.2   Patterns of activity-related low back pain in 500 primary care patients

	Male (%)	Female (%)
Pain aggravated by certain positions and relieved by moving about or changing position	17	35
Pain unrelated to physical activity	10	3
Pain aggravated by certain activities and relieved by changing or stopping activities	74	62

musculoskeletal system and they vary with physical activity.

Fiddler (1980) surveyed the members of the International Society for the Study of the Lumbar Spine (ISSLS). They described a mechanical syndrome for non-specific back pain without nerve root involvement (Box 9.1). Different authors describe these as movement disorders or activity-related spinal disorders.

These clinicians focused on what made the pain worse. However, Tables 9.1 and 9.2 show that various activities can make back pain either better or worse. Different activities may have opposite effects in different patients. It would be ideal if we could find patterns that might help to classify different types of back pain, but unfortunately no one has managed to produce any consistent results. We also found that many patients distinguished the immediate effects of activity on their symptoms and what they felt was the best long-term management for their problems. Disability varied with these mechanical characteristics. Patients who said that physical activity, walking, and physical therapy made their pain worse were more severely disabled. Their response to treatment was poorer.

PAIN RECEPTORS

Pain can only arise from structures that contain nerve endings. Most nociceptors are unmyelinated, free nerve endings. More specialized nerve endings in tendons, ligaments, and joint capsules are sensitive to mechanical stimuli. These normally serve proprioception, but they can also give pain under certain conditions.

Kellgren (1938, 1939) performed the classic experiment to find possible sources of low back pain. He injected hypertonic saline into various low back structures to produce different patterns of pain (see Figs 2.5 and 2.6). Later studies had more accurate anatomic placement, used different types of stimuli, and confirmed they could relieve the pain by local anesthetic, but they broadly confirmed Kellgren's work. On the basis of such studies, we now believe the following low back structures can give rise to pain (Bogduk & Twomey 1991, Adams et al 2002):

- *Vertebrae* – there are nociceptors in periostium and accompanying blood vessels in cancellous bone.

- *Intervertebral disk* – histology of the normal disk suggests that only the most peripheral annulus is innervated. However, granulation or scar tissue may grow into the degenerate disk, and the new blood vessels in this tissue may contain nociceptors.

- *Dura and nerve root sleeves* – this is quite separate from stimulation of the actual lumbosacral nerve root.

- *Facet joint capsules* – these have a rich supply of nociceptors.

- *Ligaments and fascia* – these also have rich innervation.

- *Muscle* – there has been long anatomic debate about muscle as a source of back pain. But anyone who claims that muscles cannot feel pain has never done hard physical exercise. Or they are being pedantic about muscle fibers vs muscles. There are mechanoreceptors in tendons and muscle insertions that can give rise to pain. There are nociceptors in the region of blood vessels and in fascia. It is doubtful if muscle fibers themselves can produce pain, but muscle spindles are highly sensitive to mechanical stimuli. If a muscle contracts under ischemic conditions, pain develops within 1 minute. Muscle activity leads to lowered oxygen tension and pH and local build-up of metabolites. These cause increased sensitivity to stretch and increased muscle tone. Disuse makes these physiologic responses more marked, while training reduces them. The question has been raised of increased muscle pressure in back pain, but this is unconfirmed. The paraspinal muscles are unique in that they are innervated by the posterior primary rami, while all other voluntary muscles in the body are innervated by the anterior primary rami. Experimental muscle pain is diffuse and aching, and may also produce referred pain and hyperalgesia in distant somatic structures (Arendt-Nielsen et al 1998).

The posterior primary rami of the lumbar nerve roots supply all these structures, with overlap between several adjacent levels. There are also links with sympathetic and parasympathetic nerves. Stimulation of most of these structures can produce pain in the lower back and referred pain into the leg(s) similar to that in patients.

However, we should interpret anatomic studies of "pain generators" with care. Identifying a sensitive site to artificial stimulation is not necessarily the same as finding the cause of the clinical problem. The anatomic site and the pathologic nature of any disorder are separate issues. Even if we do find the site of pain, that does not diagnose pathology, e.g., pain in the hip may have many causes. Conversely, even when we cannot localize an anatomic site we may still be able to understand the nature of the disorder, e.g., neurologic disease. Further, the various structures at one segmental level are closely linked, share common innervation, and function together. So even when we localize pain to one level, that may not tell which of the segmental structures is the cause of the problem. Even if one part of the segment is sensitive now, the initial disturbance may be in other linked parts of the segment. We have often blurred these issues in our search for the source of back pain.

A STRUCTURAL BASIS FOR BACK PAIN?

For more than a century, orthodox medicine, orthopedics, and biomechanics have looked for a structural cause for back pain. They have searched for disease, or injury, or damage.

Radiologic anomalies

The history of X-rays (Ch. 4) showed the temptation to attribute back pain to every incidental radiographic finding. But anatomic coincidence is not proof of cause and effect. That would be like saying: "Red hair is very uncommon, so in that sense it is not normal. It is at the site of headache. So your red hair must be the cause of your head pain. Maybe we should think about shaving your red hair to cure your headache." That is clearly absurd, but it is the same kind of logic. We must be more analytic. Back pain is very common and so are many X-ray findings. We may start from the observation that a finding is more common in people with back pain than in those without. But we must still prove that it really is a risk factor, with a cause and effect relationship, and significant effect size (Ch. 6). We should have a plausible pathologic explanation of the mechanism. Finally, anesthetic blocks or specific treatment should relieve the pain. When we apply these tests, most X-ray anomalies turn out to be incidental findings (Box 9.2).

> **Box 9.2**   Radiographic anomalies that appear to be incidental findings in adult back pain (Wiltse 1971, Van Tulder et al 1997, Nachemson & Vingaord 2000)
>
> - Transitional vertebra
> - Lumbarization, sacralization
> - Spina bifida occulta
> - Accessory ossicles
> - Schmorl's nodes
> - Disk calcification
> - Height of sacrum in pelvis
> - Lumbosacral angle
> - Lumbar lordosis
> - Mild–moderate scoliosis
> - Spondylolysis
> - Spondylolisthesis
> - Scheuermann's disease

Disk prolapse

The discovery of the disk prolapse seemed at first to end the long search for the cause of back pain. In Chapter 4, we saw how early enthusiasts claimed it was the cause of most, if not all, back pain. Many patients with a disk prolapse do have a previous history of recurrent back pain. The acute episode may start with back pain, which over days or weeks changes to nerve root pain. So back pain can be part of the natural history of disk prolapse. We know that stimulation of the posterior longitudinal ligament and dura can produce back pain, and a disk prolapse can irritate these structures. So there is a plausible pathologic mechanism. However, it is an enormous and illogical jump to claim that disk prolapse is the cause of most back pain. Sixty percent of adults have back pain each year, but only 3–5% ever develop a disk prolapse. No one would dispute that disk prolapse *can* cause back pain, but it is not the usual cause.

Disk degeneration

Although few of us now believe that disk prolapse is the cause of most back pain, the lure of the disk is still strong. Many doctors and patients find X-ray and magnetic resonance imaging (MRI) changes almost irresistible. Look at the X-ray in Figure 9.1.

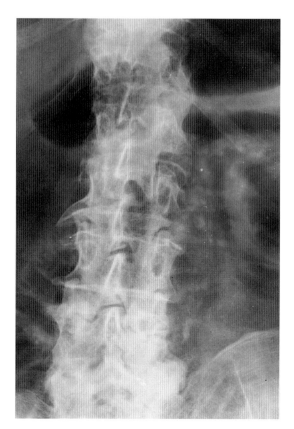

Figure 9.1   Severe degenerative changes – an incidental radiographic finding.

By any standards, this shows severe spinal degeneration. There is narrowing of the lower lumbar disks, marked osteophyte formation, loss of alignment of the spine, and facet joint osteoarthritis. It looks terrible and must be very painful. There is only one snag to this story, and the clue is the distended stomach. This is an abdominal X-ray of an 80-year-old woman with acute bowel obstruction. She never had back pain in her life.

We now know a great deal about the gross changes, histology, biochemistry, and biomechanics of the disk (Buckwalter 1995, Adams et al 2002). These changes all increase with age. They are also often described as degeneration. The problem is how to distinguish aging from degeneration. Adams et al (2002, p 67) suggested that normal aging involves biochemical and functional changes in the composition of the disk, while pathologic degeneration involves gross structural changes. But biomechanical, functional, and structural changes often go together, if to variable degree. The clinical evidence shows no such clear demarcation.

Van Tulder et al (1997) reviewed 12 studies that compared X-ray findings in people with or without symptoms. They considered there was a consistent but weak association between degenerative changes and back pain. However, it is difficult to interpret X-ray findings in an individual patient because a large proportion of asymptomatic people show the same changes. Likewise, this patient's changes are almost certainly longstanding and predate their present symptoms. Van Tulder et al also pointed out weaknesses in these studies. In particular, many of the studies compared present X-ray changes with past history of back pain and that may tell us little about present symptoms. They concluded that it is not possible to establish a cause and effect relationship between degenerative changes and clinical symptoms.

Nachemson & Vingard (2000) reviewed 14 MRI studies of the cervical and lumbar spine in normal, asymptomatic people. These sensitive tests showed disk bulging, annular tears, narrowing, degeneration, herniation, and stenosis (Fig. 9.2). Everything increased with age. They concluded that MRI was useful for "red flag" conditions, but these findings really do not help our understanding or diagnosis of back pain.

Jarvik & Deyo (2000) made one of the most careful longitudinal studies of MRI in normal, asymptomatic people. They classified the MRI findings as:

- findings with little relationship to either aging or previous low back pain, e.g., annular tears
- findings that increase with age, but have little or no association with previous low back pain, e.g., disk bulging and end plate changes
- findings related to both aging and previous low back pain, e.g., dehydration and loss of disk height
- rare findings that are fairly constant across age groups, but are directly related to previous low back pain, e.g., disk extrusions.

There are now five longitudinal studies in normal, asymptomatic people, which show that none of these findings predict future disk prolapse, back pain, or (in)capacity for work (Table 9.3). The UK occupational health guidelines were clear: "There is strong evidence that X-ray and MRI findings have

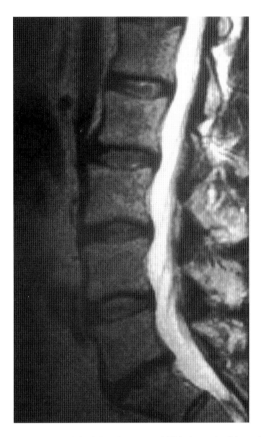

Figure 9.2   Disk bulging is *normal*. This is an incidental magnetic resonance imaging finding in a healthy 55-year-old man. The more sensitive the investigation, the higher the false-positive rate in older patients. From Dr N McMillan, with thanks.

no predictive value for future low back pain or disability" (Waddell & Burton 2000).

The problem remains how to distinguish "normal" age-related changes from fair wear and tear or a pathologic condition of "disk degeneration." To what extent are these normal biologic changes with age or the effect of cumulative exposure to physical loading? Is there accelerated or exaggerated aging, and how can we distinguish it from the wide normal distribution? Or is it a matter of perspective (and perhaps the age of the observer!) whether we regard aging itself as normal or a degenerative process?

There is good biomechanical evidence and theory how these changes can impair biomechanical function and so might explain back pain. Unfortunately, these are usually in vitro theories and are not correlated with clinical findings. Conversely, we do not

Table 9.3

Authors	Type of study	Subject	Original authors' main conclusions
Riihimaki et al (1989)	5-year prospective cohort	Clinical findings X-rays	Previous history of LBP was the best predictor of sciatica. Degenerative changes on initial X-ray did not predict sciatica after adjustment for age
Symmons et al (1991a, b)	9-year prospective population study of 1009 middle-aged women	Clinical findings X-rays	Degenerative changes on initial X-ray did not predict onset of new LBP in those with no previous history of LBP or recurrent LBP in those with a previous history of LBP. Continuing LBP was not related to deterioration of disk degeneration during follow-up. The strongest predictor of progressive degenerative changes was the presence of degeneration at onset, but that was quite separate from symptoms
Savage et al (1997)	Prospective cohort	MRI in asymptomatic subjects	No clear relationships between MRI findings and LBP. MRI findings not related to type of occupation. No change in MRI appearance in those subjects who developed new-onset LBP during 1-year follow-up. MRI findings did not predict new LBP on 1-year follow-up. Authors concluded that MRI is not suitable for pre-employment screening
Boos et al (2000)	Prospective cohort	MRI in selected asymptomatic subjects with MRI abnormalities	MRI findings did not predict significant new LBP or sciatica or work absence or medical consultation with 5-year follow-up
Borenstein et al (2001)	Prospective cohort	MRI in asymptomatic subjects	MRI did not predict the development or duration of significant new LBP or sciatica or work loss on 7-year follow-up

LBP, low back pain; MRI, magnetic resonance imaging.

have clinical investigations to make a biomechanical diagnosis in individual patients. The difficulty is when we test biomechanical theory against the clinical and epidemiologic evidence. Back trouble does not increase progressively with age, but peaks in middle life (Ch. 5). But back pain does not correlate well with degenerative changes either. There is little relation between clinical symptoms and the severity of radiographic changes in the disks. Patients with back pain and normal, asymptomatic people show similar age-related findings in their disks. Degenerative changes get progressively worse with age, but symptoms get slightly less after middle age.

Adams et al (2002) have argued that the links between back pain and mechanical loading and aging and dysfunction and degeneration are complex and should not be dismissed without further research. I fully support the need for further research in this area. But from a clinical perspective, that research must include clinical data. And I would argue from the clinical evidence that it is probably not simply a matter of structural degeneration. We must escape from the biomechanical as well as the orthopedic dynasty of the disk. In the meantime, in clinical practice, we must not be seduced by pretty pictures! We should not fall into the trap of blaming back pain on incidental radiographic findings. We are better to regard them as normal, age-related changes, like gray hair.

Facet joints

The facet joints are another potential source of pain. They are synovial joints and so can develop true osteoarthritis.

Fiddler (1980) tried to distinguish syndromes of disk, facet, and instability pain. Unfortunately, the members of ISSLS could not agree. One-third of the experts freely admitted they could not separate these syndromes. The others thought they could, but they all gave different descriptions. Scientific studies have been just as inconclusive. Jackson et al (1988) found no relation between pain on extension and pain relief by local anesthetic injection into the facets. Lilius et al (1989) found no link between initial pain relief by local anesthetic and lasting relief from cortisone injection. In a controlled trial, injections into or around the facet were no better than placebo. Both groups felt they could not identify a facet joint syndrome. The review by Van Tulder et al (1997) did not link X-ray changes in the facet joints to back pain.

Sprains and strains

The most common clinical diagnosis for non-specific low back pain, especially an acute episode with sudden onset, is a sprain or strain. We often simply assume it is an injury, even if any "accident" is a normal, everyday activity. We rarely specify the exact site or tissue, but assume it is muscle or connective tissue. The diagnosis seems plausible and may even be likely in some cases, but there is little direct evidence.

Most minor limb injuries are to the soft tissues, mainly the connective tissues. Structural damage to a muscle is quite rare, although muscle symptoms associated with use are common. By analogy, there may be similar injuries in the back, but they are more difficult to assess because the tissues are deeply placed. It is possible that we simply do not have the clinical ability or investigations to demonstrate soft-tissue injuries in the back. These cases do not come to autopsy or surgery, so we have no tissue studies. Nevertheless, for a clinical problem that is so common, we have surprisingly little direct evidence. There is still considerable doubt as to whether there is any true soft-tissue injury with structural damage, either in general or in the individual patient. At present, I would offer the old Scots legal verdict of "not proven."

Conclusion

For more than 100 years, orthodox medicine, orthopedics, and biomechanics have searched for a structural cause for back pain. They have focused on tissue damage or mechanical failure, whether due to single injury or cumulative injuries or repetitive loading. Early osteopathic concepts of displacement and early chiropractic concepts of subluxation reflected the same approach. Surgeons and engineers have undertaken research on the spine and disks, but this may just reflect their professional interests. The spine may simply be more accessible than other structures to medical investigations and laboratory experiment. This approach has been very informative for spinal injury, disk prolapse, and nerve root problems, but it has failed to find the cause of back pain. Perhaps after so much fruitless search we should question our starting assumption that non-specific low back pain is due to disease or injury or structural damage. The soft tissues of the back may be just as important as or even more important than bones, disks, and nerves. We saw in the previous chapter that physical impairment may be physiologic rather than anatomic. Let me suggest the hypothesis that disturbed function may be just as important as or even more important than structural damage as the physical basis of non-specific back pain.

BIOMECHANICS

I am indebted to Pope et al (1991) and Adams et al (2002) for much of the material in this section.

Most biomechanics starts from the concept of mechanical damage or failure and focuses on the spine. In theory, musculoskeletal damage may be caused by direct trauma, by a single overload, or by repetitive or sustained loading. Tissue strength varies with gender, age, body build, physical fitness, and fatigue. Damage may be to one or more of the musculoskeletal structures. Direct trauma may injure many tissues at the same time.

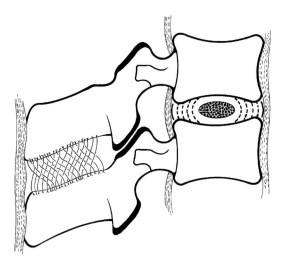

Figure 9.3   The motion segment – two adjacent vertebrae with the disk, facet joints, ligaments, and muscles between them. Drawing by Stewart Wood, with thanks.

Box 9.3   The functions of the spine

- Support
  - body
  - loads
- Movement
  - flexion–extension
  - lateral bending
  - axial rotation (twisting)
- Protection
  - central nervous system and nerve roots

Overexertion, such as lifting, usually only damages one tissue. Repeated or sustained loading is also likely to lead to fatigue failure at one site. In life, an isolated injury is followed by healing. However, with repetitive or sustained loading, continued damage and healing may occur simultaneously. Repeated or sustained loading may stimulate growth or adaptation.

We must always remember the fundamental limitations of our present biomechanical knowledge. Many of the classic studies were in the laboratory on cadaver material, and of a single motion segment of the spine (Fig. 9.3). Many studies are still on a few specimens. The tissues are no longer alive but are completely inert; there is no nutrition or neuromuscular activity; there is no biologic response or inflammation, and certainly no healing. Testing segments of the spine to failure may tell us about the mechanics of spinal fracture and disk prolapse but is of doubtful relevance to non-specific back pain. The earliest in vivo experiments measured the pressure in the intervertebral disk, and showed the load on the spine in different activities. However, once again, the disk was simply the most suitable site to measure these loads. This may not accurately reflect comparable loads on various parts of the musculoskeletal system. Biomechanical models do now often include the facet joints and the ligaments of the spine. But they usually consider

ligaments, muscles, and soft tissues mainly for their influence on the spine, rather than being of interest in their own right. This is a fundamental bias that may not reflect clinical reality.

The spine

The spine is mechanically complex because it has to serve different functions (Box 9.3). The demands on the spine are conflicting but it has to meet them all simultaneously. This inevitably involves compromise.

In biomechanics, as in embryology and mythology, the spine forms the backbone of the body. It supports the head and the trunk and the limbs. Even the internal organs are suspended from the spine. If support were its only function, the simplest and strongest mechanical solution would be a rigid spine. It is the need for mobility that causes problems. So, instead of being rigid, the spine is a flexible column of bony blocks joined by disks. The demands of support and those of mobility are always in conflict, and achieving a balance between them requires good control mechanisms. We must maintain equilibrium between the load on the spine and the tension in disks, ligaments, and muscles. If we are to stay upright, there must be a balance between the moments of all the forces acting. When we lift, the load on the back depends on the weight and the distance from the body. Pregnancy also alters posture and the loads on the back.

Panjabi (1992) suggested that stability of the spine depends on three subsystems (Fig. 9.4). The passive system is the spinal column, made up of the vertebrae, disks, facet joints, ligaments, and joint capsules. The active system includes the muscles

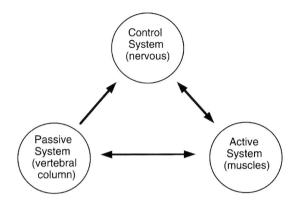

Figure 9.4   The three subsystems of spinal stability. From Panjabi (1992), with permission.

and tendons that surround and can apply forces to the spinal column. The neurologic or control system monitors the position, loading, and demands on the spine, and directs the active system to provide the required stability and action. Dysfunction in any one system leads to a response in one or both of the other systems, which may or may not compensate, or lead to failure or long-term adaptation.

The spine is a flexible column with multiple curves. The thoracic spine is splinted by the ribcage. The sacrum is more or less fixed in the pelvis and the coccyx has no mechanical function. The lumbar and cervical spines are flexible, but, of the two, the lumbar spine has to carry greater loads. The transitional regions between fixed and flexible parts of the spine have greater functional demands, which might explain why these are the areas of most symptoms.

The anterior and posterior elements of the spine serve different mechanical functions. The main anterior column of the spine is made up of the vertebral bodies and disks. These provide support and in life carry 75–80% of the load. The disks allow flexion, extension, and lateral bending and also a limited amount of rotation and glide. The flexibility of the spine, with the spinal curves and disks, allows it to act as a shock absorber so that we do not suffer concussion every time we jump down on to our heels. The posterior half of each vertebra is an arch of bone to surround and protect the spinal cord and nerves. Each arch articulates with the arch above and below by the two small facet joints. Bony processes project backwards and to each side as levers for ligament and muscle attachments.

Movement of the spine never occurs as pure flexion or extension in one plane. The spine is flexible, and must be controlled in three dimensions. In practice, there is always some movement in the other planes. Even a simple axial load causes such a coupled response. In real life we subject our backs to complex movements and loads. Consider a simple lift at work. We may start with flexion and axial loading. When we turn to lay the load down, there may be axial rotation, lateral bending, and shear forces. Then we straighten up and stretch. Each of these mechanical demands occurs at different stages of the lift and in varying combinations and sequence.

Vertebral body

The vertebral body is a honeycomb of cancellous bone that gives a high strength-to-weight ratio. There is a roughly linear relationship between the mineral content of the bone and the load at which it fails, as in osteoporosis. The trabeculae develop to withstand the forces acting on the bone, so their pattern reveals the common forces on the vertebrae. In life the vertebrae are full of blood, which may add hydraulic strength. The vertebrae are larger and stronger lower down the spine where the load of the body is greater. We tend to think of bone as rigid but that is not strictly true. Vertebrae are six times stiffer and three times thicker than the disks and only allow half the deformation, but they do have some elasticity. Microfractures may occur in the trabeculae and some authors suggest they may be a source of back pain, although there is no proof of this. Increased venous pressure in cancellous bone may occur adjacent to osteoarthritis in peripheral joints, but we do not know if this is important in the vertebrae.

Disk

The disk forms the main articulation between the vertebral bodies. The mechanical properties of the disk depend on the tissues of the annulus and the nucleus (Fig. 9.5). The annulus contains about 90 collagen lamellae, which are spiral and interdigitate like a modern car tire to give maximum strength. With age, the collagen fibers and lamellae split and break. The young nucleus is about 90% water and is

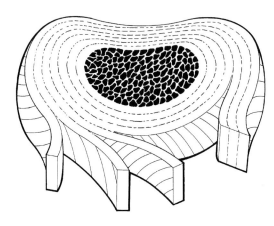

Figure 9.5 The dynasty of the disk. The disk is most accessible to experiment and investigation, but this has led to the neglect of soft tissues, which may be more important in ordinary backache. Drawing by Stewart Wood, with thanks.

an incompressible gel. With age, the water content falls and the nucleus loses much of its mechanical properties. The normal nucleus is under pressure even at rest and this increases to balance axial loads, which produces tension and slight bulging of the annulus. Disk bulging is *normal* and reflects the balance between the mechanical forces applied to the spine and the osmotic forces in the nucleus (Fig. 9.2). There is about 20% diurnal variation in disk height and volume. During the day, the load on the disk due to gravity and physical activity gradually overcomes the osmotic forces, and the disk is squashed. When we lie down at night, osmotic forces restore disk height. The pressure in the disk varies with posture and physical activity. Even distribution of stress within the disk depends on the intact nucleus and annulus, and becomes uneven with aging or degeneration.

Disks are avascular and their nutrition depends on diffusion. The permeability of the vertebral end plates decreases with age. Movement is good for the disk, improving the transport of nutrients and disk metabolism. Continuous motion is more effective than intermittent motion, and regular exercise every day is better than once or twice a week.

Facet joints

The main functional posterior elements of the spine are the facet joints. The facets stabilize the spine and limit rotation and shift. The facet joint itself is subject to compression and shearing. The facets carry 20–25% of the axial load, although this may rise to 70% with disk narrowing. The facets provide 40% of torsional and shear strength. The posterior elements may be more vulnerable to cyclic fatigue, as in spondylolysis. Small articular fractures may occur within the facet joints, though it is not clear if they are a common cause of back pain.

Panjabi (1992) suggested that the "neutral zone" is the range of normal motion within which there is no resistance from either the disk or the facet joint. Stability and movement within the neutral zone depend on muscle control. Any disturbance of muscular activity could lead to instability or injury. Beyond the neutral zone there is increasing stiffness in the disk and facet joints. The concept of the neutral zone is theoretically attractive. Unfortunately, there is little empirical evidence on its significance for dysfunction, or for therapy and rehabilitation (Thompson et al 2003).

Ligaments

Ligaments stabilize the spine and set the limits to movement. They are one of the main tensile elements acting as check reins to prevent excessive movement. They are relatively non-elastic, or more accurately they are viscoelastic: they "creep" under load. Five minutes in full flexion can reduce the motion segment's resistance to flexion by 40%. The intervertebral ligaments are very strong. Trauma may rupture collagen fibers, but complete rupture of the ligament probably only occurs with violent injury almost sufficient to dislocate the spine. Ligaments are subject to fatigue failure. Most important, ligaments can also heal, and we can see healed minor tears at autopsy. However, it is rarely possible to demonstrate such tears at the time of acute injury, and it is not clear if they are a common cause of back pain.

In general, flexion puts tension on the posterior ligaments, and extension puts tension on the anterior ligaments. Muscles can act on ligaments and fascia to alter their tension. This may indirectly modify load bearing and help to control the range of movement.

Muscles

The spine depends on muscles for stability. The muscles control and position the spine and the trunk. They provide movement and power for voluntary activity. A spine held by ligaments alone, with all the muscle excised, buckles under loads of only 2 kg (about 4 lb). Paralytic scoliosis provides a dramatic illustration of the role of the spinal muscles.

Different trunk muscles play different roles in the stability and movement of the spine (Panjabi 1992). Bergmark (1989) suggested there are two main muscle systems and this is supported by a recent study by Danneels et al (2001). The global muscle system consists of the large trunk muscles that act indirectly on the spine: the rectus abdominis, external oblique, and iliocostalis lumborum. These global muscles provide general trunk stability and the main torque for movement in flexion, lateral bending, and rotation. However, they cannot exert any direct influence on individual motion segments. The local muscle system consists of muscles that attach directly to the vertebrae: the lumbar multifidus, transversus abdominis, and internal oblique. These provide segmental stability and directly control the lumbar segments. The human lordosis is unique because of our upright posture, and the multifidus is now the largest part of the erector spinae. The trunk muscles, particularly the transversus abdominis, can also raise the pressure in the abdomen and chest and convert the entire trunk into a semirigid cylinder.

The psoas and iliacus muscles are too close to the axis of motion to bend the lumbar spine and their main function is to flex the hip. However, they exert large compressive forces and can also help to stabilize the spine and pelvis. The small segmental muscles between the spinous and transverse processes are too weak to have any mechanical function. They have a high concentration of muscle spindles and probably serve proprioception.

All the muscles work in synergy. When the anterior or posterior muscles contract symmetrically, they produce flexion or extension. When the left or right sides contract in various combinations, they produce lateral bending or rotation. When muscles contract, the antagonistic muscles must relax. Smooth movement also depends on stabilization and coordination of the various motion segments. So it is not surprising that multifidus and transversus abdominis contract first at the start of any movement.

Many muscles can move the torso, so different combinations of muscles can achieve any particular movement or task. In back pain, there is scope to compensate by modifying the pattern of muscle activity. This also makes it difficult to produce a theoretic biomechanical model of muscle action.

Standing erect, there is little electrical activity in the extensor muscles. As we bend forward, there is increasing muscle activity in the erector spinae. Beyond about 35° of trunk flexion, this activity reduces. By full flexion, the muscles are silent and the trunk is "hanging on the ligaments." This is the normal flexion–relaxation response. Coming back up, movement begins with the hip extensors. Then, as we rise further, the spinal extensors take up the load.

Different types of muscle fibers have different mechanical and metabolic properties. Slow fibers maintain posture; they activate more easily and are capable of more sustained contraction. Fast or phasic fibers give dynamic, voluntary movement; they fatigue more rapidly. Different muscles contain varying proportions of slow and fast fibers. Postural and phasic muscles are often antagonistic.

All voluntary striated muscles are highly metabolic tissues, and need a good and continuous supply of oxygen and nutrients. They fatigue: on sustained effort, electromyogram (EMG) activity diminishes with time. They take a finite time to react to sudden loads, and this time increases with fatigue. Muscle has a remarkable ability to increase or decrease its size and strength and endurance within a matter of days or a few weeks. Muscle can waste with disuse more rapidly than any other tissue. Conversely, muscle is one of the most responsive tissues to physical training.

The pelvis and sacroiliac joints

Vleeming et al (1997) pointed out that the spine, pelvis, and legs function as an integrated whole and the pelvis has an essential role that we have often neglected. The human pelvis is unique because we are the only truly erect, bipedal animal. We walk by swiveling on each leg in turn, which places great loads across the pelvis and sacroiliac joints. The glutei have developed enormously compared with any other animal to become the largest muscle mass in the human body. The iliopsoas acts across the lumbar spine, pelvis, and hips.

The thoracolumbar fascia plays an important role in load transfer between the trunk and legs. It is part of a "corset" that surrounds the trunk. The erector spinae lies within its layers. Contractions of the latissimus dorsi, gluteus maximus, and abdominal wall muscles tense the fascia, which effectively links the actions of these muscles. The biceps femoris tendon tenses the sacrotuberous ligament below. This all acts as a muscle–tendon–fascia sling that provides a functional link between the trunk, the pelvis, and the legs. This fascia also has rich innervation for both proprioception and nociception.

There is long-standing dispute about the possible role of the sacroiliac joints in back pain. The closely matched shape of these joints and the strong surrounding ligaments make it very unlikely that they are often damaged. However, the sacroiliac joints do permit a few degrees of movement and protective "give" in the pelvis. They again contain proprioceptors. So the sacroiliac joints could be subject to abnormal strains and could give rise to pain. They could play a role in the compound function or dysfunction of the lower back.

Functional anatomy

Functional anatomy, physical therapy, and rehabilitation all stress that the body functions as a whole. The entire spinal column, its muscles, and control system form a single, integrated system. The spine, pelvis, and legs function together. Indeed, most normal daily activities and work depend on whole-body function.

CLINICAL CONCEPTS OF DYSFUNCTION

Structure and function are intimately related. The previous section used structure as the starting point to understand disturbed function. Let us now approach the problem from the opposite direction and consider dysfunction per se as a possible explanation for back pain. Once again, let us start from clinical findings and then see if biomechanics and physiology can help to explain them.

Alternative medicine has more than a century of astute clinical observation of the musculoskeletal system. It is worth the effort of trying to integrate this into medical and biomechanical research. Osteopathy, chiropractic, and physical therapy each use different terms and emphasize different features, but they share many underlying ideas about back pain. The key concept is of a painful musculoskeletal dysfunction, which may occur in tissues that are structurally normal. It is a primary dysfunction arising in response to abnormal forces imposed on or generated within the musculoskeletal system. Normal function of the locomotor system includes:

- strength
- endurance
- flexibility
- coordination
- balance.

Dysfunction may involve any or all of these musculoskeletal and neuromuscular functions. Abnormal muscle function, abnormal forces acting on musculoskeletal structures, abnormal posture, or abnormal joint movement may all produce pain.

Chapman-Smith (2000) gave a modern chiropractic definition of joint dysfunction:

A motion segment in which alignment, movement integrity, and/or physiologic function are altered, although contact between joint surfaces remains intact ... Dysfunction in the musculoskeletal system may, of course, be in many tissues – muscles, connective tissue, fascia, ligaments ... Joint dysfunction has been given emphasis because of its central importance in chiropractic principle and practice.

DiGiovanna & Schiowitz (1991) gave a similar, osteopathic definition of somatic dysfunction: "Somatic dysfunction is an impaired or altered function of related components of the somatic (body framework) system: Skeletal, arthrodial and myofascial structures, and related vascular, lymphatic, and neural elements." The focus is on change in the normal functioning of a joint, or, in the case of the spine, a motion segment. It is implicit that it is a type of lesion suitable for manipulation.

These are clinical definitions, which then incorporate possible pathologic mechanisms. DiGiovanna &

Schiowitz (1991) based diagnosis of dysfunction on clinical criteria:

- *Asymmetry or vertebral malposition.* The vertebrae may lie in an asymmetric position compared with normal and the neighboring vertebrae. This is still within the normal range.
- *Restriction of movement.* Movement may be painful, stiff, limited, or abnormal. There may be barriers to normal movement, in one or more planes. The physiologic barrier is the functional limit to the range of active movement. Further passive movement may be possible. The anatomic barrier is the limit of passive movement. This restriction is due to bone, ligament, or tendon. Overcoming the anatomic barrier requires disruption of tissue.
- *Tissue changes.* There are palpable changes in the skin, fascia, or muscle around the affected joint.

MacDonald (1988a, b) gave a more extensive list of possible dysfunctions (Box 9.4). Many of these clinical findings may fit a motion segment, or segmental dysfunction at one or more levels, e.g.:

- altered patterns of movement
- altered muscle function
- soft-tissue changes due to changed autonomic function
- neurophysiologic changes
- psychophysiologic changes.

These are all integral elements of the one functional unit. Dysfunction may affect them all, perhaps to varying degrees, no matter how or where the problem started. Nociception may come from mechanoreceptors in stressed tissues or chemical changes in muscle (Williams 1997).

Altered patterns of movement

Early concepts of vertebrae or disks actually being out of place are now largely discredited. They placed too much emphasis on anatomy and structural pathology for which there is little evidence. Many manual therapists still focus on limitation of movement, but this is also now under question. We saw in Chapter 8 that the range of lumbar flexion is more or less normal in patients with chronic low back pain. Burton et al (1989, 1990) questioned the role of simple limitation of movement in back

---

Box 9.4 Musculoskeletal dysfunction (after MacDonald 1988a, b, with permission)

- Abnormalities of posture
- Abnormalities of joint movement
  - limited movement
  - hypermobility
  - abnormal patterns of movement
  - acute joint-locking (Droz-Georget 1980)
- Muscle
  - fatigue
  - weakness
  - tension: stress/anxiety
  - shortening, stretching
  - reflex muscle spasm
- Connective tissue (fascia, ligaments, joint capsule, muscle)
  - adhesions, scarring, contracture
  - "trigger points"
  - "fibrositis"
- Neuromuscular incoordination
  - muscle imbalance
  - abnormal patterns of movement
- Altered proprioceptor and nociceptor input and neurophysiologic processing

---

pain, whether segmental or total. The range of movement is one of the crudest measures of spinal function, and may miss the point. We need to consider more complex, *dynamic patterns of movement.*

Clinically, it may be possible to palpate altered patterns of movement at one or more segmental levels, either individually or in relation to each other. There may be postural disturbance with abnormal resting position of the vertebrae. There may be hyper- or hypomobility, or lack of joint play. The quality of joint movement may vary, with crepitus or altered end feel, or there may be locking. Palpation of these abnormalities may produce tenderness or pain.

Altered muscle function

Palpable changes in segmental and limb muscles in rheumatic conditions have been known for several centuries. These include hyper- or hypotonicity, fibrotic tissue, atrophy, or hypertrophy. The

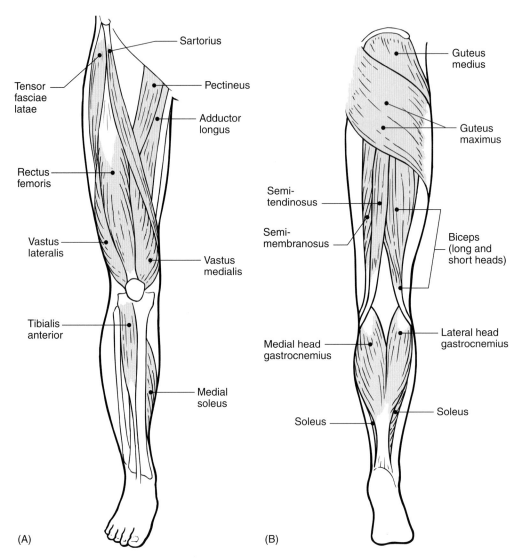

Figure 9.6 The site of tender motor points in the lower limb muscles. (A) Anterior aspect. (B) Posterior aspect. From Gunn & Milbrandt (1976), with permission.

muscle may contract or relax in response to movement. It may be possible to palpate focal areas of muscle spasm or contracture. When they are tender and painful, these are sometimes described as trigger points. In the limb muscles, these tender areas correspond to motor points (Fig. 9.6). There is little doubt about such clinical observations, though there is heated debate about their interpretation. Some medical studies suggest these clinical findings are unreliable, although that may simply reflect the lack of training and skill of physicians.

Strender et al (1997) have shown that trained manual therapists can assess such findings reliably, even if physicians cannot. Terms such as increased muscle tone, spasm, or contracture are often used loosely and interchangably. Few examiners attempt to differentiate connective tissue changes and neuromuscular effects. Pseudopathologic diagnoses include muscular rheumatism, fibrositis, or myofasciitis, to name but a few. Attempts to find an anatomic basis for trigger points have failed, consistent with disturbed physiology rather than structural pathology.

This has all led to great confusion about the nature and meaning of these findings, but does not deny their existence or importance. Logically, altered muscle tone and abnormalities of muscle function must be key elements in movement disorders.

Some of the most tender sites are the junctions of muscle, tendon, intermuscular septum, ligament, or capsule with periosteum and bone. This is because these sites are rich in nociceptors. Increased muscle tension or contracture may stress these sensitive areas. Foci of hyperirritable tissue may give myofascial, cutaneous, fascial, ligamentous, or periosteal trigger points.

Grieve (1981) suggested that dysfunction often involves muscle imbalance, which may give typical clinical patterns of postural disturbance. For example, there may be tightness of the erector spinae, iliopsoas, and hamstrings, with weakness of the abdominal muscles, glutei, and anterior tibial muscles. This produces increased lumbar lordosis, and limitation of hip and knee extension. He pointed out that postural and phasic muscles are often antagonistic. Slow fibers tend to become tight and shortened; fast fibers tend to weakness. Hypertrophy and atrophy can occur at the same time in antagonistic muscles. Increased activity of the more postural muscle may mechanically limit the range of movement of its antagonist, and also inhibit that more phasic muscle. To exaggerate this, a sedentary lifestyle leads to overuse of postural muscles, while phasic muscles become weak with disuse. This may all lead to shortening of the postural muscles and stretching of the phasic muscle. Muscle imbalance may cause abnormal loads on joints and other structures, abnormal patterns of movement, muscle fatigue, and loss of coordination.

Soft-tissue changes

DiGiovanna & Schiowitz (1991) listed a wide range of palpable changes in tissue texture, which form an important diagnostic tool. These vary between acute and chronic back pain (Table 9.4). Disturbed autonomic function causes trophic changes in the skin and subcutaneous tissues of the spinal segment (Gunn & Milbrandt 1978). Vasomotor effects cause local change in the temperature of the skin – vasoconstriction usually makes the skin palpably colder. Sudomotor effects cause increased sweating. The

Table 9.4 Tissue texture changes in acute and chronic somatic dysfunctions

Characteristic	Acute	Chronic
Temperature	Increased	Slight increase or decrease
Texture	Boggy, more rough	Thin, smooth
Moisture	Increased	Dry
Tension	Increased, rigid, board-like	Slight increase, ropy, stringy
Tenderness	Greatest	Present but less
Edema	Yes	No
Erythema test	Redness lasts	Redness fades quickly or blanching

From DiGiovannia & Schiowitz (1991), with permission.
Bogginess is a palpable sense of sponginess in the tissue, probably due to edema.
Ropiness is a palpable cord or string-like feeling.
Stringiness is a palpable tissue texture characterized by fine or string-like myofascial structures.

pilomotor reflex is often hyperactive to produce visible "goose bumps." These changes may affect a dermatome or a local band of skin innervated by the posterior primary ramus. They may be transient, and appear only when the patient undresses to expose the skin to cold, or in response to painful stimuli.

These autonomic changes also lead to subcutaneous skin edema or trophedema. The skin is tight with loss of wrinkles, and the consistency of the subcutaneous tissues is firmer. Gently squeezing an area of skin and subcutaneous tissue produces a *peau d'orange* effect (Fig. 9.7).

THE BIOMECHANICS AND PHYSIOLOGY OF DYSFUNCTION

What basic science evidence is there to support physiologic dysfunction as the basis of back pain?

Abnormal mechanical loading

Mechanical loading is good for your back, but abnormal, localized stress concentrations may cause pain in innervated tissues (Adams et al 2002). The loading does not have to be extreme nor cause

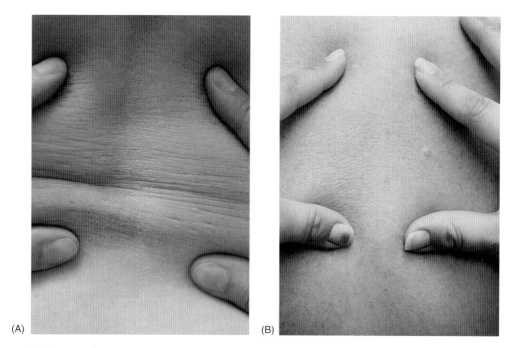

(A)   (B)

Figure 9.7   (A) Trophedema due to disturbed autonomic function in a patient with acute low back pain. (B) Normal. From Dr C C Gunn, with thanks.

tissue damage to produce pain. Relatively small forces can produce pain if concentrated into a small area. Adams et al suggest that if you doubt this, try pricking yourself gently with a pin!

Small changes in posture and spinal loading, particularly over time, might generate stress concentrations. Abnormal posture involves changes in the orientation of adjacent vertebrae. Muscle spasm and high forces in antagonistic muscles increase the compressive forces and loading on the spine. Sustained loading causes creep, which may alter anatomic relationships. Loading, posture, and creep may alter the biomechanical properties, and produce high stress concentrations in the disks, facet joints, and ligaments. However, there is little direct evidence these mechanisms are important in back pain.

Disturbed lumbar motion

Marras et al (1999) studied back motion in 335 patients with chronic low back pain and 374 healthy, asymptomatic subjects. They considered symmetric and asymmetric motion in flexion–extension, lateral bending, and rotation. They not only measured range of motion, but also velocity and acceleration. The emphasis was on the performance of tasks.

Using complex equations that reflect *patterns* of movement, they were able to discriminate patients from healthy subjects with up to 94% accuracy. They found greater differences in velocity and acceleration than in range of motion. Performance was reduced more in asymmetric tasks. Most interesting for the present discussion, they found that motion profiles were very different in low back pain of muscular vs structural origin. They then used these measures to track patients over time and against response to treatment. As pain improved, so did velocity and acceleration (but not range of motion). Patients with persistent pain did not show any such improvement.

Many other studies emphasize the importance of dynamic *patterns* of movement (Esola et al 1996, Steffen et al 1997). There may be change in the balance of lumbar and pelvic movements, or between flexion and extension. There may be different mobility in the upper and lower lumbar spine. Spinal movement occurs in three dimensions and there may be complex changes in coupled movements. Perhaps most important of all is what happens during movement and how the various musculoskeletal components work and interact, even if that is more difficult to measure.

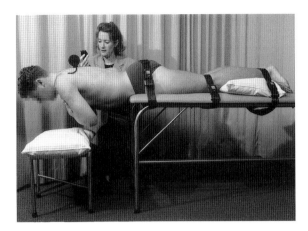

Figure 9.8   Clinical testing of muscle endurance using the Biering–Sorensen test. From Latimer et al 1999 Spine 24(20): 2087. With permission.

Davis et al (2002) studied how mental processes can affect spinal movement and loading. They measured spinal loads in 60 subjects, and the impact of simple or complex mental decisions before or during lifting. They found that simultaneous, more complex, and faster decisions led to poorer muscle coordination and greater loads on the spine. They suggested this might be a mechanism by which greater psychosocial stress could increase biomechanical load and the risk of injury or dysfunction.

Disturbed muscle function

Isokinetic and isoinertial studies provide objective, dynamic measurement of trunk strength during movement (Mayer & Gatchel 1988). These measures are reliable and valid (Newton et al 1993). They show clearly that patients with low back pain have reduced strength compared with normal, asymptomatic subjects (Fig. 18.5, Ch. 18). These tests can monitor clinical progress. At least in theory, they can provide information to direct rehabilitation to meet individual needs.

There are many studies showing loss of muscle endurance associated with low back pain. Biering-Sorensen (1984) described the most widely used clinical test (Fig. 9.8). Most studies show that it is reliable and it differentiates patients with low back pain and normal, asymptomatic subjects (Latimer et al 1999). Once again, it can monitor clinical progress and rehabilitation.

These clinical tests of strength and endurance suffer the same limitation we discussed in Chapter 8. To what extent do they reflect physiologic dysfunction or performance? One possible way round this is to record objective electrical activity in muscles. (Though, like any measure of muscle activity, it still depends ultimately on what people are *doing* with their muscles.)

Marras et al (1999) and Adams et al (2002) reviewed the extensive EMG studies in back pain. These show various disturbances in electrical activity:

- increased muscle tension and spinal loading
- asymmetric muscle activity
- altered reflexes
- loss of the normal flexion–relaxation response
- muscle deficiency
- more rapid muscle fatigue
- loss of neuromuscular coordination.

Muscle spasm is a common clinical observation associated with pain. Pain can produce reflex muscle spasm, and muscle spasm can produce pain, so psychophysiologists hypothesize there might be a pain–spasm–pain cycle. Whatever the initial cause of back pain, continued pain may be associated with increased muscle tension.

Flor and her colleagues (Flor et al 1990, Flor & Birbaumer 1994) reviewed the evidence on muscle tension. Some studies show that EMG activity in the erector spinae is higher in patients with back pain, both standing and sitting. Increased muscle tension during physical or psychological stress is probably more important than baseline activity. Increased muscle tension is local to patients' symptoms: in patients with back pain, raised muscle tension occurs in the paraspinal muscles but not in other parts of the body. It only occurs with pain or stress relevant to the individual. Muscle hyperactivity may continue after the stimulus stops, and only return slowly to baseline levels. Previous experience may lead to faster development and slower decay of the response. However, there are many limitations to this evidence. Any increase in static EMG activity in chronic low back pain is so small it is of doubtful clinical significance. The concept of pain–spasm–pain is simple and attractive, but there is little evidence that static muscle tension plays a direct role in low back pain (Roland 1986, Lund et al 1991, Orbach & McCall 1996).

This led Orbach & McCall (1996) to think about possible indirect effects of muscle tension. Even slight increases in muscle tension could be enough to reduce resting muscle length. This may start as a mechanism to protect against painful movement. Attempts to move, and so stretch the muscle, could lead to increased muscle proprioception, and muscle contraction to guard against that movement.

However, the physiologic evidence suggests that "muscle deficiency" is more important than muscle tension (Lund et al 1991, Cassisi et al 1993). This includes lower muscle strength, less total electrical activity, faster fatigue, and lower endurance. The key may be that muscles *work*, and dynamic testing is more relevant than any static findings. Also, these hypotheses are not mutually exclusive. Muscle deficiency and guarded movement may go together.

Lund et al (1991) suggested a pain-adaptation model:

- reduced maximum voluntary force
- reduced velocity and amplitude of movement
- increased antagonist activity
- reduced agonist activity.

They also questioned whether this dysfunction was a cause or effect of pain.

We now have much more EMG evidence. Adams et al (2002) showed that there can be large asymmetries in EMG activity in the muscles of patients with back pain (Fig. 9.9). One of the best documented muscle abnormalities in chronic low back pain is loss of the normal flexion–relaxation response (Ahern et al 1988, 1990, Watson et al 1997). As we have already noted, in normal people the extensor muscles go through a period of electrical silence during forward flexion. In patients with back pain, this period of muscle relaxation is reduced or even absent (Fig. 9.10).

Rapid forward bending causes reflex contraction of the extensor muscles to decelerate the upper body. Once again, this seems to involve the multifidus in particular. Adams et al (2002) reviewed the limited evidence that loss or inhibition of such reflexes might occur in back pain.

There is evidence of other disturbed neuromuscular function in patients with low back pain. Patients with low back pain have poorer position sense, possibly due to reduced paraspinal proprioception (Brumagne et al 2000, Newcomer et al 2000). Position sense deteriorates with fatigue

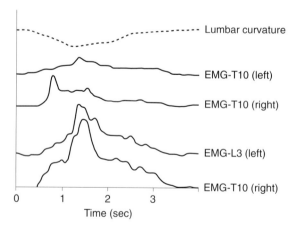

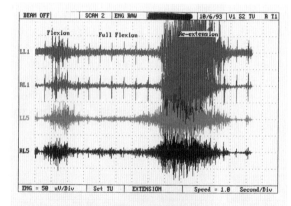

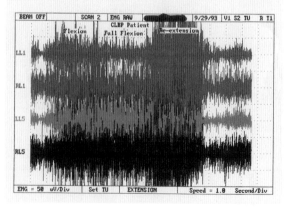

Figure 9.9 Asymmetric electromyogram activity during forward flexion in a patient with acute low back pain. From Adams et al (2002), with permission.

Figure 9.10 Loss of the normal flexion–relaxation response. From Dr P Watson, with thanks.

(Taimela et al 1999). Contraction of the transversus is delayed in patients with low back pain, and this might reflect inefficient stabilization (Hodges & Richardson 1996, 1998).

These muscle and EMG findings are objective, physiologic changes. They correspond to changes in muscle strength, fatigue, and endurance, which must therefore reflect physical dysfunction.

However, Main & Watson (1996) suggested a broader perspective on abnormal patterns of movement and muscle activity. They might start as a reflex response to pain, but then persist as physiologic dysfunction. This may correspond to clinical concepts of *guarded movement*. Abnormal patterns of movement and muscle activity may represent physiologic dysfunction, but guarded movements might also become a learned, protective habit (Box 9.5). These patterns improve with natural recovery (Haig et al 1993), rehabilitation (Ahern et al 1988), or a pain management program (Main & Watson 1995).

Studies in gait biomechanics suggest that limping may be another form of guarded movement. Keefe & Hill (1985) showed that patients with chronic low back pain walk more slowly, with shorter steps and asymmetric gait patterns. Limping again bears little relation to the severity of pain, but more to anticipation of pain and pain behavior.

Deconditioning

Health and fitness depend on continued use: "use it or lose it." Normal musculoskeletal function depends on movement, physical activity, and regular exercise. These are essential for the development, maintenance, and continued function of the musculoskeletal system throughout life. They stimulate and maintain bone and muscle mass and strength, aid nutrition, help to maintain articular cartilage and joint range, and improve endurance and coordination. They promote neuromuscular function and increase pain tolerance.

Disuse is bad for the human frame. Prolonged immobilization leads to deterioration of the musculoskeletal, cardiovascular, and central nervous systems. The ill effects of prolonged bed rest are a standard part of student teaching (Box 9.6). Bortz (1984) coined the term disuse syndrome. Mayer & Gatchel (1988) called it the deconditioning syndrome.

Most people with ordinary backache have much less extreme degrees of deconditioning, but the general principle is the same. Reduced activity, of any degree, causes loss of functional capacity. "Use it or lose it" applies just the same. The more severe systemic effects do not usually occur, although patients with severe, chronic back pain do lose some cardiovascular fitness. The more common and important effects are reduced and guarded movements, loss of muscle strength and endurance, and stiffness.

Box 9.5   Physical dysfunction

- Abnormal patterns of movement
- Abnormal patterns of muscle activity
- Abnormal patterns of neurophysiologic activity
- Disturbed posture and gait
- Abnormal patterns of physical activity and behavior

Box 9.6   Effects of prolonged bed rest

- Catabolic, poor tissue nutrition, depressed metabolism
- Progressive loss of bone mineral and bone strength
- Stiffness due to loss of joint and soft-tissue mobility, connective tissue contracture, fibrosis, and adhesions
- Muscle wasting, 3% loss of muscle strength per day, decrease in time to fatigue, reduced endurance
- Loss of neuromuscular coordination and balance
- Ligaments lose strength
- Poorer healing, increased scar tissue formation
- Systemic effects
  - loss of cardiovascular fitness
  - anemia and thrombosis
  - respiratory and renal stagnation
  - endocrine changes
  - immune system, lowered resistance
- Loss of sensory and mental acuity
- Psychological distress, depression
- Lower pain tolerance

Physical inactivity produces muscle deficiency and atrophy. The proportion of contractile tissue falls and the relative proportion of collagen rises. If a muscle is immobilized in a shortened position, it becomes stiffer, less extensible, and contracted. Muscle strength and endurance deteriorate rapidly. Joints become stiffer, partly due to changes in the muscles, but also due to connective tissue changes and joint capsule adhesions.

In patients with chronic low back pain, the erector spinae muscles are atrophied and contain an increased percentage of fat (Mooney et al 1997, Fig. 9.11). Hides et al (1994) found local wasting in the multifidus muscle, with 30% reduction in cross-sectional area. The changes were segmental and unilateral, and corresponded to the level and side of symptoms. Because this wasting was so localized and developed so rapidly, Hides et al suggested that it might be due to segmental inhibition rather than to a general effect of disuse. Acute low back pain usually resolves, but recurrent attacks are common. Even when symptoms settle, multifidus wasting may not recover spontaneously, and this might predispose to recurrence.

At the time of writing, I am aware of two randomized controlled trials of stabilizing exercises, although there are only preliminary results at 6 months. Goldby et al (2000) found some pain relief in 183 patients with chronic low back pain.

Cairns et al (2002) found no effect on pain or disability in 97 patients with recurrent low back pain. The jury is still out on the importance of multifidus and spinal stabilizing exercises.

Neurophysiology

We have already looked at how neurophysiologic changes may aggravate and perpetuate pain (Ch. 3). These changes directly affect neuromuscular activity.

Some clinicians call this increased sensitivity "neuropathic pain." Unfortunately, this may imply that the cause of pain is physical damage of a nerve, which is not necessarily correct. The key concept is simply altered neuromuscular activity – what osteopaths called the facilitated segment. There is hypersensitivity of joints and, indeed, the entire motion segment to mechanical strain and movement. Normal afferent input from mechanoreceptors may be interpreted as pain. Musculoskeletal structures may become tender to gentle pressure, and normal movements may become painful. These inputs may also lead to reflex response in muscle and autonomic activity.

This also leads to reprogramming of neuromuscular control. The central nervous system "learns" new patterns of posture, locomotion, and activities of daily living. These patterns of motor behavior become fixed and self-perpetuating.

The origin of dysfunction

From this point of view, the present state of dysfunction is more important than any original cause. Dysfunction depends on imbalance between physical stresses and individual vulnerabilities, and their interaction over time (Fig. 9.12). This imbalance may be triggered by increased physical stress, such as increased loading, or increased or unaccustomed activity. But there does not have to be an

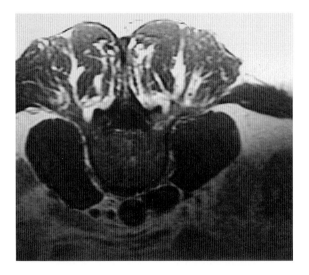

Figure 9.11 Multifidus muscle wasting in a patient with chronic low back pain. From Dr V Mooney, with thanks.

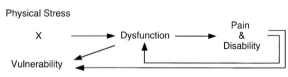

Figure 9.12 The origins of dysfunction. From Manual medicine, Osteopathic diagnosis of back pain, MacDonald R S, 3: 110–113, Fig. 2, 1988b, with kind permission from Springer-Verlag.

external cause. Any stress may increase vulnerability. Fatigue, lack of fitness, postural abnormalities, faulty movement patterns, and abnormal loads may cause imbalance and hence dysfunction. It may be only a question of degree when the normal bodily sensation of normal function becomes the discomfort or pain of dysfunction. Whatever the initial trigger, both physiologic change and change in the pattern of activity then occur, and dysfunction might become self-perpetuating.

If you still have difficulty accepting the concept of pain due to disturbed function without any structural damage, try a few simple experiments for yourself:

- *Observation 1.* Lift a weight of a few pounds (1–2 kg) in your hand and stretch your arm out at shoulder height. Hold it there. After a few minutes it begins to hurt. The weight gets heavier and heavier. The pain spreads down the muscles of your shoulder and arm. You may try different ways of coping with the pain, but sooner or later you have no choice: you lower your arm and put down the weight.

- *Observation 2.* Rest your left elbow on a table with your forearm upright. Extend your wrist and your fingers. Use your right hand to hyperextend your left middle finger as far as it will go. Hold it there. After a few minutes, your finger and then your hand and wrist become painful. Sooner or later the pain makes you release the finger and let it relax to a more normal position.

- *Observation 3.* Cramp is a good example of muscululoskeletal dysfunction. It can be very painful and disabling. The acute pain persists till we manage to break the reflex arc.

- Observation 4. If we attempt prolonged strenuous exercise when we are unfit, our muscles and joints ache. If we measure them, we find the muscles are swollen. The ache may take several days to settle.

These are all examples of pain from normal muscles and joints. You do not need structural damage. It is pain from musculoskeletal dysfunction. As a final analogy, if your electric kettle breaks down, you send for an electrician to fix the hardware. If your PC goes wrong, it is more likely to be a software problem.

This concept of dysfunction also helps us deal with the vexed question of the duration of back pain. One of the strongest criticisms of the diagnosis of a soft-tissue sprain or strain is that injury would normally be followed by healing. So symptoms should settle over expected tissue healing time. If the problem is dysfunction, however, that may be self-sustaining. So symptoms can persist indefinitely for as long as dysfunction continues. McGill (2002) described this nicely as "lingering deficits." But the other important implication is that dysfunction does not involve any permanent change, so it is always reversible. Even if dysfunction and symptoms can persist indefinitely, there is always the potential for recovery by restoring normal function.

Ability or performance?

We have still not fully resolved the recurring question about physical dysfunction. To what extent is it loss of physical capacity and ability, and how much is it a matter of performance? There is no question that there are objective physical changes in the muscles and backs of patients with low back pain (certainly by the chronic stage and probably from a much earlier stage). But much of what we measure clinically and biomechanically is performance. (Loss of) physical ability and physical performance go together and we can never separate them completely.

In an award-winning study, Mannion and her colleagues looked at the biomechanical effects of rehabilitation (Mannion et al 1999, 2001a, b, Kaser et al 2001). This was a randomized controlled trial of 148 patients with chronic low back pain. It compared active physiotherapy, muscle reconditioning on training devices, and low-impact aerobics. Pain intensity, frequency, and disability improved after all three treatments and these effects were maintained on 6-month follow-up. However, there was little difference between the three treatments.

There was a small improvement in the range of lumbar motion following treatment, but this only correlated weakly with improved pain and disability. Isometric strength and EMG activity increased after treatment, though the correlation between them was weak. Fifty-five percent of patients had loss of the normal flexion–relaxation response at baseline, but this did not improve following treatment. Endurance in the Biering-Sorensen test improved after treatment, but there was no corresponding improvement in EMG measures of fatigability. At baseline, the cross-sectional area of the paraspinal muscles and the fiber types correlated with isometric strength. Following treatment, there was little change in muscle size or fiber type. Improvement in strength did not correlate with any changes in muscle size. Altogether, physical changes in the muscles were insufficient to account for the observed improvement in muscle performance.

Treatment was clearly effective, but treatment effects appeared to be non-specific. Mannion et al (1999, 2001b) concluded that active therapy could improve physical function, but this was not due to direct improvement in muscle deficiency. Instead, the undoubted clinical improvement was mainly a matter of improved performance. Improvement in pain and disability depended more on changed perceptions and behavior. We might add that persisting muscle deficiency could explain the high recurrence rate of back pain.

AN EXPLANATION FOR PATIENTS

The reason why disk injuries are so popular is that the idea is easy to understand, plausible, and acceptable to patients. It is amazing how many people with ordinary backache believe they have a "disk out of place" or "worn disks," with or without "trapped nerves." These ideas carry all the implications about permanent damage, fear of reinjury, and the need to rest or get fixed. We desperately need an equally simple, plausible, and acceptable explanation that fits modern understanding of the physical basis of back pain. It must also support modern ideas of management. Let me try to use the ideas in this chapter to develop an alternative explanation suitable for patients.

First, back pain is a physical problem. Psychosocial factors may influence how we react to pain and how it affects us, but they do not cause the pain. Back pain is not a psychological problem. Back pain starts with a physical problem in the back.

Second, back pain is a mechanical problem. It is a movement disorder or an activity-related disorder of the musculoskeletal system.

Third, back pain is only a symptom, not a disease. The most important message is that most back pain is not a signal of any serious disease or damage to the back.

Fourth, most back pain is simply a symptom of physical dysfunction. Pain and disability are intimately related to each other. The back is not working as it should. It is out of condition, like a car engine that is out of tune. This involves all the elements of dysfunction that we have discussed. Posture may be poor. The back is not moving normally, but may be stiff or seized up. This leads to fear and guarded movements. The muscles are not working properly, but may be weak and wasted and tire easily. There may be loss of strength and endurance and coordination. Loss of fitness makes it harder to rehabilitate. Changes in the nervous system lead to increased sensitivity, which together with stress and tension leads to a vicious circle. This whole pattern of painful dysfunction is the core of the problem and becomes self-perpetuating. It is much more important that any original, long-gone trigger for the pain.

Finally, this has obvious implications for management. The original cause or site of the pain really does not matter much any more. Whatever the original trigger, pain will continue as long as there is dysfunction. Recovery and relief of pain depend on getting the back working again and restoring normal function. The answer is to get moving. This leads to a sports medicine analogy, and sports medicine principles of rehabilitation. It also depends very much on the patient taking responsibility for what he or she does, rather than depending on a doctor or therapist to "fix it."

Summary

An explanation for patients
- Back pain is a symptom, not a disease. Most back pain is not due to any serious disease or damage in your back
- Back pain is usually a symptom of *physical dysfunction*. Your back is simply not moving and working as it should. It is unfit or out of condition
- Recovery and relief of pain depend on getting your back moving and working again and restoring normal function

CONCLUSION

I am well aware that we have limited scientific evidence for many of the ideas in this chapter, but they are firmly based on clinical observation. Some are unproven hypotheses. In many areas the evidence is limited or conflicting. There are large gaps in the evidence. However, I have argued already that we must seek the basic science that helps to explain our clinical findings, instead of trying to force our patients to fit basic science.

It is encouraging that so many health professionals from such different backgrounds have reached so much common ground – and that it fits modern neurophysiology and functional biomechanics. Dysfunction is a potentially rich but as yet untapped mine of knowledge. We still need much basic science and clinical research to develop and test these ideas. We should look more closely at the soft tissues and their physiology, at physical dysfunction and the effects of inactivity. We must integrate clinical, biomechanical, and physical performance findings and concepts. I believe the traditional search for anatomic sites and structural causes of pain is simply inappropriate for non-specific low back pain. That is why it has failed. More physiologic concepts of dysfunction hold much greater promise.

References

Adams M A, Bogduk N, Burton K, Dolan P 2002 The biomechanics of back pain. Churchill Livingstone, Edinburgh

Ahern D K, Follick M J, Council J R et al 1988 Comparison of lumbar intervertebral EMG patterns in chronic low back pain patients and non-pain controls. Pain 34: 153–160

Ahern D K, Hannon D J, Goreczny A J et al 1990 Correlation of chronic low back pain behaviour and muscle function examination of the flexion–relaxation response. Spine 15: 92–95

Arendt-Nielsen L, Graven-Nielsen T, Drewes A M 1998 Referred pain and hyperalgesia related to muscle and visceral pain. International Association for the Study of Pain, Seattle. IASP Newsletter January/February 3–6

Bergmark A 1989 Stability of the spine: a study in mechanical engineering. Acta Orthopaedica Scandinavica 60 (suppl): 20–24

Biering-Sorensen F 1984 Physical measurements as risk indicators for low back trouble over a one year period. Spine 9: 106–119

Bogduk N, Twomey L T 1991 Clinical anatomy of the lumbar spine. Churchill Livingstone, New York

Boos N, Semmer N, Elfering A et al 2000 Psychosocial factors and not MRI-based disk abnormalities predict future low-back pain-related medical consultation and work absence. Spine 25: 1484–1492

Borenstein D G, O'Mara J W, Boden S D et al 2001 The value of magnetic resonance imaging of the lumbar spine to predict low back pain in asymptomatic individuals. Journal of Bone and Joint Surgery 83A: 1306–1311

Bortz W M 1984 The disuse syndrome. Western Journal of Medicine 141: 691–694

Brumagne S, Cordo P, Lysens R, Verschueren S, Swinnen S 2000 The role of paraspinal muscle spindles in lumbosacral position sense in individuals with and without low back pain. Spine 25: 989–994

Buckwalter J A 1995 Spine update: aging and degeneration of the human intervertebral disk. Spine 20: 1307–1314

Burton A K, Tillotson K M, Troup J D G 1989 Variation in lumbar sagittal mobility with low back trouble. Spine 14: 584–590

Burton A K, Tillotson K M, Edwards V A, Sykes D A 1990 Lumbar sagittal mobility and low back symptoms in patients treated with manipulation. Journal of Spinal Disorders 3: 262–268

Cairns M C, Foster N E, Wright C C 2002 Prospective, pragmatic RCT examining the effectiveness of spinal stabilisation exercises in the management of recurrent lumbar spinal pain and dysfunction: 6-month results. Poster presentation. Fifth International Forum for Primary Care Research on Low Back Pain. Montreal May 10–11, 2002

Cassisi J E M, Robinson M E, O'Connor P, MacMillan M 1993 Trunk strength and lumbar paraspinal muscle activity during isometric exercise in chronic low-back pain patients and controls. Spine 18: 245–251

Chapman-Smith D 2000 The chiropractic profession: its education, practice, research and future directions. NCMIC Group, West Des Moines, Iowa

Danneels L A, Vanderstraeten G G, Cambier D C et al 2001 A functional subdivision of hip, abdominal and back muscles during asymmetric lifting. Spine 26: E114–E121

Davis K G, Marras W S, Heaney C A, Waters T R, Gupta P 2002 The impact of mental processing and pacing on spine loading. Spine 27: 2645–2653

DiGiovanna E L, Schiowitz S (eds) 1991 An osteopathic approach to diagnosis and treatment. Lippincott, Philadelphia

Droz-Georget J H 1980 High velocity thrust and pathophysiology of segmental dysfunction. British Osteopathic Journal 12: 2–17

Esola M A, McClure P W, Fitzgerald G K, Siegler S 1996 Analysis of lumbar spine and hip motion during forward bending in subjects with and without a history of low back pain. Spine 21: 71–78

Fiddler M 1980 Back pain without direct nerve root involvement. Unpublished report to ISSLS

Flor H, Birbaumer N 1994 Acquisition of chronic pain: psychophysiological mechanisms. American Pain Society Journal 3: 119–127

Flor H, Birbaumer N, Turk D C 1990 The psychobiology of chronic pain. Advances in Behavioural Research and Therapy 12: 47–84

Goldby L, Moore A, Doust J, Trew M, Lewis J 2000 A randomised controlled trial investigating the efficacy of manual therapy, exercises to rehabilitate spinal stabilisation and an education booklet in the conservative treatment of chronic low back pain: preliminary results on 183 patients. Presented at the 7th Scientific Conference of the International Federation of Orthopaedic Manipulative Therapists Perth Australia November 6–10, 2000

Grieve G P 1981 Common vertebral joint problems. Churchill Livingstone, Edinburgh, pp 112–121

Gunn C C, Milbrandt W E 1976 Tenderness at motor points. A diagnostic and prognostic aid for low back injury. Journal of Bone and Joint Surgery 58A: 815–825

Gunn C C, Milbrandt W E 1978 Early and subtle signs in low back sprain. Spine 3: 267–281

Haig A J, Weisman G, Haugh L D, Pope M, Grobler L 1993 Prospective evidence for change in paraspinal muscle activity after herniated nucleus pulposis. Spine 18: 926–930

Hides J A, Stokes M J, Saide M, Jull G A, Cooper D H 1994 Evidence of lumbar multifidus muscle wasting ipsilateral to symptoms in patients with acute/subacute low back pain. Spine 19: 165–172

Hodges P W, Richardson C A 1996 Inefficient muscular stabilization of the lumbar spine associated with low back pain. A motor control evaluation of transversus abdominis. Spine 21: 2640–2650

Hodges P W, Richardson C A 1998 Delayed postural contraction of transversus abdominis in low back pain associated with movement of the lower limb. Journal of Spinal Disorders 11: 46–56

Jackson R P, Jacobs R R, Montesano P X 1988 Facet joint injection in low-back pain. A prospective statistical study. Spine 13: 966–971

Jarvik J G, Deyo R A 2000 Imaging of lumbar intervertebral disk degeneration and aging, excluding disk herniation. Radiological Clinics of North America 38: 1255–1266

Kaser L, Mannion A F, Rhyner A et al 2001 Active therapy for chronic low back pain. Part 2. Effects on paraspinal muscle cross-sectional area, fiber type size and distribution. Spine 26: 909–919

Keefe F, Hill W 1985 An objective approach to quantifying pain behavior and gait patterns in low back pain patients. Pain 21: 153–161

Kellgren J H 1938 Observations on referred pain arising from muscle. Clinical Science 3: 175–190

Kellgren J H 1939 On the distribution of pain arising from deep somatic structures with charts of segmental pain areas. Clinical Science 4: 35–46

Latimer J, Maher C G, Refshauge K, Colaco I 1999 The reliability and validity of the Biering–Sorensen test in asymptomatic subjects and subjects reporting current or previous non-specific low back pain. Spine 24(20): 2085–2089

Lilius G, Lassonen E M, Myllynen P, Harilainen A, Gronlund G 1989 Lumbar facet joint syndrome. A randomised clinical trial. Journal of Bone and Joint Surgery 71B: 681–684

Lund J P, Donga R, Widmer C G, Stohler C S 1991 The pain-adaptation model: a discussion of the relationship between chronic musculoskeletal pain and motor activity. Canadian Journal of Physiology and Pharmacology 6: 683–694

MacDonald R S 1988a Primary dysfunction of the spine. Holistic Medicine 3: 27–33

MacDonald R S 1988b Osteopathic diagnosis of back pain. Manual Medicine 3: 110–113

Main C J, Watson P J 1995 Screening for patients at risk of developing chronic incapacity. Journal of Occupational Rehabilitation 5: 207–217

Main C J, Watson P J 1996 Guarded movements: development of chronicity. Journal of Musculoskeletal Pain 4: 163–170

Mannion A F, Muntener M, Taimela S, Dvorak J 1999 A randomized clinical trial of three active therapies for chronic low back pain. Spine 24: 2435–2448

Mannion A F, Taimela S, Muntener M, Dvorak J 2001a Active therapy for chronic low back pain: part 1. Effects on back muscle activation, fatigability and strength. Spine 26: 897–908

Mannion A F, Junge A, Taqimela S et al 2001b Active therapy for chronic low back pain: part 3. Factors influencing self-rated disability and its change following therapy. Spine 26: 920–929

Marras W S, Ferguson S A, Gupta P et al 1999 The quantification of low back disorder using motion measures: methodology and validation. Spine 24: 2091–2100

Mayer T G, Gatchel R J 1988 Functional restoration for spinal disorders: the sports medicine approach. Lea & Febiger, Philadelphia

McGill S 2002 Low back disorders: evidence based prevention and rehabilitation. Human Kinetics, Champaign, Illinois

Mooney V, Gulick J, Perlman M et al 1997 Relationships between myoelectric activity, strength, and MRI of extensor muscles in back pain patients and normal subjects. Journal of Spinal Disorders 10: 348–356

Nachemson A, Vingard E 2000 Assessment of patients with neck and back pain: a best-evidence synthesis. In: Nachemson A, Jonsson E (eds) Neck and back pain: the scientific evidence of causes, diagnosis and treatment. Lippincott/Williams & Wilkins, Philadelphia, pp 189–235

Newcomer K L, Laskowski E R, Yu B, Johnson J C, An K-N 2000 Differences in repositioning error among patients with low back pain compared with control subjects. Spine 25: 2488–2493

Newton M, Thom M, Somerville D, Henderson I, Waddell G 1993 Trunk strength testing with iso-machines. Part II. Experimental evaluation of the Cybex II back testing system in normal subjects and patients with chronic low back pain. Spine 18: 812–824

Orbach R, McCall W D 1996 The stress–hyperactivity–pain theory of myogenic pain: proposal for a revised theory. Pain Forum 5: 51–66

Panjabi M M 1992 The stabilizing system of the spine. Part I. Function, dysfunction, adaptation and enhancement. Journal of Spinal Disorders 5: 383–389

Pope M H, Wilder D G, Krag M H 1991 Biomechanics of the lumbar spine: A. basic principles. In: Frymoyer J W (ed.) The adult spine: principles and practice. Raven Press, New York, pp 1487–1501

Riihimaki H, Wickstrom G, Hanninen K, Luopajarvi T 1989 Predictors of sciatic pain among concrete reinforcement workers and house painters – a five-year follow-up. Scandinavian Journal of Work and Environmental Health 15: 415–423

Roland M O 1986 A critical review of the evidence for a pain–spasm–pain cycle in spinal disorders. Clinical Biomechanics 1: 102–109

Savage R A, Whitehouse G H, Roberts N 1997 The relationship between the magnetic resonance imaging appearance of the lumbar spine and low back pain, age and occupation in males. European Spine Journal 2: 106–114

Steffen T, Rubin R K, Baramki H G, Antoniou J, Marchesi D, Aebi M 1997 A new technique of measuring lumbar segmental motion in vivo. Spine 22: 156–166

Strender L-E, Sjoblom A, Sundell K, Ludwig R, Taube A 1997 Inter-examiner reliability in physical examination of patients with low back pain. Spine 22: 814–820

Symmons D P M, van Hemert A M, Vandenbrouke J P, Valkenburg H A 1991a A longitudinal study of back pain and radiological changes in the lumbar spines of middle-aged women. I. Clinical findings. Annals of the Rheumatic Diseases 50: 158–161

Symmons D P M, van Hemert A M, Vandenbrouke J P, Valkenburg H A 1991b A longitudinal study of back pain and radiological changes in the lumbar spines of middle-aged women. II. Radiographic findings. Annals of the Rheumatic Diseases 50: 162–166

Taimela S, Kankaanpaa M, Luoto S 1999 The effect of lumbar fatigue on the ability to sense a change in lumbar position. Spine 24 (13): 1322–1327

Thompson R E, Barker T M, Pearcy M J 2003 Defining the neutral zone of intervertebral joints during dynamic motions. Clinical Biomechanics 18: 89–98

Van Tulder M W, Assendelft W J J, Koes B W, Bouter L M 1997 Spinal radiographic findings and non-specific low back pain. Spine 22: 427–434

Vleeming A, Mooney V, Dorman T, Snijders C, Stoeckart R (eds) 1997 Movement stability and low back pain: the essential role of the pelvis. Churchill Livingstone, New York

Waddell G, Burton A K 2000 Occupational health guidelines for the management of low back pain: evidence review. Faculty of Occupational Medicine, London

Watson P J, Booker C K, Main C J 1997 Surface electromyography in the identification of chronic low back pain patients: the development of the flexion relaxation ratio. Clinical Biomechanics 12: 165–171

Williams N 1997 Managing back pain in general practice – is osteopathy the new paradigm? British Journal of General Practice 47: 653–655

Wiltse L 1971 The effect of common anomalies of the lumbar spine upon disc degeneration and low back pain. Orthopedic Clinics of North America 2: 569–582

Chapter **10**

Illness behavior

We first looked at pain behavior in Chapter 3 on pain and disability. The chapters on epidemiology showed that we must interpret carefully what patients say and do. In all forms of physical assessment, we had to allow for performance. These are all matters of behavior. Illness behavior is a key part of our story and it is time to look at it more closely.

Illness behavior is what people say and do that expresses and communicates that they are ill. It depends on what and how they think about their illness.

We know that someone is ill, not by seeing disease or even by examining them, but by what they say and do. Consciously or unconsciously, we recognize that the way this person behaves is not well but ill.

If we drive past a traffic accident, we might see someone lying on the road in front of a car. From a distance we cannot see his broken leg. What draws our attention is the victim lying in the middle of the road. He is very still. A crowd stands around looking worried and trying to help. We automatically interpret the scene as a road accident and an injured person waiting for help. We do not need to stop and ask what happened or examine his broken leg. We can tell by how he behaves – and how those about him behave.

Your first thought might be that his behavior is simply the physical effect of his broken leg, but that is not the whole story. Suppose he only had a sprained ankle. If you knew this, you might wonder why he was lying in the middle of the road waiting for an ambulance. However, he was knocked down and must have had a terrible fright. His ankle may feel broken and he might be afraid even to try to get up. Bystanders may have told him they had sent for the ambulance and he should not move till help arrives. So his illness behavior may be out of proportion to his physical injury, but it is still easy to understand.

Now consider how two different patients cope with a sprained ankle. Let us suppose that each has a severe sprain with marked swelling and a lot of pain but no fracture or ligament instability. One patient will be completely unable to bear weight and will need crutches for a week or so. The other will laugh or be insulted at the very suggestion of crutches. Instead, he will insist on having the ankle strapped up so that he can try to get ready for an important game of football next weekend. They each have a similar physical injury, but what they do about it is very different.

Now let us move on a year. Suppose that the man with the sprained ankle is still using a cane and unable to work. His ligaments healed long ago, but his ankle is stiff and he has muscle wasting from lack of use. He is very unfit. He may even have some disuse osteoporosis. It is not surprising that his ankle is still painful, but there is no clinical or X-ray evidence of any serious damage. Yet he still spends most of the day sitting or lying about the house. He keeps his ankle warm and supports it on a cushion. He does not go out of the house much, but when he does he uses his cane and is very careful of his ankle. His social life has suffered and his friends rarely visit him to talk about his injured ankle, which is one of his main topics of conversation. He has not really considered going back to work. Indeed, when asked, he seems to be astonished by the question. Is it not obvious that he can't even begin to think about work until his ankle fully recovers? – though he cannot imagine how or when that miraculous event will occur. This whole pattern of illness behavior may have been reasonable for the first few days after the injury, but a year later it is now something more than just the physical effects of his original injury or the present state of his ankle. His pattern of illness behavior and lifestyle of invalidity are now, in themselves, a major part of his disability.

This may seem an extreme and even ridiculous example. You might say that no one becomes permanently crippled by a sprained ankle. Now substitute "back" for ankle, and "strain" for sprain.

Read that story again. That gives you a clinical history that is all too common.

EXAMPLES OF ILLNESS BEHAVIOR IN BACK PAIN

When we meet a friend who has back pain, we know if her back is troubling her again. We can tell by her awkward posture and guarded movements. She fidgets and grimaces and rubs her back. We get the message across the room before we exchange a word and without looking at her back. Not only do we know what is wrong, but the way she behaves gives us some idea of how bad she feels her back is. This is normal. Most illness behavior simply reflects the physical problem. I must stress that *illness behavior is reasonable and normal*.

The fascination of back pain is how different patients react and behave so very differently. Several years ago, purely by chance, I had two patients with back pain in the same ward (Fig. 10.1). The man

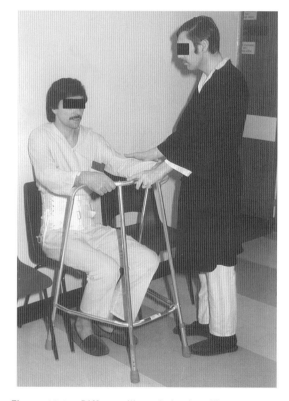

Figure 10.1   Different illness behaviors. The man standing up has just had a surgical biopsy of a spinal infection. The man sitting down was hospitalized as an emergency with ordinary backache.

standing up had a small surgical biopsy of a thoracic vertebra earlier that day. The final histology showed a low-grade infection, but at the time of this photograph we thought it was probably cancer. He had a serious disease in his spine, was in a lot of pain, and thought it was something that would probably kill him. The healthy young man sitting down had a recurrent attack of non-specific low back pain. It was so severe that he had an opioid injection from his family doctor and was hospitalized in the middle of the night. On admission he was so agitated we could hardly examine him. Within a few hours he settled and we could control his pain with non-steroidal anti-inflammatories. There is no question that his back was very painful and he had a lot of muscle spasm, but there was no evidence of any serious spinal disease or nerve root problem. Further tests were all normal. Over the next few days, the man with the spinal infection helped and encouraged the man with ordinary backache on to his feet. He used a walking frame and wore his lumbar support outside his clothes so that everyone could see how bad he was. A few days later, he was able to walk without any aids and went home, while the man with the spinal infection waited for the result of his biopsy to learn whether he would live or die.

This does not mean it is a choice between either physical pathology or a psychological problem. Both these men had a physical problem in their back. Our failure to make a precise diagnosis of non-specific back pain does not mean that the problem is psychological. Nor does physical disease preclude a psychological disturbance, any more than psychological disturbance excludes a treatable physical disease.

Look at two other less common but instructive examples. The first was a 58-year-old woman with many years' history of chronic back pain, invalidity, and depression. She had frequent medical and psychiatric hospitalization with multiple complaints. On this occasion she came in with an overdose of sleeping tablets and depression. Once again, she blamed this on her pain, but it was clear that her long-standing problems were mainly psychiatric rather than physical. When we listened carefully to her story, however, her recent attack of thoracic back pain was different from her usual chronic low back pain. Further investigation showed that she now had widespread breast metastases.

The second example was a 34-year-old man with a long history of psoriatic arthropathy (Fig. 10.2). He had been on systemic steroids for many years. He had severe arthritis of his hips, steroid-induced

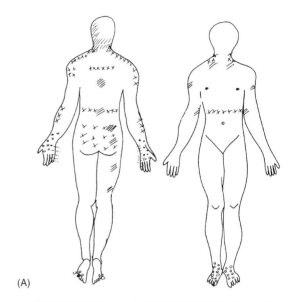

(A)

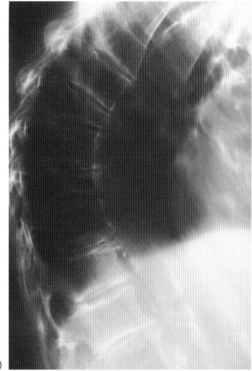

(B)

Figure 10.2 A man of 34 with marked distress and illness behavior (A) who also had severe steroid-induced osteoporosis (B).

osteoporosis, and vertebral collapse. He had a severe spinal deformity and a lot of back pain. He also had considerable psychological problems and depression. He was a very difficult patient who was very angry and uncooperative. He showed a great deal of illness behavior. He was almost completely confined to the house. He was very demanding with his family and much of his family's life revolved around his illness.

- Illness behavior is normal.
- Most patients have both a physical problem in their backs *and* varying degrees of illness behavior.

CLINICAL OBSERVATION OF ILLNESS BEHAVIOR

We were all taught as students to use the clinical history and examination to diagnose disease, but we should also use them to learn about our patients. The great clinicians of the past established their reputations from their skill in differential diagnosis, but they also had an almost uncanny ability to assess patients. Much of their skill was subconscious and they could not explain or teach it. It seemed to come from natural aptitude and long experience. I believe we should all be able to dissect, teach, and learn this vital clinical skill. Perhaps these great clinicians were actually observing illness behavior – they just did not realize what they were doing. Modern professional training is all about the symptoms and signs of disease and we pay little attention to assessing the person. We leave that to clinical impression and assume that we will learn somehow by osmosis and experience. Unfortunately, these impressions are unreliable, and we should instead learn how to assess illness behavior. There are a number of ways of doing this. They form a homogeneous group of clinical observations and tell us a great deal about a patient's illness behavior.

The pain drawing

The pain drawing is the simplest example of illness behavior (Ransford et al 1976). Patients readily record their pain on an outline of the body. They regard it as a simple question about the

physical pattern of their pain. However, the *way* in which they describe their pain also depends on how they react to the pain.

Figure 10.3 shows two pain drawings. Patient A is giving an anatomic description of her S1 pain and paresthesia from a disk prolapse. Patient B is not paraplegic. He also has a disk prolapse, but he is trying to tell us about the severity of his pain and how much he is suffering. This is a cry for help. The simplest signal is the sheer quantity of drawing – how large an area and how densely they fill it in. Pain may be widespread or non-anatomic. It may expand to other areas of the body. It may even spread outside the body outline. Some patients put excessive detail into the drawing. They may add emphasis or comments on the severity of their pain. All these features reflect the patient's psychological state. Thus, the simple pain drawing gives us both physical information about the pain and psychological information about the patient. Once again, these are not alternatives. It is not a question of whether this is a physical drawing or a

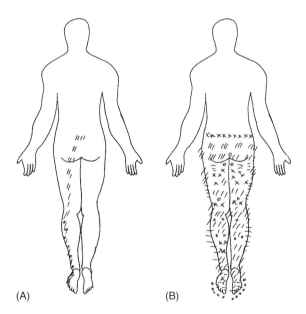

(A)　　　　(B)

Figure 10.3 The pain drawing tells us about the physical and emotional characteristics of the pain. Patient A describes the anatomic pattern of S1 pain and paresthesia from a disk prolapse. Patient B is not paraplegic but also has a disk prolapse. This pain drawing is communicating distress. Many patients do both to varying degrees. //, pain; 0, pins and needles; ×, ache; =, numbness.

psychological drawing. Remember that patients A and B both had a disk prolapse. Both had some degree of emotional reaction to the pain. Most pain drawings include both physical and psychological information, although one or other may dominate the picture. And sometimes, like in patient B, illness behavior may obscure the underlying physical problem.

We may look at the McGill Pain Questionnaire in the same way (Table 3.3). The physical drawing of pain is like the sensory adjectives: shooting, throbbing, and burning. The drawing also shows the emotional characteristics of the pain experience, rather like the emotional adjectives: tiring, sickening, or fearful. In both the questionnaire and the drawing, most patients describe their pain in some mixture of sensory and emotional terms.

We must not overinterpret the pain drawing. It is crude and cannot give a complete psychological profile or diagnosis. That is why I have not described detailed methods of scoring it. All that is important is to recognize that the patient's description of pain includes both sensory and emotional elements. The pain drawing may be the first clue that you should assess this patient in more depth.

However, you cannot rely on the pain drawing alone. Most patients with an exaggerated pain drawing are distressed, but 50% of patients with distress will give a normal pain drawing.

Behavioral symptoms

Clinical diagnosis depends on recognizing common patterns of symptoms and signs. Most patients with back pain describe their symptoms in a way that fits anatomy and mechanics. The symptoms often do not fit exactly, but they do make some kind of physical sense. However, patients occasionally describe their symptoms in a way that does not fit clinical experience. These symptoms are vague and ill-localized. They lack the normal relationship with time and activity. Indeed, they seem to cross anatomic boundaries and contradict normal mechanics.

We tried to find those symptoms that seem to have more to do with illness behavior than physical disease (Waddell et al 1984a, b). We found more than 30 possible symptoms from a literature review and pilot studies in our own Problem Back Clinic. We tested these symptoms carefully. We did reliability studies. We looked at the symptoms in 180 patients with back pain and compared them with normal painfree people. We had to discard many of the symptoms because they were unsatisfactory. Some were too rare for routine use, such as fainting with pain and written lists of symptoms. Some were common in normal people, such as involuntary jumping of the leg. Some were not reproducible between different doctors, such as flattery or manipulative behavior. We then looked to see which symptoms correlated with psychological factors. Our final result was a group of seven non-anatomic or behavioral descriptions of symptoms:

1. *Pain at the tip of the tailbone* (Fig. 10.4). Coccydynia can occur after direct injury. In a patient with non-specific back pain it generally occurs together with other behavioral symptoms.

2. *Whole-leg pain* (Fig. 10.5). The whole leg becomes painful in a stocking distribution. It usually affects a body image segment from the groin down or below the knee. You should distinguish this from the usual pattern of nerve root pain, which at least approximates to a dermatome and does not affect the entire circumference of the leg. Whole-leg pain is also quite different from the sclerotomal pattern of referred leg pain. Do not be confused by multiple nerve root

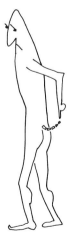

Figure 10.4 Pain at the tip of the tailbone. Drawing by Mr J C Semple, with thanks.

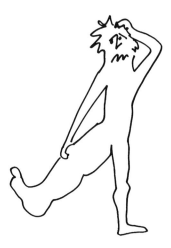

Figure 10.5   Whole-leg pain. Drawing by Mr J C Semple, with thanks.

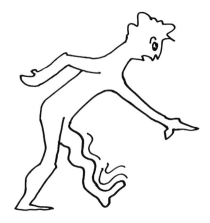

Figure 10.7   Whole leg giving way. Drawing by Mr J C Semple, with thanks.

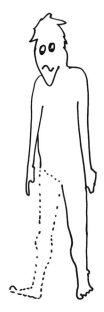

Figure 10.6   Whole-leg numbness. Drawing by Mr J C Semple, with thanks.

involvement, particularly in patients who have had spinal surgery.

3. *Whole-leg numbness* (Fig. 10.6). This again affects the whole leg in a stocking distribution. It usually only occurs at times. Some patients describe this as their whole leg going dead.

4. *Whole leg giving way* (Fig. 10.7). The whole leg gives way or collapses, although few patients actually fall to the ground. Again, the key feature is that the whole leg gives way, although at other times it works quite normally. Like whole-leg numbness, it is intermittent. This is quite different from local muscle weakness, such as going over on the ankle due to L5 weakness.

5. *Complete absence of any spells with very little pain in the past year*. Some patients insist they have never been free of pain for a minute, for years on end. They may report that their pain is so severe it could not possibly be any worse, yet it gets even worse on each consultation.

6. *Intolerance of, or reactions to, many treatments*. Most of our treatments for back pain are quite ineffective, so we should never blame the patient if they do not help. Side-effects are also quite common, even if most are minor. A few patients, however, say that almost every treatment caused side-effects or complications or that they could not tolerate it for one reason or another. Every tablet caused either dyspepsia or an allergy. They could not wear the corset because it made their asthma worse. And that therapist made the pain unbearable! This kind of patient is telling you more about their reaction to treatment than about their physical problem.

7. *Emergency admission to hospital with ordinary backache*. This is not from a road accident or a spinal fracture, but emergency hospitalization because of the severity of ordinary backache. This may

be inappropriate behavior on the part of those who sent the patient to the hospital, or those who admitted her. But it is a measure of what the patient is doing about the problem and of the pressure on those around her to do something. There are striking variations in the number of such admissions in different areas depending on local attitudes.

You can also record these symptoms using a questionnaire:

- Specific questions
  - do you get pain at the tip of your tailbone?
  - does your *whole* leg ever become painful?
  - does your *whole* leg ever go numb?
  - does your *whole* leg ever give way?
  - in the past year have you had *any* spells with very little pain? (Score No = positive)
- Data gathered in routine history
  - intolerance of or reactions to treatments (>1)
  - emergency admission(s) to hospital with ordinary backache.

This group of behavioral symptoms is clearly separate from the common mechanical symptoms of back pain. We first developed these behavioral symptoms and signs in our Problem Back Clinic, where our aim was to clarify assessment of nerve root problems and decisions about surgery. This is the simplest and clearest example. But the same principles apply to mechanical low back pain and referred leg pain (Table 10.1).

We can assess these behavioral symptoms simply and reliably as part of our routine clinical history. Patients offer these descriptions in response to the standard clinical questions. It is simply a matter of recognizing the patterns and realizing that they provide information about illness behavior.

Non-organic or behavioral signs

In the same way, we have standardized a group of non-organic signs or, more accurately, behavioral responses to examination (Waddell et al 1980).

We often assume that physical signs on clinical examination are objective. They *are* objective in the sense that they are assessed by an independent observer, but that does not necessarily mean they

Table 10.1   The spectrum of clinical symptoms and signs

	Physical disease	Illness behavior
Pain		
Pain drawing	Localized Anatomic	Non-anatomic Regional Magnified
Pain adjectives	Sensory	Emotional
Symptoms		
Pain	Musculoskeletal or neurologic distribution	Whole-leg pain Pain at the tip of the tailbone
Numbness	Dermatomal	Whole-leg numbness
Weakness	Myotomal	Whole leg giving way
Time pattern	Varies with time and activity	Never free of pain
Response to treatment	Variable benefit	Intolerance of treatments Emergency hospitalization
Signs		
Tenderness	Musculoskeletal distribution	Superficial Non-anatomic
Axial loading	Neck pain	Low back pain
Simulated rotation	Nerve root pain	Low back pain
Straight leg raising	Limited on formal examination No improvement on distraction	Marked improvement with distraction
Motor	Myotomal	Regional, jerky, giving way
Sensory	Dermatomal	Regional

Adapted from Waddell et al (1984a).

are purely physical and independent of the patient. Some physical findings, like structural deformities, may remain the same even under general anesthesia. But with many signs in the back, we deliberately try to produce pain and see how the patient responds. In the assessment of impairment, we found that tenderness, lumbar movement, and straight leg raising (SLR) all depend to some extent on how the patient reacts. However, there are other signs that appear to depend much more on the patient's behavior during examination than on his or her physical disorder. These are the behavioral signs.

Once again we carried out a literature search and pilot studies to find nearly 30 possible signs. We tested them in the same way, and had to discard many of the signs because they were unreliable or prone to observer bias. Observer bias is a particular problem with these signs. Too many examiners fall into the trap of making judgments rather than dispassionate clinical observations. Our studies produced a final group of seven behavioral signs, in four categories:

- tenderness
  — superficial
  — non-anatomic
- simulation
  — axial loading
  — simulated rotation
- distraction
  — straight leg raising
- regional
  — weakness
  — sensory disturbance

You can add or substitute other signs, but that makes little difference. This is a simple but comprehensive group of tests suitable for routine clinical use. It is easy to learn and quick to perform, and you can include it unobtrusively in your routine clinical examination. The tests work equally well in North America and in the UK.

Tenderness

You often cannot localize physical tenderness exactly but in most clinical practice you can usually find some kind of musculoskeletal pattern. Non-organic tenderness is widespread, spreading far beyond any musculoskeletal anatomy. It may be superficial or non-anatomic (Fig. 10.8).

Superficial tenderness   The lumbar skin is tender to light pinch over a wide area. Nerve irritation can cause a local band of tenderness in the distribution of the posterior primary ramus, which is physical.

Non-anatomic tenderness   This is deep tenderness over a wide area that crosses musculoskeletal

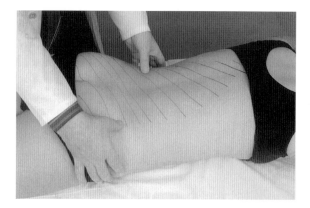

Figure 10.8   Superficial and non-anatomic tenderness.

boundaries. It may extend from the occiput to the coccyx and round to the mid-axillary line on both sides.

Simulation tests

These give the impression that you are performing a test when you are not. It is usually simulation of a movement that causes pain. When you carry out a certain movement on formal examination, the patient reports pain. You then simulate the movement but it is not really taking place. If the patient still reports pain on the simulated test, this is due to expectation of pain rather than actual movement. The wording is important and you must avoid suggestion. You should ask, "What do you feel when I do that?" and not "Is that painful?"

Axial loading   Apply a few pounds of pressure to the top of the patient's skull with your hands (Fig. 10.9). This often produces neck pain, which is physical, but to test the lower back you can then repeat the test on the shoulders. Low back pain on axial loading is surprisingly rare even in the presence of serious spinal pathology. If axial loading produces low back pain in a patient with ordinary backache or root pain, it is behavioral.

Simulated rotation   Spinal rotation does often cause back pain. Now get the patient to stand relaxed with hands at the sides. Hold the patient's hands against the pelvis and passively rotate the trunk. Move the shoulders and pelvis together so

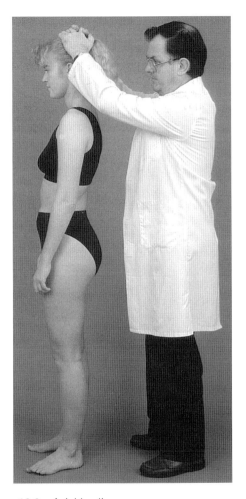

Figure 10.9   Axial loading.

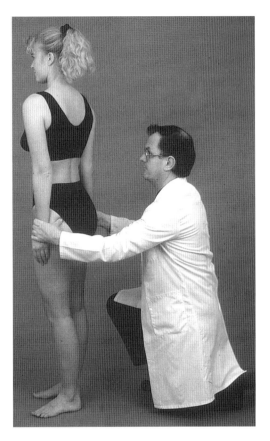

Figure 10.10   Simulated rotation.

that they stay in the same plane (Fig. 10.10). There is no rotation taking place in the spine and any low back pain is behavioral. If the patient has nerve irritation, this test can produce nerve root pain, which is physical.

Distraction tests

Demonstrate a finding in the routine manner and then check the finding while the patient's attention is distracted. Distraction must be non-painful, non-emotional, and non-surprising. In its simplest and most effective form, simply observe patients all the time they are in your presence, while they are not aware of being examined. This includes dressing and undressing, getting off the couch at the end of examination, and walking out of the office or clinic. When you are examining any one part, you should also observe what the patient is doing with the rest of his or her body. Any finding that is present at all times, during formal examination and when distracted, is likely to be physical. Findings that are present only on formal examination, but disappear at other times, have a large behavioral element.

Straight leg raising   SLR is the most useful distraction test (Fig. 10.11). SLR is part of the standard clinical examination, but if SLR is limited on formal examination you should always check it later while the patient is distracted. There are several ways to do this test. You may simply ask the patient to sit up on the couch, or you may sit the patient on the side of the couch with the legs hanging over the edge. Test the knee and ankle reflexes and then lift their leg to examine the knee

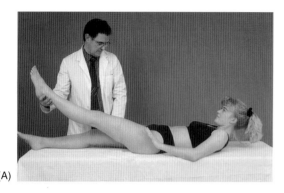

(A)

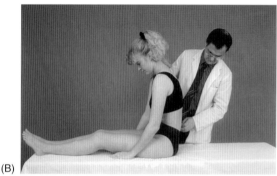

(B)

Figure 10.11 Straight leg raising apparently limited on formal examination (A), and improving with distraction (B).

or test the plantar reflex. This is the flip test. Let me sound a note of caution. There is 10–20° difference in SLR in the lying or sitting position due to a change in lordosis and the position of the pelvis, so only count this test positive if there is at least 40° change between formal SLR and SLR on distraction. If SLR becomes normal when the patient is distracted then the apparent restriction on formal examination was not due to any physical limitation or nerve irritation. Distraction SLR is then positive and the original restriction was behavioral. This is also important to the physical examination and diagnostic triage. Distraction SLR may invalidate what you first thought was a sign of nerve irritation.

This is a suitable point to stress that improvement in SLR with distraction does not necessarily mean the patient is faking or trying to deceive you. Many patients know the SLR test and have learned from experience that it is painful. They anticipate pain and try to protect themselves by tensing and resisting SLR. They are in pain and

your examination may already have made the pain worse. Remember that at this stage you are simply observing their pattern of response and behavior and must not overinterpret its possible cause.

Regional changes

Regional changes involve a widespread area. They often fit a body image or body segments such as the whole leg or from the knee down.

Regional weakness Neurologic weakness approximates to a myotome. You may overcome a weak muscle with hand pressure, but resistance is steady and even. Non-organic weakness is much more widespread. It involves many muscle groups that do not fit any neurology. Quite unlike physical muscle weakness, non-organic weakness is jerky, "giving way." One minute there is more or less normal power but then there is sudden collapse of muscle resistance. If you test hip extension by lifting the patient's leg and telling him or her to keep it down on the couch, you may find almost no resistance. Instead, you may find that the patient is actually lifting the leg himself! Despite apparent severe weakness of many leg muscles on formal testing, the patient is then able to walk. However, test for regional weakness with caution. Patients may give way simply because of pain, and this often inhibits hip flexion or extension. If there is nerve irritation, you should ask the patient to flex the hips and knees to relieve the tension on the nerve before you test ankle and toe strength.

Regional sensory change The best way to test for regional sensory change is with light touch. Classic hysterical anesthesia is now rare. There is usually only slight alteration in sensation so you can detect it best by comparison with the other leg. The key finding is the "stocking" rather than dermatomal pattern (Fig. 10.12). Giving way and sensory changes often affect the same area. In patients with spinal surgery or spinal stenosis, take care not to mistake multiple nerve root damage for a regional disturbance.

It is important to look at the whole group of symptoms and signs, and at the whole pattern of behavior. In all our studies we found that most patients

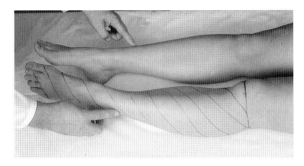

Figure 10.12   *Regional sensory change.*

had either 0–1 behavioral signs or showed a constellation of three or more. Multiple behavioral
symptoms and signs are reliable and consistent
over time and correlate with other features of illness behavior. Isolated symptoms and signs are
quite common in normal people with straightforward physical pathology and no other evidence of
illness behavior. All clinical diagnosis depends on
patterns of illness rather than isolated findings.
You would not diagnose a disk prolapse from an
isolated depressed ankle reflex without any other
clinical features. In the same way you cannot
assess illness behavior from one or two symptoms
or signs. You must not overinterpret isolated
behavioral symptoms or signs.

There are three situations where you cannot
use the behavioral signs. You should ignore even
multiple signs in these patients:

1. Patients with possible serious spinal pathology or
    widespread neurology. You must carry out diag-
    nostic triage and exclude these first. Behavioral
    symptoms and signs are only "inappropriate" to
    mechanical low back pain and sciatica.

2. Patients over about 60 years of age. These
    responses are common in elderly patients, who
    behave differently when they are ill. I do not
    know how to interpret these findings in elderly
    patients and it is better to ignore them.

3. Patients from ethnic minorities. There are wide
    cultural variations in pain behavior. We have
    only standardized the behavioral symptoms
    and signs in white patients. If you want to use
    these tests in other groups you will need to stan-
    dardize them for your patients. This merits
    further research.

**Box 10.1   Overt pain behavior (from Keefe &
Block 1982, with permission)**

- Guarding – abnormally stiff, interrupted, or
  rigid movement while moving from one
  position to another
- Bracing – a stationary position in which a
  fully extended limb supports and maintains
  an abnormal distribution of weight
- Rubbing – any contact between hand and
  back, i.e., touching, rubbing, or holding the
  painful area
- Grimacing – obvious facial expression of pain
  that may include furrowed brow, narrowed
  eyes, tightened lips, corners of mouth pulled
  back, and clenched teeth
- Sighing – obvious exaggerated exhalation of
  air, usually accompanied by the shoulders
  first rising and then falling. They may expand
  their cheeks first

Overt pain behavior

Our original description of the behavioral signs
included overreaction to examination. All experienced doctors and therapists recognize this. We
see it during physical examination or minor procedures such as venepuncture. We are all aware of
how some patients react, but this is a very subjective
judgment. It is unreliable and prone to observer bias.

Keefe & Block (1982) developed a much better
way of looking at this. They studied the expressions and body actions made by patients that communicate they are in pain. They called this overt
pain behavior (Box 10.1). They showed these signs
are reliable and free from observer bias. They
found the same pain behaviors in other conditions
such as cancer and rheumatoid arthritis. We have
shown that doctors and therapists can assess overt
pain behavior during a routine examination
(Waddell & Richardson 1992). These findings are
common during the examination of patients with
back pain. They are much less common but even
more significant if they occur spontaneously during interview. They do require careful training and
standardized methods of observation. Of all the
clinical tests that we use, they are the hardest to

perform properly. Prkachin et al (2002) recently confirmed that it is possible to assess overt pain behavior reliably in a standard physical examination. However, they also found it difficult, and used a separate observer.

Once again, we should be cautious not to over-interpret overt pain behavior. Labus et al (2003) reviewed 29 studies that showed there is only a moderate association of about 0.26 between overt pain behavior and self-reports of pain intensity.

History of illness behavior in daily life

These methods of assessing pain, behavioral symptoms and signs, and overt pain behavior are all measures of illness presentation in the context of a clinical history and examination. They provide useful information, but may be peculiar to the health care situation and may be colored by patient–professional communication. We now have several other powerful measures of illness behavior in daily life. These are all illness behaviors in *chronic* back pain and sciatica. They are of much less significance for a few days in an acute attack. They are obviously not a matter of illness behavior in patients with serious spinal pathology or widespread neurology.

Use of walking aids

This includes use of one or two canes, crutches, or even a wheelchair because of chronic back pain (Fig. 10.13). These patients do not have any gross structural instability or major neurology. There is no physical reason why they are unable to walk. Indeed, when you examine them, they do usually walk more or less normally for a short distance. This is a behavioral response to pain.

Down-time

Down-time is the amount of time spent lying down most days because of chronic pain (Fig. 10.14). You may take this as the average number of hours lying down between 7 a.m. and 11 p.m.

Help with personal care

Frequent and wide-ranging help from a partner or family with bodily care, e.g., washing hair, dressing,

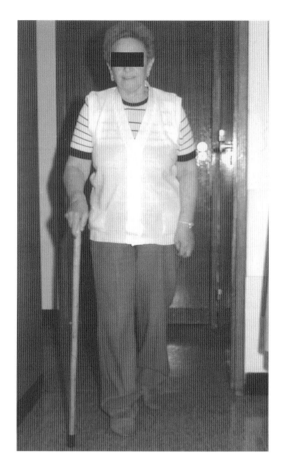

Figure 10.13   Illness behavior in daily life. Use of walking aids for chronic back pain.

and putting on footwear (Fig. 10.15). More extreme examples include helping to turn over in bed during the night. Again, there is no physical reason why these patients cannot do these personal tasks, although they may have to modify the way they do them. This is a behavioral response to pain.

Observations of illness behavior

- pain drawing
- pain adjectives and description
- non-anatomic or behavioral descriptions of symptoms
- non-organic or behavioral signs
- overt pain behavior
- use of walking aids
- down-time
- help with personal care.

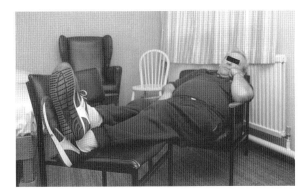

Figure 10.14   Illness behavior in daily life. Chronic down-time: the average number of hours lying down between 7 a.m. and 11 p.m.

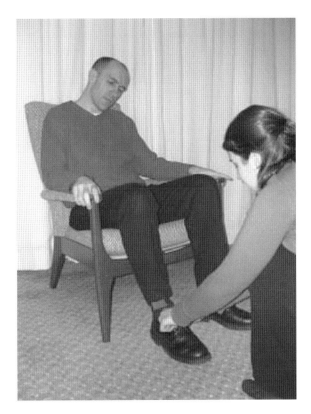

Figure 10.15   Illness behavior in daily life. Family assistance with personal care such as dressing.

UAB pain behavior scale

Richards et al (1982) developed the University of Alabama (UAB) pain behavior scale independently (Box 10.2). It includes various aspects of

> **Box 10.2   UAB pain behavior scale (from Richards et al 1982, with permission)**
>
> - Vocal complaints: verbal
> - Vocal complaints: non-verbal (moans, groans, gasps, etc.)
> - Down-time because of pain (none; 0–60 min; >60 min/day)
> - Facial grimaces
> - Standing posture (normal; mildly impaired; distorted)
> - Mobility: walking (normal; mild limp or impairment; marked limp or labored walking)
> - Body language (clutching, rubbing site of pain)
> - Use of visible physical supports (corset, stick, crutches, lean on furniture, transcutaneous electrical nerve stimulation (TENS) – none; occasional; dependent, constant use)
> - Stationary movement (sit or stand still; occasional shift of position; constant movement or shifts of position)
> - Medication (none; non-narcotic as prescribed; demands for increased dose or frequency, narcotics, analgesic abuse)
>
> Score each item as follows: none, 0; occasional, 0.5; frequent, 1. This gives a total score of 0–10.

illness behavior. They designed it for inpatients in a chronic pain clinic, but it is a simple method suitable for routine clinical use. Nurses or other staff can administer it in 5 minutes, and it gives reliable results and is sensitive enough to measure progress. Ohlund et al (1994) found that the UAB scale and some of our clinical methods of assessing illness behavior gave similar results.

Important caveats

These methods of observing illness behavior are powerful tools, but like most powerful tools they can be dangerous if you misuse them. You must use them with care and compassion, and must not overinterpret or misinterpret your clinical observations. This is equally true in clinical practice and medicolegal assessment. So there are some important caveats to their use (Main & Waddell 1998, Waddell 1999):

- Always carry out diagnostic triage first. Exclude serious spinal pathology or a widespread neurologic disorder before even thinking about illness behavior.

- Clinical observation of illness behavior depends on careful technique. It is important to avoid observer bias.

- Isolated behavioral symptoms and signs do not mean anything. Many normal patients show a few such features. Only multiple findings, preferably of several different kinds, are significant.

- Behavioral symptoms and signs do not tell us anything about the initial cause of the pain. They certainly do not mean that the patient does not have "real" physical pain, and they do not mean that the pain is psychogenic or hysteric. Most back pain starts with a physical problem in the back. Illness behavior is only one aspect of the patient's current clinical presentation.

- It is not a differential diagnosis between physical disease and illness behavior. Most patients have *both* a physical problem in their backs and varying degrees of illness behavior. The fact that we cannot demonstrate the physical basis of the pain does not mean that the pain is psychogenic, any more than the presence of illness behavior excludes a treatable physical problem. Recognizing psychological problems and illness behavior depends on positive psychological and behavioral findings.

- Illness behavior is not a diagnosis. Clinical observations of illness behavior do not provide a complete psychological assessment and do not give you a psychological or psychiatric diagnosis. They are only a screening tool. They alert you to the need for a more thorough assessment of this patient, and of how he or she is reacting and behaving with back pain.

- Behavioral symptoms and signs are not lie-detector tests, but observations of normal human behavior in illness. They do not necessarily mean that the patient is acting, faking, or malingering. Most illness behavior occurs in pain patients who are not in a compensation or adversarial legal situation.

We summarized this in the original article (Waddell et al 1980):

> It is safer to assume that all patients complaining of back pain have a physical source of pain in their back. Equally, all patients with pain show some emotional and behavioral reaction. Physical pathology and nonorganic reactions are discrete and yet frequently interacting dimensions; they are not alternative diagnoses but should each be assessed separately.

Summary

How often do I have to say this to stop people misquoting my work?

- I believe back pain is a physical problem
- Non-organic signs are simply one part of the current clinical presentation
- Non-organic signs do not tell us anything about the original cause of the pain
- Non-organic signs do not mean that the pain is not "real," psychological, or faked.

THE CONCEPT OF ILLNESS BEHAVIOR

Up to now, we have looked at the clinical features of illness behavior. Let us now consider the theoretic concept. It originally came from medical sociology, for illness is a social event. Halliday (1937), one of the pioneers of social medicine, described illness as "a mode of behavior of a person or community." Mechanic (1968) defined illness behavior as "the ways in which given symptoms may be differentially perceived, evaluated and acted (or not acted) upon by different kinds of persons and in different social situations." They stressed the role of mental events and of attitudes and beliefs in illness behavior. What people do depends very much on how and what they think about their symptoms and their illness.

Although beliefs about illness, psychological processes, and actual illness behavior are all important and all interact, we should make a clear distinction between them. The dictionary defines behavior as acts, manners, and conduct. Behavioral psychologists, after Fordyce (1976), emphasize that behavior is overt actions and conduct that we can observe. Illness behavior is what patients actually do and how they react to pain and clinical examination. This is not to deny the reality or importance of inner mental events. It simply recognizes that we cannot observe directly such subjective experiences but must rely on the patient's own report of them. We can only observe behavior. This is a pragmatic approach, and we must always remember that the behavior we observe is only the outward manifestation of these inner mental and emotional events. It is only one clinical perspective on the whole pattern of illness. Its particular value is that it is one of the few objective, external observations of pain. Against that background, we can define illness behavior as "observable and potentially measurable actions and conduct that express and communicate the individual's own perception of disturbed health" (Waddell et al 1989).

Illness behavior is a normal part of human illness, and back pain is no different from any other illness. In most patients, illness behavior is in proportion to their physical problem. In some patients, however, illness behavior gets out of proportion and reflects these psychological and behavioral processes more than the underlying physical disorder. Illness behavior may then aggravate and perpetuate pain and suffering and disability. It becomes counterproductive and is then part of the continuing problem. However, this does not mean that there is normal and abnormal illness behavior. All illness behavior is part of human illness. It is a spectrum, and it does not help to label it normal or abnormal. It is more important to try to understand how each patient is reacting to and dealing with his or her illness.

The physical basis of illness behavior

Illness behavior generally reflects the severity of the underlying physical problem (Table 10.2). Some doctors seem to have the idea that if patients show illness behavior, then they do not have anything physically wrong with them. Or at least nothing much. In fact, that is the opposite of the truth. Illness behavior expresses and communicates the severity of pain and physical impairment. The more severe the physical problem, the more ill the patient, and the more illness behavior he or she displays.

However, physical severity only explains about 20–25% of illness behavior. In some patients, illness behavior clearly gets out of proportion to their physical problem. So there is something more to illness behavior than just an expression of severity.

Psychological factors in illness behavior

There is strong clinical evidence that these clinical observations can also give us information about illness behavior (Table 10.2). We can clearly separate the behavioral symptoms and signs, both clinically and statistically, from the symptoms and signs of physical disease or impairment. They often spread far beyond any likely neurophysiologic mechanism and tend to a body image distribution. They are closely related to other observations of illness behavior. Illness behavior is closely related to emotional arousal and distress. As a first oversimplification, we might regard illness behavior as the clinical equivalent or expression of distress.

Pilowsky (1978) integrated sociologic concepts of illness behavior with psychiatric observation of hypochondriasis. The key feature of hypochondriasis is a persistent preoccupation with health or disease. It is out of proportion to any physical pathology, and it persists despite investigation and reassurance. Illness behavior is closely related to disease conviction. Some patients are overwhelmed by pain and disability and become convinced they have a serious physical illness, despite all the evidence to the contrary. They reject any suggestion that their mental or emotional reactions may play any part in their continuing pain problem. Their illness behavior is to some extent simply a magnified or more emphatic presentation of their pain. These patients are trying to get the message across that they really do have a physical problem. They are concerned about the problem, and feel it is all getting out of control. They are distressed about its severity and persistence and the failure of treatment, and are trying to get help. From their experience up to now, these worries will not settle with simple reassurance. From this point of view, illness behavior is a powerful form of communication between patient and health professional. Up to a point, it may serve a useful purpose. Unfortunately, beyond a certain point it may become counterproductive, both for the patient and for communication with health professionals.

Illness behavior is closely linked to disturbed function, performance, and disability. Illness behavior is what you do, or do not do, and how you behave. Depending on how you look at it, disability *is* illness behavior and illness behavior *is* disability.

Illness behavior is associated with chronic pain and disability, the amount of failed treatment, and "problem patient" status. These all lead to increased illness behavior, but the cause and effect relationship is not entirely clear. Illness behavior is not only the consequence of chronic pain and disability. It occurs at an earlier stage than we previously thought, and it may be involved in the process of developing chronic pain and disability. Patients who show marked illness behaviors have a lower success rate of any kind of treatment. Beliefs, distress, and illness behavior all get better or worse with the success or failure of physical treatment. This may become a vicious circle, which we will consider again from different perspectives in the following chapters.

Illness behavior does not just happen: it is learned. It is not fixed, but is a dynamic process over time, and health care may play a key role in its development. The information and advice we give may color patients' beliefs about their illness and what they should do about it. Traditional treatment of back pain was often direct advice to stop or restrict normal activities and to behave in a more ill manner. We may prescribe sick certification. In more extreme cases, doctors or therapists may offer or support the use of walking aids, and the patient's partner or family may encourage and support illness behavior. Chronic pain patients often have repeated consultations and examinations and learn what to say and do for health professionals. They learn what to expect, and what is expected of them, and this modifies how they react and behave. Conflicting opinions and advice, failed treatment, disappointment, and frustration all lead them to press their case more strongly. We teach, and they learn, illness behavior in their clinical presentation. All of this is unconscious, learned behavior. Sadly, traditional health care for back pain may have done more to cause than to prevent illness behavior.

Clinical observation of illness behavior is clearly only one facet of a complex phenomenon. We must assess the whole clinical picture before we can begin to understand illness behavior. That will be the task of the next four chapters.

HOW ILLNESS BEHAVIOR AFFECTS CLINICAL MANAGEMENT

Before we consider psychological issues in more detail (Chs 11–12), we should note the value of observing illness behavior in routine practice.

If you recognize illness behavior, this helps to clarify your clinical assessment and removes a potential source of great confusion. Too often, in our Problem Back Clinic, we see patients with failed back surgery who have whole-leg pain, apparent limitation of SLR that improves with distraction, and regional weakness. If we look carefully at their records, we find they had these features before surgery. Unfortunately, their surgeon did not recognize that these were symptoms and signs of illness behavior and made a clinical diagnosis of a disk prolapse. The severity of pain and distress led to great pressure to do something and the magnetic resonance imaging (MRI) showed a bulge. So, surprise, surprise, they had a negative surgical exploration and that made them worse. If the surgeon had recognized the illness behavior, he or she would have seen that these symptoms and signs were not of nerve root pain, nerve irritation, and combined L5 and S1 weakness, and the patient had no specific symptoms or objective signs of a disk prolapse. There was never any clinical indication for surgery. The incidental findings on the MRI only completed the trap. Dr P Dudley White was President Eisenhower's personal physician, though it is not clear whether this political background led to his clinical insight! "The doctor who cannot take a good history and the patient who cannot give one are in danger of giving and receiving bad treatment."

In both assessment and management, it is not a question of *either* physical disease *or* illness behavior. Rather, we must recognize which symptoms and signs are behavioral in nature and which tell us about the physical problem. We must assess both. Recognizing illness behavior helps to clarify your physical assessment, but also alerts you to the need for further psychological assessment. These patients may require both physical treatment of their physical disorder and more careful assessment and management of the psychosocial and behavioral aspects of their illness.

This is not only important for surgery. The concept of illness behavior is fundamental to understanding low back pain and disability and its clinical management. It is one of the keys to treating people rather than spines. Our aim is better understanding of the clinical presentation. It is not a question of credibility. We should believe both physical and behavioral observations, but each gives us different information about the patient and his or her illness. Illness behavior must not lead to moral judgments or to rejecting these patients. It is our job as health professionals to care for our patients, both their physical disorders and their illness behavior. The aim of recognizing illness behavior is to manage them more appropriately.

Summary

- Methods of assessing illness behavior are a powerful aid to understanding the clinical presentation of back pain. It is important to distinguish the symptoms and signs of illness behavior from those of physical disease
- This distinction clarifies the assessment of the physical problem
- These findings of illness behavior should also alert you to the need for more detailed psychosocial assessment. They do not, on their own, give a diagnosis of psychological disturbance, or of exaggeration in a compensation or medicolegal context
- These patients may require *both* physical treatment of their physical problem *and* more careful management of the psychosocial and behavioral aspects of their illness
- Health care may have a profound influence on illness behavior

Table 10.2   The scientific evidence on the non-organic signs

Normal subjects Waddell et al (1980) Waddell et al (1982)	Non-organic signs are not present in asymptomatic white subjects age <60 years
Battery of non-organic signs Waddell et al (1980) Lehmann et al (1983) Waddell et al (1984b) Korbon et al (1987) Waddell & Richardson (1992)	Four out of five studies show that the non-organic signs form a homogeneous group, although the exact list of signs included varies (partly depending on the incidence in different cohorts). Korbon et al (1987) found the signs were loaded on three different factors[a]
Test–retest and interobserver reliability Waddell et al (1980) Korbon et al (1987) Reesor & Craig (1988) McCombe et al (1989) Spratt et al (1990)	Four out of five studies show that a group of non-organic signs has acceptable test–retest and interrater reliability, at least comparable to most clinical information. Individual signs may be more variable. The only study that found the signs to be unreliable (McCombe et al 1989) had a very low incidence of non-organic signs and did not assess the signs as a group[a]
Relationship to self-reported severity of pain Fishbain et al (2003) found 14 studies	I agree with Fishbain et al that there is reasonably consistent evidence that non-organic signs are associated with more severe pain, though the strength of the relationship varies. However, pain is not a purely physical measure but also depends on psychological factors (Ch. 3). By definition, self-reports of pain intensity may be regarded as another

Table 10.2   (Continued)

		expression of pain behavior. It is therefore difficult to interpret this relationship. Does more severe pain cause more illness behavior? Or are self-reports of more severe pain simply another reflection of illness behavior? See Chapters 3 and 14 for further discussion
Relationship to physical impairment Waddell et al (1980) Waddell et al (1984b) Waddell et al (1992)		These three studies show that non-organic signs are associated with clinical measures of physical impairment. Physical severity generally explains about 20–25% of the non-organic signs. See also Chapter 8 for a discussion of the limitations and interpretation of clinical assessment of physical impairment
Relationship to physical performance Fishbain et al (2003) found seven studies		I agree with Fishbain et al that there is reasonably consistent evidence that non-organic signs are associated with poorer physical performance. However, performance, like pain, is influenced by physical, psychological, and behavioral issues. These studies do not provide any evidence on the nature or direction of the relationship between illness behavior and performance. This is the key to the whole problem. See Chapter 14 for further discussion
Relationship to psychological distress Waddell et al (1980) Main & Waddell (1982) Lehmann et al (1983) Waddell et al (1984b) Korbon et al (1987) Doxey et al (1988) Reesor & Craig (1988): positive (but not significant after allowing for physical severity) Lacroix et al (1990): relationship not significant Maruta et al (1997) (men only) Vendrig et al (1998) (men only) Novy et al (1998)		Most of these studies show that non-organic signs are associated with various measures of psychological distress. The relationship may be stronger in men than in women. We have never suggested that non-organic signs are related to *psychiatric* disorders (Fishbain et al 1991 negative, Streltzer et al 2000 positive)[a]
Relationship to catastrophizing Reesor & Craig (1988)		There is one study which shows the non-organic signs are related to catastrophizing (Ch. 12). This is unconfirmed
Relationship to other measures of illness behavior Waddell et al (1980) Waddell et al (1984b) Reesor & Craig (1988) Waddell et al (1989) Waddell & Richardson (1992) Chan et al (1993) Ohlund et al (1994)		These studies show consistently that non-organic signs are associated with other clinical measures of illness behavior such as the pain drawing, overt pain behavior, behavioral descriptions of symptoms, the UAB pain behavior scale, and various scales of the Illness Behavior Questionnaire. The strength of the association varies, but correlation coefficients are generally 0.20–0.40[a]
Change over time with treatment Waddell et al (1986) Cooke et al (1992) Main et al (1992) Werneke et al (1993) Polatin et al (1997) Friedrich et al (1998)	Surgery Lumbar dynamometry Pain management Rehabilitation Functional restoration Rehabilitation	These studies show consistently that non-organic signs are not fixed but can decrease or increase over time with medical treatment and improvement or deterioration in the clinical condition[b]

Table 10.2   (Continued)

Prediction of clinical outcome

McCulloch (1977)	+	Most but not all of these prospective studies show
Porter & Hibbert (1983)	+	that non-organic signs predict clinical outcomes of
Lehmann et al (1983)	+	conservative and surgical treatments and rehabilitation.[a]
Dzioba & Doxey (1984)	+	Several studies raise the possibility that non-organic
Waddell et al (1986)	+	signs may be less predictive at the acute than at the chronic stage.
Doxey et al (1988)	+	Non-organic signs may no longer be predictive in
Bradish et al (1988)	−	rehabilitation programs that specifically address
Klenerman et al (1995)	+(at 2 months)	psychosocial issues (Polatin et al 1997)
Flynn et al (2002)	−	

Prediction of return to work

Dzioba & Doxey (1984)	+	These studies provide inconsistent and conflicting results,
Waddell et al (1986)	−	so non-organic signs should not be used as predictors of
Bradish et al (1988)	−	return to work
Doxey et al (1988)	−ve surgery cases, +ve non-surgery	
Lacroix et al (1990)	2 samples: 1 +ve; 1 −ve	
Lancourt & Kettelhut (1992)	+	
Werneke et al (1993)	+	
Ohlund et al (1994)	+(weak)	
Kummel (1996)	−(larger group of signs +ve)	
Polatin et al (1997)	−	
Karas et al (1997)	+	
Gaines & Hegmann (1999)	+	
McIntosh et al (2000)	+	
Fritz et al (2000)	−	
Kool et al (2002)	+	
Hunt et al (2002)	−	

[a]Conclusions opposite to those reached by Fishbain et al (2003), mainly because of their misclassification of studies under each topic, double counting, selective data extraction, and unfounded conclusions.

[b]In an earlier draft, Fishbain et al (2003) actually tried to use studies showing change over time after treatment to attack test–retest reliability!

Fishbain et al (2003) reviewed further evidence that the non-organic signs do not distinguish "organic" from "non-organic" pain, and lack any relationship to self-esteem or workers' compensation status. However, we have always made it clear that the non-organic signs do *not* differentiate "organic" from "non-organic" pain (which is not a valid concept anyway) and are not confined to workers' compensation patients. Note that workers' compensation status is *not* equivalent to "secondary gain," "malingering," or the legal issue of credibility. Self-esteem is an irrelevance.

Based on the final manuscript of Fishbain et al (2003).

APPENDIX 10A A RESPONSE TO CRITICS

You might want to skip this section first time round. I have added it to this edition by popular demand, but by its nature you may find it heavier-going. It is not essential to the line of my main argument.

It is almost 25 years since I first wrote up the non-organic signs (Waddell et al 1980), and none of my research has caused so much controversy. It continues to this day. So let me say straight out that I still stand by the non-organic signs, *provided* we are careful to define what they are and what they are not. We must recognize their strengths and their limitations. That is what I have tried to do in this chapter. But why have they provoked such a strong reaction? Perhaps it is the fate of any new idea that raises questions about accepted practice? At least, it may show some kind of balance that they have been attacked with equal ferocity from both extremes. The opposing criticisms also counter each other. If either were correct, that would demolish the other!

Some eminent pain specialists have attacked my interpretation of the non-organic signs as being contrary to modern neurophysiologic and clinical understanding of chronic pain. Dr Harold Merskey has been a constant critic throughout. Pat Wall profoundly disagreed and Fishbain et al (2003) recently published a zealous attack.

Criticism from the other extreme is legal rather than scientific. Many medical and legal experts swear in court that non-organic signs are conscious and deliberate attempts to deceive the examiner, and evidence of faking or malingering. Any attempt to offer a psychological explanation is some kind of left-wing, intellectual or moral weakness.

If the importance of an idea can be judged by powerful enemies, the non-organic signs and illness behavior seem to have touched some very raw nerves. Perhaps the strength of the reaction means they really are addressing something fundamental.

CHRONIC PAIN

The first criticism is that modern neurophysiologic and clinical understanding of chronic pain provides an alternative explanation for the non-organic signs (Merskey 1988, Margoles 1990, Fishbain et al 2003).

So my interpretation as illness behavior is invalid. There are two main lines to this argument:

1. neurophysiologic mechanisms
2. improved clinical diagnosis of the causes of chronic pain.

First, a large number of animal experiments show that neurophysiologic mechanisms can produce spread of pain. The central nervous system is plastic: it changes with damage and sensory input and time. Pain thresholds may rise or fall and receptive fields may enlarge. So a neurone may respond to different stimuli or stimuli from a wider area, or a localized stimulus may excite more neurones. Light touch or pressure may become pain or there may be reduction in sensation, and neurologic activity may persist after the stimulus stops. Pain, tenderness, altered sensation, and muscle inhibition may spread outwith the nerve territory.

We now have an animal model for neuropathic pain if we ligate the lumbar nerve roots in the rat. This physical pain has non-organic features:

- spontaneous pain
- persistent, intense, burning pain
- pain from innocuous stimuli such as light touch or pressure
- intense pain from normally painless stimuli.

These rats also show pain behavior. We can then reverse these changes by sympathectomy.

Thus, neurophysiologic mechanisms can produce and explain non-dermatomal, non-anatomic, or regional patterns of pain, tenderness, hypersensitivity, or altered sensation, all from a local lesion. There are reports of patients with serious neurologic diseases that are consistent with such mechanisms.

Second, clinical studies show that patients with fibromyalgia, myofascial pain syndrome, and complex regional pain syndrome often have non-organic signs. These findings are related to perceived pain and pain-associated phenomena. Recent advances in demonstrating "pain generators", functional MRI (fMRI) changes, and pain imaging in the brain now provide a physical basis for chronic pain and these associated phenomena. Even when clinicians cannot diagnose traditional pathology, there may be occult damage that we are simply unable to recognize. Thus, we can never exclude a physical basis for chronic pain. Future advances are likely to explain most of these findings.

I accept the neurophysiologic evidence – up to a point, of course pain has a physical basis. Of course there can be some spread of pain and tenderness, hypersensitivity, altered sensation, and inhibition of motor activity. Clinical localization is never exact. At best, symptoms and signs only approximate to musculoskeletal or neuroanatomy. They often include referred patterns. So common clinical findings do fit modern ideas of neurophysiology. Moreover, poorly localized symptoms, non-anatomic tenderness, and regional findings can occur in isolation in patients with no other evidence of illness behavior. That is why we must interpret our clinical findings with caution. That is why we must not overinterpret isolated symptoms or signs. But there is the constant danger of applying basic science to clinical practice. Unless there is actual nerve damage, it is rarely possible to prove neurophysiologic change in the individual patient. The behavioral symptoms and signs I have described often spread far beyond any likely neurophysiologic mechanism and fit better with body image patterns. Anyone who has actually examined patients can recognize that these findings are quite different in character from the usual referred patterns. They form part of a constellation of other illness behaviors that even the most ardent neurophysiologist accepts have a large psychological component.

I find the clinical evidence much more open to debate. We have always stressed that it is important to exclude serious neurologic disease before even considering illness behavior. The clinical syndromes offered by the critics are much more questionable. Applying a pseudopathologic label to a clinical syndrome does not prove its purely physical basis. The counter argument is that these clinical findings raise the question of a psychological element to some of these syndromes. I fully agree that behavioral symptoms and signs are related to perceived pain and pain-associated phenomena but I interpret that differently. I fully agree there may be a physical basis for chronic pain beyond expected healing times, such as physiologic dysfunction (Ch. 9) and neurophysiologic changes (Ch. 3). However, that does not mean that chronic pain cannot also be aggravated and maintained by psychological

and behavioral mechanisms. We should not fall into the trap of trying to force every clinical symptom and sign into a *purely* physical or neurophysiologic explanation.

That returns to the old mind–body dichotomy, which we all decry (Ch. 3). It pretends that medical science can explain everything in bodily terms. (Or will be able to, some day. But invoking future discoveries is a sign of desperation.) We should remember that neurophysiology is only the electrochemical substrate: it fails to account for what is happening in the mind. All human activity and behavior depends ultimately on neurophysiologic mechanisms, but also on mental events. Imagine I commit a murder. I might offer a neurophysiologic explanation: the active areas of my brain; the motor activity from brain to anterior horn of the spinal cord; the peripheral nerves; the neuromuscular transmission that makes my index finger pull the trigger. Do you think the jury would be interested? The court would still want to know why I committed this act.

We cannot observe the underlying physical disease or neurophysiologic events directly. The clinical presentation that we observe is behavior. Neurophysiology may help us to understand the *mechanisms* of pain, but we must also look at pain psychology and behavior if we want to understand the *meaning* of our clinical findings.

At the time of writing this chapter, Fishbain et al (2003) are in the process of publishing a highly critical review of the non-organic signs. They attack their entire scientific basis. But we should be clear where they come from. They do not offer an independent, unbiased review. Drs Fishbain and Rosomoff have been critics of the non-organic signs for more than a decade (Rosomoff et al 1989, Fishbain et al 1991). They present it as a kind of systematic review and attempt to blind the reader with pseudoscience, but it is riddled with fatal methodologic flaws (Box 10.3). It appears to me that they have simply tried to dream up every possible way they could attack the non-organic signs and support their own argument that the signs can be explained entirely in terms of physical pathology and neurophysiologic mechanisms (Rosomoff et al 1989, Fishbain et al 1991). This leads them to some mutually contradictory conclusions. For example, they are very critical of the reliability and

Box 10.3   Methodologic flaws to Fishbain et al (2003)

- Search and retrieval of studies incomplete
- Reference to abstract or conference proceedings
- Double and treble counting of studies
- Misclassification of studies under each topic
- Selective reporting of results
- Inappropriate quality criteria
- Unfounded conclusions
- Mutually contradictory conclusions

psychometric properties of the signs. But when it suits their case, they forget that and decide the signs show a 100% consistent relation to pain and physical performance.

Let me try to redress the balance. My review of the same literature (Table 10.2) reaches some opposing conclusions to theirs (Fishbain et al 2003, footnotes to Table 10.2). On other points we agree on the evidence, though our interpretations differ. You might suspect me of bias also, but I am confident enough to leave you to decide which is the fairer review. Place the two reviews side by side, and see how they compare and differ. Where we disagree on important points, look at the argument and the evidence and make up your own mind.

CREDIBILITY

The second criticism is that non-organic signs are a conscious and deliberate attempt to exaggerate symptoms and disability, and to deceive the examiner. Thus, non-organic signs provide evidence of faking or malingering. So my interpretation as illness behavior is invalid.

The scientific evidence in this area is weak. There is a great deal of clinical confusion about secondary gain. Most studies compare workers' compensation patients with non-compensation patients, but that is a very different issue (Ch. 13). Whether or not patients improve with treatment does not prove or disprove secondary gain. Indeed, contrary to common belief, litigation appears to be a quite separate matter from clinical progress (again, see Ch. 13). Table 10.3 summarizes the limited evidence that is

available, but I agree with Fishbain et al (1999, 2003) that it is not possible to draw any conclusions.

However, this is not really a scientific or a clinical issue. It is a legal matter. The debate is in court and judgment is based on legal evidence. The medical evidence is only one part of this. There are two positive and one negative lines to this argument:

1. non-organic signs are conscious reactions to examination
2. non-organic signs correlate with other evidence on lack of credibility
3. rejection of a psychological basis for illness behavior.

Nearly everyone agrees that malingering, in the sense of faking illness that does not exist, is rare. It is usually a question of whether there is exaggeration of symptoms and disability from more minor injury. The legal issue is one of credibility – whether the claimant is an honest witness whose account of his or her illness should be accepted. If symptoms and disability are out of proportion to the physical injury (whatever the clinical limitations of assessing that), then the legal debate is about whether this is due to conscious or unconscious (i.e., psychological) mechanisms.

First, I agree that non-organic signs do sometimes represent a conscious and deliberate attempt to exaggerate the problem. Second, I agree that non-organic signs do sometimes occur in claimants with other evidence that they lack credibility. It is naive to deny that some claimants exaggerate their symptoms and disability for financial gain: that is human nature. In addition to non-organic signs, there may be other inconsistencies in the medical evidence, surveillance, or other non-medical evidence, or legal reasons why a court rejects their credibility.

However, the fact that non-organic signs *can* be produced consciously does not mean that their presence is *necessarily* proof of faking. There is a wealth of clinical evidence, and legal evidence too, that illness behavior can also be due to unconscious, psychological mechanisms. In clinical practice, non-organic signs are common in patients who have no legal claim and no question of financial gain. Thus, non-organic signs do not, *in themselves*, provide sufficient evidence to prove lack of credibility. In the clinical setting, non-organic signs are a screening tool that indicates the need for more

Table 10.3   Scientific evidence on whether non-organic signs relate to credibility

Study	Findings	
Waddell et al (1980)	Nonorganic signs do not correlate with the validity scales of the MMPI[a]	−ve
Lehmann et al (1983)	Non-organic signs do not correlate with the validity scales of the MMPI.[a]	−ve
	Patients with multiple non-organic signs are more likely to have a lawyer	+ve
Waddell et al (1984b)	Litigation status accounts for 9.2% of the variance of non-organic signs	Weakly +ve
Korbon et al (1987)	Non-organic signs correlate with the Somatic Amplification Rating Scale (SARS).	
	However, SARS is simply an expanded version of our non-organic signs	Meaning less
Reesor & Craig (1988)	Non-organic signs are not related to litigation status	−ve
Chan et al (1993)	Non-organic signs are not related to litigation status	−ve
Hayes et al (1993)	Non-organic signs correlate with inconsistency scores on various psychological questionnaires	+ve
Rucker et al (1996)	Non-organic signs correlate with an index made up of functional capacity evaluation estimates of level of effort and MD exaggeration questions	+ve
Novy et al (1998)	Non-organic signs do not correlate with the validity scales of the MMPI[a]	−ve
Gracovetsky et al (1998)	This was an experimental study in which normal subjects and patients with back pain were instructed to simulate or dissimulate back pain. Physical examination was repeated, including the non-organic signs, although it is not clear how far judgment was based on them. This gave 85% concordance for "honest" subjects but only 38% for the simulators/dissimulators, who succeeded in deceiving expert examiners	Clinical examination is a poor method of detecting deception

[a]Though Chapman & Brena (1990) found that "inconsistency in statements and/or behaviors" did not correlate with the validity scales of the Minnesota Multiphasic Personality Inventory (MMPI) either.
Fishbain et al (2003) confused the issue of credibility with workers' compensation and with whether patients respond to treatment.

detailed psychological assessment. So, in the legal setting, non-organic signs may raise the question of credibility, but they do not provide an answer. That judgment depends on a much more thorough assessment of all the evidence. That may *either* be other evidence on credibility, *or* medical and psychological evidence of a psychological basis for the claimant's illness behavior. Legal judgments are on the balance of all that evidence.

I said that we must not overinterpret the non-organic signs clinically, but should consider them as one part of the whole clinical picture. Equally, we must not overinterpret the non-organic

signs legally, but should consider them as one part of the whole medical and other evidence (Table 10.4).

Despite all that I have tried to say since 1980, the non-organic signs have often been misused. The most serious abuse has been because of the misconceptions that the patient has nothing physically wrong or is not genuine. They have been used by some surgeons to deny some patients further investigation or treatment. I try to rationalize this, because such patients are probably safer to escape from surgeons who have such lack of understanding of illness behavior. More seriously,

Table 10.4   Medicolegal assessment of illness behavior and credibility

Compare the claimant's subjective report of symptoms and disability with the objective medical evidence of injury, diagnosis, and physical impairment	When they are all more or less in proportion, the medical evidence supports the claimant's own account. There is no dispute about the medical evidence
When there is significant discrepancy between the claimed severity of symptoms and disability, and the objective medical evidence	Is there evidence of illness behavior?
If there is evidence of illness behavior	Is there clinical or psychological evidence of unconscious psychological mechanisms for this? Is there other medical or non-medical evidence that casts doubt on the claimant's credibility? (Or occasionally both)

The final judgment of credibility is a judicial or administrative decision

they have been used unscrupulously by defense "experts" and lawyers to deny some patients the compensation to which they are entitled. That shows a lack of knowledge of illness behavior that destroys their claim to expertise in this field. I condemn these abuses absolutely. All health professionals are supposed to try to understand and help patients, not to make moral judgments or condemn them if they do not behave as we think they should.

CONCLUSION

Some of the critics seem uncomfortable with the whole idea of illness behavior. I know from my own experience that illness behavior can be threatening and disturbing. It is no longer enough to know about anatomy and pathology and mechanics and neurophysiology. It opens a whole new perspective about how people react and behave when they are ill. But most of us are not trained or skilled at dealing with such difficult human problems. Opening this Pandora's box reveals the limitations of our treatment for back pain and of our professional skills. It exposes us to the difficulties and stress of dealing with emotions – both our patients' and our own. Professional life is much simpler if we stick to the physical treatment of disease. But patients are not just cases of disturbed pathology or mechanics or neurophysiology: they are suffering human beings. This is what health care is all about.

References

Bradish C F, Lloyd G J, Aldam C H et al 1988 Do nonorganic signs help to predict the return to activity of patients with low back pain? Spine 13: 557–560

Chan C W, Goldman S, Ilstrup D M, Kunselman A R, O'Neill P I 1993 The pain drawing and Waddell's nonorganic physical signs in chronic low back pain. Spine 18: 1717–1722

Chapman S L, Brena S F 1990 Patterns of conscious failure to provide accurate self-report data in patients with low back pain. Pain 6: 178–190

Cooke C, Menard M R, Beach G N, Locke S R, Hirsch G H 1992 Serial lumbar dynamometry in low back pain. Spine 17: 653–662

Doxey N C, Dzioba R B, Mitson G L, Lacroix J M 1988 Predictors of outcome in back surgery candidates. Journal of Clinical Psychology 44: 611–622

Dzioba R B, Doxey N C 1984 A prospective investigation into the orthopedic and psychologic predictors of outcome of first lumbar surgery following industrial injury. Spine 9: 614–623

Fishbain D A, Goldberg M, Rosomoff R S, Rosomoff H 1991 Chronic pain patients and the nonorganic physical sign of nondermatomal sensory abnormalities (NDSA). Psychosomatics 32: 294–303

Fishbain D A, Cutler R, Rosomoff H L, Rosomoff R S 1999 Chronic pain disability exaggeration/malingering and submaximal effort research. Clinical Journal of Pain 15: 244–274

Fishbain D A, Cole B, Cutler R B, Lewis J, Rosomoff H L, Rosomoff R S 2003 A structured, evidence-based review of the meaning of nonorganic physical signs: Waddell signs. Pain Medicine (in press)

Flynn T, Whitman J, Wainner R et al 2002 A clinical prediction rule for classifying patients with low back pain who demonstrate short-term improvement with spinal manipulation. Spine 27: 2835–2843

Fordyce W E 1976 Behavioural methods for chronic pain and illness. Mosby, St Louis

Friedrich M, Gittler G, Halberstadt Y, Cermak T, Heiller I 1998 Combined exercise and motivation program: effect on the compliance and level of disability of patients with chronic low back pain: a randomized controlled trial. Archives of Physical Medicine and Rehabilitation 79: 475–487

Fritz J M, Wainner R S, Hicks G E 2000 The use of nonorganic signs and symptoms as a screening tool for return-to-work in patients with acute low back pain. Spine 25: 1925–1931

Gaines W G Jr, Hegmann K T 1999 Effectiveness of Waddell's nonorganic signs in predicting a delayed return to regular work in patients experiencing acute occupational low back pain. Spine 24: 396–400

Gracovetsky S A, Newman N M, Richards M P et al 1998 Evaluation of clinician and machine performance in the assessments of low back pain. Spine 23: 568–575

Halliday J L 1937 Psychological factors in rheumatism: a preliminary study. British Medical Journal 1: 213–217, 264–269

Hayes B, Solyom C A, Wing P C, Berkowitz J 1993 Use of psychometric measures and nonorganic signs testing in detecting nomogenic disorders in low back pain patients. Spine 18: 1254–1259

Hunt D G, Zuberbier O A, Kozlowski A J et al 2002 Are components of a comprehensive medical assessment predictive of work disability after an episode of occupational low back trouble? Spine 27: 2715–2719

Karas R, McIntosh G, Hall H, Wilson L, Melles T 1997 The relationship between nonorganic signs and centralization of symptoms in the prediction of return to work for patients with low back pain. Physical Therapy 77: 354–360

Keefe F J, Block A R 1982 Development of an observation method for assessing pain behavior in chronic low back pain patients. Behavioral Therapy 13: 363–375

Klenerman L, Slade P D, Stanley M et al 1995 The prediction of chronicity in patients with an acute attack of low back pain in a general practice setting. Spine 20: 478–484

Kool J P, Oesd P R, DeBe R A 2002 Predictive tests for non-return to work in patients with chronic low back pain. European Spine Journal 11: 258–266

Korbon G A, DeGood D E, Schroeder M E, Schwartz D P, Shutty M S Jr 1987 The development of a somatic amplification rating scale for low back pain. Spine 12: 787–791

Kummel B M 1996 Nonorganic signs of significance in low back pain. Spine 21: 1077–1081

Labus J S, Keefe F J, Jensen M P 2003 Self-reports of pain intensity and direct observations of pain behavior: when are they correlated? Pain 102: 109–124

Lacroix J M, Powell J, Lloyd G J et al 1990 Low back pain: factors of value in predicting outcome. Spine 15: 495–499

Lancourt J, Kettelhut M 1992 Predicting return to work for lower back pain patients receiving workers' compensation. Spine 17: 629–640

Lehmann T R, Russell D W, Spratt K F 1983 The impact of patients with nonorganic physical findings on a controlled trial of transcutaneous electrical nerve stimulation and electroacupuncture. Spine 8: 625–634

Main C J, Waddell G 1982 Chronic pain, distress and illness behavior. In: Main CJ (ed.) Clinical psychology and medicine: a clinical perspective. Plenum Press, New York, pp 1–52

Main C J, Waddell G 1998 Behavioral responses to examination. A reappraisal of the interpretation of "nonorganic signs". Spine 23: 2367–2371

Main C J, Wood P L R, Hollis S, Spanswick C C, Waddell G 1992 The distress and risk assessment method: a simple patient classification to identify distress and evaluate the risk of poor outcome. Spine 17: 42–52

Margoles M S 1990 Letter to the editor. Pain 42: 258–259

Maruta T, Goldman S, Chan C W et al 1997 Waddell's nonorganic signs and Minnesota Multiphasic Personality Inventory profiles in patients with chronic low back pain. Spine 22: 72–75

McCombe P F, Fairbank J C T, Cockersole B C, Pynsent P B 1989 Reproducibility of physical signs in low back pain. Spine 14: 908–918

McCulloch J A 1977 Chemonucleolysis. Journal of Bone and Joint Surgery 59-B: 25–52

McIntosh G, Frank J, Hogg-Johnson S, Bombardier C, Hall H 2000 Prognostic factors for time receiving workers' compensation benefits in a cohort of patients with low back pain. Spine 25: 147–157

Mechanic D 1968 Medical sociology. Free Press, New York

Merskey H 1988 Regional pain is rarely hysterical. Archives of Neurology 45: 915–918

Novy D M, Collins H S, Nelson D V et al 1998 Waddell signs: distributional properties and correlates. Archives of Physical Medicine and Rehabilitation 179: 820–822

Ohlund C, Lindstrom I, Areskoug B et al 1994 Pain behavior in industrial subacute low back pain. Part I. Reliability: concurrent and predictive validity of pain behavior assessments. Pain 58: 201–209

Pilowsky I 1978 A general classification of abnormal illness behaviours. British Journal of Medical Psychology 51: 131–137

Polatin P B, Cox B, Gatchel R J, Mayer T B 1997 A prospective study of Waddell signs in patients with chronic low back pain. When they may not be predictive. Spine 22: 1618–1621

Porter R W, Hibbert C 1983 Neurogenic claudication treated with calcitonin. Presented to the 10th annual meeting of the International Society for the Study of the Lumbar Spine. Cambridge

Prkachin K M, Hughes E, Schultz I, Joy P, Hunt D 2002 Real-time assessment of pain behavior during clinical assessment of low back pain patients. Pain 95: 23–30

Ransford A O, Cairns D, Mooney V 1976 The pain drawing as an aid to the psychological evaluation of patients with low back pain. Spine 1: 127–134

Reesor K A, Craig K D 1988 Medically incongruent chronic back pain: physical limitations, suffering, and ineffective coping. Pain 32: 35–45

Richards J S, Nepomuceno C, Riles M, Suer Z 1982 Assessing pain behavior: the UAB pain behavior scale. Pain 14: 393–398

Rosomoff H L, Fishbain D A, Goldberg M, Santana R, Rosomoff R S 1989 Physical findings in patients with chronic intractable benign pain of the neck and/or back. Pain 37: 279–287

Rucker K S, Metzler H M, Kregel J 1996 Standardization of chronic pain assessment: a multiperspective approach. Clinical Journal of Pain 12: 94–110

Spratt K F, Lehmann T R, Weinstein J N, Sayre H A 1990 A new approach to the low-back physical examination: behavioral assessment of mechanical signs. Spine 15: 96–102

Streltzer J, Eliashof B A, Kline A E, Goebert D 2000 Chronic pain disorder following physical injury. Psychosomatics 41: 227–234

Vendrig A A, deMey H R, Derksen J J, van Akkerveken P F 1998 Assessment of chronic back pain patient characteristics using factor analysis of the MMPI-2: which dimensions are actually assessed? Pain 76: 179–188

Waddell G 1999 Nonorganic signs or behavioral responses to examination in low back pain. Hippocrates' Lantern 6: 1–5

Waddell G, Richardson J 1992 Clinical assessment of overt pain behavior by physicians during routine clinical examination. Journal of Psychosomatic Research 36: 77–87

Waddell G, McCulloch J A, Kummel E, Venner R M 1980 Non-organic physical signs in low back pain. Spine 5: 117–125

Waddell G, Main C J, Morris E W et al 1982 Normality and reliability in the clinical assessment of backache. British Medical Journal 284: 1519–1523

Waddell G, Bircher M, Finlayson D, Main C J 1984a Symptoms and signs: physical disease or illness behavior? British Medical Journal 289: 739–741

Waddell G, Main C J, Morris E W, Di Paola M P, Gray I C M 1984b Chronic low back pain, psychologic distress, and illness behavior. Spine 9: 209–213

Waddell G, Morris E W, DiPaola M P, Bircher M, Finlayson D 1986 A concept of illness tested as an improved basis for surgical decisions in low-back disorders. Spine 11: 712–718

Waddell G, Pilowksy I, Bond M R 1989 Clinical assessment and interpretation of abnormal illness behavior in low back pain. Pain 39: 41–53

Waddell G, Somerville D, Henderson I, Newton M 1992 Objective clinical evaluation of physical impairment in chronic low back pain. Spine 17: 617–628

Werneke M W, Harris D E, Lichter R L 1993 Clinical effectiveness of behavioral signs for screening chronic low back pain patients in a work oriented rehabilitation program. Spine 18: 2412–2418

Chapter 11

Emotions

Chris J. Main   Gordon Waddell

Think again about the two patients in Figure 10.1. It should be clear by now that how people think and feel about back pain is central to what they do about it and how it affects them. Let us look first at feelings.

Pain is a "passion of the soul." Our modern definition of pain describes it as "an unpleasant sensory and emotional experience." Pain is highly personal and subjective, and always has an emotional dimension that we must allow for. This is obvious in its clinical presentation and management:

- individual patients seem to experience very different pain from apparently similar injuries
- anxiety and depression can make pain feel worse
- distraction can make pain feel better
- placebos can give good pain relief
- psychosocial factors play a major role in the development of chronic pain and disability.

Emotional changes accompanying pain vary in different people and at different times. Acute pain raises natural fears and anxiety about its cause and prognosis. It leads to increased awareness and preoccupation with the pain and urgent search for a remedy. People with acute pain are often more irritable and less tolerant than usual. Pain may distract them and cause poor concentration and faulty judgment. This may lead to strained relations with family and fellow workers.

As pain becomes chronic, emotions change in nature and degree. Chronic pain implies failed treatment and that colors the emotions. Patients may still be anxious, but the focus changes to fear of persistent pain and disability. There is increasing conviction that the pain reflects a serious problem, and skepticism about attempts at reassurance. This sometimes leads to a desperate and unrealistic search for anyone who can offer a diagnosis or a cure. Repeated failures to find an answer may cause anger, distrust, and hostility. There is pessimism about the future and the prospect of continued pain and disability. Some patients with chronic pain become helpless, hopeless, and depressed. Drugs and surgery may cause physical and emotional side-effects and some chronic pain patients develop analgesic or alcohol dependence. Chronic pain and its associated emotions may lead to progressive withdrawal from social activities. Chronic pain can have a profound impact on family relationships and work. Many patients with chronic back pain eventually lose their jobs, with all the economic, social, and emotional consequences of unemployment.

These emotional changes have wide-ranging effects on how patients think and feel about their pain (Box 11.1). They influence pain behavior and disability. They are also important for clinical management. Robinson & Riley (1999) provide an excellent review of the relationship between emotion and pain. Gatchel & Turk (1999) give a more general overview of psychosocial factors in pain. Main & Spanswick (2000) and Linton (2002) offer further discussion of how psychological factors influence the clinical presentation and management of pain.

EARLY PSYCHOLOGICAL STUDIES IN BACK PAIN

Disk surgery gives good results in 80–90% of carefully selected patients, but the "human wreckage" of failure is equally dramatic. Early studies of failed back surgery recognized the importance of psychological factors, and that these could affect the outcome of further surgery.

A classic study by Wiltse & Rocchio (1975) showed that psychological tests could actually predict how patients with disk prolapse would respond to treatment (Table 14.6, Ch. 14). There was no question that these patients had physical pathology, yet psychological factors influenced the outcome of physical treatment. Further studies showed that psychological factors influence how patients respond to every form of conservative or surgical treatment.

These findings stimulated research into the role of psychological factors in back pain. The first goal was to predict how patients would respond to surgery, to improve selection for surgery. But it was then realized that psychological issues are of much more fundamental importance. Psychological factors influence how patients react to back pain, the development of chronic pain and disability, and clinical management.

Box 11.1   The influence of psychological factors on pain and disability

- Fundamental mechanisms
- Clinical recovery vs development of chronic disability
- Seeking health care
- Response to treatment
  - patient expectations
  - placebo response
  - compliance with treatment
  - outcome of treatment
  - taking responsibility for own continued management

(Adapted from Main & Spanswick 2000 p 21)

Personality

Most of the early psychological studies focused on the personality of patients who had chronic pain. The findings were assumed to be fixed characteristics of the person's psychological make-up – personality traits. It was thought that people with certain types of personality might be more likely to develop chronic pain. These patients were then described as "neurotic" or "low back losers." So the fault lay in the patient rather than our unsuccessful treatment. Even worse, because these traits were fixed, there was little the patient or anyone else could do about it.

Further studies showed that was too pessimistic. People can change. Prospective studies of normal people show that most of the findings develop after they get back pain. Studies of patients with acute episodes of back pain show that most people do get better. So these findings really reflect patients' *present* emotional state, and their current clinical situation. Despite years of research, no one has been able to identify a personality type that predisposes to back pain. People with back pain are no different from the rest of us, which is hardly surprising as we are all likely to get it at some time!

Personality, in the sense of our individual psychological make-up due to our unique combination of nature and nurture, clearly does influence how we respond if we develop back pain. It is the pond into which the stone of back pain drops to produce emotional ripples. It sets our psychological style, the defense mechanisms we use, and the ways in which we try to cope. Understanding patients' psychological make-up may help us to understand their clinical presentation, their methods of communication, and their responses to health care. But the most important psychological changes are in how patients think and feel and react emotionally to their current clinical situation.

You may be misled by some reports from pain clinics which suggest that 30–50% of chronic pain patients do have some kind of "personality disorder" (Polatin et al 1993, Weisberg & Keefe 1997). We do not dispute these findings. However, these specialized clinics deal with highly selected patients. Many of them have a history of physical or sexual abuse, alcohol and drug problems. These are very different patients from those in primary care or other clinical settings. So we must be careful about extrapolating these findings. And we need to be careful with the diagnosis of "personality disorder," which can be applied to about 10% of normal people! So we must not overinterpret these findings. It is doubtful if they help us to understand the average patient with back pain or the development of disability.

MISCONCEPTIONS

Before we go any further, we should clear away some common misconceptions. We accept that some of our more knowledgeable readers may regard this as oversimplified and dogmatic, but we feel it is important to start this discussion with a clean slate.

First, back pain is usually not psychogenic – it is not "in your head." Emotional changes, psychological disturbance, and illness behavior do not tell us anything about the original cause of the pain. Most back pain starts with a physical problem in the back, even if it is only the ordinary backache that we all get at some time. Most psychological changes occur secondary to pain and influence how people adjust to it. Psychological factors may make a person more aware of back pain or more likely to seek health care. They may aggravate and perpetuate the pain, or even help to turn ordinary backache into chronic pain and disability. Physical treatment alone may not then solve the problem, and by that stage we may also need to deal with any psychological disturbance as well.

Second, we cannot divide pain into physical or psychological, organic or non-organic, real or imaginary. The IASP definition (Ch. 3) states that pain is an unpleasant sensory *and* emotional experience. Despite this, many doctors and therapists wrongly act as if pain is *either* physical *or* psychological. If there are few physical findings to explain continued pain, then they assume the pain is psychogenic. Clinical experience and many scientific studies show this is false. Sensory and emotional dimensions are integral to pain itself. Physical pain and emotional changes are not alternatives: they are two sides of the same coin. Our failure to identify the physical source of back pain does not mean the pain is psychogenic, any more than the presence of emotional changes excludes a treatable physical problem. In clinical practice it is more realistic to accept that back pain has a physical cause. It is also safer and more helpful. Nothing destroys the patient–professional relationship faster than questioning the physical basis of back pain. Our inability to find the source of back pain is not the patient's fault, but rather reflects our limited knowledge. We should not diagnose psychological events by exclusion, but must assess the patient's emotional state on positive psychological and behavioral features.

Third, as we have already discussed, most ordinary patients with back pain do not have any personality disorder.

Fourth, some patients with chronic back pain may become depressed, but they are usually not mentally ill. Most patients who present with back pain do not have a *primary* psychiatric illness, and attempts at formal psychiatric diagnosis are inappropriate. This is why referral to traditional mental health services is usually not much help. The psychiatrist simply responds, correctly, that the problem is in the patient's back and not head. Clinicians should avoid pseudopsychiatric diagnoses. The terms hysteria and hypochondriasis have been so variously used, misused, and abused that we are glad to see they are now disappearing from the literature on back pain.

Finally, this is not just about malingering. Most of these psychological changes and illness behavior occur in the absence of any claim for compensation. Patients cannot help how they react to pain. They do not want to have pain and they do not choose to be emotional or disabled. Emotions are generally outside our conscious control and most illness behavior is involuntary. Our job as health professionals is not to sit in judgment, but to understand the problem with compassion and to provide the best possible management for each patient.

THE NATURE OF STRESS AND DISTRESS

Stress is a normal human emotion that is part of everyday living. It is how we become energized, and a certain level of stress is necessary for us to perform to our best. In situations requiring a high level of performance or concentration, the body releases chemicals and stress hormones. Biologically, we may think of this as a method of mustering our resources to cope with threat or danger. Animals react by "fight or flight." We rarely face physical danger in our modern lives, but we still react to any kind of stressful situation with the same kinds of biologic and psychological responses. When faced with an unpleasant or threatening stress, our normal first reaction is to try and escape from the situation. However, escape is not always possible or it may not be an acceptable option. When we face severe or prolonged stress from which we cannot escape, we may become stressed. Too much stress can be counterproductive. Instead of raising our performance, it may make it worse. We become fatigued or "burnt out." We may become distressed.

We should distinguish *distress* from *stress*. "Stress" has now become a popular diagnosis, but it is used very loosely. In ordinary speech, we sometimes use the word stress to refer to the event that is stressful, such as bereavement, a difficult situation at work, or financial worries. Strictly, such events are *stressors*, and we all have many of these in life. We also use the word stress for reactions to a stressor, or for symptoms such as irritability, difficulty sleeping, or sweating. Strictly, these are *stress responses*. However, these can occur without the person being distressed. Sometimes a person does not realize he or she is under stress, even though it may be obvious to family and friends. We should only use the term *distress* for excessive or abnormal stress responses. At its most severe, distress may require formal psychiatric treatment, but most pain patients do not require that. Good information and advice, and simple reassurance will often be enough to reduce distress (Main & Watson 2002, Main & Williams 2002).

People react to stress in different ways. The most common emotions are anxiety, depression, and anger. These are not mutually exclusive, and some patients show features of them all. Some patients wear their emotions on their sleeve. They recognize and talk about their anxiety, depression, and frustration. It is important to spend time listening to such patients. If they feel they have had the opportunity to express their view, and that someone has listened to their difficulties, this may be a major step in their management.

However, other patients do not find it easy to talk about their feelings. They may instead present what appear to be straightforward physical symptoms that actually communicate distress. In our research, we found that the most common presentations of distress in patients with back pain are increased awareness of bodily symptoms and depressive symptoms (Main 1983, Main & Waddell 1984, Main et al 1992).

Distress may also present as changes in the patient's usual behavioral patterns. Altered sleep patterns; sexual interest or activity; food, alcohol and drug consumption; and personal relationships or social activities may indicate distress.

Clinically, we can define distress as "a disturbance of emotion and mood in which psychological and physical symptoms occur." It is similar in nature, if not in scale, to the normal stress response. It is a normal human reaction to pain, a state of emotional arousal, of disturbed emotions and suffering. Croft et al (1995) found that 15–30% of people with back pain may have some degree of distress, sufficient to influence their perception of pain and their decision to seek health care.

It is now clear that many of the psychological and behavioral changes that we used to associate with chronic pain can appear much earlier. Burton et al (1995) found that 18% of patients had significant distress when they first presented in primary care. Roberts (1991) found distress at 3 weeks in an acute attack. Ohlund et al (1994) found pain behavior by 6 weeks. It is clear, then, that these emotional and behavioral changes can develop within 3–6 weeks.

Generalized vs specific distress

Once you recognize that a patient is distressed, you should try to find the reason why. This is not always as straightforward as it might appear. Your clinical history may begin to give some insight into how much stress or "hassle" this patient faces in life generally, either at present or in the recent past. You may think about a "distress profile" of their current back trouble:

- pain
- restricted activities
- sleep disturbance
- quality of life and relationships
- impact on work
- background: previous episodes and treatment
- other life stresses.

But be careful: your interview must be sensitive. Many patients are reluctant to disclose what they feel are personal details that they consider to be irrelevant to their back pain. Why should this background be so important? Simply put, experience may color patients' views of their current difficulties. People's general emotional reactions to stress may cast light on their current reaction to their back pain and disability. Some people may show a general tendency to become distressed or even depressed in the face of stress, while others shrug things off.

There is no doubt that back pain can be a powerful stressor. However, the effects of pain – the resulting disability – may be even worse than pain itself. And some patients may have other, unrelated difficulties that are confounding the current problem. These may need separate consideration and may need to be dealt with in their own right. Recent bereavement is an example. Sometimes a major marital problem predates the onset of the back trouble. More extreme examples may need professional psychological assessment and treatment. But any such life events may limit the range of therapeutic options or affect the outcome of treatment for back pain.

Four examples of a stress history merit special attention:

1. First, a small but important group of chronic pain patients have a history of physical and sexual abuse, either in childhood or as part of their continuing problem. It is often assumed that such abuse is more common in women, but it is now clear that similar problems also occur in men. If you find such a history, it is important to decide immediately whether the patient requires more specialized assessment and treatment. An abused patient should have the option of talking to a skilled professional of the same sex, if he or she so wishes. This is no area for the amateur. Traumatizing physical or sexual abuse needs delicate handling.

2. Second, if a patient has been involved in a serious accident, you should think about the possibility of posttraumatic stress (Box 11.2). Severe or persisting symptoms may need special investigation or treatment. It is important to identify such symptoms and to assess their significance before deciding on the management of back pain.

Box 11.2   Posttraumatic stress disorder (Mendelson 1988)

- An event outside the usual range of experience that would markedly distress almost anyone
- Persistent re-experiencing of the traumatic event, e.g., distressing recollections, dreams, reliving
- Avoiding thoughts, activities, or situations associated with the trauma
- Symptoms of physiologic arousal and psychological distress
- Duration of symptoms >1 month

3. Third, some patients may have become distressed about seeing doctors or other health professionals. By the time you see them, they may have received a whole range of opinions, which may be conflicting. They may want a diagnosis, but never got any clear answer. They may not have understood what they were told, or may feel they were not taken seriously. Other doctors may have implied that their pain is trivial or even imaginary, and may have seemed unsympathetic. Such experience colors and shapes the patient's attitude towards consultation. They may be angry. Before you blame the patient, listen carefully to the history. You may find that they have good reason to be angry and distressed. Part of your job is to put your patient at ease. In order to understand and help your patient, you need to establish a rapport.

4. Finally, adversarial legal proceedings may be a stressor for some patients. Although this often causes some distress, that rarely requires professional help. However, ongoing litigation often influences recovery and clinical management.

In summary, the stress history should assess the importance of other life stresses facing the patient, quite apart from those related to back pain. At times it may be difficult to judge the relative importance of back pain among these other problems. You must set priorities, and make judgments about the place and value of treatment for the symptom of back pain.

CLINICAL PRESENTATIONS

Most studies show that the main emotions associated with back pain are anxiety, increased bodily awareness, fear, depression, and anger. These are all negative emotions. They can all be part of the emotional experience and impact of pain. There is no sharp divide between acute and chronic pain. It is now clear that some of these changes can develop earlier than we used to think.

There is overlap and interaction between all these emotions. They are all part of the normal human response to pain and stress. Patients with back pain may show a complex but variable mixture of these emotions and the mix will vary according to individual make-up and background. Apart from depression, individual emotions rarely

reach the level of true psychiatric illness. Rather, these patients are emotionally aroused by their pain and disability and failed treatment. In some patients, these emotional changes may be more severe and prolonged and get out of control. This rich emotional broth may then aggravate and perpetuate pain and disability, and may itself become part of the problem. It may interfere with treatment and reduce its chances of success. At root, however, patients with back pain are quite simply distressed by their continued pain and disability and by our failure to solve their problem.

Anxiety

We all experience anxiety at times, but excessive or prolonged anxiety can become harmful. We all respond differently to stress and we all vary in how prone we are to anxiety. Some of us become anxious in response to a wide range of stressors; others may only be anxious about a particular situation. Anxiety can range from a mild emotional reaction to a crippling psychiatric illness. Autonomic activity may produce physiologic and emotional changes and symptoms. Different patients emphasize physical or emotional symptoms. Some patients describe feelings of being "tense," "wound up," or "on edge." They may be anxious, nervous, or suffer panic attacks. Others may complain of physiologic symptoms such as sweating, nausea, dry mouth, tremor, or palpitations. They may describe their symptoms more dramatically as "butterflies in the stomach," shortness of breath or choking. The anxious person is restless and unable to relax or settle for any length of time. Disturbances of sleep and appetite are common. High levels of anxiety typically present as poor concentration, worry, irritability, and disturbed sleep.

Anxiety is one of the most basic emotions in illness, and has a major impact on consulting and health care (Leigh & Reiser 1980). However, in the context of back pain, anxiety is probably less important than specific fears and seldom merits treatment in its own right.

Increased bodily awareness

We all receive a constant stream of bodily sensations from our somatic and autonomic nervous systems, but usually we are unaware of it. Most of us spend most of our lives blithely paying little conscious attention to our bodies, although some people are by nature and upbringing much more introspective. Usually, however, it is only when something goes wrong that we pay attention. It is then normal to become more aware of and concerned about bodily symptoms. Pain, anxiety, and stress all lead to sympathetic activity and emotional arousal. This heightened emotional state produces sensitizing to bodily sensations and physiologic events. We may then interpret these sensations as discomfort or malaise and we are more likely to seek health care (Brosschot & Eriksen 2002, Eriksen & Ursin 2002).

Main (1983) explored the concept of somatic awareness. Most patients with back pain are naturally anxious and concerned about their pain. Some describe symptoms of increased sympathetic activity, which are closely allied to anxiety, but few meet the criteria for anxiety neurosis. Many show an understandable focus on their physical problem, but few meet the criteria for hypochondriasis. The common theme seems to be that they are simply more aware of their bodily sensations and function. Main (1983) then developed a Modified Somatic Perception Questionnaire (MSPQ; Fig. 11.1). Usually, this is best understood as a normal emotional reaction to illness rather than a psychological disturbance or psychiatric illness.

Fear and uncertainty

Back pain can be frightening, especially if you do not know what caused it or what is happening to you and no one seems to have an answer. There are overtones to do with back pain coming from behind, where we cannot see it and feel vulnerable. There is implied threat to our very backbone and physical capability. We all know that back pain can be due to serious disease and can lead to chronic disability and incapacity for work. So we may have very real and realistic fears about the possible meaning of the pain and its consequences for our lives.

Patients with back pain often have specific areas of concern:

- fear of pain
- fear of hurt and harm

- fear of disability
- fear of loss of control
- fear of surgery
- fear of effect on family and relationships
- fear of impact on work, incapacity, loss of earnings.

Health professionals are often not very good at allaying these fears. Too often, we give inadequate or conflicting information and advice, which undermines any reassurance. Most of our treatment for back pain has a low success rate and recurrences are common, which undermines faith and confidence. To reduce the chances of misunderstanding and dissatisfaction, we should be clear what the patient wants from the consultation:

- relief of pain or cure
- a clearer diagnosis
- reassurance
- legitimization of symptoms
- to express distress, frustration, or anger.

Clinical management should aim to relieve these anxieties, fears, and bodily concerns and prevent them interfering with treatment and recovery.

Depressive symptoms

Depression is probably the most common psychological disturbance in chronic pain. Various studies show that 30–80% of patients at a pain clinic have some depressive symptoms, and up to 20% meet the criteria for a major depressive disorder (Sullivan et al 1992, Banks & Kerns 1996). Although pain clinic patients are not representative, most patients with chronic back pain probably have some lesser degree of depression (von Korff et al 1993, Croft et al 1995, Ohayon & Schatzbrg 2003).

However, we need to be clear what we mean by depression. In ordinary speech, we use the word depression for anything from a minor emotional reaction such as feeling fed-up to a crippling psychiatric illness or even suicide. It is important to distinguish depressed mood from actual depressive illness. Patients with chronic pain often have depressed mood and describe depressive symptoms, but this is seldom severe enough to meet the criteria for a depressive illness. It is important to identify those patients who are psychiatrically ill, and to refer them for appropriate treatment

Please describe how you have felt during the PAST WEEK by making a check mark (√) in the appropriate box. Please answer all questions. Do not think too long before answering.

	Not at all	A little/slightly	A great deal/ quite a lot	Extremely/could not have been worse
Heart rate increasing				
Feeling hot all over*	0	1	2	3
Sweating all over*	0	1	2	3
Sweating in a particular part of the body				
Pulse in neck				
Pounding in head				
Dizziness*	0	1	2	3
Blurring of vision*	0	1	2	3
Feeling faint*	0	1	2	3
Everything appearing unreal				
Nausea*	0	1	2	3
Butterflies in stomach				
Pain or ache in stomach*	0	1	2	3
Stomach churning*	0	1	2	3
Desire to pass water				
Mouth becoming dry*	0	1	2	3
Difficulty swallowing				
Muscles in neck aching*	0	1	2	3
Legs feeling weak*	0	1	2	3
Muscles twitching or jumping*	0	1	2	3
Tense feeling across forehead*	0	1	2	3
Tense feeling in jaw muscles				

The questionnaire as given to patients does not include the scoring.
Only those items marked with an asterik (*) are scored and added to give a total score.

Figure 11.1   Modified Somatic Perception Questionnaire (MSPQ). From Main (1983), with permission.

(Rush et al 2000). For most patients with back pain, however, depressed mood is simply one more facet of their chronic pain. We must not ignore depression just because it is associated with chronic pain, but the best treatment is usually to help them cope with their pain.

Depression involves negative beliefs, lowered mood, and clinical symptoms. Different patients show different patterns. The key feature of depression is a negative view of oneself, of the world, and of the future. There is loss of interest and energy and slowing of mental function. Mental symptoms include a sense of loss, sadness, hopelessness, and pessimism about the future. There may be disturbances of appetite, sleep, and sexual function. Physical symptoms such as headache, constipation, weakness, aches, and pain are also common. Simon et al (1999) found that about 50% of patients with major depression have multiple unexplained bodily symptoms. Many of them present with somatic symptoms but acknowledge psychological symptoms when asked about them. Eleven percent deny any psychological symptoms, even on direct questioning. In patients with chronic low back pain, the most common depressive symptoms include sleep disturbance, loss of energy, chronic fatigue, and persistent worrisome thoughts (Rush et al 2000). (See Main & Spanswick 2000 p 203 for the ICD-10 and DSM-IV diagnostic criteria for depression and other psychiatric conditions.)

The above description of depression is true, as far as it goes. However, recent research suggests that the relationship between depression and pain is more complex than this (Averill et al 1996, Banks & Kerns 1996, Wilson et al 2001, Clyde & Williams 2002). Part of the difficulty is that many of the bodily symptoms of chronic pain are very similar to those of depression. So chronic pain itself may meet some of the usual diagnostic criteria for depression, and we need to be more careful how we diagnose depression in these patients (Robinson & Riley 1999, Wilson et al 2001, Slesinger et al 2002). Pain and depression are often *associated* with each other, but the link can work in various ways. Patients who are depressed report more pain, and some pain may be a symptom of depression. Depression may aggravate pain of physical origin. And, not surprisingly, chronic pain and failed treatment may cause depression. So it can be a vicious circle. Most research shows that in chronic pain patients, depression develops secondary to the pain (Magni et al 1994, Rush et al 2000, Ohayon & Schatzbrg 2003). So we need to interpret these symptoms in the context of chronic pain. Perhaps we can describe it best as learned helplessness in the face of severe and chronic pain, which the patient cannot control, and which impacts on the patient's whole life.

Once again, we must set priorities for treatment (Rush et al 2000). A few patients need to be referred for specialized help. For most patients, the best way to relieve pain-associated depression is to help them regain some measure of control over their pain and disability.

Anger and hostility

Many patients with chronic low back pain get angry and frustrated (Fernandez & Turk 1995, Main & Watson 2002). They are angry at the pain. Why should they have to suffer like this? They may blame what they think is the cause of their problem, which may be their work or an accident. If treatment fails and back pain becomes chronic and disabling, they may blame doctors and therapists who have failed to find the cause or provide a cure. When each doctor and therapist gives them a different story, they become confused, suspicious, and angry. Loss of their job and financial hardship make them angrier still at the injustice of it all. If they have a legal dispute, they become angry at "the system," the lawyers, or medical examiners.

We must confess that doctors and therapists also become angry with patients with chronic back pain. These patients fail to meet our disease stereotypes and fail to get better as they should with our treatment. They try our professional skills and expose our limitations. It is tempting and more comfortable to blame the patient rather than ourselves, and we get angry at patients for putting us in this predicament.

So patients, doctors, and therapists may all get angry. Patients may express their anger openly as hostility, or it may be inhibited and result in non-cooperation with treatment. Doctors and therapists may lose sympathy and patience. There may be a breakdown in communication. All of these undermine the patient–professional relationship. All health care depends on mutual trust and cooperation, which may not survive anger and hostility. Anger may lead to failed treatment, which then makes the patient angrier still, trapping them in a self-perpetuating rut of failure and frustration.

Please indicate for each of these questions which answer best describes how you have been feeling recently.

	Rarely or none of the time (less than 1 day per week)	Some or little of the time (1–2 days per week)	A moderate amount of time (3–4 days per week)	Most of the time (5–7 days per week)
1. I feel downhearted and sad	0	1	2	3
2. Morning is when I feel best	3	2	1	0
3. I have crying spells or feel like it	0	1	2	3
4. I have trouble getting to sleep at night	0	1	2	3
5. I feel that nobody cares	0	1	2	3
6. I eat as much as I used to	3	2	1	0
7. I still enjoy sex	3	2	1	0
8. I notice I am losing weight	0	1	2	3
9. I have trouble with constipation	0	1	2	3
10. My heart beats faster than usual	0	1	2	3
11. I get tired for no reason	0	1	2	3
12. My mind is as clear as it used to be	3	2	1	0
13. I tend to wake up too early	0	1	2	3
14. I find it easy to do the things I used to do	3	2	1	0
15. I am restless and can't keep still	0	1	2	3
16. I feel hopeful about the future	3	2	1	0
17. I am more irritable than usual	0	1	2	3
18. I find it easy to make a decision	3	2	1	0
19. I feel quite guilty	0	1	2	3
20. I feel that I am useful and needed	3	2	1	0
21. My life is pretty full	3	2	1	0
22. I feel that others would be better off if I were dead	0	1	2	3
23. I am still able to enjoy the things I used to	3	2	1	0

The questionnaire as given to patients does not include the scoring.
All items are scored as marked and added to give a total score.

Figure 11.2   Modified Zung depression questionnaire. From Zung (1965), Main & Waddell (1984), with permission from Macmillan Press Ltd.

It is important to identify the focus of anger and hostility and attempt to defuse it (Box 11.3).

Psychological questionnaires

Questionnaires can be used as a simple screen for distress. Two of the most important emotional changes in low back pain are increased bodily awareness and depressive symptoms. So we recommend the MSPQ (Fig. 11.1) and the Modified Zung Depression Inventory (Fig. 11.2; Zung 1965, Main & Waddell 1984). These also form the basis of the Distress and Risk Assessment Method (DRAM; Main et al 1992). The DRAM is a simple and straightforward method of classifying patients into those showing no psychological distress, those at risk, and those who are clearly distressed (Table 11.1).

The DRAM may help to identify patients who should be referred for more formal psychological assessment. Those showing no distress can have routine clinical management, without much concern for psychological issues. Those who are at risk can also be managed routinely, but with awareness and monitoring of the possible development of distress. Management of those who are clearly

---

Box 11.3   Strategies for dealing with distress and anger

- Give the patient time
- Signal that it is permitted to be upset
- Find out gently the patient's particular focus of concern
- Find out why they are telling you
- Distinguish distress associated with pain and disability from more general distress
- Identify iatrogenic misunderstandings
- Identify mistaken beliefs and fears
- Try to correct misunderstandings
- Identify iatrogenic distress and anger
- Listen and empathize
- Above all, don't get angry yourself!

(Adapted from Main & Watson 2002 and Main & Williams 2002)

Table 11.1   The Distress and Risk Assessment Method (DRAM) of assessing psychological distress

Classification	Zung and MSPQ scores
Normal	Modified Zung < 17
At risk	Modified Zung 17–33 and MSPQ < 13
Distressed, somatic	Modified Zung 17–33 and MSPQ > 12
Distressed, depressive	Modified Zung > 33

MSPQ, Modified Somatic Perception Questionnaire.
From Main et al (1992).

---

distressed must address both physical and psychological issues. These patients need more than just physical treatment. They may need more comprehensive psychological assessment to decide if they also require formal pain management. Burton et al (1995) showed that the DRAM predicted 1-year outcomes in primary care patients (Table 11.2). We have found that it also predicts response to a pain management program.

Before you consider using psychological tests, you should be aware of their strengths and limitations (Table 11.3). Questionnaires have some advantages over clinical interview. They are carefully designed and tested. They eliminate observer variation and bias. They can give a precise and detailed assessment of a particular psychological

---

Table 11.2   Distress and Risk Assessment Method (DRAM) prediction of 1-year outcome in primary care patients

DRAM at presentation	DRAM at 1 year		
	Normal	At risk	Distressed
Normal (79)	87% (69)	9% (7)	4% (3)
At risk (59)	46% (27)	44% (26)	10% (6)
Distressed (34)	18% (6)	35% (12)	47% (16)

Numbers in brackets refer to the numbers of patients in each group.
Based on data from Burton et al (1995).

Table 11.3   The advantages and disadvantages of clinical interview and questionnaires

Clinical interview	Questionnaires
Advantages	
Can be adapted to individual patient	Quick, easy to administer
Incorporates clinical experience and judgment	Standardized
Link to goals for treatment	Easy to score
Disadvantages	
May be time-consuming	Require reading and language skills
Potential observer bias	Limited perspective
May be misleading unless skilled	May be too sensitive and susceptible to patient bias

feature, allowing it to be measured in numbers. They are reproducible, so they can observe change over time or with treatment. But questionnaires also have weaknesses. They are based entirely on the patient's self-report. They usually focus on particular psychological features that we know are important in most patients, but they will miss less common features that may be important in a few patients. Patients must be fluent in the language, have sufficient mental ability, and be able to read and write. They must be cooperative and honest, or the questionnaires may be liable to bias.

Questionnaires must also be interpreted with care. Numbers sometimes give an illusion of accuracy. It is not possible to diagnose psychiatric illness from psychological questionnaires alone. Nor can questionnaires turn a clinician into an amateur psychologist. If you do decide to use these questionnaires, you should probably first seek advice from a clinical psychologist. That will also give you a contact for help when you need it. Even at best, questionnaires are only a first-stage screening test, either to support clinical impression or to alert you to the need for more thorough psychological assessment.

So questionnaires may supplement, but can never replace, the clinical interview. Questionnaires may be most useful in particular settings, such as patients with chronic pain and disability, before surgery, or when planning a rehabilitation or pain management program.

Distress

Stress, anxiety, increased somatic awareness, fear and uncertainty, depressive symptoms, anger: at the simplest level, we might think of these all as aspects of distress. However, these emotional changes are not unique to low back pain. They seem to be similar in whiplash or any other form of chronic pain. They form a characteristic cluster of psychological symptoms and responses to pain (Peebles et al 2001).

Patients with back pain may become emotionally aroused and show mood disturbances, but we must repeat that most of them are not psychiatrically ill. This is a normal human reaction to an unresolved stressor from which they cannot escape. The problem is that, as pain becomes chronic, these emotional changes may become counterproductive.

They may then aggravate and perpetuate pain and disability. And interfere with clinical management.

CLINICAL MANAGEMENT

Emotions are only one aspect of the psychology of pain, but understanding distress is a reasonable starting point in clinical practice.

We should be clear about our aims. All health professionals should have sufficient understanding of psychological issues to provide understanding, reassurance, and support for the patient with back pain. We should be able to recognize those few patients who require referral for more thorough psychological assessment and possible treatment. But we must also recognize our limitations. Most health professionals who treat back pain do not have the background or experience to provide specialized help. Fortunately, very few patients with back pain, even chronic pain and disability, need formal psychological or psychiatric treatment. But emotional issues are so common that every doctor and therapist should be aware of them and must deal with them.

Understanding

Most doctors and therapists rely on clinical impression of the patient's emotional state. Despite our experience in this field, we have both learned to distrust our "gut feelings" – they are often wrong.

The starting point is to make a more conscious effort to be aware of emotions and distress. Start with the patient's description of pain. Listen to the adjectives they use. How strong is the emotional content? Listen to their description of their symptoms and the impact on their lives. Obviously, patients describe their physical problems, but are they also describing emotional problems? Ask outright how they feel about the pain. What are their hopes and fears and worries? Don't assume that you know what they are worried about: ask them! Find out gently their particular focus of concern.

Encourage them to talk and make sure you listen. Pay attention not only to *what* they say, but also *how* they say it. Watch their body language and illness behavior. Too often, it may seem easier and more efficient to focus on physical symptoms and disease. A brief clinical consultation may become "rushing in with a diagnosis, and rushing out with a treatment." We must give patients the opportunity and the time to talk about *their* problems. With most patients, it only takes a moment to get a more balanced picture that helps you to provide better management and saves time in the long run. In a few patients, this may open an unexpected can of worms that you cannot possibly deal with in a few minutes. These patients may need another, longer consultation at a more convenient time, and they may need further help. However, these are the very patients in whom we should aim to recognize psychological problems as early as possible, so that we can manage them better or refer them for appropriate help.

Box 11.3 lists some key issues in the clinical assessment of distress. Main & Spanswick (2000) and Main & Williams (2002) give more detailed discussions.

Communication

Good clinical practice is built upon the patient–professional relationship (Box 11.4). That depends on communication skills, which now are (or should be) a basic part of every health professional's training. This is not the place for a detailed account, and Table 11.4 only gives the briefest of summaries. But throughout this chapter we have tried to show that effective communication is the key to better assessment and management of the psychological issues associated with back pain.

Main & Spanswick (2000), Main & Watson (2002), and Main & Williams (2002) provide more detailed accounts of how to handle psychological issues in clinical practice.

> **Box 11.4   The doctor–patient relationship (Balint 1964)**
>
> - Listening and taking time to listen are important
> - Warmth: demonstrate an unconditional positive regard for the patient as a human being; do not judge or like/dislike
> - Accurate empathy: convey to patients that you have an accurate understanding of their problem and experience
> - Genuineness: be yourself; do not hide behind a professional facade. This does not mean disclosing personal details about yourself
> - Provide continuity of support over time
> - Draw the line between support and counseling and do not try to be an amateur psychiatrist

Table 11.4   Communication

Factors affecting the quality of communication	Factors influencing self-disclosure	Style of communication
Communication characteristics	Expectations	Suspend judgment
Verbal	Misunderstandings	Listen and observe
Simple, non-technical language	Nature of previous consultations	Show empathy but not collusion
Clarity of message	Distress	Encourage self-disclosure
Non-verbal	Fear	Explain what you can and cannot do
General demeanor	Anger and hostility	Re-establish confidence
Eye contact		Kick-start self-control
Signaling continuing attention		
The therapeutic relationship		
Practical considerations		
Familiarity		
Liking and trust		

Adapted with permission from Main & Spanswick (2000) pp 56–58.

Summary

- Back pain arises from a physical problem in the back. It is usually not psychogenic.
- We cannot divide back pain into physical or psychologic.
- Most patients with back pain are no different from the rest of us:
  - they are not personality-deficient
  - they do not have a psychiatric disorder
  - they are not malingering.

In summary, patients with back pain are not mad or bad or psychologically different from the rest of us. Most of them are normal people with pain in their back.

References

Averill P M, Novy D M, Nelson D V, Berry L A 1996 Correlates of depression in chronic pain patients: a comprehensive examination. Pain 65: 93–100

Balint M 1964 The doctor, his patient, and the illness. International Universities Press, New York

Banks S M, Kerns R D 1996 Explaining high rates of depression in chronic pain: a diathesis-stress framework. Psychological Bulletin 119: 95–110

Brosschot J F, Eriksen H R (eds) 2002 Special issue on somatization, sensitization and subjective health complaints. Scandinavian Journal of Psychology 43: 97–196

Burton A K, Tillotson K M, Main C J, Hollis S 1995 Psychosocial predictors of outcome in acute and subacute low-back trouble. Spine 20: 722–728

Clyde Z, Williams A C deC 2002 Depression and mood. In: Linton S J (ed.) New avenues for the prevention of chronic musculoskeletal pain and disability. Pain research and clinical management, vol. 12. Elsevier, Amsterdam, pp 105–121

Croft P R, Papageorgiou A C, Ferry S et al 1995 Psychological distress and low back pain: evidence from a prospective study in the general population. Spine 20: 2731–2737

Eriksen H R, Ursin H 2002 Sensitization and subjective health complaints. Scandinavian Journal of Psychology 43: 189–196

Fernandez E, Turk D C 1995 Clinical review: the scope and significance of anger in the experience of chronic pain. Pain 61: 165–175

Gatchel R L, Turk D C (eds) 1999 Psychosocial factors in pain. Guildford Press, New York

Leigh H, Reiser M F 1980 The patient: biological, psychological and social dimensions of medical practice. Plenum, New York, pp 39–69

Linton S J (ed.) 2002 New avenues for the prevention of chronic musculoskeletal pain and disability. Pain research and clinical management, vol. 12. Elsevier, Amsterdam

Magni G, Moreschi C, Rigatti-Luchini S, Merskey H 1994 Prospective study on the relationship between depressive symptoms and chronic musculoskeletal pain. Pain 56: 289–297

Main C J 1983 The modified somatic perception questionnaire. Journal of Psychosomatic Research 27: 503–514

Main C J, Spanswick C C 2000 Pain management: an interdisciplinary approach. Churchill Livingstone, Edinburgh

Main C J, Waddell G 1984 The detection of psychological abnormality in chronic low back pain using four simple scales. Current Concepts in Pain 2: 10–15

Main C J, Watson P J 2002 The distressed and angry low back pain patient. In: Gifford L (ed.) Topical issues in pain, vol. 3. CNS Press, Falmouth, pp 175–200

Main C J, Williams A C 2002 ABC of psychological medicine: musculoskeletal pain. British Medical Journal 325: 534–537

Main C J, Wood P L R, Hollis S, Spanswick C C, Waddell G 1992 The distress and risk assessment method: a simple patient classification to identify distress and evaluate the risk of poor outcome. Spine 17: 42–52

Mendelson G 1988 Psychiatric aspects of personal injury claims. CC Thomas, Springfield, IL, pp 122–123

Ohayon M M, Schatzbrg A F 2003 Using chronic pain to predict depressive morbidity in the general population. Archives of General Psychiatry 60: 39–47

Ohlund C, Lindstrom I, Areskoug B, Eeek C, Peterson L-E, Nachemson A 1994 Pain behavior in industrial subacute low back pain. Part I. Reliability: concurrent and predictive validity of pain behavior assessments. Pain 58: 201–209

Peebles J E, McWilliams L A, MacLennan R 2001 A comparison of Symptom Checklist 90 – revised profiles from patients with chronic pain from whiplash and patients with other musculoskeletal injuries. Spine 26: 766–770

Polatin P G, Kinney R K, Gatchel R J, Lillo E, Mayer T G 1993 Psychiatric illness and low back pain. Spine 18: 66–71

Roberts A 1991 The conservative treatment of low back pain. MD thesis, University of Nottingham

Robinson M E, Riley J L III 1999 The role of emotion in pain. In: Gatchel R L, Turk D C (eds) Psychosocial factors in pain. Guildford Press, New York, pp 74–88

Rush A J, Polatin P, Gatchel R J 2000 Depression and chronic low back pain: establishing priorities in treatment. Spine 25: 2566–2571

Simon G E, von Korff M, Piccinelli M, Fullerton C, Ormel J 1999 An international study of the relation between somatic symptoms and depression. New England Journal of Medicine 341: 1329–1335

Slesinger D, Archer R P, Duane W 2002 MMPI-2 characteristics in a chronic pain population. Assessment 9: 406–414

Sullivan M J L, Reesor K, Mikail S, Fisher R 1992 The treatment of depression in chronic low back pain: review and recommendations. Pain 50: 5–13

von Korff M, Resche L L, Dworkin S F 1993 First onset of common pain symptoms: a prospective study of depression as a risk factor. Pain 55: 251–258

Weisberg J N, Keefe F J 1997 Personality disorders in the chronic pain population. Pain Forum 6: 1–9

Wilson K G, Mikail S F, D'Eon J L, Minns J E 2001 Alternative diagnostic criteria for major depressive disorder in patients with chronic pain. Pain 91: 227–234

Wiltse L L, Rocchio P D 1975 Pre-operative psychological tests as predictions of success of chemonucleolysis in the treatment of the low back syndrome. Journal of Bone and Joint Surgery 57A: 478–483

Zung W W K 1965 A self-rated depression scale. Archives of General Psychiatry 32: 63–70

Chapter 12

Beliefs about back pain

Chris J. Main   Gordon Waddell

How people think and feel about back pain is central to what they do about it and how it affects them (Fig. 12.1). In Chapter 11 we looked at feelings and emotions. It is now time to look at how people *think* about back pain – their beliefs about the pain, about what they should do about it, about health care, about work, and about what it means for their future.

THE NATURE OF BELIEFS

Man, above all else, is the thinking animal. The power of human thought can move mountains and transform our lives. It is our strength and our weakness, which sets us apart from all the other beasts. Beliefs are the mental engine that drives

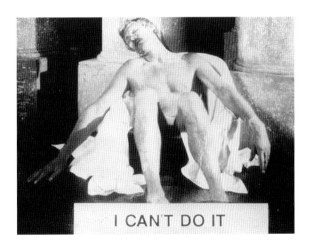

Figure 12.1   "I can't do it."

human behavior, and may raise us to the skies or cast us down to the depths of hell.

Beliefs are basic and relatively stable ideas about the nature of reality. They help us to understand our lives and our experience. Beliefs are ideas written in stone. They can become fixed and sometimes the only way to change them may be to break the mold.

Beliefs are shaped from childhood onwards and are the product of experience and learning and culture. We each develop our individual beliefs, but share them to a greater or lesser extent with our families, our peer groups, and our fellow workers. Some beliefs are very general, but others are highly specific to a particular situation. Personal experience molds our beliefs, but once they are established they may then persist despite contrary experience. Beliefs shape our perceptions of further experiences and determine our behavior.

Beliefs about pain and illness

Pain beliefs are patients' own ideas about their pain and what it means for them. To put this in context, it may help to start with beliefs about illness. There appear to be four main elements to patients' beliefs about illness (DeGood & Tait 2001, see also Petrie & Weinman 1998):

1. The nature of the illness – beliefs about the cause and meaning of the illness and symptoms
2. The future course of the illness – beliefs about its likely duration and outcome
3. Consequences – expected effects of the illness and its impact on the individual's life and work
4. Cure or control – beliefs about how to deal with the illness, including personal responsibility and expectations of health care.

These beliefs provide a framework for us to make sense of illness and how to deal with it. They influence our decisions about health care and sickness absence from work. Every patient brings a set of beliefs to the consulting room. Indeed, the fact that they consult at all shows certain beliefs about health care. Earlier psychological studies focused on general beliefs, and we have only recently begun to appreciate the importance of specific beliefs about back pain. Beliefs play an important role in the persistence of pain and how we adapt to it (Pincus & Morley 2002).

Pain beliefs range from the very general to the highly specific. They range from broad philosophic perspectives to very specific beliefs about the nature of *my* back trouble and *this* treatment. The most general beliefs are basic assumptions about pain and disability and work. These are personal beliefs but at the same time they are strongly rooted in a particular culture. They are often inconsistent and contradictory, and they are very difficult to change. More individual beliefs include basic personal characteristics such as introspection about health, self-confidence, and ability to cope. Finally, there are specific beliefs about this particular pain and how I should deal with it, or what others can and should do to help. These are the "nuts and bolts" that directly influence what each patient does about their problem. They help to determine illness behavior and disability. They are specific to the particular pain context. Patients' beliefs about their particular pain may be quite distinct from their knowledge and ideas about pain in general. These specific beliefs are also more open to positive or negative influence by health professionals.

Beliefs are not simply the product of the pain experience. Rather, beliefs about the pain, its course, its likely impact on life, and how to get adequate help lie at the heart of the chronic pain problem. Box 12.1 shows some common beliefs about chronic pain.

Psychosocial factors play an important part in the *process* of developing chronic pain and disability. They not only develop earlier than we previously thought, they also contribute to the process at an early stage.

Beliefs about damage

Pain is the most universal physical and emotional stress that human beings experience. Thirty-five percent of patients regard their pain as the most stressful event in their lives (at least at the point in time and in the context of clinical care). The emotional impact of any stress depends not only on the intensity and duration of the threat, but also on the extent to which we feel we can deal with it or that it may tax and exceed our resources.

Box 12.1   Common beliefs about chronic pain and treatment (adapted from DeGood & Tait 2001)

- Etiology of pain
  - pain as symptom of disease vs pain as a benign condition
  - somatic cause vs interaction of multiple factors
  - external vs internal, e.g., accident vs personal fitness
  - "someone is to blame" vs unfortunate, natural, or chance event
- Diagnostic expectations regarding
  - medical history
  - clinical examination
  - laboratory tests, especially X-rays and scans
  - consideration of psychosocial issues
- Treatment expectations
  - medical and physical treatment vs self-management issues
  - patient active vs passive, e.g., exercise and personal responsibility vs medication or surgery
  - "fix" or repair vs rehabilitation
- Outcome goals
  - "cure" vs partial relief or control of pain
  - rapid vs gradual improvement
  - 100% vs partial freedom from pain
  - pain vs disability
  - return to work vs quality of life

Table 12.1   Specific worries about back pain

The wrong movement might cause a serious problem with my back	64%
My body is indicating that something is dangerously wrong	50%
I might become disabled for a long time due to back pain	47%
I am unable to do all the things normal people do, because it is too easy to be injured	44%
My back pain may be due to a serious disease	19%

Based on data from Von Korff & Moore (2001).

Von Korff & Moore (2001) found that patients with back pain have a number of fears (Table 12.1). Most people seek to understand the cause of their problem. There is obvious concern about damage that may already have occurred, but there is also concern about the risk of future damage. Human beings are probably the only animals that can imagine and worry about the future. Fear of what may happen to us in the future can be even more important than present pain.

Tarasuk & Eakin (1994) interviewed people who claimed workers' compensation for back injuries. They focused on the workers' own perceptions and experience of what their back injury meant to them. How did their experience of back pain influence how they viewed their bodies, their work, and their future? A central feature was that many of these workers felt their back problems were permanent. This belief sometimes arose from their current experience of persisting pain, combined with other aspects of their current life situation. For most of them, however, it was linked to a belief that their backs were permanently vulnerable to reinjury. Even some who had a simple back strain a few weeks previously were convinced they would have back problems for life. Others feared their condition would get worse as they got older and lead eventually to permanent disability. Even if their back pain settled completely, many still had a fear of reinjury. Many had a sense of fragility (with echoes of spinal irritability). These beliefs had a strong influence on return to work.

Symonds et al (1995, 1996) looked more closely at beliefs about the future course and inevitability of back pain. They developed a short, simple Back Beliefs Questionnaire (Fig. 12.2). It is suitable for patients with back pain and also for workers with or without back pain. They found that workers with a previous history of back pain were more likely to believe their backs would give continuing problems. They were also more negative about their ability to control the pain and to take personal responsibility. The greater the number of previous spells and the longer the amount of time off work with back pain, the more negative their beliefs. Those who had back pain at the time of the study had more negative beliefs than those who were painfree. People who believed they would inevitably have continuing back trouble were more negative in their approach to rehabilitation and return to work.

We are trying to find out what people think about low back trouble. Please indicate your general views towards back trouble, *even if you have never had any.*
Please answer ALL statements and indicate whether you *agree* or *disagree* with each statement by circling the appropriate number on the scale.

1 = COMPLETELY DISAGREE, 5 = COMPLETELY AGREE

1	2	3	4	5
Completely disagree				Completely agree

		Disagree				Agree
1	There is no real treatment for back trouble	1	2	3	4	5
2	Back trouble will eventually stop you from working	1	2	3	4	5
3	Back trouble means periods of pain for the rest of one's life	1	2	3	4	5
4	Doctors cannot do anything for back trouble	1	2	3	4	5
5	A bad back should be exercised	1	2	3	4	5
6	Back trouble makes everything in life worse	1	2	3	4	5
7	Surgery is the most effective way to treat back trouble	1	2	3	4	5
8	Back trouble may mean you end up in a wheelchair	1	2	3	4	5
9	Alternative treatments are the answer to back trouble	1	2	3	4	5
10	Back trouble means long periods of time off work	1	2	3	4	5
11	Medication is the *only* way of relieving back trouble	1	2	3	4	5
12	Once you have had back trouble there is *always* a weakness	1	2	3	4	5
13	Back trouble *must* be rested	1	2	3	4	5
14	Later in life back trouble gets progressively worse	1	2	3	4	5

The inevitability scale uses nine of these statements: items 1, 2, 3, 6, 8, 10, 12, 13, 14.
Calculate the scale by reversing the scores (i.e. 5, 4, 3, 2, 1) and adding the nine scores.
©1993 University of Huddersfield, UK

Figure 12.2   The Back Beliefs Questionnaire (BBQ). From Symonds et al (1995), with permission.

Szpalski et al (1995) also found that patients who believed that low back pain is a lifetime problem sought more health care, took more bed rest, and used more medication.

Fear of hurt and harm

Fear is a basic instinct throughout the animal kingdom. Some fears, such as fear of the dark or of snakes, may be biologic and can occur even without personal experience. Other fears are learned. Pain is aversive and frightening, as it is commonly a warning signal of actual or impending tissue damage. This fear has an important and useful purpose. If a child touches something hot, it will burn itself. The sudden pain leads the child instinctively to withdraw its hand, thus minimizing tissue damage. The child does not think about withdrawing its hand. There is no time. In many such situations, pain is biologically useful, but because it is unpleasant and linked to such experiences, we become afraid of it.

There is increasing evidence that fear of pain, and fear of hurt and harm, is a fundamental mechanism in low back pain and disability (Vlaeyen & Linton 2000, 2002). In the first instance, most people's reaction to back pain is instinctive and automatic: they try to avoid what seemed to be the cause of the pain. However, fear may then lead to continued attempts to avoid that situation. Up to a point this is reasonable. Unfortunately, depending on circumstances, patients may develop all sorts of misunderstandings about back pain. The intensity of fear depends on the context of the pain, and particular situations will be more likely to cause painful memories and fear (Turk et al 1996). Fear may become associated not only with recurrent injury, but also with pain itself. Such fears may develop into fixed beliefs about hurt and harm.

If patients wrongly believe that pain from unfit muscles means continuing damage, it may seem natural and indeed logical that they should avoid exercise. If they believe that pain *always* means further damage is taking place, they may avoid any

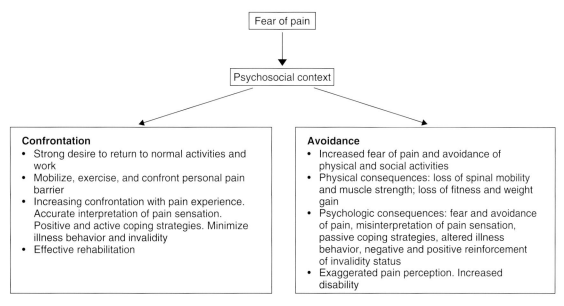

Figure 12.3   Fear avoidance: confronters and avoiders. In reality, of course, many people fall between these two extremes. Adapted from Lethem et al (1983).

treatment that involves pain, e.g., trying to mobilize. They may even give up treatment or rehabilitation altogether. Inappropriate fears about back pain, based on misunderstandings or on painful emotional memories, are an important obstacle to treatment and rehabilitation.

However, pain does not always produce fear or anxiety. For example, athletes accept pain as a normal part of training, especially when unfit or when recovering from injury. This may be a useful analogy for patients with back pain.

Fear–avoidance beliefs

With experimental pain in the laboratory, forewarning of pain may reduce its impact. Subjects cope better if they feel they have some control over what is happening. Lack of control makes pain feel more intense. In clinical pain also, expectations and fear of pain affect the intensity of pain, emotions, and pain behavior.

Fear is a powerful negative drive in humans and in animals, closely allied to pain. Fear is to some extent an innate, inborn instinct, but to a greater extent it is learned. We learn from experience to fear situations or stimuli that have caused us stress or pain, and we then try to avoid them. If we avoid

the situation and do not have pain, this may reinforce our belief and fear about the cause of the pain, and reward our efforts to avoid it.

Patients who believe that physical activity may aggravate their pain, whether from their past experience or because of their understanding of the pain, will expect and fear more pain if they are active. Note that this is all a matter of fears and expectations about what *might* happen. Schmidt (1985) showed that patients with chronic low back pain do not do as much on a treadmill task and have lower pain tolerance when they immerse their forearm in ice water. However, it is not simply a question of the intensity of pain during the task. They found that treadmill performance depended more on previous reports of pain than on pain at the time. Cold tolerance depended more on beliefs about how well they could cope. Al-Obaidi et al (2000) again showed that physical performance on lumbar isometric strength testing depended on anticipation of pain and fear-avoidance beliefs, rather than on actual pain during testing or beliefs about disability.

Lethem et al (1983) and Troup et al (1987) used these ideas to develop a "fear avoidance model of exaggerated pain perception" in chronic low back pain (Fig. 12.3). Their main focus was on patients' beliefs as the driving force for behavior. They drew

Here are some of the things which other patients have told us about their pain. For each statement please circle any number from 0 to 6 to say how much physical activities such as bending, lifting, walking or driving affect or would affect your back pain.

	COMPLETELY DISAGREE			UNSURE			COMPLETELY AGREE	
1 My pain was caused by physical activity	0	1	2	3	4	5	6
2 Physical activity makes my pain worse	0	1	2	3	4	5	6
3 Physical activity might harm my back	0	1	1	3	4	5	6
4 I should not do physical activities which (might) make my pain worse	0	1	2	3	4	5	6
5 I cannot do physical activities which (might) make by pain worse	0	1	2	3	4	5	6

The following statements are about how your normal work affects or would affect your back gain.

	COMPLETELY DISAGREE			UNSURE			COMPLETELY AGREE	
6 My pain was caused by my work or by an accident at work	0	1	2	3	4	5	6
7 My work aggravated my pain	0	1	2	3	4	5	6
8 I have a claim for compensation for my pain	0	1	2	3	4	5	6
9 My work is too heavy for me	0	1	2	3	4	5	6
10 My work makes or would make my pain worse	0	1	2	3	4	5	6
11 My work might harm my back	0	1	2	3	4	5	6
12 I should not do my normal work with my present pain	0	1	2	3	4	5	6
13 I cannot do my normal work with my present pain	0	1	2	3	4	5	6
14 I cannot do my normal work until my pain is treated	0	1	2	3	4	5	6
15 I do not think that I will be back to my normal work within 3 months	0	1	2	3	4	5	6
16 I do not think that I will ever be able to go back to that work	0	1	2	3	4	5	6

Figure 12.4   The Fear-Avoidance Beliefs Questionnaire (Waddell et al 1993).

attention to the central role of fear of pain leading directly to pain-avoidance behavior.

Measuring fear-avoidance beliefs

We used these ideas to develop the Fear-Avoidance Beliefs Questionnaire (FABQ), which measures beliefs about physical activity and work (Fig. 12.4; Waddell et al 1993). People with back pain may believe that physical activity or work could increase their pain, injure their back, or damage their back. These beliefs are closely allied to their conviction that they should not or cannot do these activities. We showed that these fear-avoidance beliefs help to explain self-reported disability in activities of daily living and loss of time from work. Table 12.2 shows how much fear-avoidance beliefs *add* to disability, over and above the effects

Table 12.2   The influence of pain and fear-avoidance beliefs on disability

	Disability in activities of daily living (%)	Work loss (%)
Pain		
Anatomic pattern		
Time pattern	14	5
Severity		
Fear-avoidance beliefs	+32	+26
Total identified	56	31

These are the additive effects, after allowing for severity of pain. It is usually only possible to identify a modest proportion of any biologic relationship.
Based on data from Waddell et al (1993).

of pain itself. Indeed, we found that low back disability depends more on fear avoidance than on pain or physical pathology. *Fear of pain may be more disabling than pain itself.*

In our study, fear-avoidance beliefs about work were more powerful than fear-avoidance beliefs about physical activity in general.

The development of fear-avoidance beliefs

It may seem at first that fear-avoidance beliefs are a natural interpretation of pain as a signal of injury, but that is only part of the story. In fact, by the time pain becomes chronic, there is very little relation between fear-avoidance beliefs and pain itself. In our study, fear-avoidance beliefs about physical activity were only weakly related to the severity of pain. Fear-avoidance beliefs about work bore no relation to any measure of pain. None of the fear-avoidance beliefs was related to duration of pain. Fear-avoidance beliefs seemed to relate more to the uncertainty of diagnosis than to the severity of the physical problem.

Fear-avoidance beliefs may start from experience that physical activity or work aggravates back pain, although even this may have more to do with the patient's understanding or expectation than with reality. Only 36% of patients with low back pain say that physical activity such as walking makes their pain worse. When you question them carefully, 45% say it makes no difference and 16% say it

actually makes their pain better. Even if physical activity does aggravate pain, that is quite different from being the cause of the pain. Temporary aggravation may also be quite different from any long-term effect. To use the sports analogy again, training may cause temporary musculoskeletal aches but still lead to long-term benefit. Moreover, patients' perceptions of physical activity and its relation to pain are often inaccurate. Several studies have shown that patients with back pain overestimate the physical demands of their job compared with healthy fellow workers. Patients tend to overpredict the pain they will get on exercise. Treadmill endurance of patients with chronic low back pain is only 75% that of normal controls, even when this form of exercise does not increase their pain (Schmidt 1985). Both groups rate their exertion similarly, but the patients with back pain actually show lower levels of physiologic demand. They stop because they overestimate their exertion rather than because of increased pain. Exercise to the limit of pain tolerance is very dependent on feedback. In the absence of feedback, chronic pain patients increase their performance on an incremented exercise program at the same rate as normal, painfree subjects.

Fear-avoidance beliefs may start from experience, but all the evidence suggests that those beliefs then develop lives of their own which may diverge from reality. The crucial point is that fear of pain is more about expectancy of future pain than about current reality. Avoidance behavior may reduce nociception at the acute stage. Later, these avoidance behaviors may persist in anticipation of pain rather than as a response to it. If we do not attempt the activity and do not get increased pain, we may get false reinforcement. There is then no need for any external reinforcement to maintain the behavior. Avoidance behavior itself reinforces fear-avoidance beliefs in a vicious circle. It is like the dog that barks every time the postman appears. The postman never has and never will break into the house, but the dog believes that is because it has chased him away. The very fact that the threat never materializes encourages the dog to go on barking every time the postman appears.

Vlaeyen et al (1995a,b) looked at more specific fears that physical activity or work may cause (re-) injury. They found that patients who were

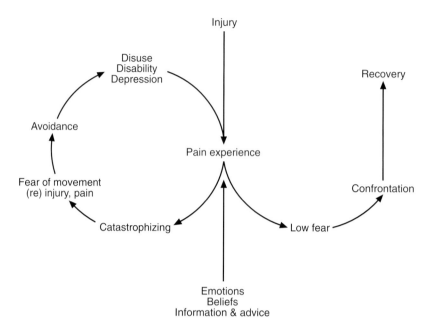

Figure 12.5 The fear-avoidance model. Fear of movement and reinjury can determine how some people recover from back pain while others go on to chronic pain and disability. Adapted from Vlaeyen, personal communication (2002).

afraid of reinjury showed more fear and avoidance behavior when they were asked to do a simple movement. Patients with high fear levels and avoidance behavior performed less well at motor tasks. This fear was more closely linked to depressive symptoms and catastrophizing than to pain itself.

The effect of fear-avoidance beliefs

From the fear-avoidance model, Lethem et al (1983) described patients as confronters or avoiders (Fig. 12.3). These are obviously the extremes, but they illustrate the principle. Confronters may have severe pain, but they have little fear of pain. They remain positive and confident and able to confront their pain. They gradually increase their activities even if they have some temporary aggravation of pain. They gain confidence in their ability to cope with the pain and to maintain daily activities despite some persisting symptoms. Success reinforces their positive beliefs and their ability to cope. Avoiders have similar pain, but they also have a strong fear of pain. This leads them to avoid activities that are painful, or that they think might be painful. Indeed, they do everything possible to avoid the experience of pain, fearing reinjury and

further damage. They rest a lot and wait for the pain to get better. Avoidance behavior maintains and exacerbates fear, which may even become a phobia.

Longitudinal studies by Klenerman et al (1995) and Burton et al (1995) showed that these fears act at an early stage and contribute to the development, not just the maintenance, of chronic pain and disability. Klenerman et al (1995) studied 300 patients attending their family doctor with acute low back pain, and found that fear-avoidance beliefs at the acute stage predicted outcome at 2 and 12 months. Some patients ignored their pain, carried on, and took physical exercise, while others took analgesics and rested. Those who used the more active coping strategies had less pain and disability and sick leave at 2 and 12 months. Fritz et al (2001) confirmed that fear-avoidance beliefs were present within 5 days, and predicted disability and work status at 4 weeks. Thus, fear-avoidance beliefs are important at the acute stage, and not just in chronic pain and disability.

It is always difficult to restart physical activity or work after sickness absence. The longer the lay-off, the greater the loss of physical fitness, and the worse the deconditioning, the harder it will be. Return to work may then lead to some temporary increase in low back pain, which reinforces fear-avoidance beliefs. If the patient goes off sick again, this failure will further reinforce these negative beliefs. Fear-avoidance beliefs about work are most important in patients with work-related back pain and compensation claims.

Vlaeyen & Linton (2000, 2002) have reviewed the latest research on pain-related fear and chronic disability. Figure 12.5 shows their fear-avoidance model.

Summary

There are many aspects to fear

- Beliefs about injury and damage
- Pain and fear; expectations and fear of future pain and reinjury
- The assumption that hurt means harm
- Fear avoidance: "confronters" and "avoiders"
- Increased pain behavior and disability
- Barriers to rehabilitation

Personal responsibility and control

Psychologists have shown that, from early childhood, one of our main goals is to try to gain some control over our world. The attempt to reduce uncertainty and establish control seems to be one of the most fundamental human drives. One of the key aspects of personality is the strength of this drive and the balance between our personal needs for control and the needs of others. These beliefs are probably not innate, but more likely a product of learning and social conditioning. Our self-confidence is related in part to the extent to which we can establish sufficient control over our environment to meet our needs. If our needs are frustrated we become angry and unsettled, and try to regain control. We all differ in our tolerance for lack of control.

As a result of this life experience, we all form beliefs about the extent to which we are able to get control of our lives. At one extreme are those who believe they are powerless to affect their own future. Their lives and human affairs are predetermined by fate or the stars. It does not matter what they do; the die is already cast. They are passive and wait for life or other people, including health professionals, to take control for them. At the other extreme are those who believe they can and indeed must exercise control over every aspect of their lives. They are hell-bent on establishing control. Not only do they have confidence that they can establish control, but they try at every opportunity to do so, and become various sorts of "control freaks." We might describe these extremes as being either *externally* or *internally* controlled.

Of course, it is easy to caricature such personality types. Most people fall somewhere between these extremes. But this concept of control has an important influence on how people react to adversity and illness (Williams & Keefe 1991, Jensen et al 1994). In particular, it influences how people seek and respond to treatment. *Internals* seek less health care, and respond well to management approaches in which they can play an active part. *Externals* seek more health care. They are more likely to be passive and to rely on health professionals to make them better.

Clinical impression and psychological studies suggest that patients who accept personal responsibility for their pain do better than those who leave it to others. Those who feel it is entirely up to doctors or therapists or someone else to cure them do worse. Accepting personal responsibility is closely allied to feelings of control. People who feel in control of their own destiny are more able to take responsibility for their own health and do better than those who feel that they cannot do much about it.

Gaining control over back pain means actually mastering the pain and ordinary activities of daily living. Confidence to do so depends on the individual's own judgment of their capabilities. Psychologists call this self-efficacy – the belief that you can *successfully* perform a particular act. People are more likely to attempt and complete activities that they believe they are able to do. We do not attempt the daily tasks that constitute low back disability without thinking about them first. We evaluate the tasks and our own ability against our fear of possible pain or harm. This inner debate largely determines our performance, when we decide to stop, or whether we even try. Lackner et al (1996) showed that patients with chronic low back pain could predict quite accurately their performance at a set of lifting, carrying, pushing, and pulling tasks. Indeed, patients' own rating of their expected ability was more closely related to their performance than pain, fear of pain, or fear of reinjury. Estlander et al (1994) found that back patients' beliefs in their ability to endure physical activity were the best predictor of isokinetic performance. Anthropometric measures, pain, and disability levels were all less important.

People who regard themselves as capable have more confidence in their own ability. They try harder, they persevere despite their symptoms, and they show fewer signs of anxiety. People who regard themselves as less able do not try as hard, are less persistent, get frustrated, and give up more easily. They show more distress and they do not cooperate as well with treatment and advice. Patients with strong beliefs in their own abilities commit themselves more firmly to their tasks and are more highly motivated to complete them despite temporary setbacks. They also function better psychologically and show less distress. They are less likely to become disabled.

Many of the beliefs described in previous sections may influence patients' own expectations of what they can do. Self-efficacy may then be one of the most important links between intensity of pain and beliefs vs behavior, performance, and disability (Arnstein et al 1999). People with high self-efficacy are more confident in their ability to achieve control of their pain, and live up to their own expectations. They are less likely to become depressed.

Large & Strong (1997) studied 19 people who were successfully coping with chronic low back pain. These people were well, leading active lives and not receiving current health care. This was a selected group of people, but they offered several insights into coping.

- They stressed *authenticity*: the coper must be genuine and sincere and have a real physical disorder.
- Coping involves *mastery*: control and relief are obtained through learning, solving problems, and through suffering.
- They were stoical: "carrying on regardless" and "not lying down to things."
- They were cheerful: "staying positive," keeping their "pride" and keeping hope.

- They saw coping as a method of maintaining social interactions and appearances and of gaining acceptance.
- They would still prefer to be painfree, but saw coping as a necessary evil that enabled them to get on with their lives.

Beliefs about treatment

Patients vary widely in their beliefs about health care and their expectations about the outcome of treatment (Main & Spanswick 2000, DeGood & Tait 2001). Some patients may arrive with a straightforward and realistic understanding of their problem and realistic expectations. Others may believe their spine is crumbling, that they will end up in a wheelchair, and that no one can do anything to prevent it. You should always try to find out what each patient expects in terms of treatment and its likely outcome. These beliefs about treatment obviously also depend on what patients believe about the nature and cause of their pain. You must correct misunderstandings, if the patient is to accept and benefit from treatment. You must also give a clear and honest account of the range of possible treatment options. Do not be tempted into offering second-rate treatment just because the patient is distressed and you feel sorry for them. Patients must have realistic expectations of treatment if they are to make sensible choices and not be disappointed. Patients and health professionals must share the same beliefs and expectations concerning treatment if they are to work in harmony to a common goal. This is also one of the keys to satisfaction with care.

Beliefs about work

Beliefs about back pain and its relation to work are fundamental for rehabilitation and return to work (Dehlin et al 1981, Feuerstein 1991, Main 2002). Basic beliefs set the scene: about whether back pain should be treated by rest or staying active. Some patients – or their wives or doctors or therapists or employers – believe they should not return to work till their pain is 100% cured. Unfortunately, from the natural history of back pain as a persistent or recurring problem, that is unrealistic. In reality, most people do continue working or get back to work while they still have some pain.

Table 12.3 The impact of patients' beliefs about return to work on the outcome of a multidisciplinary treatment program

	Outcome of program	
	Did return to work	Did not return to work
Beliefs before treatment:		
will return to work	31 (81%)	7
will not return to work	12 (46%)	14

Based on data from Hildebrandt et al (1997).

Sandstrom & Esbjornsson (1986) found that patients' own expectations were the best predictor of return to work after rehabilitation. They questioned patients before a rehabilitation program, and those who believed they would not be able to return to work were much less likely to do so. One of the most important statements was: "I am afraid to start working again, because I don't think I will be able to manage." Carosella et al (1994) found that patients' own expectations about return to work were the best predictor of whether they were likely to drop out of an intensive rehabilitation program. It was a better predictor than severity of pain, patients' perceptions of their work environment, or time off work. Hildebrandt et al (1997) also found that poor expectations were one of the strongest predictors of failure to return to work after a multidisciplinary treatment program (Table 12.3). Expectations about return to work reflect self-efficacy. Patients who are convinced they will continue to have back pain and remain disabled are likely to fulfil their own prophecy. And that is quite apart from their physical condition. Changing attitudes like this is fundamental to successful rehabilitation.

Modern approaches to the management of musculoskeletal symptoms in the workplace focus on obstacles to recovery (Main 2002). Among the most important are workers' or patients' beliefs about their condition, about their work and the workplace. Patients may believe that their back pain was caused by injury at work, and that they are vulnerable to reinjury. They may attribute fault and blame to their employer, which undermines cooperation about return to work. DeGood & Kiernan (1996) showed that patients who blamed their employer reported similar levels of pain and disability, but they had more distress and poorer response to treatment. They were much less likely to return to work. Vowles & Gross (2003) suggest that specific fears about work-related injury are most important for rehabilitation and return to work.

COPING WITH PAIN AND DISABILITY

Coping is the way in which we deal with problems. More precisely, coping strategies are the purposeful mental efforts we make to manage or reduce the impact of stress (Lazarus & Folkman 1984). But coping is not only a matter of how we think. It includes what we do, so it is also a matter of behavior. Coping is how we try to prevent problems from taxing or exceeding our resources and endangering our mental well-being.

People cope with stress or adversity or pain in many different ways. Broadly speaking, coping strategies either confront (in an attempt to deal with) the stress, or try to escape from or avoid the situation. *Problem-focused* coping aims to control the pain, e.g., by avoiding situations or activities that cause or increase the pain, or by doing things that reduce it. *Emotion-focused* coping aims to reduce its emotional impact, e.g., by trying not to think about the pain. This does not mean that we only use one or other kind of coping strategy. We all use varying combinations of problem-focused and emotion-focused strategies to cope.

Ideally, the most effective coping strategy is to avoid a stressful situation entirely. For example, it may be possible to avoid certain activities that cause or aggravate back pain. We might think of such accommodation as a set of successful coping strategies. Unfortunately, avoidance is not always possible or may have a cost, and we have seen that sometimes the cost is high. You may try to reduce the aggravation of back pain by avoiding lifting, but that may cost you your job. If sitting is painful, you may avoid travel and certain social situations, but that may impair your quality of life. Avoiding sex lest it increase back pain may put strain on a valued relationship. The balance of costs and benefits of avoidance is a matter for the individual. It depends on the person's circumstances and needs. If avoidance causes too much disruption to family life or work, other coping strategies will be required.

In fact, back patients employ a wide range of behaviors and coping strategies to limit the effects of pain. Much coping may be trial and error, or based on information and advice from friends, relatives, or health professionals. The choice of strategy will be based on the patient's understanding of the problem. As we discussed previously, the strategies people choose depend on their beliefs about the pain, its cause, and its likely outcome. This choice also depends on their confidence in being able to influence events, and their repertoire of coping skills and behaviors.

Coping with back pain

Most people with back pain, even chronic pain, cope with the pain, adjust, and continue to lead more or less normal lives. Chronic pain is not synonymous with disability and depression. So how is it that some people cope with the pain successfully while others become disabled? What are the different mental strategies they use to cope with the stress (Jensen et al 1991, Main & Spanswick 2000)?

Coping strategies may be active or passive (Snow-Turek et al 1996). Active coping strategies are positive attempts to manage the pain, e.g., exercising, staying active, and ignoring the pain. Passive strategies succumb to the pain, e.g., withdrawal, giving up control, rest, and analgesics. Active coping strategies help to reduce pain, depression, and disability, whereas passive strategies are associated with increased pain, depression, and disability. Passive coping strategies also predict poorer outcomes over time.

The most widely used measure of coping is the Coping Strategies Questionnaire (Figure 12.6; Rosenstiel & Keefe 1983). This measures helpful and unhelpful coping strategies, which influence the outcome of treatment. The most harmful or maladaptive coping strategy in patients with back pain is catastrophizing. Catastrophizing is negative and distorted thinking and worrying about the pain and one's inability to cope. We might summarize it as "fearing the worst" or "looking on the dark side." This may be clearer in some examples from the Coping Strategies Questionnaire:

Cognitive coping strategies

1. *Diverting attention*: thinking of things that serve to distract one away from the pain.
   Sample item: I count in my head or run a song through my head.

2. *Reinterpreting pain sensations*: imagining something which, if real, would be inconsistent with the experience of pain.
   Sample item: I just think of it as some other sensation, such as numbness.

3. *Coping self-statements*: telling oneself that one can cope with pain, no matter how bad it gets.
   Sample item: I tell myself to be brave and carry on despite the pain,

4. *Ignoring pain sensation*: denying that pain hurts or affects one in any way.
   Sample item: I tell myself it doesn't hurt.

5. *Praying or hoping*: telling myself to hope and pray that the pain will get better someday.
   Sample item: I pray to God that it won't last.

6. *Catastrophizing*: negative self-statements, catastrophizing thoughts and ideation.
   Sample item: I worry all the time about whether it will end.

Behavioral coping strategies

1. *Increasing activity level*: engaging in active behaviors which divert one's attention away from pain.
   Sample item: I do something active, like household chores or projects.

2. *Increasing pain behavior*: overt pain behaviors that reduce pain sensations.
   Sample item: I take my medication.

Effectiveness ratings

1. Control over pain

2. Ability to decrease pain

Figure 12.6 The Coping Strategies Questionnaire. From Rosenstiel & Keefe (1983), with permission.

- "It is terrible and I feel it is never going to get any better."
- "It is awful and it overwhelms me."
- "I worry all the time about whether it will end."
- "I feel I can't stand it any more."
- "I feel like I can't go on."

Catastrophizing is maladaptive: it is irrational and harmful and leads to psychological and physical dysfunction.

Widely differing beliefs and coping strategies help to explain the very different outcomes of back pain. People tend to cope either quite well or quite badly. People who catastrophize do particularly badly. This fits with clinical experience that most people cope well with low back pain and get on with their lives more or less normally despite the pain. A few become chronic back cripples from ordinary backache.

Beliefs, emotions, and the development of disability

There are complex links between beliefs, coping strategies, and pain behavior. Beliefs frame our mental image of the pain problem; they have a direct effect on mood and may lead to depression. They also affect how we try to cope. Coping strategies link beliefs and behavior. A sense of personal control and self-efficacy are associated with positive and active coping strategies and better mental adjustment. Negative thoughts and coping strategies lead to maladaptive behavior. They impair psychological and physical adjustment to pain and increase chronic pain and illness behavior. Lack of personal control and feelings of helplessness are associated with passive coping strategies and catastrophizing. Catastrophizing is closely related to maladaptive beliefs and depression.

There is a huge amount of recent interest and research in this field (Kerns et al 1997, Petrie & Weinman 1998, Main & Spanswick 2000, Turner et al 2000, Sullivan et al 2001). Much of this psychological research is quite technical and there is a lot of overlap between different measures. Despite that, there is emerging agreement on a number of key themes:

- Beliefs about pain and coping strategies can influence the perception of pain and its impact.
- Such beliefs develop from a wide variety of sources.
- Patients often get "mixed messages" from health care providers.
- Patients may develop mistaken beliefs about back pain and treatment.
- Some coping strategies are more useful or effective than others.
- Individuals differ in the coping strategies they use.
- There are close links between fear, catastrophizing, and depression.
- Dysfunctional beliefs and negative coping strategies can aggravate illness behavior and disability.
- Such beliefs can be thought of as obstacles to recovery and to rehabilitation.

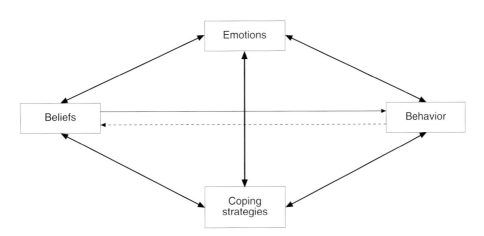

Figure 12.7   The relationship between beliefs and behavior.

Flor et al (1990) stressed the role of learning in the development and maintenance of chronic pain and disability. Chronic pain and inactivity lead to preoccupation with physical symptoms. Withdrawal, distress, and depression increase bodily awareness and aggravate the pain. Pain patients often misinterpret their sensations. They develop maladaptive beliefs about the cause and meaning of their pain, and what they should do about it. Once these beliefs become fixed, they are very resistant to change, even when they are clearly inaccurate and unhelpful. Avoidance learning and passive coping strategies may be particularly important and difficult to reverse, especially if they lead to physiologic changes:

$$\text{Learning} \iff \begin{array}{c}\text{Changed}\\\text{behavior}\end{array} \iff \begin{array}{c}\text{Physiologic}\\\text{changes}\end{array}$$

HEALTH CARE

How beliefs affect health care

Beliefs about back pain determine what we do about it, including the health care we seek and how we respond to treatment.

Most patients, like most doctors and therapists, work on a simple Cartesian model of pain. They start from the belief that pain is a warning signal that something is wrong with their bodies. If it is severe or if it does not settle, they believe they should seek health care to diagnose and treat the underlying problem. That may be an appropriate response to trauma or acute illness. However, if expectations of diagnosis and cure are not met, fear soon rears its ugly head. If pain becomes chronic and they do not get a clear diagnosis or cure, or, even worse, if they receive conflicting diagnoses and advice, they become confused. They do not understand why pain persists or recurs, and may express a desire to "have the bit which hurts cut out." Health care is now confounded by a morass of experience, beliefs, and coping strategies. Some of these may be reasonable but others are likely to be mistaken or positively harmful.

We have reviewed the spectrum of beliefs and coping strategies that affect health care for back pain. At one end of the spectrum are people with back pain who are not unduly concerned about it.

Although they have pain, which may be persistent or recurring, they do not believe it is a serious problem. They have little fear and do not worry about long-term consequences. They accept it is up to them to deal with the problem, they take control, and they get on with their lives despite the pain. They do not seek much health care. If they do decide to see a doctor to make sure there is nothing seriously wrong, they are easy to reassure. They then only seek health care occasionally to help control more acute episodes or for short-term sick certification.

At the other end of the spectrum are patients to whom back pain is a serious problem that takes over their attention and their lives. Fear dominates their approach. They are convinced it is due to some serious disease, which no one has yet been able to identify. They are pessimistic about the future, believing they will continue to have back pain permanently and that sooner or later it will disable them. They feel it is all out of their control, and there is nothing they can do about it. It is up to health professionals to find out what is wrong and to cure them. Their beliefs are fixed and difficult to change. They do not accept reassurance easily, and may seek repeated reassurance or alternative opinions. They have low expectations of treatment and poorer outcomes. They may be depressed, which distorts their beliefs and coping strategies, and makes them even more hopeless and helpless. And harder to help. One of the most striking features of some patients with chronic pain is maladaptive beliefs about medical diagnosis and treatment. Despite repeated negative investigations, they still demand more tests in their desperate search for a cause for their pain. Despite multiple failed treatments, they are still pathetically ready to undergo more of the same, even if there is little realistic hope that it will help. Indeed, their own experience should show it is more likely to make them worse. Such wishful thinking may be an understandable result of desperation, but such beliefs and behavior are maladaptive. They are unrealistic and harmful, and may trap these patients into a hopeless cycle of treatment, preventing them from seeking a more realistic and effective approach.

Fortunately, few chronic pain patients reach that sorry state. In most patients with back pain, specific beliefs about treatment may be more powerful than these general beliefs. Kalauokalani et al

(2001) found little difference between acupuncture and massage in a randomized controlled trial. More interesting, however, they also looked at patients' expectations of treatment at the start of the trial. Patients who believed that acupuncture was more effective did better with acupuncture. Patients who believed that massage was more effective did better with massage. Thus, patient expectations of treatment may have a greater influence on outcome than any physical effect of the treatment. Once again, they found that specific beliefs about treatment appear to be more important than general optimism or faith about health care.

Fear avoidance of movement and physical activity and exercise is one of the major obstacles to physical therapy and rehabilitation.

How health care influences beliefs about back pain

The information and advice we give to our patients can have a profound effect on their beliefs. Too often, this effect is negative. The harmful effect of medical "labeling" was first shown in hypertension. A population survey found people with asymptomatic hypertension. Before the survey they were unaware of their condition, had no symptoms, and were not ill. After they were told they had hypertension, they developed symptoms and became ill. There was no change in their blood pressure, but labeling them sick made them ill and turned them into patients. There is some evidence this is equally true in back pain.

Tarasuk & Eakin (1994) explored how workers' sense of permanent vulnerability in their back was related to their health care. Many of these patients' beliefs seemed to come from, or at least be reinforced by, health professionals. This was partly due to the information and advice they received: your back is injured, it is damaged, it is vulnerable to reinjury.

It is not only patients who have fear-avoidance beliefs. Linton et al (2002) studied 60 family doctors and 71 physical therapists. More than two-thirds said they would advise patients to avoid painful movements. More than a quarter believed that sick leave was a good treatment for back pain. More than one-third believed that reduction of pain was a prerequisite for return to work. Health professionals who held such negative, fear-avoidance beliefs were more likely to give poor information and advice, and more passive management. Fear-avoidance beliefs can be infectious!

Some of the messages are more subtle. Medical uncertainty and the absence of a definite diagnosis or prognosis cast doubt on the possibility of full recovery. Conflicting opinions and treatments imply that no one will be able to find the answer. Deyo & Diehl (1986) found that patients' most frequent reason for dissatisfaction with medical care was failure to get an adequate explanation for their back pain. Fifteen percent of patients did not believe that doctors and nurses understood their pain problem. Patients who felt that their explanation was inadequate wanted more diagnostic tests, did not cooperate as well with treatment, and had poorer outcomes at 3 weeks.

Think about some of the things we tell patients with ordinary backache. Take the example of normal, age-related changes on lumbar spine X-rays. "You have wear and tear in your spine" or (even worse) "degenerate disk disease." To patients, this means serious deterioration; it is irreversible, and will get even worse as they get older. If I am like this now what will I be like in 10 years? Will I end up in a wheelchair? It is no use then saying: "But it is nothing to worry about!" The damage is done. We have labeled them with a disease that may make them ill.

Our advice on management is just as bad. Too many doctors and therapists give the implicit message: "Pain is a signal that you are damaging your back, so you should stop whatever you are doing." Unfortunately, this often includes daily activities and work. Advice to change your lifestyle and even your job confirms that your disability will be permanent. This all promotes fear avoidance, illness behavior, and disability. And we are surprised at our patients' beliefs? It is then too late to tell them to stop worrying and that it is time to get active again.

Health professionals are also guilty of taking over. Patients bring their problems to us and we take responsibility for diagnosis and treatment. Unfortunately we have no magic cure for backache, but we take over anyway. Instead of advising patients on how they themselves can best deal with their problem, we prescribe our treatment. If patients get better, there is no problem, but if they do not get better quite quickly they are trapped.

Box 12.2   Interview prompts (adapted with permission from Main & Williams 2002)

- What do you understand caused your pain?
- What are you expecting will help you?
- How are other people reacting to your back pain (family, co-workers, employer)?
- What are you doing to cope with your pain?
- How are you coping at work?

Instead of patients taking responsibility and coping with their own situation, they have handed over responsibility, lost control, and now wait helplessly to be "fixed," with all the negative effects on disability and outcomes.

Clinical management

Patients who are convinced that the doctor takes their pain seriously are more likely to accept information and advice. Unfortunately, the converse is more common. Patients who feel a doctor dismisses or underrates their pain are less likely to disclose their feelings and fears. They are also less likely to accept reassurance or adhere to treatment.

The vital first step is simply to be more aware of patients' own beliefs (Box 12.2). If back pain persists or is becoming a problem, you should look carefully at this patient's individual beliefs about the pain and its management. They will have discussed it with families and friends and fellow workers, and gathered lay information and advice. You should appreciate the power of folklore and old wives' tales. Popular magazines are full of advice about back pain, and hardly a month passes without another miracle cure. Nowadays, they may also have looked on the internet. So it is essential to find out just what your patient believes. Once again, do not assume that you know what they think: ask them! What have other doctors or therapists told them – or rather, what have they understood from what they were told? What does their partner think? What about their employer and fellow workers?

We should try to identify mistaken beliefs and dysfunctional coping strategies. These may include beliefs about the cause of the pain, its likely progress and outcome, or its relation to activity and work. What is this patient looking for from this consultation? What are their expectations of treatment? Are they realistic? How are they coping with the pain – what are their coping strategies and are they successful? Are they catastrophizing or depressed? Mistaken beliefs and dysfunctional coping strategies not only aggravate and perpetuate disability, they may also form obstacles to treatment.

Beliefs are not hard-wired – they can be changed. So we can try to correct misunderstandings and mistaken beliefs. For many patients, accurate information is enough, but it must be honest and reliable. False reassurance will surely return to haunt you. For some patients, reassurance may need to be repeated and continuing. Information and advice may be supplemented by written material. It is important that all members of the team – doctors and therapists – tell the same story even if they use different words. But remember the aim is not just to impart information. The purpose of the exercise is to address and change dysfunctional beliefs.

Fixed beliefs and dysfunctional coping strategies are likely to be resistant to simple information and advice. Personal experience is then a more powerful intervention. We will discuss this further when we look at rehabilitation.

We should pay particular attention to specific beliefs about back pain and work. It is important to get across the message that the best treatment for back pain is to stay active, continue ordinary activities as normally as possible, and get on with your life. This is much more positive and acceptable than bald advice to "get back to work." Getting active and back to work does *not* lead to reinjury, but actually reduces the chance of recurrent problems. You do *not* need to wait till the pain is 100% gone. Indeed, the sooner you get active, the faster you will get better.

Building patients' confidence and self-efficacy and changing their expectations about return to work are fundamental to successful rehabilitation.

Back pain is often a persistent or recurring problem, and it is vital for patients to accept responsibility for their own management to deal with future problems. The role of the doctor or therapist is to assist and enable the patient to regain control. At the same time, most of us need support and encouragement at times, particularly when we face difficulties. Patients also appreciate positive reinforcement of their progress.

Beliefs about back pain 237

Box 12.3   Factors associated with chronicity and outcome (reproduced with permission from Main & Williams 2002)

Distress
- Symptom awareness and concern
- Depressive reactions, helplessness

Beliefs about pain and disability
- Significance and controllability
- Fears and misunderstanding about the pain

Behavioral factors
- Guarded movements and avoidance behavior
- Coping style and strategies

Box 12.4   Psychological principles of clinical management (adapted with permission from Main & Williams 2002)

- Listen carefully to the patient
- Observe the patient's behavior and body language
- Atttend not only to what is said but also to how it is said
- Try to understand how the patient feels
- Offer encouragement to disclose feeling and fears
- Offer reassurance that you accept the reality of the pain
- Try to correct misunderstandings about back pain
- Offer appropriate challenges to unhelpful beliefs and coping strategies
- Try to understand the patient's family, work, and economic circumstances

Box 12.5   Enhancing positive beliefs and coping strategies

- Identify negative beliefs, emotions, and coping strategies
- Identify and correct misunderstandings
- Encourage thinking positively and relaxation
- Change behavioral responses to pain
- Pace activities
- Pick achievable goals
- Build confidence
- Recognize and reinforce progress
- Encourage self-efficacy and a sense of self-control

CONCLUSION

Treating pain and physical problems in the back is only one-half of the story. Patients' beliefs and their ability to cope play an equally important role in the development of chronic pain and disability (Box 12.3). They may also form obstacles to recovery. So, addressing patients' beliefs, distress, and coping strategies is an integral part of good management (Main & Williams 2002). Clinical assessment (Box 12.4), information and advice, and clinical management (Box 12.5) must take account of these issues. We should always be conscious that what we say and how we say it may affect our patients' beliefs. This may be more important than any direct effect of our advice on their physical condition.

We should have more faith in the power of human thought and in our patients' own capabilities. Beliefs *can* move mountains.

References

Al-Obaidi S M, Nelson R M, Al-Awadhi S, Al-Shuwaie N 2000 The role of anticipation and fear of pain in the persistence of avoidance learning in patients with chronic low back pain. Spine 25: 1126–1131

Arnstein P, Caudill M, Mandle C L, Norris A, Beasley R 1999 Self-efficacy as a mediator of the relationship between pain intensity, disability and depression in chronic pain patients. Pain 80: 483–491

Burton A K, Tillotson M, Main C J, Hollis S 1995 Psychosocial predictors of outcome in acute and subchronic low back trouble. Spine 20: 722–728

Carosella A-M, Lackner J M, Feuerstein M 1994 Factors associated with early discharge from a multidisciplinary work rehabilitation program for chronic low back pain. Pain 57: 69–76

DeGood D E, Kiernan B 1996 Perception of fault in patients with chronic pain. Pain 64: 153–159

DeGood D E, Tait R C 2001 Assessment of pain beliefs and pain coping. In: Turk D C, Melzack R (eds) Handbook of pain assessment, 2nd edn., Guilford Press, New York, pp 320–345

Dehlin O, Berg S, Andersson G B J, Grimby G 1981 Effect of physical training and ergonomic counselling on the psychological perception of work and on the subjective assessment of low back insufficiency. Scandinavian Journal of Rehabilitation Medicine 13: 1–9

Deyo R A, Diehl A K 1986 Patient satisfaction with medical care for low back pain. Spine 11: 28–30

Estlander A-M, Vanharanta H, Moneta G B, Kaivanto K 1994 Anthropometric variables, self-efficacy beliefs, and pain and disability ratings on the isometric performance of low back pain patients. Spine 19: 941–947

Feuerstein M 1991 A multidisciplinary approach to the prevention, evaluation and management of work disability. Journal of Occupational Rehabilitation 1: 5–12

Flor H, Birbaumer N, Turk D C 1990 The psychobiology of chronic pain. Advances in Behavioural Research and Therapy 12: 47–84

Fritz J M, George S Z, Delkitto A 2001 The role of fear-avoidance beliefs in acute low back pain: relationships with current and future disability and work status. Pain 94: 7–15

Hildebrandt J, Pfingsten M, Saur P, Jansen J 1997 Prediction of success from a multidisciplinary treatment program for chronic low back pain. Spine 22: 990–1001

Jensen M P, Turner J A, Romano J M, Karoly P 1991 Coping with chronic pain: a critical review of the literature. Pain 47: 249–283

Jensen M P, Turner J A, Romano J M, Lawler B K 1994 Relationship of pain-specific beliefs to chronic pain adjustment. Pain 57: 301–309

Kalauokalani D, Cherkin D C, Sherman K J, Koepsell T D, Deyo R A 2001 Lessons from a trial of acupuncture and massage for low back pain: patient expectations and treatment effects. Spine 26: 1418–1424

Kerns R D, Rosenberg R, Jamison R N, Caudill M A, Haythornewaite J A 1997 Readiness to adopt a self-management approach to chronic pain: the Pain Stages of Change Questionnaire (PSOCQ). Pain 72: 227–234

Klenerman L, Slade P D, Stenley I M et al 1995 The prediction of chronicity in patients with an acute attack of low back pain in a general practice setting. Spine 20: 478–484

Lackner J M, Carosella A M, Feuerstein M 1996 Pain expectancies, pain, and functional self-efficacy expectancies as determinants of disability in patients with chronic low back disorders. Journal of Consulting Clinical Psychology 64: 212–220

Large R, Strong J 1997 The personal constructs of coping with chronic low back pain: is coping a necessary evil? Pain 73: 245–252

Lazarus R A, Folkman S 1984 Stress, appraisal and coping. Springer, New York

Lethem J, Slade P D, Troup J D G, Bentley G 1983 Outline of a fear avoidance model of exaggerated pain perception. Behavioral Research and Therapy 21: 401–408

Linton S J, Vlaeyen J, Ostelo R 2002 The back pain beliefs of health care providers: are we fear-avoidant? Journal of Occupational Rehabilitation 12: 223–232

Main C J 2002 Concepts of treatment and prevention in musculoskeletal disorders. In: Linton S J (ed.) New avenues for the prevention of chronic musculoskeletal pain and disability. Pain Research and Clinical Management 12. Elsevier, Amsterdam, pp 47–63

Main C J, Spanswick C C 2000 Pain management: an interdisciplinary approach. Churchill Livingstone, Edinburgh

Main C J, Williams A C 2002 ABC of psychological medicine: musculoskeletal pain. British Medical Journal 325: 534–537

Petrie K J, Weinman J A (eds) 1998 Perceptions of health and illness: current research and applications. Harwood Academic, Amsterdam

Pincus T, Morley S 2002 Cognitive appraisal. In: Linton S J (ed.) New avenues for the prevention of chronic musculoskeletal pain and disability. Pain research and clinical management, vol. 12. Elsevier, Amsterdam, pp 123–141

Rosenstiel A K, Keefe F J 1983 The use of coping strategies in chronic low back pain patients: relationship to patient characteristics and current adjustment. Pain 17: 33–44

Sandstrom J, Esbjornsson E 1986 Return to work after rehabilitation. The significance of the patient's own prediction. Scandinavian Journal of Rehabilitation Medicine 18: 29–33

Schmidt A J 1985 Cognitive factors in the performance level of chronic low back pain patients. Journal of Psychosomatic Research 29: 183–189

Snow-Turek A L, Norris M P, Tan G 1996 Active and passive coping strategies in chronic pain patients. Pain 64: 455–462

Sullivan M J L, Rodgers W M, Kirsch I 2001 Catastrophizing, depression and expectancies for pain and emotional distress. Pain 91: 147–154

Symonds T L, Burton A K, Tillotson K M, Main C J 1995 Absence resulting from low back trouble can be reduced by psychosocial intervention at the workplace. Spine 20: 2738–2745

Symonds T L, Burton A K, Tillotson K M, Main C J 1996 Do attitudes and beliefs influence work loss due to low back pain? Occupational Medicine 48: 3–10

Szpalski M, Nordin M, Skovron M L, Melot C, Cukier D 1995 Health care utilization for low back pain in Belgium. Influence of sociocultural factors and health beliefs. Spine 20: 431–442

Tarasuk V, Eakin J M 1994 Back problems are for life: perceived vulnerability and its implications for chronic disability. Journal of Occupational Rehabilitation 4: 55–64

Troup J D G, Foreman T K, Baxter C E, Brown D 1987 The perception of back pain and the role of psychophysical tests of lifting capacity. Spine 12: 645–657

Turk D C, Okifuji A, Starz T W, Sinclair J D 1996 Effects of type of symptom onset on psychological distress and disability in fibromyalgia syndrome patients. Pain 68: 423–430

Turner J A, Jensen M P, Romano J M 2000 Do beliefs, coping and catastrophizing independently predict functioning in patients with chronic pain? Pain 85: 115–125

Vlaeyen J W S, Linton S J 2000 Fear-avoidance and its consequences in chronic musculoskeletal pain: a state of the art. Pain 85: 317–332

Vlaeyen J W S, Linton S J 2002 Pain-related fear and its consequences in chronic musculoskeletal pain. In: Linton S J (ed.) New avenues for the prevention of chronic musculoskeletal pain and disability. Pain research and clinical management, vol. 12. Elsevier, Amsterdam, pp 83–103

Vlaeyen J W S, Kole-Snijders A M J, Boeren R G B, van Eek H 1995a Fear of movement/(re)injury in chronic low back pain and its relation to behavioral performance. Pain 62: 363–372

Vlaeyen J W S, Kole-Snijders A M J, Rottevel A, Ruesink R, Heuts P H T G 1995b The role of fear of movement/ (re)injury in pain disability. Journal of Occupational Rehabilitation 5: 235–252

Von Korff M, Moore J C 2001 Stepped care for back pain: activating approaches for primary care. Annals of Internal Medicine 134: 911–917

Vowles K E, Gross R T 2003 Work-related fears about injury and physical capability for work in individuals with chronic pain. Pain 101: 291–298

Waddell G, Somerville D, Henderson I, Newton M, Main C J 1993 A fear avoidance beliefs questionnaire (FABQ) and the role of fear avoidance beliefs in chronic low back pain and disability. Pain 52: 157–168

Williams D A, Keefe F J 1991 Pain beliefs and the use of cognitive-behavioral coping strategies. Pain 46: 185–190

Chapter 13

Social interactions

We often talk loosely about "psychosocial" factors, but we should distinguish psychological from social. Psychological issues, e.g., beliefs and emotions, are individual and *internal*, within our heads. Social issues are *external* relationships or interactions with other people, whether individually, in a group, or collectively with society (Table 13.1).

Aristotle, in the fourth century BC, recognized that "man is by nature a social animal" and laid out the principles of social interactions. The poet John Donne put it nicely: "No man is an island". We act out our lives on a social stage, in concert with our fellow man – and woman. Social interactions are the stuff of drama and tragedy. Halliday (1937), the father of social medicine, pointed out that is just

Table 13.1

Basic social issues	Social influences	Can all affect
The social context	Culture	Reporting of back pain
Social learning	Family	Pain behavior
Social support	Social class/ occupation/ education	Disability
The sick role		Health care and sick certification
	Job satisfaction and psychosocial aspects of work	Sickness absence
	Unemployment	Social security claims and benefits
	Early retirement	Early retirement
	Workers' compensation	
	Litigation	
	Social security	

as true of illness as of any other human behavior. Illness is very much a social phenomenon, molded by its social context. Back pain always occurs in a particular social setting, which affects its impact. Physical and psychological issues may have most influence on pain, but social issues may have even more influence on disability and sickness absence. Social interactions are two-way: individual low back pain and disability may impact on other people and on society; how other people react and the provisions society makes may impact on the individual's illness behavior.

It is not possible to be human except as an integrated member of society. A child raised in isolation is not truly human. He will look human, and will have the same mental abilities, but he will not have learned to *be* human. Quite apart from lack of speech, he will not know how to act or behave like a human being. We start with a clean slate, with great potential abilities but few innate skills or instinctive knowledge. It is our capacity to learn through an extended childhood that lets us acquire the knowledge and experience of past generations to take our place in human society. This social and cultural heritage has enabled the human race to evolve over the last 10 000 years far faster than any possible biologic change. But this need to learn also means that our social and cultural background has a powerful influence on how we think, what we believe, and how we behave.

Thus, social issues are important in back pain, as in any other illness. The biologic imperatives of a disease such as cancer may set the physical limits of health and mortality, but there is much scope for how we behave when we are ill and even for the manner of our dying. With a more subjective health complaint like back pain, there is even greater scope for what we do about it. The less we understand and the more frightening the experience, the greater the scope for social influences on how we think and behave: "When reality is unclear, other people become a major source of information" (Aronson 1984).

BASIC SOCIAL ISSUES

The social context

Beecher (1959) first pointed out how the context of pain influences its meaning. He observed that battle casualties on the Anzio beachhead in World War II seemed to need very little analgesia for serious injuries compared with civilian casualties. He suggested that their injuries represented an honorable escape from danger and stress, and so caused less pain and distress than a civilian accident. I must confess to some doubt about this classic observation. In my experience, most road traffic accident victims with serious injuries do not require much analgesia at the acute stage either. However, once again, this may simply reflect my particular clinical situation and expectations.

Torstensen (1996) and Vikne (1996) looked at back pain in top Norwegian athletes, and compared them with chronic low back pain patients in the general population (Table 13.2). About 10% of all athletic injuries involve the spine, and 25–40% of these are serious problems such as fractures or spondylolysis. But chronic disability due to a simple back strain is rare in athletes. Even among elite soccer players who get frequent musculoskeletal injuries, early retirement because of back pain is almost unknown.

Patients with chronic low back pain and disability in the general population present a very different picture:

- 74% do strenuous physical work
- 59% are unsatisfied with their work
- 30% want to change their work
- 55% are dissatisfied with their leisure activities
- 38% are generally dissatisfied with their lives.

Athletes, on the other hand, love their sport and are highly motivated to get back to it as fast as possible. They seem to have very different expectations about back pain and what they should do about it. They also receive very different health care (Table 13.3).

The outcomes and impact of back pain in these two groups are very different, but we should not overinterpret this example. This was a very selected group of elite athletes and also a selected group of workers with chronic pain and disability. Most workers with back pain also recover quite rapidly. Suffice to say that even in a homogeneous cultural group, the social setting can affect attitudes to back pain and the development of chronic disability.

We all know the importance of the social context of pain and illness from our own experience.

Table 13.2   A comparison between top athletes with back pain and chronic low back pain (LBP) patients in the general population

	Top athletes	Chronic LBP patients in the general population
Age	15–30 years	Peak 40 years
Higher education	52%	13%
Smokers	12%	54%
Physical activity	100% enjoy physical activity and feel physically healthy	9% physically active; 90% unsatisfied with their physical health

From Vikne (1996) and Torstensen (1996), with permission.

Table 13.3   Organization of health care for top athletes and the general population with back pain in Norway

General population	Top athletes
Weak organization, 15-minute GP assessment	Good organization, medical team
Waiting lists for treatment	Immediate access
Poor communication between health professionals	Good communication within team
Health professionals focus on symptomatic treatment. Little interest or focus on rehabilitation or return to work?	Health professionals highly motivated to rehabilitate and retrain
Common goal – return to work?	Athletes and professionals share common goal of return to sport as rapidly as possible

After Torstensen (1996), with permission.

We have all had a bad cold or flu. If your partner asks you to do a household chore that you have been putting off for a while, your symptoms feel worse and you do not feel up to it. When you are watching an exciting ball game on television, however, your symptoms make a magic, if temporary, recovery. Even my dog Misty responds the same way. She once had a sore paw. When my daughters showed their concern, examining her leg and patting her, she limped around the room on three legs. Real pathetic. Then I offered the magic command "walk" and she rushed to the door without a trace of a limp. On the walk the limp gradually reappeared as she got tired, but it was never as dramatic as in the family setting. It is perfectly normal for pain and illness behavior to vary with social context.

Social learning

Obviously, we must learn this kind of social behavior. It is part of socialization and growing up. We probably learn it mostly in childhood, both consciously and unconsciously. As in most social learning, the family is the first and most powerful learning situation. Balague et al (1995) looked at how school children report pain. They found little evidence that family background actually affects the occurrence of back pain, but it did seem to influence children's attitudes, reporting of symptoms, and behavior. As we grow up, our social peer groups may become equally or even more influential.

There are three interrelated processes to learning or changing social behavior (Aronson 1984):

- communication
- feedback
- conforming.

All social intercourse depends on communication and humans have the richest means of communication of any animal. The most sophisticated is language, and linguistic studies cast light on each culture's views of pain and its expression. Sayings such as "the backbone of …" or "a pain in the neck" reflect cultural beliefs about the spine and spinal pain. Non-verbal communication is equally important, the human face being particularly expressive. We all subconsciously pay as much attention to *how* someone tells as something as to *what* they say. When the non-verbal message conflicts with the verbal message, we will probably not believe what they say. We saw in Chapter 10 that overt pain behavior is a powerful form of communication. We use it with little conscious thought. We recognize it and interpret it with ease. More complex illness behaviors such as failing to meet social duties or staying off work, and resting or lying down, make an even stronger social statement.

Because of the nature of human society, there is always feedback. Social communication is a two-way interaction. By definition, it is an exchange of ideas, thoughts, and feelings. Talk of pain, pain behavior, and illness behavior are almost impossible to ignore and we have to make some kind of response. Even if we deliberately ignore them, this gives a powerful message. Every aspect of our communication contributes to the patient's thinking about the pain. As we have seen, the impact on their beliefs and feelings is probably more important than the actual information or advice.

Several factors may affect the strength of this feedback. The more entrenched the patient's own ideas and attitudes, the harder they will be to change. The more important the person who provides the feedback, in the sense of social importance to the patient, the stronger will be the influence. So the spouse or partner and immediate family are likely to have most influence. They also provide some of the earliest feedback before ideas become entrenched. The influence of health professionals will depend on what the patient thinks of them. The more immediate, relevant, and personal the feedback, the stronger it will be.

Fordyce (1976) first applied behavioral principles to pain. He suggested there is always positive or negative social reinforcement of pain behavior, which influences whether or not that behavior will continue. Attention, sympathy, and social support encourage expressions of pain and feelings about it, and continued pain behavior. Ignoring pain expressions and behavior, rejecting emotions, withholding social support, and expecting the person to fulfill social duties all discourage the communication of pain.

Underlying this is strong social pressure to conform. Human society can only survive if we all share a large measure of common attitudes, beliefs, and behavior. This effect is most powerful in small, intimate social groups such as the family or peer groups. Our opinions and behavior are strongly influenced by real or imagined pressure from other members of the group. This will depend on the strength and importance of these common ideas, the unanimity of opinion, and on who holds the opinions. But if we identify with our group, we must in large measure identify with these ideas and adopt them as our own.

This all leads to a social role (Coulter 1993). Social roles are part of the social structure of society. They provide the social norms that guide our behavior and fit us into society. They are also part of our personal beliefs about ourselves and expectations about how we should behave. This set of expectations are our own, other people's, and society's. We may not always live up to the role, but the expectations may be more important than actual behavior. Society consists of a network of related social roles: you cannot be a doctor or a therapist without patients. We each fill several roles, and these roles may change over time. There is a massive change from the role of a healthy, active member of society, a productive worker, and breadwinner of a family, to the role of a patient with chronic low back pain and disability. It involves a radical shift in your beliefs and feelings and expectations about yourself. It changes your needs and duties in relation to your family, work, and society. It also means that your partner and family, your fellow workers and employers, your friends and society at large take a very different view of you and your place in society.

Social support

One of the major strengths of human society is the social support that it provides, particularly in times of difficulty. In general, social support helps us to cope with crisis and adapt to change, and provides protection against stress. It reduces distress, improves our ability to cope, aids recovery, and improves general health.

The most important source of social support is a partner or confidante – someone you can share your life and your problems with. Psychologists call this your "significant other." Is there someone you can talk to about problems like illness, money, or personal relationships? Do they live close at hand and can you see and speak to them easily? Can you discuss your most intimate problems with them, and do they trust you equally with their problems? We also get support from a wider network of family, friends, and fellow workers. How many people do you feel that you know and can talk to about your problems among your family, neighbors, friends, and fellow workers?

Note that this is all about how you feel. It is not a question of material support or services. It is more the feedback you get from others, which leads you to believe that you are cared for, esteemed, and loved. It is a common and shared network of communication and mutual obligation. More than anything else, it is about emotional support.

The sick role

The onset of illness always triggers a social process involving the patient, other people, and society. The sick role is not a medical condition or diagnosis. It is a status granted to the individual by other members of society, and may bear a variable relationship to their medical condition. The individual must accept and assume the sick role, and usually becomes a patient. Often, particularly for chronic illness or financial support, they must receive medical certification to legitimize the role.

Parsons (1951) considered illness as a social phenomenon and tried to define the social rights and duties of the person in the sick role. He started from the assumption that sickness is something unfortunate that occurs outside our control and involves some degree of helplessness. The sick role applies equally to a non-specific symptom like back pain or to a clear-cut pathology like cancer.

- Rights
  — exempt from responsibility for incapacity
  — relieved from normal social duties and responsibilities
  — entitled to special attention and support.

On the other hand, anyone who claims these rights when they are not "really" sick will be judged to be malingering.

- Duties
  — accept that to be sick is undesirable, and that there is an obligation to try to get well
  — an obligation to seek professional help and to cooperate in the process of getting well.

So health professionals and society will disapprove of those who do not try to get well.

The concept of the sick role immediately takes illness beyond the presence of disease. It treats illness as part of the much broader relationship between the individual and society. Health professionals should not regard themselves as somehow being above or outside this system. "Doctor" or "therapist" and "patient" are mutually dependent social roles. So it is not surprising that we interpret and enforce the sick role and its conditions more rigidly than other members of society.

Parsons (1951) based these ideas on acute physical illness. We must modify his analysis for chronic pain and disability, which we cannot understand purely in terms of physical disease and treatment. With chronic illness we must modify our expectations of health care and getting well. Nor does this analysis fit well with chronic disability, where the person's beliefs and behavior may be part of the problem. Waddell et al (1989) offered a modified analysis of the sick role for chronic pain and disability:

- Rights
  — The sick person is not held responsible for the original physical problem.
  — The sick person may modify normal social obligations to a degree that is proportionate to their health condition.

- Duties
  — The sick person should recognize that to be ill is undesirable and there is an obligation to minimize illness behavior and disability.
  — The sick person must share responsibility for his or her own health and disability.

This analysis recognizes that the sick role is not static but dynamic. It may change with time and the stage of the illness. There is scope for adapting and coping. What is a normal sick role in acute illness, as in Parsons' original model, may even become dysfunctional in chronic illness. It means some shift in responsibility from health professionals to the individual. It raises questions about the relative rights and duties of the sick role, and society's views and obligations to the chronically sick person.

Many of these questions are now in flux. New understanding of low back pain and disability and their management undermines the old Parsonian sick role of a simple social perspective on physical disease (Kleinman 1988). It does not diminish the importance of these issues, but may make them

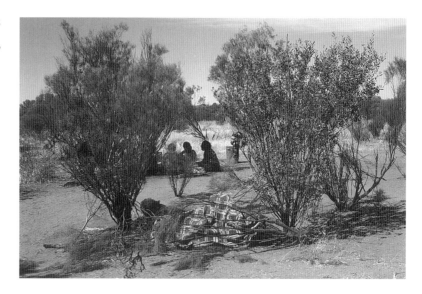

Figure 13.1 Australian aboriginals lead very "public" lives even today. They get back pain but it is "private" and they do not express or communicate their pain.

even more important. Society will need to rethink the sick role.

SOCIAL INFLUENCES

Waddell & Waddell (2000) reviewed the literature about social influences on back pain and disability.

Culture

Culture is "the collective attitudes, beliefs and behavior that characterize a particular social group over time". (See also Fabrega & Tyma 1976.) The group may range from western society, to a country, an ethnic group, a social class, or a particular work force. Zborowski (1952) made the classic observation of how ethnic background affects the expression of pain. He studied 103 patients – all men – in a US veterans' hospital; 87 had chronic pain, mainly spinal. He compared 31 men of Jewish background, 24 Italian, 11 Irish, and 26 "old American" WASPs (white Anglo-Saxon protestants). Pain threshold is more or less the same irrespective of nationality, sex, or age, but Zborowski found that his different groups expressed their pain in very different ways. Italians and Jews showed a more emotional response. They gave free expression to their feelings in words, sounds, and gestures, and were not ashamed of this, wanting support and company. However, their underlying concerns varied. The Italians' main concern was about their

present pain and its immediate impact. They wanted analgesics and had faith in doctors. The Jews' main concern was about the meaning of the pain and its effect on their future. They refused analgesics, were skeptical of doctors, and pessimistic about the future. The old Americans simply reported their pain and did not express their emotions. They were concerned with the meaning of the pain. They were very health-conscious, though in a mechanistic way, and optimistic about a "fix." They behaved well as patients and cooperated with the treatment team but withdrew from intimate contact.

These patterns of behavior varied with the degree of americanization, socioeconomic background, education, religion, and occupation. Zborowski thought that culture had more effect on attitudes and beliefs about pain, but that individual background and peer pressure had more effect on actual behavior.

Looking at very different cultures shows the impact of social and cultural learning on pain and illness behavior even more dramatically. Honeyman & Jacobs (1996) studied back pain in Australian aboriginals (Figure 13.1). On close questioning, nearly one-third of the men and half the women admitted to long-term back pain. However, they kept their pain private, not communicating it to others or seeking health care. In that society, there are strong cultural pressures about tolerating and not displaying pain. This is reflected in painful and mutilating initiation rights. Volinn (1997) reviewed the prevalence of back pain in different countries and found that urbanization and rapid industrialization were associated with increased reports of back pain.

Back pain is common to all societies, but different cultural groups do not perceive or respond to this pain in the same way. Social and cultural attitudes and beliefs, pressures, and learning all seem to be important. This is just as true of smaller social groups as of large ethnic groups. There is cultural variation in attitudes, expectations, and the meanings we attach to pain. Levels of distress vary. Culture influences how we express pain and emotions, our pain behavior, and how we communicate our pain to others, including health professionals. It affects whether and how we seek and respond to treatment. However, there is a risk to this kind of stereotyping. Cultural patterns are not fixed but fluid. Zborowski (1952) found that as his different patients became americanized, they changed their attitudes and behavioral patterns to conform to their new society. Stereotyping also ignores the great individual variation in learning and experience about pain and illness within each cultural group.

Despite the importance of cultural influences on back pain, we do not know which cultural issues are most important, how they operate, or how they can be modified.

The family

The family is the primary social unit of society. Families involve another whole set of social roles and rights and duties.

The influence of back pain on the family

The lives of family members are closely bound together, so back pain inevitably affects all members of the family to some extent. Chronic pain and disability have a major social and financial impact. Halmosh & Israeli (1982) gave a graphic description of the wife of an injured worker, whom they described as the "associate victim."

During the first acute stage, when the patient is under active treatment, family and friends rally round and there is little or no immediate financial impact. Everyone is optimistic about rapid recovery.

After a few weeks or months, however, the support of family and friends begins to wane. The wife is put under growing strain to maintain the family and home. She has to take on more of the patient's normal duties. Sooner or later, financial problems begin to arise. At this stage, the patient may at first still feel he is doing fine. He is freed of his normal duties. His wife, on the other hand, becomes tense and tired, but inside she also feels angry and guilty. As time passes, the patient becomes aware of these changes in his wife, but may misinterpret them as concern that he is more severely injured than he has been told. Both may find it difficult to communicate.

Gradually, progress seems to grind to a halt and both patient and spouse sooner or later come face to face with hard reality. This happens on several levels of consciousness and with very different perspectives for husband and wife. Active treatment comes to an end or is clearly not getting anywhere. The patient becomes worried and concerned about his lack of progress and pessimistic about his future recovery. They are both thrown back on their resources, and these resources often diminish as income drops and family and friends reduce their support to get on with their own lives. If the patient is unable – or feels unable – to return to work, that raises serious questions about his whole existence. Not only how they will cope financially, but also who is he now and what is he worth? He may express this anxiety in several ways. He may increase his physical complaints, which means that as long as he still has pain he can postpone these difficult questions. Continued pain legitimizes his situation. His wife shares these doubts and worries, and is under increasing strain. She begins to question herself, more or less consciously. Is this the life I am going to lead from here on? What is going to become of *me*? What is going to become of *us*? There may be further breakdown of communication, increase in marital stress, and mutual recriminations.

The duration of the marriage, the strength of the relationship, and past experience all help to determine the outcome. Tragically, some marriages fail and both partners are then forced to make a fresh start in their lives. Most couples join forces, face up to the difficult questions of rehabilitation, retraining or re-employment, and survive a traumatic phase of their lives. At the other extreme, some couples put the blame on outside forces such as the accident, slow healing, and unsuccessful health care. They focus their anger and frustration on a common enemy in their fight for cure or compensation.

The influence of the family on back pain

The family and partner provide the most immediate and most powerful social feedback and pressure. How we think about and deal with back trouble depends on formal and informal consultation with family members. The family is where 70–90% of all episodes of illness are dealt with, without any professional health care.

Family duties and obligations influence what we do about back pain. The sole breadwinner with a family to support may be under pressure to remain at work or to return to work as soon as possible, despite continued back pain. A lone parent with children under school age may have contrary pressures towards the home, sickness absence, and even long-term incapacity. However, these examples should not lead us to oversimplify. Marital and family status is complex and often involves conflicting pressures.

We have already seen the importance of social support. Waddell & Waddell (2000) reviewed 15 studies of family support for patients with neck or back pain. As you would expect, it does not seem to make any difference to the occurrence of back pain or work-related injury. When back pain does occur, family support generally leads to faster recovery and return to work. It reduces the risk of chronic pain and disability. For most people with ordinary backache, family support is positive and beneficial.

However, the chronic pain literature shows that family support can go badly wrong (Flor et al 1987, Kerns 1999). Chronic pain patients are more likely to come from families with a history of pain and illness. Families may act in several ways:

- Family members may act as models for health/illness behaviors, particularly for children.
- Family members may reinforce pain behavior.
- Physical and sexual abuse may increase the risk of developing chronic pain problems, though the mechanism is unclear.

Most patients with chronic, intractable pain have a "partner in pain" (Sharp & Nicholas 2000)

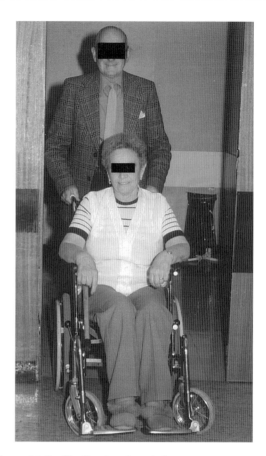

Figure 13.2   The "partner in pain."

(Fig. 13.2). The more extreme forms of chronic low back pain and disability are probably not possible without such support. The partner is intimately involved in the "pain game." Chronic pain patients and their partners play active, mutually supporting roles, and the pain may become a major focus in their whole relationship. Their whole social milieu may become pervaded by pain and disability, illness and invalidity, and health care. Chronic pain and caring may become more or less full-time careers, with both partners equally committed.

In summary, different aspects of family support and reinforcement may have positive or negative effects. They may either promote wellness behavior and the continuance of a fully active life, or promote illness behavior and incapacity. For most routine patients with back pain, good family and social support aid recovery. But for a small minority, dysfunctional family support may increase the risk of chronic pain and disability. Most routine patients with back pain probably require minimal family support, but for a minority of chronic pain patients, the influence of the family may be much stronger. Unfortunately, despite the importance of family issues, we do not know exactly which family influences are most important, how they operate, or how they can be modified.

Social class/occupation/education

In Chapter 6 we considered social class as a risk factor for back pain. We found relatively little difference in the prevalence of symptoms, and only in men. There was a stronger association with disability and work loss. So it might make more sense to look on social class as a social influence or modifier of what happens after you get back pain.

Social class is a crude measure that reflects a constellation of social characteristics such as occupation, education, and income. These are closely linked to each other and we can never really separate them. Social class may also reflect very different lifestyles and cultures. Attitudes to health, health behaviors, and health care vary with social class. A Belgian study found that people with back pain in lower social classes lie down more, seek more health care, take more medication, and are more likely to have X-rays and surgery.

Social class is based on occupation, which may be why it usually shows stronger findings in men than in women. There is a major division between manual and non-manual jobs, and disability and work loss are much greater in men in manual work. The physical demands of work may make little difference to the chances of getting back pain (Ch. 6) but they certainly affect its impact. When you do have back pain, it is more difficult to continue a heavy physical job. That is especially true where there is little help or freedom to modify the nature or speed of your work. It is also more difficult to restart work, and the longer you are off, the harder it will be. But psychosocial aspects of work also vary across social class, and these too influence work loss.

Social class reflects socioeconomic status, so it serves as a proxy for various facets of social disadvantage, in both men and women. There is now wide recognition that poverty, social disadvantage, and social exclusion lead to inequalities in health (Black 1980, Acheson 1998). There is a social class gradient for all aspects of health status and morbidity, and even mortality.

There have been a few attempts to measure socioeconomic influences on back pain. Volinn et al (1991) showed that age less than 40 years, low wages, and lack of family support (widowed or divorced with no children) all produced a modest increase in chronic work loss due to back pain. The South Manchester Study (Papageorgiou et al 1997) found that perceived inadequacy of income, poor work satisfaction, and problems getting on with fellow workers were all associated with a very slight increase in back pain. Income was more important in men, while problems getting on with fellow workers were more important in women. Lower social status (social classes IV and V) and perceived inadequacy of income were strong predictors of seeking health care for back pain. However, these social factors only seemed to account for about 5% of back pain. Remember that these social measures are quite crude, and complex social factors may be much more important in individual cases.

Education is a weak risk factor for the onset of back pain, but almost every study shows a stronger association with the impact of back pain (Dionne et al 2001). There is a stronger effect on the duration and/or recurrence of back pain than on onset of symptoms. Lower education is associated with poorer functional outcomes and more disability. Dionne et al (2001) suggested several possible mechanisms:

- variation in environmental and behavioral risk factors with education level (e.g., smoking)
- occupational differences
- compromised "health stock" (social disadvantage)
- different access and use of health care services
- differences in stress and coping.

In summary, the relationship between back pain and social class is complex. Few studies try to unravel the interrelation between social class, education, and heavy manual work. There is strong and consistent evidence that people of lower social class and in heavy physical jobs have more low back disability and time off work. The problem is what this means. It is not purely physical demands causing back pain. Social class covers a host of social, educational, occupational, economic, lifestyle, and psychosocial factors, and corresponding social and health attitudes and behavior. Any or all of these might influence disability and work loss associated with back pain. It is probably partly a matter of manual work, particularly in men. It is probably also a matter of social disadvantage in both men and women, though it is not clear exactly which aspects of that disadvantage are important or how they affect back pain.

WORK

In current western society, work occupies a major place in our lives. It provides our financial status and security, and it defines who we are and our role in society (Box 13.1). If we are asked to describe ourselves, it is one of the first things that most of us say. "I'm Dr. Waddell" immediately puts me in a particular social role and evokes a particular set of social responses.

Job satisfaction and psychosocial aspects of work

We considered psychosocial aspects of work as a risk factor for onset of back pain in Chapter 6 (Box 13.2). We found strong evidence that certain psychosocial aspects of work, such as low job satisfaction and poor social support at work, are associated with a higher prevalence of back pain. However, the effect is quite weak, and it is not clear whether they actually *cause* back pain. They may simply influence *reporting* of back pain.

In principle, it seems likely that psychosocial aspects of work may also influence what people do about back pain after it occurs and whatever its cause. Indeed, given the strength of other social influences, we might expect this to be a more powerful effect.

We looked at this as part of the unpublished background to Waddell & Waddell (2000). We reviewed 69 studies on job satisfaction and psychosocial aspects of work in patients with neck and back pain. The results surprised us. The findings about reported work-related injury or claims seem to be broadly comparable to those about back pain. We found strong evidence that job satisfaction and high job demand/intensity are significantly associated

> **Box 13.1   The value of work**
>
> - Income (should this come first or last?)
> - Activity
> - Occupies and structures our time
> - Creativity/mastery
> - Social interaction
> - Sense of identity
> - Sense of purpose
>
> All workers get these to varying degrees, although their relative importance varies with the individual and the job.

> **Box 13.2   Psychosocial aspects of work**
>
> - Job satisfaction
> - Work-related "stress"
> - Job demands/intensity
>   - work under time pressure
> - Job content
>   - decision latitude
>   - job control and autonomy
>   - monotonous work
> - Social support
>   - from co-workers
>   - from employers

with seeking health care and sick listing. But the effect sizes are even weaker than with back pain itself (relative risk or odds ratios generally about 1.5). The various other psychosocial aspects of work generally show non-significant or very weak associations with claims, seeking health care, or sick listing. Contrary to what we expected, we did not find that psychosocial aspects of work have much impact on what people do about their back pain. It appears that some writers in the 1990s overstated the importance of psychosocial aspects of work in back pain.

Once again, the limitation is that we looked at each psychosocial aspect of work in isolation. It is possible that there could be more complex interactions that we missed. Also, most of the findings are averages from groups of workers. It is possible that psychosocial aspects of work may have a much more powerful influence in individual workers.

There is one local but potentially devastating influence – downsizing. There are isolated reports that major organizational change, such as threat of lay-offs, may cause worker disaffection, sickness absence, and early retirement (Hadler 1999, Kivimaki et al 2001). This might temporarily overwhelm every other factor in that workforce.

Incapacity for work

Capacity and incapacity for work depend on complex interactions between the worker's medical condition and physical capabilities, ergonomic demands of the job, and psychosocial factors (Feuerstein 1991). The factors that influence stopping work may be different from those that influence staying off and going back to work.

The relations between sickness, incapacity for work, employment, and social benefits are complex. Consider three possible scenarios. First, back pain may be the direct cause of time off work, job loss, and unemployment, leading to sick certification and sickness benefits. Second, the physical, psychological, and social ill effects of unemployment may interact with and aggravate back pain and disability. Third, people with back pain who lose their job (for whatever reason) may be more likely to receive sick certification and benefits. These correspond broadly to three routes of entry to invalidity benefits identified in a Department of Social Security (DSS) study in the UK (Ritchie & Snape 1993):

1. *Condition-led entry.* The nature and severity of the illness and disability lead to long-term or permanent incapacity. Coming off benefits depends on the nature of the incapacity and treatment received and the availability of employment.

2. *Employment-led entry.* Restricted employment opportunities combined with illness/disability (and often also age) cause loss of employment or inability to gain work and hence the start of benefits. The main barriers to coming off benefits are employment opportunities, availability of rehabilitation or retraining, and age.

3. *Self-directed entry.* Some interaction between the person's condition, employment opportunities, and motivation to continue or gain employment results in sickness benefits being seen as a possible option. This could be either with the support

> **Box 13.3   Models of absence from work (adapted from Briner 1996)**
>
> - Medical model: the main cause of absence from work is injury or sickness
> - Deviance model: absent employees are somehow different in their attitudes and behavior, e.g., they lack commitment or are lazy
> - Withdrawal model: absent employees are withdrawing from unpleasant or unsatisfactory work conditions
> - Economic model: non-work and leisure activities are valued more highly and are therefore more attractive
> - Cultural model: identifies the cause of absence within the social context and cultural attitudes of the organization rather than in the individual employee

of the family doctor or negotiated with the family doctor. The main barriers to coming off benefits are age, low motivation, and restricted employment opportunities, often related to their condition. Coming off benefits largely depends on external triggers, usually an independent medical review by the DSS or the family doctor's decision to stop sick certification.

Ritchie et al (1993) found that many complex factors influenced family doctors' judgments of their patient's capacity for work when giving sick certificates. The patient's medical condition and its impact on employment potential were always high on the list, but they were almost immediately linked to a whole range of non-medical factors. These included the patient's prospects of finding work, age, motivation to find work, the financial and psychological consequences of returning to unemployment or job search, and the potential for rehabilitation or training.

The social process of becoming disabled and starting sickness benefits may occur insidiously and unconsciously rather than as a conscious decision. Once the person is assigned to benefit status, however, that may be almost irreversible in the current economic climate. This is especially the case if the person is approaching retirement age anyway.

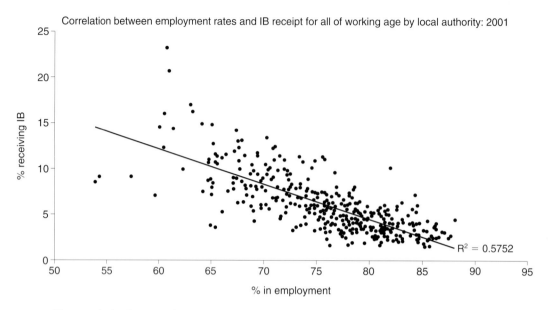

Figure 13.3 The correlation between incapacity-related benefits and local employment. Based on 2001 data for the working age population of UK, provided by the Department for Work and Pensions.

Briner (1996) reviewed absence from work and pointed out that may not be the same as incapacity. On one level, absence is easy to define and measure. It is simply non-attendance at work by an employee when attendance is expected by the employer. Despite that apparent simplicity, work absence is a complex phenomenon which resists simple explanations. It may reflect different circumstances and behaviors, so understanding and management require careful distinction between different types of absence (Box 13.3). "Sickness" may simply be a convenient label that covers the real reason for work absence.

Unemployment

As work is such an important part of our modern social fabric, it is not surprising that loss of work and unemployment are catastrophic. Unemployment causes loss of all the social and emotional benefits of work. It undermines our whole social position and status and is one of the greatest personal failures in a material society. Welfare status involves loss of social standing, loss of (self-)respect, and isolation. So it is not surprising that unemployment causes hopelessness, helplessness, and depression. Unemployment leads to poorer physical and mental health, with increased suicide and mortality rates (Janlert 1997, Acheson 1998). Lack of work causes loss of physical fitness and increased weight, psychological distress and depression, and loss of work-related attitudes and habits. We have seen that all of these characteristics are common to low back disability.

Waddell et al (2002) reviewed the literature on unemployment and back pain. In earlier times of low unemployment (<5–6%), there appeared to be an inverse relationship. Four longitudinal studies showed that higher unemployment rates were associated with lower sickness absence and claims rates. In more recent times of higher unemployment, the relationship appears to be the opposite. Three more recent longitudinal analyses and numerous cross-sectional analyses show that increased unemployment rates are associated with increased numbers of social security claims (Fig. 13.3). This suggests that unemployment may have different effects in different situations. In earlier times of low unemployment, when unemployment rose and job security fell, there may have been more pressure on workers to stay at work when they felt unwell. This perhaps reduced absenteeism associated with a subjective health complaint like back pain. However, in times of high unemployment the individual may be more vulnerable to market forces outwith their control. Those with poorer health might be disadvantaged at retaining work or re-entering the labor force. Once someone is under threat of lay-off or loses their job, there are social and financial incentives to sickness and disability benefits. These might tend to increase sick certification and claims for incapacity and disability benefits.

Over the past decade or two, there has been a change in attitudes to disability, which has become much more socially acceptable. This has been supported by policy attempts to improve the social facilities and status of people with disabilities. For people with disabilities, that has clearly been helpful. It means, however, that entry to disability status has also become more socially acceptable. Indeed, sickness and disability now appear to be more socially acceptable than unemployment. Over the same period, pain per se has also become acceptable as a basis for chronic disability and benefits (Fordyce 1995). Enterline (1966) commented that "the right not to go to work when *feeling* ill appears to be part of a social movement that has swept across Europe" (my italics). Recent US statistics suggest that is now equally true in North America.

Higher unemployment rates produce greater competition for available work and higher selection criteria by employers. More jobs are also now shorter-term with greater turnover of labor, which increases the frequency with which workers must seek and gain jobs. Any degree of mental or physical impairment, whether due to age, health complaints, or a poor sickness record, may make it harder to get or to hold work than in better economic times when work was more readily available. A mild degree of incapacity may then lead someone to adopt the sick role, who would otherwise have been able to continue working without their symptoms being a health problem.

There is very little difference in the prevalence of back pain between the employed and the unemployed (Table 13.4). The unemployed seek more health care for back pain, but the most dramatic increase is in sick certification. Social security data from the UK show that about half of all incapacity benefits now go to people who were not employed when they started benefits. Sickness benefits in all countries are financially higher than unemployment benefits, continue longer, and have less social

Table 13.4 Relationship of back pain to lack of employment

	Employed (%)	Not employed (%)
Prevalence of back pain		
Point prevalence	11	9
1-year prevalence	37	42
Lifetime prevalence	65	62
Medical care for back pain in the past year	13	20
Sick certification for the last 4 weeks because of low back pain	1	20

Based on data from Mason (1994) and Department of Social Security data.

stigma. There is a strong suspicion that many doctors try to help their patients by giving sick certificates for social rather than medical reasons.

Chew-Graham & May (1997, 1999) looked at the dilemma faced by the family doctor in this situation. They suggested that back pain might be a social resource for some patients, which has major implications for how patient and doctor approach the consultation. They pointed out that:

- chronic low back pain permits withdrawal from normal social obligations
- patients recognize that their doctor is not able to help, but view the doctor as a resource through which their social and economic inactivity might be legitimized
- patients and doctors recognize the relation between psychosocial factors and pain
- chronic low back pain involves both the patient and the doctor negotiating conflicting roles.

Once again, these social relationships are complex. Unemployment may be only a marker for a whole set of social and occupational characteristics that influence back pain, incapacity, and health care.

Early retirement

Early retirement on health grounds is probably the single greatest problem facing all social security systems (Waddell et al 2002). In the UK, 51% of incapacity benefit recipients are now aged more than 50 years and most of them will stay on benefits till they reach the official retirement age. Back pain is one of the most common reasons given, together with other musculoskeletal and mental health conditions.

There is a paradox. People are living longer, and staying healthier longer, yet more and more retire earlier. Only 30% of men in Europe now work beyond age 60, and <40% of women beyond age 55 years, though this varies greatly in different countries. Pensions were first introduced for workers who had worked 40–50 years or more, and who died within a few years of retirement. Some people now have an active retirement and draw a pension for longer than they worked and contributed to their pension scheme. Demographic trends and economics dictate that we should work longer, but instead the trend is to retire earlier.

Over the past few decades, there has been a dramatic change in attitudes to work and retirement. Many people now want and expect to retire before the official retirement age. Scales & Scase (2000) looked at social, occupational and economic trends among UK adults in their 50s, with fascinating insights:

- We are redefining "old." Most people in their 50s now enjoy good health. They are now much more comparable in their attitudes, activities, and behavior to people in their 30s and 40s. They no longer regard themselves as older and it is only in their 60s that they begin to age.

- The position of people in their 50s now varies greatly, depending on type of employment, occupational pensions, marital status, and financial commitments such as children and mortgages. They are likely to polarize into affluent early retirees and those compelled to continue working because of financial necessity.

- For many professionals in their 50s, early retirement is by choice, based on access to an occupational or private pension. Half of them remain financially comfortable and 80% are satisfied with life. However, for blue-collar workers, early retirement is more likely to be on grounds of ill health. Incapacity and disability pensions may be the only financial mechanism available to them to bridge the gap between early retirement and age retirement pensions. Less than 20% of them are financially comfortable and their overall satisfaction with life is low.

- Moving out of employment reduces stress and improves health for those in managerial and professional occupations. It increases stress and is associated with deteriorating health for those in manual unskilled occupations. Professional women who remain in employment are likely to show increased stress.

Figure 13.4 summarizes various possible routes from work to retirement.

Health is clearly part of the picture, but it is not the whole story. Over the last two decades, during which there has been a marked increase in early retirement with back pain, there has been no change in back pain, and the number of people in heavy manual jobs has fallen. Erens & Ghate (1993) studied 1545 new recipients of long-term sickness benefits in the UK.

Among recipients aged 50+, their health condition appeared to be only one of several considerations in determining their attitudes towards returning to work. Attitudes to work appear to change quite dramatically around age 50. It would appear that personal considerations and labor market conditions play a prominent role in shaping the attitudes of recipients aged 50+.

There is a fundamental question about the extent to which early retirement is forced upon people by labor market forces or is a matter of personal choice. In practice, it is probably never entirely one or the other. The decision more likely depends on a variable balance between health, personal attitudes and expectations, labor market forces, and pension and social security provisions. This raises questions about how long people should be expected to work, and about the social and financial mechanisms society should provide for retirement. There is a particular question whether subjective health complaints like low back pain should be acceptable grounds for early retirement. Other forces may also intervene. For example, in the 1990s, some countries encouraged early retirement as more politically acceptable than rising unemployment. Whichever, back pain may be caught in the middle of a social and political debate to which there is no medical answer.

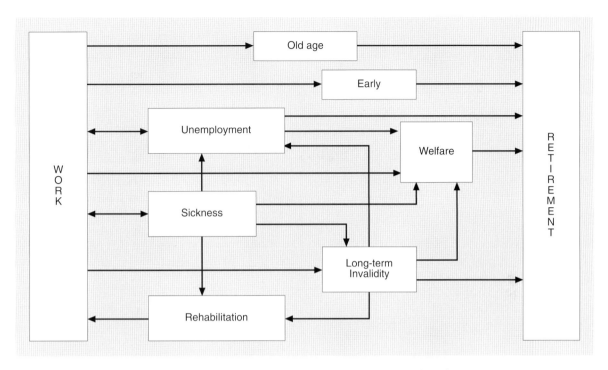

Figure 13.4   Alternative routes from work to retirement. Adapted from Aarts et al (1996).

Waddell et al (2002) reviewed the literature on early retirement and back pain. Although back pain is one of the most common reasons for early retirement, the trend seems to be more social than biologic. Older people may have more difficulty coping with back pain, with heavy physical work, or especially with a combination of the two. However, the worker's medical condition appears to be only one and often not the most important element in early retirement on health grounds. Early retirement attributed to back pain is often associated with comorbidities, psychological problems, and social factors, including psychosocial aspects of work. On the present data, we cannot determine the relative importance of these various mechanisms linking employment status, low back disability, and early retirement. It is probable that each is important in some people. More than one mechanism may operate simultaneously. Back pain and disability may contribute to incapacity for work and job loss. Conversely, physical demands and psycho-social aspects of work may influence back complaints and how workers cope. The physical, mental, and social ill effects of loss of employment may interact

with and aggravate low back pain and disability. There may be social and financial pressures towards sick certification and sickness benefits. Or the common bodily symptom of back pain may be used to cover other reasons for sickness absence or early retirement. On the available evidence, the balance of probabilities is that the physical state of the worker's back is often the least important.

SOCIOECONOMIC ISSUES

Workers' compensation

Few issues around back pain give rise to more heated debate than the question of compensation.

Before we go any further, we should stress that true malingering – the fabrication of symptoms and disability that do not exist – is rare. Boden (1996) estimated that, at most, 3% of injured workers in the US fall into this category. Most workers have entirely genuine physical pain, even if reasonable people may reasonably disagree about the appropriate duration of sickness absence, or the level of (in)capacity for work.

At the same time, we must recognize that money is a major motivating force in a material society. We all respond to financial incentives and disincentives.

Secondary gain is a vague term that suggests individuals are somehow rewarded economically, socially, or emotionally as a result of their injury or illness (Fishbain 1994, Fishbain et al 1995). All illness involves some secondary gains in terms of relief from social duties or receipt of social support or benefits. Too often, however, discussions about secondary gain focus on money and imply malingering. Any benefit such as disability payments or a concerned family member then casts suspicion on the patient's credibility. If treatment fails, secondary gain makes a good excuse. This is a circular argument, which may say more about the bias of the observer than the motivation of the patient. No one raises questions of secondary gain about the patient with a stroke. Before we cast any stones, we should also recognize that all health professionals make much greater secondary gains from back pain than any patient ever did.

These discussions usually neglect the fact that secondary gains are balanced by secondary losses (Fishbain 1994). Money is only one part of stopping work and going sick, and probably not the most important. Loss of all the other social benefits of working, loss of social status, and the change from a working role to a sick role are probably more important. Emotional losses usually outweigh any emotional gains. Even if we confine the argument to money, we should not overestimate the value of compensation. Most people on workers' compensation are financially much worse off than when they were working, particularly in the longterm. Those few who are better off are usually part-time or poorly paid workers whose wages were so low that they gave little financial incentive to work at all. Looking at their whole social situation, most people off work with back pain are much worse off in many ways. Workers' compensation or other sickness benefits are a very inadequate replacement.

Incapacity for work, health care, and compensation are closely linked. Health care is a requirement of the sick role and legitimizes incapacity. Sick certification is an integral part of clinical management, and provides the gateway to compensation. Clinical assessment and management may be subtly different in workers' compensation patients. Taylor et al (1996) suggested it might even influence the decisions taken by US patients and professionals about back surgery. Conversely, clinical decisions have a major impact on health care costs, and on the duration and costs of compensation. Before we pass moral judgment on how compensation incentives influence workers, we should also consider how they influence employers, health professionals, and lawyers.

Nevertheless, financial incentives do modify workers' behavior after a back injury. Miller (1976) was one of the first to calculate that benefits of much over 50% of wages led to an increase in the duration of disability claimed by insured persons. There have been many such studies, reviewed by Loeser et al (1995). The evidence is not fully consistent, and not all studies show any effect. However, the best available literature suggests that a 10% increase in workers' compensation benefits produces a 1–11% increase in the number of claims, and a 2–11% increase in the average duration of claims. That is an average increase of 2–5 days off work. Wage replacement levels clearly influence behavior, but the effect is modest. Too often, this is overstated. It is also important to note that these effects are similar for verifiable injuries like fractures, as well as more subjective, soft-tissue injuries.

However, the level of compensation is probably a very small factor in the decision to stop work, and only one factor in maintaining the sick role. As we have already noted, there have been great changes in attitudes to work and disability and compensation over recent decades. There is rapid change in conditions of employment, with much more unemployment, job insecurity, and job turnover. The average job tenure in the US is now less than 3 years. This has inevitably changed attitudes to work, employers, and unemployment. These changed attitudes are all probably more important than the actual level of compensation.

Clinical studies of workers' compensation show a striking dichotomy. At one extreme, some pain clinic studies and experts say there is no clinical difference between workers' compensation and non-compensation patients. At the other extreme, some medicolegal experts, who are mainly orthopedic surgeons, imply that many of the claimants they see are little short of frank malingerers. The difference seems to be a combination of case selection and observer bias, in both directions.

Rohling et al (1995) reviewed 32 studies from pain clinic settings, though most were retrospective and cross-sectional. They had usable data on 3802 compensated and 3849 non-compensated patients. Compensation patients consistently reported more intense pain, although the difference was only about 6%. The outcomes of conservative treatment, back surgery, and chronic pain rehabilitation programs were consistently poorer in compensation patients. However, there was conflicting evidence on the size of this effect, with estimates ranging from 0 to 30%. Nor is it clear whether compensation delays return to work or the lack of compensation pressures patients into faster return to work, or which of these is medically ideal. Many studies show there is little difference in the physical findings and levels of distress in compensation patients. Some studies suggest that compensation patients are more depressed. There are three prospective studies that confirm these findings (Rainville et al 1997, Atlas et al 2000, Taylor et al 2000).

There appear to be different patterns of sickness absence after work-related back injuries (Nagi & Hadley 1972, Burns et al 1995, Galizzi & Boden 1996). Most patients with back injuries return to work quickly and actually do better than most non-back injuries. Social factors are less important in these patients. A subgroup of patients with simple back strains who are off work >1 month do relatively badly, and return to work much more slowly than non-back injuries. These are the patients in whom social influences are important. In patients with severe spinal injuries such as fractures, there is little difference between workers' compensation and non-compensation patients.

It is too easy to assume this is all a direct effect of compensation, but that does not allow for other differences in these patients. Leavitt (1992) pointed out that workers' compensation patients usually have heavier physical jobs. They are generally younger, male, less educated, and from lower social classes. They form a very different occupational, social, and economic group. By definition, workers' compensation patients have had an injury at work, while most non-compensation patients have non-specific back pain. Their selection and referral patterns are different. These differences may have much greater impact on their clinical progress and return to work than compensation itself.

There is conflicting evidence on the relative influence of workers' compensation, occupation, job demands, and work status (Dworkin et al 1985, Leavitt 1992, Sanderson et al 1995). Perhaps that is because they are all inextricably linked. Suter (2002) made one of the most careful studies of both adversarial workers' compensation and work status. He looked at 200 patients with chronic low back pain and followed them over 15–24 months. They fell into four groups: working or not and litigating or not. Patients who were litigating had higher levels of pain, depression, and disability. Patients who were working had lower levels. Suter suggested that litigation increased patients' perception and reporting of symptoms and disability. There was an interaction over time with settlement of legal proceedings and with return to work. The cause and effect relation between symptoms and work was not entirely clear. However, Suter felt the results were most consistent with work being beneficial.

Tito (2000) pointed out this is all a very "professional" view of workers' compensation. Clinical and administrative data tell part of the story, but they fail to acknowledge the injured worker's experience of the compensation system. When a previously healthy worker is suddenly injured, and does not recover quickly and get back to work, he or she enters a very strange, frightening, and difficult world. Tito painted a graphic picture of confusion and alarm; of disempowerment; of anger and frustration; of health care systems that often do not deliver the best possible care; of administrative systems that give injured people mixed messages; and of compensation arrangements that create obstacles to early recovery. The lack of expected correlation between apparently minor injury and prolonged time off work leads to suspicion. The "system" explicitly or implicitly questions the injured worker's credibility or motivation. The worker, in turn, becomes defensive. But most injured workers want to work and only a small minority deliberately abuse the system. Too often, the system is designed to discourage or punish the injured worker, but this is ineffective and may be counterproductive. "The interface between health care and compensation is intimate and complex: a marriage of convenience out of different cultures, with all the

---

Box 13.4 Effects of compensation

Effect of compensation level on claims
- There is no evidence that compensation changes the actual injury rate
- 10% increase in compensation level produces 1–11% increase in claims rate
- 10% increase in compensation level produces 2–11% increase in duration of disability
- This affects verifiable injuries like fractures as much as more subjective, soft-tissue injuries

Effect of compensation on clinical outcomes
- Compensation patients have poorer clinical outcomes and more disability
- These findings have been criticized:
  - these men often have heavier physical jobs
  - they have many other psychosocial differences
  - they may get different treatment

Effect of compensation on rehabilitation outcome
- Compensation patients respond less well to pain management and rehabilitation
- These findings have been criticized:
  - there are methodologic flaws in many of these studies. They are often small samples of highly selected patients with poor diagnostic criteria. Follow-up is poor. There is failure to allow for other factors such as job demands
  - differences are small

Despite all of this, 75–90% of workers' compensation patients do respond well to health care, recover, and return to work rapidly.

---

conflict, tension and interest this can create." "A crucial challenge for health professionals and compensation administrators is how to minimize the additional disabling impact of the compensation process, so that all injured people have to deal with is the original injury."

In summary, there is little doubt that compensation affects what people do when they have back pain (Box 13.4). It influences clinical progress, rehabilitation, and return to work. But it is only one, and probably one of the less powerful, social influences on what they do to get out of that situation.

We should not exaggerate the impact of workers' compensation. Remember that most compensation patients do respond to treatment, make a good recovery, and return to work quite quickly.

Litigation

It is accepted clinical wisdom that patients who have an attorney or who are involved in adversarial legal proceedings have poorer clinical outcomes. The belief is that ongoing legal proceedings reinforce illness behavior and disability.

Many of the quoted articles are actually of workers' compensation and not litigation. Waddell & Waddell (2000) were only able to find 14 studies of litigation in patients with neck or back pain, which provide limited and conflicting evidence. We should distinguish the legal and clinical situations. There is certainly legal evidence that a medicolegal context may provoke conscious or unconscious exaggeration of reported symptoms and disability and of the clinical presentation. There may even be deliberate intent to deceive. But that does not seem to carry over into routine clinical practice. There, litigation does not appear to be associated with any increase in pain intensity or distress. Contrary to general belief, there is insufficient evidence to show whether or to what extent litigation is associated with any difference in clinical outcomes, disability, or return to work.

Social security

There is now general agreement that social security is one of the hallmarks of modern society (Waddell et al 2002). It provides for the traditional risks of sickness, disability, old age, and unemployment. It makes variable provision to alleviate poverty. However, that agreement is a recent historic development, and it is only in western society. It depends on a set of assumptions and beliefs about the individual's and society's rights and duties. Over the last 20–30 years, an increasing number of people now receive more generous social benefits such as sick pay and pensions through their employment. But there is a large minority of people in poorer jobs or on the margins of the labor force who will always depend on the state to provide cover. We are all willing to pay taxes to support those who are "really" disabled. (Even if that immediately raises a whole set of practical questions.) But this is expensive, and now accounts for 12–18% of gross domestic product in different countries. And these costs show a constant tendency to rise, which leads to a continuing welfare debate. Nevertheless, people in all European countries are proud of their welfare systems, which seem to form an important part of the culture of each country (Ploug & Kvist 1996). All US surveys also show strong public support, even if there is concern that benefits may be inadequate or unfair (Kingson & Schulz 1997, Lazar & Stoyko 1998). Whatever its problems and weaknesses, the welfare state is remarkably resilient. Its record since World War II confirms its social and economic value.

However, the welfare state is not perfect. Hill (1990) suggested that there are now three social welfare classes. The first class is people who are in well-paid and secure employment. When they are sick they receive sick pay, which may provide full salary for 6–12 months, and when they retire they have generous pensions. They do not really depend on the state social security system, even though they pay contributions and draw benefits when they are entitled. They are less likely to become unemployed, and if they do it is usually only for a short period (though this is less true today). Even if they are paid off, that is usually cushioned by generous redundancy and early retirement provisions. Some women in this class, however, depend on their husband's entitlement and may be vulnerable if the marriage breaks up.

The second social welfare class is the traditional working class. These were the people for whom the social security system was originally designed, and it still works for them. For short-term sickness, they receive some form of statutory sick pay from their employer. If they are paid off, they receive some form of social security benefits, which provide a reasonable long-term income. However, these benefits depend on having built up sufficient entitlement. They have some cover for unemployment, at least in the short term. When they retire they receive a state pension, possibly with some employment-related supplement. The combination of social security benefits and employment-related entitlement works reasonably well for many members of the second class. However, women in this class may have much poorer cover, particularly if they are in part-time or low-paid

jobs. Long-term sickness or unemployment may demote both men and women to the third class. Some "fall through the cracks in the system."

The third social welfare class contains the socially disadvantaged. They have low education and skills, a poor and low-paid employment record, and limited financial resources. They also have more sickness. When they are sick, their employers pay the statutory minimum of sick pay and they are likely to be paid off. They have often built up limited entitlement to social insurance benefits. When they are sick or unemployed, it is more likely to be prolonged. When they retire, they receive the basic state retirement pension or less if their employment record is poor. Social insurance fails for this class and instead many of them are dependent on the means-tested safety net to stave off poverty. A few people in the first class and more in the second class may fall into this third class as a result of long-term sickness or unemployment. Most people in the third class face many social, employment, and financial barriers that trap them there.

The welfare debate always raises the question of "moral hazard": the idea that social security benefits act as a disincentive to work. This is usually raised by the well-off and applied to the poorly paid. It argues that behavior is influenced by the relative costs and benefits of working, of sickness absence, of workers' compensation and of social security benefits. (Though there are both financial and other social costs and benefits.) Clearly, this is an important part of the story. However, I doubt if many people actually think this out consciously at the time of stopping work and going off sick with back pain. At that point, most patients are more concerned with their acute symptoms. They expect to get better and return to work quite quickly, and they do not think about the long-term financial implications. Economic incentives probably become more important in chronic disability and have more influence on return to work. There may also be a number of benefit traps that act as obstacles to return to work.

Waddell et al (2002) reviewed social security arrangements and trends in various countries. They concluded that:

- There is no doubt that social security systems influence sick certification, claims, and trends of sickness and disability benefits.

- Everyone responds to economic incentives and disincentives: money matters. However, the structure and control mechanisms of the social security system may be even more important. The ease or difficulty of getting benefits seem to have a greater impact than the financial value of the benefits received.

- One of the greatest problems faced by all social security systems is early retirement on health grounds. Disability pensions now account for most of the sickness and incapacity trends and costs. Back pain is one of the most common reasons given, even though we have seen that there has been no change in back pain over the period of these trends. However, this is not unique to back pain, but forms part of a much larger social issue.

- Low back pain and disability, sick certification, and sickness and disability benefits are also associated with social disadvantage. This is hardly surprising, given the basic purpose of social security to alleviate misfortune and poverty. Again, this is not unique to back pain, but forms part of a much larger social issue.

- Some of these issues may be equally relevant to other social security problem areas, such as musculoskeletal, mental health and stress-related disorders, and medically unexplained symptoms.

- We cannot consider sickness and disability benefits in isolation. They are only one element of a much broader social framework.

HEALTH CARE

Health care has reappeared throughout this chapter. The World Health Organization defines health as a state of complete physical, mental, and social well-being, and not simply the absence of disease or infirmity. The ultimate social role of health care is to make patients healthy and enable them to take their place in society.

We must consider our own role as health professionals in this process (Bennet 1979, Coulter 1993). Patients and health professionals have an intimate social relationship, because we are equally involved, in our very different ways, in illness. We each have very different needs and demands and duties. Patients face illness as a personal and threatening experience. At a clinical level, health professionals may take a more detached view, but illness also provides us with our livelihood and identity. Society takes a much broader view of the social and economic impact of illness, and of health care. These views are very different, but they are simply different perspectives on a common problem. How these views blend or collide affects the quality and success of health care.

Doctors and other health professionals also play a key social role in disability and the provision of social support. We certify and legitimize the process, often with little insight into the consequences for the patient, their family, their work, and society.

It is naive to think that all we do is treat disease to make our patients better. It should be clear by now that, quite apart from the treatment we offer, we are

Table 13.5 The evidence on social influences on low back disability and work loss

Strength of association	Weak	Moderate	Strong
Culture			C
Family	Acute B +ve	Chronic pain patients B −ve	
Social class		A	
Education	B		
Job satisfaction		A	
Psychosocial aspects of work		A	
Industrial relations		C	
Unemployment			B
Early retirement			A
Workers' compensation		B	
Adversarial legal proceedings	C		
Social security			
− availability			B
− benefit level		B	

Levels of evidence
A Strong evidence: provided by generally consistent findings in systematic review or in two or more high-quality studies.
B Moderate evidence: provided by generally consistent finding in one high-quality and one or more low-quality studies, or generally consistent finding in multiple low-quality studies.
C Limited evidence: one high-quality study or inconsistent findings in multiple studies.

a powerful *social change agent* (Phillips 1994). We must consider and allow for all these social factors and consequences in our management of the patient with back pain. We must be sure that our contribution is to the patient's overall benefit. From a social perspective, that is what this whole book is about.

CONCLUSION

Table 13.5 gives a summary of the evidence on these social issues and back pain. Or rather, on the resulting disability and work loss. It offers my rating of the strength of the evidence and the importance of each social influence. It appears that some of these influences are powerful and at times may be more important than the physical problem in the back. This supports the view that the trend of chronic low back disability at the end of the 20th century was a social epidemic. Equally, understanding social issues may be the key to controlling the epidemic.

Unfortunately, these social factors are complex and our understanding is limited. On the evidence available at present, we might suggest that the most important areas are: individual, group and general societal attitudes and beliefs about work; about back pain and its relationship to work; about sickness absence; about welfare benefits; and about (early) retirement. Perhaps we might summarize this best as the culture of back pain. However, we have difficulty defining and measuring the precise social factors, never mind understanding how they work or how to modify them. We must be careful not to make moral judgments, which often reflect our own social views and values more than anything about our patient's situation. With all these caveats, I still believe this is one of the most promising but unexplored fields for back pain research.

We should end this chapter with a note of caution. Back pain is real and due to a physical cause in the back. Social issues may *influence* back symptoms and what people do about them, but that does not imply that the symptoms are not real, or that they are imaginary or faked.

References

Parts of this chapter are adapted with permission from Waddell & Waddell (2000) and Waddell et al (2002), which provide more comprehensive reviews and full bibliographies for social and social security issues

Aarts L J M, Vurkhauser R V, de Jong P R 1996 Curing the Dutch disease: an international perspective on disability policy reform, vol. I. International Studies of Social Security, Aldershot, Avebury, p 16

Acheson D 1998 Inequalities in health report. Stationery Office, London

Aronson E 1984 The social animal, 4th edn. Freeman, New York

Atlas S, Chang Y, Kammann E, Keller R B, Deyo R A, Singer D E (2000) Long-term disability and return to work among patients who have a herniated lumbar disc: the effect of disability compensation. Journal of Bone and Joint Surgery 82A: 4–15

Balague F, Skovron M-L, Nordin M, Dutoit G, Waldburger M 1995 Low back pain in school children. A study of familial and psychological factors. Spine 20: 1265–1270

Beecher H K 1959 Measurement of subjective responses: quantitative effect of drugs. Oxford University Press, New York

Bennet G 1979 Patients and their doctors. Baillière Tindall, London

Black D 1980 Inequalities in health. Report of a working group chaired by Sir Douglas Black. Her Majesty's Stationery Office, London

Boden L I 1996 Work disability in an economic context. In: Moon S, Sauter S L (eds) Psychosocial aspects of musculoskeletal disorders in office work. Taylor & Francis, London, pp 287–294

Briner R B 1996 Absence from work. British Medical Journal 313: 874–877

Burns J W, Sherman M L, Devine J, Mahoney N, Pawl R 1995 Association between workers' compensation and outcome following multidisciplinary treatment for chronic pain: roles of mediators and moderators. Clinical Journal of Pain 11: 94–102

Chew C A, May C 1997 The benefits of back pain. Family Practice 14: 461–465

Chew-Graham C, May C 1999 Chronic low back pain in general practice: the challenge of the consultation. Family Practice 16: 46–49

Coulter I D 1993 The physician, the patient and the person: the humanistic challenge. Journal of Chiropractic Humanities 1: 9–20

Dionne C E, Von Korff M, Koepsell T D et al 2001 Formal education and back pain: a review. Journal of Epidemiology and Community Health 55: 455–468

Dworkin R H, Handlin D S, Richlin D M, Brand L, Vannucci C 1985 Unraveling the effects of compensation, litigation and employment on treatment response in chronic pain. Pain 23: 49–59

Enterline P E 1966 Social causes of sick absence. Archives of Environmental Health 12: 467–473

Erens B, Ghate D 1993 Invalidity benefit: a longitudinal study of new recipients. Department of Social Security research report no. 20. HMSO, London

Fabrega H, Tyma S 1976 Language and cultural influences in the description of pain. British Journal of Medical Psychology 49: 349–371

Feuerstein M 1991 A multidisciplinary approach to the prevention, evaluation and management of work disability. Journal of Occupational Rehabilitation 1: 5–12

Fishbain D A 1994 Secondary gain concept: definition, problems and its abuse in medical practice. American Pain Society Journal 3: 264–273

Fishbain D A, Rosomoff H L, Cutler R B, Rosomoff R S 1995 Secondary gain concept: a review of the scientific evidence. Clinical Journal of Pain 11: 6–21

Flor H, Turk D C, Rudy T E 1987 Pain and families: parts I and II. Pain 30: 3–45

Fordyce W E 1976 Behavioral methods for chronic pain and illness. Mosby, St Louis

Fordyce W E 1995 Back pain in the workplace. Report of an International Association for the Study of Pain Task Force. IASP Press, Seattle

Galizzi M, Boden L I 1996 What are the most important factors shaping return to work? Evidence from Wisconsin. Workers' Compensation Research Institute, Cambridge, MA

Hadler N M 1999 Occupational musculoskeletal disorders. Lippincott, Williams & Wilkins, Philadelphia

Halliday J L 1937 Psychological factors in rheumatism, a preliminary study. British Medical Journal 1: 213–217

Halmosh A F, Israeli R 1982 Family interactions as modulator in the post-traumatic process. Medicine and Law 1: 125–134

Hill M 1990 Social security policy in Britain. Edward Elgar, Aldershot

Honeyman P T, Jacobs E A 1996 Effects of culture on back pain in Australian aboriginals. Spine 21: 841–843

Janlert U 1997 Unemployment as a disease and diseases of the unemployed. Scandinavian Journal of Work and Environmental Health 23 (suppl. 3): 79–83

Kerns R D 1999 Family therapy for adults with chronic pain. In: Gatchel R J, Turk D C (eds) Psychosocial factors in pain: critical perspectives. Guildford Press, New York, pp 445–456

Kingson E R, Schulz J H (eds) 1997 Social security in the 21st century. Oxford University Press, New York

Kivimaki M, Vahtera J, Ferrie J E, Hemingway H, Pentti J 2001 Organizational downsizing and musculoskeletal problems in employees: a prospective study. Occupational and Environmental Medicine 58: 811–817

Kleinman A 1988 The illness narratives: suffering, healing and the human condition. Basic Books, New York

Lazar H, Stoyko P 1998 The future of the welfare state. International Social Security Review 51: 3–36

Leavitt F 1992 The physical exertion factor in compensable work injuries. A hidden flaw in previous research. Spine 17: 307–310

Loeser J D, Henderlite S E, Conrad D A 1995 Incentive effects of workers' compensation benefits: a literature synthesis. Medical Care Research and Review 52: 34–59

Mason V 1994 The prevalence of back pain in Great Britain. Office of Population Censuses and Surveys, Social Survey Division (now office of National Statistics). Her Majesty's Stationery Office, London

Miller J H 1976 Preliminary report on disability insurance. Public Hearings before the Subcommittee on Social Security of the Committee on Ways and Means of the US House of Representatives. US Government Printing Office, Washington, DC, pp 115–153

Nagi S Z, Hadley L W 1972 Disability behavior, income change and motivation to work. Industrial and Labor Relations Review 25: 223–233

Papageorgiou A C, Macfarlane G F, Thomas E, Croft P R, Jayson M I V, Silman A J 1997 Psychosocial factors in the workplace – do they predict new episodes of low back pain? Spine 22: 1137–1142

Parsons T 1951 The social system. Free Press, New York

Phillips R B 1994 Social theory of chiropractic. In: Leach R A (ed.) The chiropractic theories: principles and clinical applications, 3rd edn. Williams & Wilkins, Baltimore, pp 365–371

Ploug N, Kvist J 1996 Social security in Europe: development or dismantlement? Kluwer Law International, The Hague

Rainville J, Sobel J B, Hartigan C, Wright A 1997 The effect of compensation involvement on the reporting of pain and disability by patients referred for rehabilitation of chronic low back pain. Spine 22: 2016–2024

Ritchie J, Snape D 1993 Invalidity benefit: a preliminary qualitative study of the factors affecting its growth. Social and Community Planning Research, London

Ritchie J, Ward K, Duldig W 1993 A qualitative study of the role of GPs in the award of invalidity benefit. Department of Social Security Research report number 18. Her Majesty's Stationery Office, London, pp 1–72

Rohling M L, Binder L M, Langhinrichsen-Rohling J 1995 Money matters: a meta-analytic review of the association between financial compensation and the experience and treatment of chronic pain. Health Psychology 14: 537–547

Sanderson P L, Todd B D, Holt G R, Getty C J M 1995 Compensation, work status, and disability in low back pain patients. Spine 20: 554–556

Scales J, Scase J 2000 Fit and fifty? A report prepared for the Economic and Social Research Council. University of Essex Institute for Social and Economic Research, Essex pp 1–59

Sharp T J, Nicholas M K 2000 Assessing the significant others of chronic pain patients: the psychometric properties of significant other questionnaires. Pain 88: 135–144

Suter P B 2002 Employment and litigation: improved by work, assisted by a verdict. Pain 100: 249–257

Taylor V M, Deyo R A, Ciol M, Kreuter W 1996 Surgical treatment of patients with back problems covered by workers' compensation versus those with other sources of payment. Spine 21: 2255–2259

Taylor V M, Deyo R A, Ciol M et al 2000 Patient-oriented outcomes from low back surgery. A community based study. Spine 25: 2445–2452

Tito F 2000 The consumer's perspective. In: Law, money and medicine – forum on compensable disability. Royal Australian College of Physicians, Sydney

Torstensen T A 1996 Comparing likes and un-likes of non-athletes with low back pain versus elite athletes. Presented to Sports Medicine Symposium, Telemark, Norway

Vikne J 1996 What are the characteristics of top elite athletes? MSc thesis. Norwegian University of Sport and Physical Education, Oslo

Volinn E 1997 The epidemiology of low back pain in the rest of the world, a review of surveys in low and middle income countries. Spine 22: 1747–1754

Volinn E, Koevering D V, Loeser J D 1991 Back sprain in industry: the role of socioeconomic factors in chronicity. Spine 16: 542–548

Waddell G, Waddell H 2000 Social influences on neck and back pain and disability. In: Nachemson A, Jonsson E (eds) Neck and back pain: the scientific evidence of causes, diagnosis and treatment. Lippincott, Williams & Wilkins, Philadelphia, pp 13–55

Waddell G, Pilowsky I, Bond M 1989 Clinical assessment and interpretation of abnormal illness behaviour in low back pain. Pain 39: 41–53

Waddell G, Aylward M, Sawney P 2002 Back pain, incapacity for work and social security benefits: an international literature review and analysis. Royal Society of Medicine Press, London

Zborowski M 1952 Cultural components in responses to pain. Journal of Social Issues 8: 16–30

Chapter **14**

The biopsychosocial model

We have looked at many aspects of low back pain and disability, and it is time to fit them all together. Let us step back and try to see the whole picture. It should be clear by now that the traditional disease model is inadequate to understand low back pain and disability. We need a new model that includes all the biopsychosocial influences on pain and disability (Engel 1977, Waddell 1987).

Models are simply attempts to crystallize ideas on paper. They help to clarify our thinking and communicate with others. But models also constrain our thinking. For example, if you think back pain is a sign of disease, your answer is better medical investigation and treatment. If you think back pain is an ordinary body sensation rather than a disease, you will deal with it very differently. If you think back pain is a work-related problem, your answer may be occupational interventions. And if you think that many of the restrictions suffered by people with disabilities are imposed by the way society is organized, your answer may be political and social change. So models matter.

I must emphasize that this is not a causal model. Let me repeat once more that back pain is a physical problem that arises from musculoskeletal and neurophysiologic processes. But that is only the start. What we are trying to understand is how some patients develop chronic pain and disability. The model we choose then has implications for how we should manage the problem.

Box 14.1

- Recognize patterns of symptoms and signs   History and examination
- Infer underlying injury or disease   Diagnosis
- Treat underlying injury or disease   Therapy
- Expect the patient to recover   Cure (or residual impairment and disability/rehabilitation)

THE DISEASE MODEL

For more than a century, western health care has been based on the disease model (Virchow 1858, Hadler 1995; Box 14.1).

This disease model is deeply entrenched in the way patients, doctors, and therapists think. Despite all the advances in the neurophysiology of pain and better understanding of the relation between pain and disability, it still dominates routine clinical practice. From the disease model, we assume that:

- pain = tissue injury
- tissue damage ⟶ impairment ⟶ disability ⟶ incapacity for work
- if we cure the pain, then disability will also recover.

This whole approach has worked well for clear-cut pathology such as a spinal fracture or a disk prolapse. History and epidemiology show that it has failed for ordinary backache. I believe that is because some of the basic assumptions of the disease model do not apply to non-specific low back pain:

- Back pain is a common bodily symptom, which most people deal with themselves most of the time (Ch. 5). Ursin (1997) suggested that we should regard much back pain as a "subjective health complaint" rather than a medical condition.
- We cannot identify any structural lesion in most patients (Ch. 9). (Though that is not to deny its physical basis.)
- Pain is not the same as tissue injury. The Cartesian model fails to explain many clinical observations of pain. Compare it with modern ideas about the neurophysiology of pain (Ch. 3).
- Pain, disability, and incapacity for work are not the same thing. They are related, but more weakly than most patients, doctors, and therapists

Summary

A historic perspective (Ch. 4)
- Human beings have had back pain all through history, and it is no more common or severe than it has always been
- What has changed is how we understand and manage the symptom of pain in the back
- Three key ideas in the 19th century laid the foundation for 20th-century management:
  - back pain comes from the spine and involves the nervous system
  - it is due to injury
  - the back is irritable and should be treated by rest
- These ideas were brought together into a marketable package by the discovery of the ruptured disk
- The epidemiology shows an epidemic of chronic disability attributed to ordinary backache in all western countries
  - even if there is now some evidence this may be changing, at least in some countries and some settings
- The traditional biomedical approach has not solved the problem, and may even have contributed to it

assume (Fig. 14.1). We must distinguish pain and disability conceptually and in clinical practice (Ch. 3).
- Different people respond very differently to back pain. How we think and feel has a profound influence on pain and disability (Chs 11–12), on our illness behavior (Ch. 10), on clinical progress (Ch. 7) and on how we respond to treatment.
- Social issues have a powerful influence on illness behavior and disability (Ch. 13).

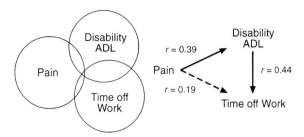

Figure 14.1 The relation between severity of low back pain, disability in activities of daily living (ADL), and incapacity for work. r is the correlation coefficient; $r = 0$ means there is no relationship, $r = 1$ means 100% correlation. Approximately, $r = 0.30$ means 10% and $r = 0.50$ means 25% in common.

I believe traditional treatment of back pain according to the disease model failed because the approach is fatally flawed. The disease model offers a simplistic view of low back pain and disability in terms of spines and physical disease. It does not allow for complex human responses to pain and disability, or for human behavior.

Pain and disability (Ch. 3)

- Pain and disability are not the same. We must make a clear distinction between them, both conceptually and in clinical practice.
- Pain is a complex sensory and emotional experience. It is much more than just a signal of tissue damage
  — pain signals do not pass unaltered to the cerebral cortex; they are always and constantly modulated at all levels of the CNS before they reach consciousness;
  — pain, emotions, and pain behavior are all integral parts of the pain experience;
  — the CNS is plastic in nature, and there may be neurophysiologic changes over time with the development of chronic pain.
- Disability is restricted activity.
- Clinical assessment depends on the patient's *report* of pain and disability, which depends on how the patient thinks and feels, and communicates the experience.

THE BIOPSYCHOSOCIAL MODEL

We will construct the biopsychosocial model in four stages. First, we will review the individual clinical

elements of the model. Second, we will consider the key question of how physical and psychological processes interact. Third, we will construct a cross-sectional outline of the biopsychosocial model, at one point in time. Finally, we will look at a more dynamic model and the development of chronic pain and disability over time.

The clinical elements of the biopsychosocial model

Let us review briefly the key clinical elements we need to build this model:

- physical dysfunction
- beliefs and coping
- distress   } pain and disability
- illness behavior
- social interactions

Physical dysfunction (Ch. 9)

The symptom of back pain arises from nociception in the back. I have argued that non-specific low back pain is mainly a matter of *dysfunction* or physiologic impairment. Dysfunction depends on the level of demand or stress, the capacity of the musculoskeletal system to cope, and the (im)balance between them. There is always a background of subconscious and conscious sensation from normal musculoskeletal function, and any symptoms depend on how we perceive them against this background. Further, if back pain is due to disturbed function then it always has at least the potential to recover. As the epidemiology shows, most back pain should be benign and self-limiting, even if recurrent pain is common.

Painful musculoskeletal dysfunction

- may occur in structurally normal tissues
- a primary dysfunction arising in response to abnormal forces imposed on or generated within the musculoskeletal system
- abnormal patterns of muscle function, abnormal forces acting on musculoskeletal structures, abnormal posture or abnormal joint movement may all produce pain
- segmental soft-tissue changes; neurophysiologic and psychophysiologic changes.

Beliefs about back pain (Ch. 12) How patients think and feel about back pain is central to what they do about it and how it affects them. Anticipation of pain, anxiety, and attention, the meaning and context of the pain, suggestion and placebos, past experience, prior conditioning, and health care all play a part. These beliefs partly reflect the physical condition of the back, but they have more to do with how the individual thinks about it. Beliefs determine behavior.

Beliefs
- Beliefs about damage and disease
- Fear of hurt and harming
- Fear-avoidance beliefs
- Personal responsibility, control, and self-efficacy
- Beliefs and expectations about treatment

Coping
- Active or passive
- Catastrophizing
- Beliefs affect health care: health care affects beliefs

Fear of pain and what we do about pain may be more disabling than back pain itself.

Distress (Ch. 11) Pain is commonly accompanied by emotional arousal and distress. Distress may raise awareness of bodily sensations, increase the severity of pain, and lower pain tolerance. It makes us more concerned about the pain and more likely to seek health care.

- anxiety
- increased bodily awareness
- fear and uncertainty
- depressive symptoms
- anger and hostility.

Illness behavior (Ch. 12) Beliefs about the pain, coping strategies, and distress all affect what we do – our illness behavior. Illness behavior reflects the severity of the physical problem, but in its final expression it may reflect these psychological processes more than the underlying physical problem.

Observations of illness behavior

- pain drawing
- pain adjectives and description

- non-anatomic or behavioral descriptions of symptoms
- non-organic or behavioral responses to examination
- overt pain behavior
- use of walking aids
- down-time
- help with personal care.

There is now a great deal of evidence that beliefs, distress, and illness behavior are powerful influences on low back disability (Tables 14.1 and 14.2 and Fig. 14.2).

Social interactions (Ch. 13) with other people, either individually, in a group or collectively with

Table 14.1 Fear of pain may be more disabling than pain itself

Main elements of illness	Extent to which these account for chronic low back disability	
	In activities of daily living (%)	In loss of time from work (%)
Severity of pain	14	5
Fear-avoidance beliefs	+32	+26
Total identified	46	31

These are the additive effects, after allowing for severity of pain. It is unusual to be able to identify such a high proportion of any biologic relationship.
Based on data from Waddell et al (1993).

Table 14.2 Distress and illness behavior may be as disabling as physical impairment

Main elements of illness	Extent to which these account for chronic low back disability	
	In activities of daily living (%)	In loss of time from work (%)
Physical impairment	40	22
Distress		
Illness behavior	+31	+7
Social interactions	?	?
Total identified	71	29

These are the additive effects of distress and illness behavior, after allowing for physical impairment.
Based on data from Waddell et al (1984).

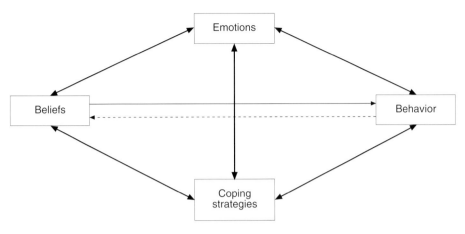

Figure 14.2   *The complex relationship between beliefs, emotions, and behavior.*

Table 14.3   Social influences on back pain and disability

Social influences	Can all affect
Culture	Reporting of back pain
Family	Pain behavior
Social class/occupation/	Disability
education	Health care and sick
Job satisfaction and	certification
psychosocial aspects	Sickness absence
of work	Social security claims and
Unemployment	benefits
Early retirement	Early retirement
Workers' compensation	
Litigation	
Social security	

society. Illness and the sick role are social phenomena. Low back pain and disability occur in a particular social setting. Family, work, and wider social networks influence beliefs, coping strategies, and illness behavior. Chronic low back disability requires sanction and support from the family and society. The availability, nature, and strength of these social influences may either reinforce or discourage illness behavior and disability. In turn, pain and pain behaviors are powerful means of communication with other people, including health professionals. Ultimately, the impact of back pain may reflect the prevailing culture of (back) pain and illness and disability in society (Table 14.3).

The relation between physical and psychological dysfunction

How do these various elements relate? It is not a question of *either* physical *or* psychological mechanisms. Rather, disability depends on the combination of physiologic and psychological processes and how they interact over time.

The neurophysiology of pain

Pain is both a sensory and an emotional experience. The gate control theory (Melzack & Wall 1965) and modern neurophysiology suggest mechanisms by which both neurophysiologic and psychological processes can modulate pain (Fig. 14.3). They help to explain the complexity of clinical pain. They bridge the mind–body dichotomy.

Psychological and neurophysiologic processes may *sensitize* patients to common bodily symptoms

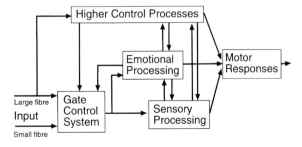

Figure 14.3   How the gate control system links the psychological and neurophysiologic aspects of pain. After Melzack & Casey (1968), with permission.

(Brosschot & Eriksen 2002, Eriksen & Ursin 2002). Emotions, attitudes, and beliefs may turn these symptoms into subjective health complaints. Ferrari & Schrader (2001) describe a similar brew of "expectations, amplification and attribution" in the late whiplash syndrome. See Hadler (1996, 2001) for further discussion on medicalization.

Physical function, performance and illness behavior

Clinical assessment of (dys)function, (dis)ability and (in)capacity is largely a matter of *performance*. Even clinical examination of impairment cannot be divorced from performance. They all depend on the physical condition and function of the back. They all attempt to assess physical (in)capacity. But in practice assessment is based on observation of performance. Performance is a matter of what the patient does. It is behavior. So we can never wholly separate physical function from behavior, either conceptually or in practice.

- Non-specific low back pain seems to be mainly a matter of disturbed function or painful musculoskeletal dysfunction.

- Disability is reduced function. Ideally, we would like to measure capacity but in practice we measure reduced activity. So disability is a matter of what we do (or do not do) and of altered performance.

- Pain behavior or illness behavior is also a matter of what we do (or do not do).

- Disability involves both physical dysfunction and illness behavior, which in a sense are simply two sides of the same coin. Behavior always involves motor and physiologic activity; and physiologic processes often have behavioral expressions. Behavior changes at both subjective and physiologic levels.

- As an oversimplification:
  — capacity is determined by physiologic limits.
  — performance is determined by psychological factors.

This combination of dysfunction and behavior is the crux of the problem (Fig. 14.4). It is not a question of whether physical dysfunction or altered behavior comes first or which is more important,

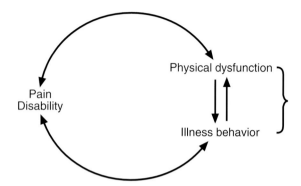

Figure 14.4 Physical dysfunction and illness behavior are intimately linked to each other. They lie at the heart of the process of developing chronic low back pain and disability. Low back pain leads to physical dysfunction and altered behavior, which in turn aggravate and perpetuate the pain. Physical dysfunction and illness behavior lead to low back disability or, in another sense, *are* disability.

but rather how they interact and reinforce each other. What is the effect of pain and disability on mental and psychological processes, which in turn affect behavior? How do these psychological processes and altered behavior then aggravate and perpetuate musculoskeletal dysfunction?

Psychophysiology

Psychological events can affect physiologic processes by several mechanisms.

Guarded movements appear to be particularly important, and are closely linked to psychological processes (Main & Watson 1996, Watson et al 1998). Guarded movements depend more on fear avoidance than on current pain intensity. Fear of pain or reinjury, perceptions of ability – or lack of ability – to perform movements and activities, and catastrophizing can all lead to guarded movements. Exacerbations of back pain are common and reinforce this conditioning. These patterns may start as a reflex physiologic response to injury or primary dysfunction, but persist due to psychophysiologic rather than physiologic processes alone. Guarded movements become a learned, protective habit and then persist as physiologic dysfunction (Fig. 14.5).

Physiologic dysfunction

- abnormal patterns of movement
- abnormal patterns of muscle activity

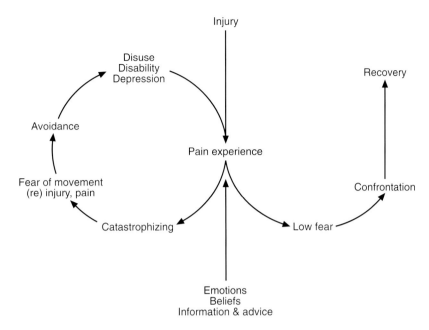

Figure 14.5   The fear-avoidance model. Fear of movement and reinjury can determine how some people recover from back pain while others go on to chronic pain and disability. After JWS Vlaeyen, personal communication (2002).

- abnormal patterns of neurophysiologic activity
- disturbed posture and gait
- abnormal patterns of physical activity and behavior.

Guarded movements and lack of normal use lead in turn to physical and psychological deconditioning. This "disuse syndrome" is the direct consequence of reduced activity and illness behavior (Bortz 1984, Mayer & Gatchel 1988). Disuse has a profound effect on the physical condition of the back, which aggravates and maintains physical dysfunction, and leads directly to more severe disability. As well as this physical or physiologic loop, there is feedback and reinforcement of behavior. What we do, our activity level, and illness behavior all reinforce our beliefs about the pain and the coping strategies we use to deal with it. Illness behavior, disability, and sickness absence reinforce distress and depression, which increase illness behavior and disability. Illness behavior and reduced activity aggravate and perpetuate physiologic dysfunction and deconditioning. These are all interlocking, vicious circles.

Reduced activity, deconditioning, and illness behavior

- reduced physical activity
- circulatory, tissue nutrition, and metabolic changes
- muscle wasting, loss of strength and endurance
- loss of neuromuscular coordination
- muscle imbalance
- guarded movements
- physical dysfunction and illness behavior.

The biopsychosocial model

It is now widely accepted that low back pain and disability can only be understood and managed by a biopsychosocial model (Engel 1977, Waddell 1987, 2002, Turk et al 1988; Fig. 14.6).

This biopsychosocial model allows for all the physical, psychological, and social elements that we have discussed. This is not a causal model, but rather a cross-section of the clinical presentation at one point in time. It illustrates key psychological and behavioral factors that may help to understand current levels of pain and disability.

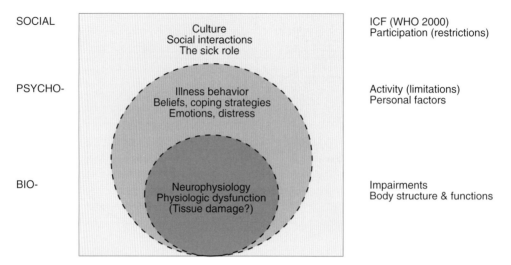

Figure 14.6   A biopsychosocial model of low back pain and disability. ICF, *International Classification of Functioning, Disability and Health*; WHO, World Health Organization.

This is a model of human illness, rather than of disease or pain. Back pain is a physical problem and pain arises from nociception in the back, but its clinical expression and human impact involve all of these other aspects. Patients and health professionals alike see that physical symptom as if through a series of filters. When we observe its clinical presentation, we can only look directly at illness behavior, which we must analyze more carefully to infer underlying biologic events. And we must allow for superimposed social influences.

However, there is no sharp division between the biopsychosocial elements, which overlap and interact. Pain is both a physical sensation and an emotional experience. Illness behavior and the sick role reflect psychological events but are also social events. These various elements not only interact, they develop together over the time-course of illness. This is also a model of illness rather than wellness. It does not consider how most people manage to cope with back pain and get on with their lives more or less normally, while others become severely and even permanently disabled.

The development of chronic pain and disability

- The symptom of back pain arises from a physical process in the back and nociception.

- The key to chronic pain and disability may be failure to recover as it should, rather than the development of a different syndrome.
- As pain becomes chronic (and this process may start within 3–8 weeks), attitudes and beliefs, distress and illness behavior play an increasing role in the development of chronicity and disability.
- This all occurs within a social context, and leads to social interactions with others, including in particular family, work, and health care.

This is a clinical model, but it has deeper historic roots (Glouberman et al 2000, Glouberman 2001). The entire debate on medical or biopsychosocial models reflects philosophies of health. These fall into three main types:

1. those that focus on the individual as an organism
2. those that stress the environment (both physical and social)
3. those that recognize the importance of the interaction between the organism and the environment.

The first is a mechanistic view of health as a function of the human body. It is also quite recent, from the Cartesian model and the development of medical science in the 19th century. The second is a much

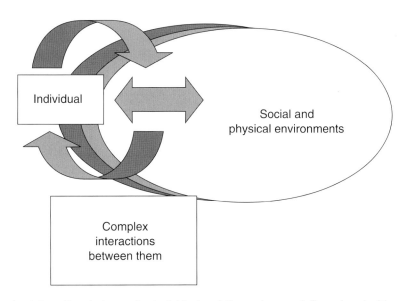

Figure 14.7   Complex interactions between the individual and the environment. Reproduced with permission from Glouberman (2001).

more ancient and philosophic view from the time of Aristotle and Hippocrates. It believes that health and sickness depend on lifestyle, healthy behavior, and the social and physical environment, rather than biological status or medical care. Public health shows that is still valid today. Preventive and therapeutic interventions have limited impact on the over-all health of the population. There is still a social gradient in health (Acheson 1998, Bush 2001). As argued throughout this book, current trends of disability appear to have more to do with social and cultural factors rather than with any biologic change.

Glouberman (2001) also pointed out that this has many of the characteristics of a *complex system* (Fig. 14.7). Such a system cannot be reduced to the sum of its parts. The interactions produce new properties, characteristics, and effects. So what appears to be a simple intervention on one element does not necessarily have a direct and predictable effect. Rather, any intervention may influence the system in complex and unforeseen ways.

Changes over time

Disability is not static. It is a dynamic process that evolves over time.

The factors that influence the development of chronic pain and disability, recovery, and return to

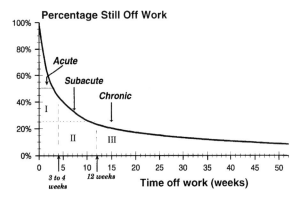

Figure 14.8   Three stages in the development of chronic disability. Reproduced with permission from Frank et al (1996).

work, and their relative importance, all vary over time. The passage of time and particularly the duration of sickness absence are fundamental to this process. Frank et al (1996, 1998) and Krause & Ragland (1994) described the clinical and occupational stages every patient must pass through on the way to chronic disability (Fig. 14.8 and Table 14.4). This also reflects increasing difficulty in clinical management, rehabilitation, and return to work.

Each phase involves a different set of interactions. Capacity for work deteriorates, and the obstacles to rehabilitation and return to work increase.

Table 14.4   Stages of disability

Acute: 0–4 weeks (a medical condition with social implications)	Natural history is benign and self-limiting Prognosis is good, irrespective of health care 90% of acute attacks settle within 6 weeks, at least sufficient to return to work, even if many people still have some persistent or recurrent symptoms Minimize health care, avoid medicalization, avoid iatrogenic disability Avoid labeling and culture of disability and incapacity
Subacute: 4–12 weeks (the critical stage for intervention)	Most people have returned to work, even if they still have some residual pain Those still off work now have 10–20% risk of going on to chronic pain and incapacity Psychosocial issues become more important. "Yellow flags" – risk factors for chronicity Active interventions to control pain and improve activity levels are effective and cost-effective The opportunity for timely health care, rehabilitation, and administrative interventions
Chronic: >12 weeks (a disability problem with medical elements)	This 10% of patients accounts for 80% of health care use and 90% of social costs Nonspecific low back pain has now become a source of chronic incapacity Major impact on every aspect of their lives, their families, and their work Psychosocial issues are always important Poor prognosis: likelihood of return to work diminishes with time Medical treatment, rehabilitation, and vocational rehabilitation are difficult and success rate is low Many patients lose their jobs and attachment to the labor force. Retraining and replacement become much more difficult

Adapted from Frank et al (1996) and Krause & Ragland (1994).

Psychosocial concerns, expectations, and behavior are very different at the acute, subacute, and chronic stages. Social, employment, and economic status changes, at some points quite dramatically. The outcome of any intervention may be quite different in each phase, so the timing of health care or rehabilitation interventions is critical.

SOCIAL MODELS OF DISABILITY

Over the past few decades, the main focus of the biopsychosocial model has been on psychological issues. We all paid lip service to the importance of social issues, but then ignored them. Too often, it was assumed that social really meant economic incentives and compensation. Perhaps we thought that social issues were outwith the scope of health care, and there was nothing we could do about them. Whatever the reason, there was little research into social issues around back pain. In practice, they got very little clinical attention either.

Over the past 5 years, I have become more and more convinced of the importance of social issues. Psychological issues may be more important for understanding chronic pain. When it comes to understanding disability and especially incapacity for work, then social issues are probably even more important.

The social model

There is now greater recognition of the needs and rights of people with disabilities, enshrined in disability discrimination legislation. As part of the fight for disabled rights, and as a reaction against the limitations of the medical model, disability groups proposed a "social model of disability" in the 1970s (Finkelstein 1996, Duckworth 2001). The social model argues that many of the restrictions suffered by people with disabilities do not really lie in the individual's impairment. Rather, they are imposed by the way society is organized for

Table 14.5 Models of disability: comparing the medical, biopsychosocial, and social models

Medical model	Biopsychosocial model	Social model
People with disabilities are directly disadvantaged by their impairments	Disability may start with impairment, but the extent of the resulting disability also depends on psychological and social factors	People with disabilities are disadvantaged by society's failure to accommodate everyone's abilities
The medical condition causes secondary social consequences	Interactions between the individual's physical and mental health and situation are important	The social situation is the problem
People with disabilities are pitied as the victims of personal tragedy	People with disabilities suffer social disadvantage and exclusion, and society should make provision to accommodate them	People with disabilities are oppressed by current social and economic institutions
Disability is best overcome through medical treatment or rehabilitation	Disability is best overcome by an appropriate combination of health care, rehabilitation, personal effort, and modification of the social situation	Disadvantage is best overcome by society adapting itself to everyone's abilities

Reproduced with permission from Waddell (2002).

able-bodied living. Society fails to make allowance and arrangements that would enable people with disabilities to fulfill the potential they retain. Physical settings such as lack of wheelchair access are obvious, but social attitudes are equally important. The social model is based on the personal experience of people with disabilities. Whatever it lacks in scientific evidence, it has wide social and political acceptance and reality.

The social model has very different implications. This is a political model. It is about social disadvantage and exclusion. With most obvious political overtones, it is a "social oppression model." Management of disability now requires social action and is the collective responsibility of society. Disability becomes a political rather than a medical issue. People with disabilities now join other minority groups in the context of equal opportunities and human rights.

Rowlingson & Berthoud (1996) compared the medical and social models of disability. However, they presented it as either a purely medical problem with medical answers or a purely social problem with social answers. They did not allow for any compromise. Table 14.5 shows how the biopsychosocial model can combine and balance the medical and social models of disability.

Other social models

A moment's thought will show that *the* social model described above is only one of a number of social perspectives.

Politicians and policy makers often prefer an economic model (Waddell 2002). Economists talk of the hypothetical "economic man" whose actions are influenced by the balance of incentives and risks. Although expressed most simply in financial terms, this covers much wider social incentives and costs. Nor should we confuse natural self-interest with selfishness or greed. Advocates of the economic model quote three lines of evidence (Ch. 13):

- The rising trend of disability benefits over the past few decades coincides with more generous benefits.
- The financial level of benefits influences the number and duration of claims.
- There is a close link between local unemployment rates and sickness and disability claims.

No one can deny that financial and other (dis)incentives influence human behavior. But this is again only one perspective that should not be overemphasized.

Perhaps both *the* social model and the economic model are too simplistic. They certainly reflect very different and opposing views. In reality, trends of low back pain and disability occur against a much broader background of social attitudes and practices. Culture is "the collective attitudes, beliefs and behavior that characterize a particular social group over time." Over the last few decades there have been major shifts in thinking about back pain and its management, disability, work and incapacity, employment patterns, (early) retirement, and social benefits. Perhaps what we need is a cultural model, however enigmatic that might be.

There is obviously some truth in all of these social models, but each offers a single perspective. And all of us who have had back pain can bear witness that it is not just a social phenomenon! Once again, this time arguing from the opposite direction, only a biopsychosocial model can allow for all the elements and influences on pain and disability.

THE BIOPSYCHOSOCIAL MODEL IN PRACTICE

Implications for clinical management

The successes and failures of treatment for spinal disorders reflect the value and the limitations of the disease model, and the need for a biopsychosocial approach. The success of physical treatment depends on accurate diagnosis of a treatable lesion, as Spangfort (1972) showed in surgery for disk prolapse (Table 14.6). However, the classic study by Wiltse & Rocchio (1975) showed that

psychological factors also affect how patients respond to surgery (Table 14.7). Many other studies have shown this to be true of all conservative therapies, surgery, pain management programs, and rehabilitation. It is true whether the patient has a clear physical pathology such as a disk prolapse, or non-specific back pain.

We studied the interaction between physical and psychological factors in a prospective surgical series of 195 patients (Waddell et al 1986). We found that the physical outcome of surgery depended on physical factors: accurate diagnosis of a surgically treatable lesion, good surgery, and avoiding complications. If surgery was successful, then the patient's distress and illness behavior also got better. But if surgery failed, everything got worse. Psychological factors could affect outcome in two ways. They could affect pain and disability directly and so affect the patient's and the surgeon's judgment of outcome. They could also influence surgical decisions and hence affect outcomes indirectly. Most often, distress led to pressure to "do something." Most dangerous of all, illness behavior could lead to inappropriate surgery. The patient was desperate, conservative treatment had failed, and the surgeon wanted to help. Surgery carried out for the wrong reasons led to predictably poor results. It not only failed to provide relief, but could also make the patient's pain and distress worse, which in turn led to more illness behavior and disability.

These are surgical examples, because that is where my story started, but the same applies to any

---

Table 14.6   Relief of sciatica and back pain according to the degree of herniation found at surgery

Operative findings	Relief of sciatica		Relief of back pain (%)
	Complete (%)	Partial (%)	
Complete herniation	90	9	75
Incomplete herniation	82	16	74
Bulging disk	63	26	54
No herniation	37	38	43

Based on data from Spangfort (1972).

Table 14.7   Psychological distress predicting symptomatic outcome of chemonucleolysis for disk prolapse

Preoperative Hs and Hy scores on the MMPI[a]	Excellent or good symptomatic relief
5+	10
75–84	16
65–74	39
55–64	72
54–	90

[a] The mean score for normal people is 50.
MMPI, Minnesota Multiphasic Personality Inventory.
Based on data from Wiltse & Rocchio (1975).

treatment. Management of a subjective complaint like back pain depends more than we realize on non-physical factors (Table 14.8).

Of course, it is not a question of *either* physical treatment *or* dealing with psychosocial issues. We must treat the whole person. That demands dealing with patients as individual human beings in all their complexity. We must distinguish the underlying physical problem from the patient's reaction and illness behavior. We should direct physical treatment to the physical problem. We must also recognize and deal with their hopes and fears, how they react and cope and behave. We must consider how our information and advice and our whole management affect their beliefs and feelings and behavior. We should recognize, and try to change, mistaken beliefs and fears at an early stage to prevent chronicity. We must always keep in mind that the ultimate goal and outcome of health care are not only to relieve, or at least control, pain, but also to help our patients to get on with their normal lives.

The biopsychosocial model forces us to rethink the role of health care in dealing with a problem like back pain (Table 14.9).

This may all seem a bit philosophic, but it has had some very practical results. Within a decade, this changed thinking has led to a complete reversal of our basic strategy of management for back pain. Traditional management was a negative strategy of rest and activity limitation, based on the disease model of back injury. The scientific evidence shows that it may actually have prescribed iatrogenic disability (Table 14.10, Waddell et al 1997, Hagen et al 2000). Modern management is a positive strategy of advice and helping patients to stay active. It is based on the biopsychosocial model and supported by strong scientific evidence (Table 14.11, Waddell et al 1997, Abenhaim et al 2000, van Tulder 2003). Despite some rearguard actions, this battle is now won!

Chapter 15 will consider clinical guidelines for back pain based on the biopsychosocial model.

Implications for rehabilitation

The traditional goal of health care is to make patients better. The goal of rehabilitation is to enable them to return to their normal activity levels and get on with their lives. The biopsychosocial

Table 14.8 The influence of different elements of illness on the amount of conservative treatment that patients receive for low back pain

Identifiable influences	Extent to which these account for the amount of treatment received (%)
Duration of symptoms	14
Physical severity	+11
Distress	+9
Illness behavior	+15
Total identified	50%

These are additive.
From Waddell et al (1984), with permission from the BMJ Publishing Group.

Table 14.9 The implications of the medical and biopsychosocial models

Medical model	Biopsychosocial model
Pain, disability, incapacity for work, and sickness absence are more or less entirely a consequence of injury or disease and of impairment	Pain, disability, incapacity for work, and sickness absence are *partly* a matter of the health condition, but *also* of how the individual thinks and feels and behaves
They are therefore outwith the individual's control and he or she bears little or no responsibility	The individual must therefore share some responsibility
The health condition and recovery are a matter of health care	The health condition and recovery are *partly* a matter of health care, but *also* of the individual's own efforts and behavior
The patient is the passive recipient of health care	The individual must be an active participant in his or her own rehabilitation and recovery
Relief of pain will automatically cure disability	Management must both relieve pain and at the same time prevent disability

Table 14.10 Randomized controlled trials demonstrating that bed rest is ineffective

Authors	Journal
Back pain	
Wiesel et al (1980)[a]	Spine 5: 324–330
Rupert et al (1985)	ICA Int Rev Chiropract 58–60
Gilbert et al (1985)	Br Med J 291: 791–794
Deyo et al (1986)	N Engl J Med 315: 1064–1070
Pal et al (1986)	Br J Rheumatol 25: 1181–1183
Evans et al (1987)	Physiother Can 39: 96–101
Postachini et al (1988)	Neuro-Orthoped 6: 28–35
Szpalski & Hayez (1992)	Eur Spine J 1: 29–31
Wilkinson (1995)	Br J Gen Pract 45: 481–484
Malmivaara et al (1995)	N Engl J Med 332: 351–355
Rozenberg et al (2002)	Spine 27: 1487–1493
Sciatica	
Coomes (1961)	Br Med J 1: 20–24
Vroomen et al (1999)	N Engl J Med 340: 418–423
Hofstee et al (2002)	J Neurosurg 96 (suppl. 1): 45–49

[a] This is the only RCT to suggest that bed rest was effective, but it was a selected group of army recruits in an unrepresentative situation.

Table 14.11 Randomized controlled trials providing strong scientific evidence on the value of staying active

Authors	Journal
Lindequist et al (1984)	Scand J Rehab Med 16: 113–116
Fordyce et al (1986)	J Behav Med 9: 127–140
Linton et al (1989)	Pain 36: 197–207
Phillips et al (1991)	Behav Res – Ther 29: 443–450
Lindstrom et al (1992)	Phys Ther 72: 279–291; Spine 17: 641–652
Linton et al (1993)	Pain 54: 353–359
Wilkinson (1995)	Br J Gen Pract 45: 481–484
Malmivaara et al (1995)	N Engl J Med 332: 351–355
Indahl et al (1995)	Spine 20: 473–477; Spine 23: 2625–2630
Burton et al (1999)	Spine 24: 2484–2491
Moore et al (2000)	Pain 88: 145–153
Linton & Andersson (2000)	Spine 25: 2825–2831
Linton & Ryberg (2001)	Pain 90: 83–90
Buchbinder et al (2001)	Br Med J 322: 1516–1520; Spine 26: 2535–2542

Table 14.12 Components of a rehabilitation program: overcoming obstacles to recovery

	Obstacles to recovery	Components of rehab program
Bio	Activity level vs job demands	Graded activity
Psycho	Beliefs and behavior	Cognitive-behavioral
Social	Employment	Occupational intervention; communication

model of pain *and* disability brings these goals together. It means that *every* doctor and therapist who treats back pain should be interested in rehabilitation (Liebenson 1996).

But rehabilitation is not only a medical matter (Wade & de Jong 2000). The biopsychosocial model provides a framework for a problem-oriented approach to rehabilitation (Table 14.12). Medical, psychological, and social obstacles to recovery and return to work are all important. Overcoming the psychosocial obstacles and changing behavior are just as important as physical reconditioning. Rehabilitation must also be set firmly in an occupational and social setting. This leads to a multidisciplinary approach to rehabilitation.

Principles of rehabilitation (Ch. 18)

- Key principles:
  - good clinical management is fundamental
  - the primary goal of patients and health care is pain relief but
  - for patients who do not recover quickly, health care alone is not enough
- The three key components of rehabilitation:
  - reactivation and progressive increase in activity levels
  - address dysfunctional beliefs and behavior
  - an occupational component and/or setting
- In addition:
  - patient, health professional(s), and employer must communicate and work together to common, agreed goals
  - identify and address obstacles to return to work
  - the main goal is job retention and (early) return to work.

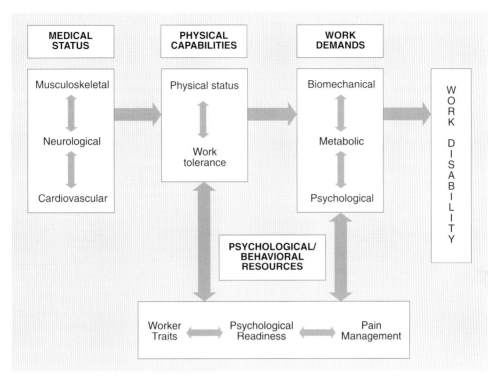

Figure 14.9   The Rochester model of work disability. Reproduced with permission from Feuerstein (1991).

Rehabilitation is so important that it is the subject of Chapter 18.

Implications for occupational health

Modern approaches to occupational health are firmly based on the biopsychosocial model. The Rochester model (Fig. 14.9) is one example (Feuerstein 1991, Feuerstein & Zastowny 1999). It includes the patient's health condition, physical capabilities, psychological and behavioral resources, and ability to meet the physical and psychological demands of work. It also emphasizes the importance of psychological factors in rehabilitation and successful return to work. This model serves as a framework to:

- guide clinical evaluation and management
- identify obstacles to return to work
- develop targeted interventions to overcome these barriers, and
- design effective rehabilitation services.

Chapter 17 will consider occupational health guidelines for back pain based on the biopsychosocial model.

Implications for disability

Whatever the biologic basis of illness and disability, they are ultimately expressed in a social context. The sick or disabled role is a social status adopted by the individual and supported by society (Parsons 1951). It is therefore subject to social rules, one of which usually demands a medical condition. The new *International Classification of Functioning* (WHO 2000) is based on the biopsychosocial model. It emphasizes that disability encompasses all of these interrelated and interacting dimensions (Box 14.2). Disability depends on interactions between the individual and his or her social context (Fig. 14.7). (In)capacity for work depends on interactions between the worker's health condition, his or her physical and mental capabilities, the demands of the job, and other psychosocial factors (Rowlingson & Berthoud 1996).

Box 14.2 International Classification of Functioning (ICF) classification of functional states (WHO 2000)

- **Body functions** are the physiologic and psychological functions of body systems
- **Impairments** are problems in body function or structure such as a significant deviation or loss
- **Activity** is the execution of a task or action by an individual
- **Participation** is involvement in a life situation
- **Activity limitations** are difficulties an individual may have in executing activities. (This is equivalent to the previous definition of disability, i.e., "restricted activity" but removes the assumption that it is "resulting from an impairment")
- **Participation restrictions** are problems an individual may experience in involvement in life situations. (This is equivalent to the previous definition of handicap)
- **Environmental factors** are external features of the physical, social, and attitudinal world, which can have an impact on the individual's performance in a given domain

From this model, disability evaluation requires holistic assessment. Chronic disability due to non-specific low back pain is never simply a matter of physical pathology. Medical diagnosis or clinical assessment of impairment is no longer enough (Cocchiarella & Andersson 2000). Nor is a label like chronic pain syndrome an adequate substitute. A medical condition and sick certification are prerequisites for long-term social support, but incapacity for work is essentially a social phenomenon. This is why medical diagnosis and treatment alone cannot solve the problem of chronic incapacity. But doctors do play a vital role in the interactions among the individual, employment, society, and legal systems.

The implications of the biopsychosocial model for social policy are beyond the scope of this clinical book. They are discussed elsewhere (Fordyce 1995, Glouberman et al 2001, Hadler 1996, 2001, Waddell 2002).

CONCLUSION

The common ideal of all our health professions is to help patients and to relieve human suffering. The biopsychosocial model simply provides a framework or set of tools for putting these ideals into clinical practice. It helps us to treat patients rather than just their spines. To do that, we must address *all* the biopsychosocial dimensions of their pain and disability if we are to deal with them effectively.

That means we must also remember that back pain starts with a physical problem in the back. Some critics reasonably argue that the emphasis on psychosocial issues may have gone too far (Borkan et al 2002). They accept that non-specific back pain has been overmedicalized and needs to be demedicalized – "First, do no harm" (Hippocrates). They accept that overzealous pursuit of elusive physical lesions has at times been counterproductive. It was the need to correct such excesses of the medical model that led to the biopsychosocial model. But some patients do have identifiable physical conditions that are amenable to treatment – and "it ill behoves the skilled physician to mumble charms that crave the knife" (Sophocles). We must not abandon the search for better understanding and treatment of different clinical patterns of non-specific back pain. Hopefully, the time will come when we can offer many of these patients more effective treatments that will prevent many of these psychosocial problems developing. In the meantime, we must adopt a flexible approach to *both* the physical and the psychosocial problems of each individual patient.

The biopsychosocial model does not deny the need for health care, but it aims at better care. Patients with back pain need relief of pain and physical treatment for their physical problems. But they may also need support and help to return to their ordinary activities and to get on with their lives. Perhaps that sums it up: we need to shift the clinical paradigm from treatment to *care* (Vernon 1991). Treatment is an integral part of health care, but it is only the means to a greater end, not an end in itself.

References

Abenhaim L, Rossignol M, Valat J-P, Nordin M 2000 The role of activity in the therapeutic management of back pain. Spine 25: 1S–33S

Acheson D 1998 Inequalities in health report. Stationery Office, London

Borkan J, Van Tulder M, Reis S, Schoene M L, Croft P, Hermoni D 2002 Advances in the field of low back pain in primary care: a report from the Fourth International Forum. Spine 27: E128–E132

Bortz W M 1984 The disuse syndrome. Western Journal of Medicine 141: 691–694

Brosschot J F, Eriksen H R (eds) 2002 Special issue on somatization, sensitization and subjective health complaints. Scandinavian Journal of Psychology 43: 97–196

Bush President G W 2001 Fulfilling America's promise to Americans with disabilities. US presidential proposal

Cocchiarella L, Andersson G B J (eds) 2000 Guides to the evaluation of permanent impairment, 5th edn. American Medical Association, Chicago

Duckworth S 2001 The disabled person's perspective. In: New beginnings: a symposium on disability. UNUM, London, pp 39–64

Engel G L 1977 The need for a new medical model: a challenge for biomedicine. Science 196: 129–136

Eriksen H R, Ursin H 2002 Sensitization and subjective health complaints. Scandinavian Journal of Psychology 43: 189–196

Ferrari R, Schrader H 2001 The late whiplash syndrome: a biopsychosocial approach. Journal of Neurology, Neurosurgery and Psychiatry 70: 722–726

Feuerstein M A 1991 Multidisciplinary approach to the prevention, evaluation and management of work disability. Journal of Occupational Rehabilitation 1: 5–12

Feuerstein M, Zastowny T R 1999 Multidisciplinary management of work related musculoskeletal pain and disability. In: Gatchel R J, Turk D C (eds) Psychological approaches to pain management: a practitioner's handbook. Guildford Press, New York, pp 458–485

Finkelstein V 1996 Modelling disability. Available online at: http://www.leeds.ac.uk/disability-studies/archiveuk/finkelstein/models/models.htm

Fordyce W (ed.) 1995 Back pain in the workplace. Report of an IASP task force. IASP Press, Seattle

Frank J W, Kerr M S, Brooker A-S et al 1996 Disability resulting from occupational low back pain. Spine 21: 2908–2929

Frank L, Sinclair S, Hogg-Johnson S et al 1998 Preventing disability from work-related low-back pain. New evidence gives new hope – if we can just get all the players on side. Canadian Medical Association Journal 158: 1625–1631

Glouberman S 2001 Towards a new perspective on health policy. Canadian Policy Research Networks Study no H I 03. Available online at: http://www.cprn.org/cprn.htm 2001

Glouberman S, Kisilevsky S, Groff P, Nicholson C 2000 Towards a new concept of health: three discussion papers. Canadian Policy Research Networks Study no H I 03. Available online at: http://www.cprn.org/cprn.htm

Hadler N M 1995 The disabling backache: an international perspective. Spine 20: 640–649

Hadler N M 1996 The disabled, the disallowed, the disaffected and the disavowed. Journal of Occupational and Environmental Medicine 38: 247–251

Hadler N M 2001 Regional musculoskeletal injuries: a social construction. Available online at: www.rheuma21st.com/archives/cutting_edge_hadler_muscul_injuries.html

Hagen K B, Hilde G, Jamtvedt G, Winnem M 2000 Bed rest for acute low back pain and sciatica (Cochrane review). In: The Cochrane Library, Issue 4, 2000. Oxford: Update Software. Spine 25: 2932–2939

Krause N, Ragland D R 1994 Occupational disability due to low back pain: a new interdisciplinary classification based on a phase model of disability. Spine 19: 1011–1020

Liebenson C 1996 Rehabilitation of the spine. Williams & Wilkins, Baltimore, pp 13–31

Main C J, Watson P J 1996 Guarded movements: development of chronicity. Journal of Musculoskeletal Pain 4: 163–170

Mayer T G, Gatchel R J 1988 Functional restoration for spinal disorders: the sports medicine approach. Lea & Febiger, Philadelphia, pp 1–321

Melzack R, Casey K L 1968 Sensory, motivational and central control determinants of pain: a new conceptual model. In: Kenshalo D (ed.) The skin senses. C C Thomas, Springfield, IL, pp 423–443

Melzack R, Wall P D 1965 Pain mechanisms: a new theory. Science 150: 971–979

Parsons T 1951 The social system. Free Press, New York

Rowlingson K, Berthoud R 1996 Disability, benefits and employment. Department of Social Security Research Report no. 54. HMSO, London

Spangfort E V 1972 The lumbar disc herniation. A computer aided analysis of 2504 operations. Acta Orthopaedica Scandinavica 142(suppl.): 1–95

Turk D C, Rudy T E, Stieg R L 1988 The disability determination dilemma: toward a mutiaxial solution. Pain 34: 217–229

Ursin H 1997 Sensitization, somatization, and subjective health complaints: a review. International Journal of Behavioural Medicine 4: 105–116

van Tulder M (Chairman) 2003 Preliminary draft of European guidelines for the management of acute non-specific low back pain in primary care. Cost action B13 European Commission, Research Directorate-General, Department of Policy, Co-ordination and Strategy, Brussels. Available online at: www.backpaineurope.org

Vernon H 1991 Chiropractic: a model of incorporating the illness behavior model in the management of low back pain patients. Journal of Manipulative and Physiological Therapeutics 14: 379–389

Virchow R 1858 Die cellular Pathologie in ihrer Begrundurg auf physiologische und pathologische. A Hirschwald, Berlin

Waddell G 1987 A new clinical model for the treatment of low back pain. Spine 12: 632–644

Waddell G 2002 Models of disability: using low back pain as an example. Royal Society of Medicine Press, London

Waddell G, Bircher M, Finlayson D, Main C J 1984 Symptoms and signs: physical disease or illness behaviour? British Medical Journal 289: 739–741

Waddell G, Morris E W, Di Paola M P, Bircher M, Finlayson D 1986 A concept of illness tested as an improved basis for surgical decisions in low back disorders. Spine 11: 712–719

Waddell G, Somerville D, Henderson I, Newton M, Main C J 1993 A fear avoidance beliefs questionnaire (FABQ) and the role of fear avoidance beliefs in chronic low back pain and disability. Pain 52: 157–168

Waddell G, Feder G, Lewis M 1997 Systematic reviews of bedrest and advice to stay active for acute low back pain. British Journal of General Practice 47: 647–652

Wade D T, de Jong B A 2000 Recent advances in rehabilitation. British Medical Journal 32: 1385–1388

Watson P J, Booker C K, Main C J 1998 Evidence for the role of psychological factors in abnormal paraspinal activity in patients with chronic low back pain. Journal of Musculoskeletal Pain 5: 82–86

WHO 2000 International classification of functioning, disability and health (ICF). World Health Organization, Geneva

Wiltse L L, Rocchio P D 1975 Pre-operative psychological tests as predictions of success of chemonucleolysis in the treatment of the low back syndrome. Journal of Bone and Joint Surgery 57A: 478–483

Chapter 15

Clinical guidelines

Gordon Waddell   Maurits van Tulder

This is the age of evidence-based medicine and every doctor and therapist should be aware of the scientific evidence base for clinical practice. However, the literature is now so extensive that none of us have time to read it all for ourselves and to keep up to date. The answer is clinical guidelines, which describe good practice for the typical patient with a common clinical problem (Institute of Medicine 1992). Their aim is to improve standards of care and clinical effectiveness. All health professionals have always tried to apply the best and most up-to-date knowledge to clinical practice. Guidelines are simply a way of presenting this knowledge in a form that is accessible and easy to use.

Guidelines are based on two main principles:

1. the best scientific evidence that is currently available
2. the widest possible professional and patient consultation and consensus.

Guidelines are not rigid protocols that we must follow slavishly. They are just what they say: guidance. They simply provide a background or framework for practice. We must always tailor clinical management to suit the individual patient, their clinical problem, and their situation. But when we depart from the guidelines, we should do so consciously and deliberately, not accidentally or in ignorance. And we should be able to justify why we treated a particular patient differently.

In this chapter we present a selection of the best and most up-to-date guidelines for the clinical management of acute back pain. They range from very basic, single-sheet presentations or algorithms

> **Box 15.1   Clinical management of acute low back pain**
>
> - Exclude serious disease
> - Reassurance
> - Simple symptomatic measures
> - Avoid overinvestigation, labeling, and medicalization
> - Continue ordinary activities as normally as possible
> - Early return to work
> - 4–6 weeks: intensive reactivation and rehabilitation.

to a comprehensive review of the scientific evidence base. The basic messages (Box 15.1) are the same in every country (Koes et al 2001). We simply offer samples of what is available, and leave it to you to decide if and how you want to use them. Which presentation you prefer depends on your situation and needs and personal taste.

We have included:

- Appendix **15A** The scientific evidence base: a table of the Cochrane reviews now available on therapy for low back pain (www.cochrane.iwh.on.ca).

You may also want to look at:

Nachemson A, Jonsson E (eds) 2000 Neck and back pain: the scientific evidence of causes, diagnosis and treatment. Lippincott, Williams & Wilkins, Philadelphia.

Van Tulder M W, Koes B W 2002 Low back pain and sciatica: acute. Clinical Evidence 8: 1156–1170.

Van Tulder M W, Koes B W 2002 Low back pain and sciatica: chronic. Clinical Evidence 8: 1171–1187. Available online at: www.clinicalevidence.com.

Cherkin et al (2003) for a recent review of manipulation, massage, and acupuncture.

- Appendix **15B** RCGP 1999 *Clinical Guidelines for the Management of Acute Low Back Pain*. Royal College of General Practitioners, London. Available online at: www.rcgp.org.uk.

This is the second edition of the UK guideline that has been recognized around the world as one of the best examples. It is simple and concise, on two sides of an A4 sheet. Although it is commonly referred to as the RCGP guideline, it is actually the official national guideline of all primary care health professionals dealing with back pain in UK.

Two algorithms designed to accompany the first edition of the RCGP guideline, and an algorithm from the New Zealand Guide (www.acc.org.nz) are also included.

You may also want to look at:

Breen A C, Langworthy J, Vogel S et al 2000 Primary care audit tool kit: acute back pain. [This is an audit pack designed to accompany the RCGP guideline.] Institute for Musculoskeletal Research and Clinical Implementation, Bournemouth. Available online at: www.imrci.ac.uk.

- Appendix **15C** Working Backs Scotland (2000) national education campaign. These are very simple sheets summarizing the key messages and designed for wide distribution to all health professionals who treat back pain. All of the material is available online at: www.workingbacksscotland.com.

- Appendix **15D** The draft European COST Action B13 *Guidelines for the Management of Acute Non-specific Low Back Pain in Primary Care*. Cost B13 Management Committee 2002: available (www.backpaineurope.org). These are up-to-date guidelines that give details of the scientific evidence base and European consensus.

You may also want to look at:

www.icsi.org/guide/LBP.pdf and www.guideline.gov.index.asp for a selection of US guidelines. (There are no recent official national guidelines in the US.)

The Dutch physiotherapy guideline for low back pain (Bekkering et al 2003).

Koes et al (2001) for a review of international guidelines.

- Appendix **15E** The New Zealand *Guide to Assessing Psychosocial Yellow Flags in Acute Low Back Pain* (Kendall et al 1997; available online at: www.acc.org.nz). This is still the classic.

References

Bekkering G E, van Tulder M W, Hendriks H J M et al 2003 Dutch physiotherapy guideline for acute low back pain. Physiotherapy 89: 82–96

Cherkin D C, Sherman K J, Deyo R A, Shekelle P G 2003 A review of the evidence for the effectiveness, safety and cost of acupuncture, massage therapy and spinal manipulation for back pain. Annals of Internal Medicine (in press)

COST B13 Management Committee 2002 European guidelines for the management of low back pain. Acta Orthopedica Scandinavica 73 (suppl. 305): 20–25

Institute of Medicine (Field M J, Lohr K N, eds) 1992 Guidelines for clinical practice. From development to use. National Academy Press, Washington, DC

Kendall N A S, Linton S J, Main C J 1997 Guide to assessing psychosocial yellow flags in acute low back pain. Accident Rehabilitation and Compensation Insurance Corporation and National Advisory Committee on Health and Disability, Wellington, NZ. Available online at: www.acc.org.nz

Koes B W, van Tulder M W, Ostelo R, Burton A K, Waddell G 2001 Clinical guidelines for the management of low back pain in primary care: an international comparison. Spine 26: 2504–2513

APPENDIX 15A THE SCIENTIFIC EVIDENCE BASE

COCHRANE REVIEWS OF TREATMENT FOR LOW BACK PAIN

Review	Journal
Acupuncture for acute and chronic low-back pain	Spine 1999; 24: 1113–1123
Advice to stay active as a single treatment for low back pain and sciatica	Spine 2002; 27: 1736–1741 See also the attached editorial comment on this review
Back schools for non-specific low-back pain	–
Bed rest for acute low-back pain and sciatica	Spine 2000; 25: 2932–2939
Behavior therapy for chronic low-back pain	Spine 2000; 25: 2688–2699
Exercise therapy for low-back pain	Spine 2000; 25: 2784–2796
Injection therapy for sub-acute and chronic benign low-back pain	Spine 2001; 26: 501–515
Lumbar supports for prevention and treatment of low-back pain	Spine 2001; 26: 377–386
Massage for low-back pain	Spine 2002; 27: 1896–1910
Multidisciplinary biopsychosocial rehabilitation for sub-acute low-back pain among working age adults	Spine 2001; 26: 262–269
Multidisciplinary rehabilitation for chronic low back pain	BMJ 2001; 322: 1511–1516
Non-steroidal anti-inflammatory drugs for low-back pain	Spine 2000; 25: 2501–2513
Rehabilitation after lumbar disc surgery	Spine 2003; 28: 209–218
Surgery for degenerative lumbar spondylosis	Spine 1999; 24: 1820–1832
Surgery for lumbar disc prolapse	Spine 1999; 24: 1820–1832
Transcutaneous electrical nerve stimulation (TENS) for chronic low back pain	Spine 2002; 27: 596–603

These reviews are all in the Cochrane Library, Issue 4, 2002.
See www.cochrane.iwh.on.ca for abstracts and up-to-date information on completed reviews.

APPENDIX 15B CLINICAL GUIDELINES FOR THE MANAGEMENT OF ACUTE LOW BACK PAIN

ACUTE LOW BACK PAIN

DIAGNOSTIC TRIAGE

Diagnostic triage is the differential diagnosis between:

- Simple backache (non specific low back pain)
- Nerve root pain
- Possible serious spinal pathology

Simple backache: *specialist referral not required*

- Presentation 20–55 years
- Lumbosacral, buttocks & thighs
- "Mechanical" pain
- Patient well

Nerve root pain: *specialist referral not generally required within first 4 weeks, provided resolving*

- Unilateral leg pain worse than low back pain
- Radiates to foot or toes
- Numbness & paraesthesia in same distribution
- SLR reproduces leg pain
- Localised neurological signs

Red flags for *possible serious spinal pathology: consider prompt investigation or referral (less than 4 weeks)*

- Presentation under age 20 or onset over 55
- Non-mechanical pain
- Thoracic pain
- Past history – carcinoma, steroids, HIV
- Unwell, weight loss
- Widespread neurological symptoms or signs
- Structural deformity

PRINCIPAL RECOMMENDATIONS

- *Assessment*
  - Carry out diagnostic triage (see left).
  - X-rays are not routinely indicated in simple backache.
  - Consider psychosocial "yellow flags" (see over).

SIMPLE BACKACHE

- *Drug Therapy*
  - Prescribe analgesics at regular intervals, not p.r.n.
  - Start with paracetamol. If inadequate, substitute NSAIDs (e.g. ibuprofen or diclofenac) and then paracetamol–weak opioid compound (e.g. codydramol or coproxamol). Finally, consider adding a short course of muscle relaxant (e.g. diazepam or baclofen).
  - Avoid strong opioids if possible.
- *Bed Rest*
  - Do not recommend or use bed rest as a treatment.
  - Some patients may be confined to bed for a few days as a consequence of their pain but this should not be considered a treatment.

EVIDENCE

- *   Diagnostic triage forms the basis for referral, investigation and management.
- *   Royal College of Radiologists Guidelines.
- *** Psychosocial factors play an important role in low back pain and disability and influence the patient's response to treatment and rehabilitation.

- **   Paracetamol effectively reduces low back pain.
- *** NSAIDs effectively reduce pain. Ibuprofen and diclofenac have lower risks of GI complications.
- **   Paracetamol–weak opioid compounds may be effective when NSAIDs or paracetamol alone are inadequate.
- *** Muscle relaxants effectively reduce low back pain.

- *** Bed rest for 2–7 days is worse than placebo or ordinary activity and is not as effective as alternative treatments for relief of pain, rate of recovery, return to daily activities and work.

Cauda equina syndrome: *emergency referral*

- Sphincter disturbance
- Gait disturbance
- Saddle anaesthesia

• *Advice on Staying Active*

◆ Advise patients to stay as active as possible and to continue normal daily activities.

◆ Advise patients to increase their physical activities progressively over a few days or weeks.

◆ If a patient is working, then advice to stay at work or return to work as soon as possible is probably beneficial.

• *Manipulation*

◆ Consider manipulative treatment for patients who need additional help with pain relief or who are failing to return to normal activities.

• *Back Exercises*

◆ Referral for reactivation/rehabilitation should be considered for patients who have not returned to ordinary activities and work by 6 weeks.

The evidence is weighted as follows:

*** Generally consistent finding in a majority of acceptable studies.

** Either based on a single acceptable study, or a weak or inconsistent finding in some of multiple acceptable studies.

* Limited scientific evidence, which does not meet all the criteria of "acceptable" studies.

*** Advice to continue ordinary activity can give equivalent or faster symptomatic recovery from the acute attack and lead to less chronic disability and less time off work.

*** Manipulation can provide short-term improvement in pain and activity levels and higher patient satisfaction.

** The optimum timing for this intervention is unclear.

** The risks of manipulation are very low in skilled hands.

*** It is doubtful that specific back exercises produce clinically significant improvement in acute low back pain.

** There is some evidence that exercise programmes and physical reconditioning can improve pain and functional levels in patients with chronic low back pain. There are theoretical arguments for starting this at around 6 weeks.

KEY PATIENT INFORMATION POINTS

- **Simple Backache**
  - *give positive messages*

- There is nothing to worry about.
  Backache is very common.
- No sign of any serious damage or disease.
  Full recovery in days or weeks – but may vary.
- No permanent weakness.
  Recurrence possible – but does not mean re-injury.
- Activity is helpful, too much rest is not.
  Hurting does not mean harm.

- **Nerve Root Pain**
  - *give guarded positive messages*

- No cause for alarm. No sign of disease.
- Conservative treatment should suffice – but may take a month or two.
- Full recovery expected – but recurrence possible.

- **Possible Serious Spinal Pathology**
  - *avoid negative messages*

- Some tests are needed to make the diagnosis.
- Often these tests are negative.
- The specialist will advise on the best treatment.
- Rest or activity avoidance until appointment to see specialist.

PATIENT BOOKLET

The above messages can be enhanced by an educational booklet given at consultation. *The Back Book* is an evidence-based booklet developed for use with these guidelines, and is published by The Stationery Office (ISBN 011 702 0788).

These brief clinical guidelines and their supporting base of research evidence are intended to assist in the management of acute low back pain. It presents a synthesis of up-to-date international evidence and makes recommendations on case management.

Recommendations and evidence relate primarily to the first six weeks of an episode, when management decisions may be required in a changing clinical picture. However, the guidelines may also be useful in the sub-acute period (6–12 weeks).

These guidelines have been constructed by a multi-professional group and subjected to extensive professional review.

They are intended to be used as a guide by the whole range of health professionals who advise people with acute low back pain, particularly simple backache, in the NHS and in private practice.

- **Psychosocial "Yellow Flags"**

When conducting assessment, it may be useful to consider psychosocial "yellow flags" (beliefs or behaviours on the part of the patient which may predict poor outcomes). The following factors are important and consistently predict poor outcomes:
- a belief that back pain is harmful or potentially severely disabling
- fear-avoidance behaviour and reduced activity levels
- tendency to low mood and withdrawal from social interaction
- expectation of passive treatment(s) rather than a belief that active participation will help

Contributing Organisations
Royal College of General Practitioners
Chartered Society of Physiotherapy
British Osteopathic Association
British Chiropractic Association
National Back Pain Association

Algorithm 15B.1   Diagnositc triage of a patient presenting with low back pain with or without sciatica.

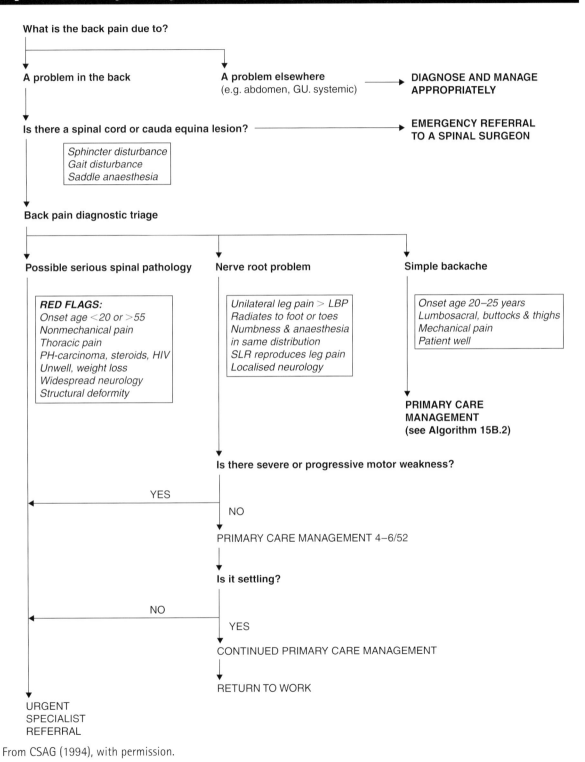

What is the back pain due to?

A problem in the back

A problem elsewhere
(e.g. abdomen, GU. systemic) ⟶ **DIAGNOSE AND MANAGE APPROPRIATELY**

Is there a spinal cord or cauda equina lesion? ⟶ **EMERGENCY REFERRAL TO A SPINAL SURGEON**

> *Sphincter disturbance*
> *Gait disturbance*
> *Saddle anaesthesia*

Back pain diagnostic triage

Possible serious spinal pathology

Nerve root problem

Simple backache

> **RED FLAGS:**
> *Onset age <20 or >55*
> *Nonmechanical pain*
> *Thoracic pain*
> *PH-carcinoma, steroids, HIV*
> *Unwell, weight loss*
> *Widespread neurology*
> *Structural deformity*

> *Unilateral leg pain > LBP*
> *Radiates to foot or toes*
> *Numbness & anaesthesia*
> *in same distribution*
> *SLR reproduces leg pain*
> *Localised neurology*

> *Onset age 20–25 years*
> *Lumbosacral, buttocks & thighs*
> *Mechanical pain*
> *Patient well*

PRIMARY CARE MANAGEMENT
(see Algorithm 15B.2)

Is there severe or progressive motor weakness?

YES

NO

PRIMARY CARE MANAGEMENT 4–6/52

Is it settling?

NO

YES

CONTINUED PRIMARY CARE MANAGEMENT

RETURN TO WORK

URGENT
SPECIALIST
REFERRAL

From CSAG (1994), with permission.

Algorithm 15B.2 Primary care management of simple backache.

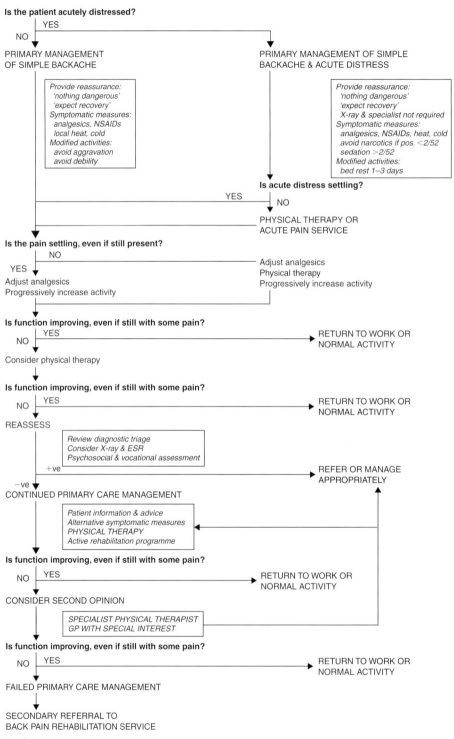

From CSAG (1994), with permission.

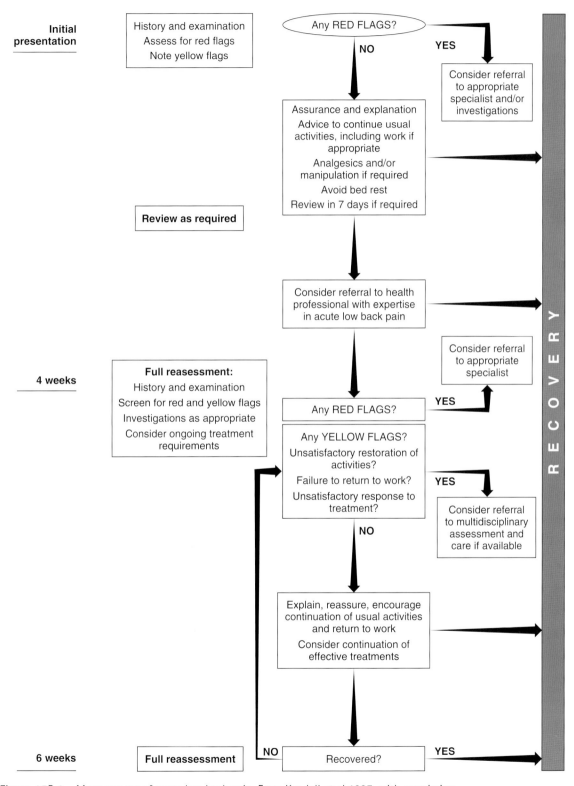

Figure 15B.1 Management of acute low back pain. From Kendall et al 1997, with permission.

APPENDIX 15C WORKING BACKS SCOTLAND EDUCATIONAL SHEETS

Low back pain evidence-based recommendations

General practitioners

(www.workingbacksscotland.com)

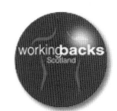

ANALGESIA

Diagnostic triage - exclude red flags.

Reassure no serious disease and that most low back pain settles quickly.

Provide adequate analgesia.

A cold pack or local heat can be used for short-term symptomatic relief.

ACTIVITY

Advise to stay active and continue as normally as possible.

Enquire about the patient's occupational duties.

Encourage the patient to remain at work if possible or return to work within a few days or weeks. They do not need to wait until they are completely pain free.

ACTION

Consider manual therapy (manipulative treatment) for patients who need additional help with pain relief or who are failing to return to their normal activities.

If the patient is still off work by four weeks there is a 10–40% chance they will not return to work within one year. Re-check red flags and consider obstacles to recovery (yellow flags).

By about six weeks the patient should be back to their normal activities or have commenced active rehabilitation.

If the patient is not back at work by about six weeks establish a dialogue with the employer and/or therapist and discuss strategies for return to work.

From Working Backs Scotland, with permission.

Low back pain evidence-based recommendations

Therapy providers

(www.workingbacksscotland.com)

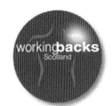

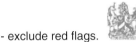

Diagnostic triage - exclude red flags.

Reassure no serious disease and that most low back pain settles quickly

Is analgesia adequate?

A cold pack or local heat can be used for short-term symptomatic relief.

Passive modalities (traction, lumbar corsets and electrotherapy) may be used to facilitate active management but do not provide lasting benefit and must not delay more active treatment.

Advise to stay active and continue as normally as possible.

Enquire about the patient's occupational duties.

Encourage the patient to remain at work if possible or return to work within a few days or weeks. They do not need to wait until they are completely pain free.

Consider manual therapy (manipulative treatment) for patients who need additional help with pain relief or who are failing to return to their normal activities.

If the patient is still off work by four weeks there is a 10-40% chance they will not return to work within one year. Re-check red flags and identify and help address obstacles to recovery (yellow flags).

By about six weeks the patient should be back to their normal activities or have commenced active rehabilitation.

If the patient is not back at work by about six weeks establish a dialogue with the GP and/or employer and discuss strategies for return to work.

From Working Backs Scotland, with permission.

Low back pain evidence-based recommendations

Pharmacists

(www.workingbacksscotland.com)

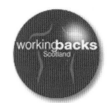

ANALGESIA

- Assess symptoms - refer to GP if warning signs exist.

- Reassure that back pain affects nearly everyone at some time but most low back pain settles quickly.

- Provide adequate analgesia.

- A cold pack or local heat can be used for short-term symptomatic relief.

ACTIVITY

- Advise to stay active and continue as normally as possible. The evidence shows that it is best to remain] at work if possible or return to work within a few days or weeks. They do not need to wait until they are completely pain free.

ACTION

- Patients who need additional help with pain relief or who are failing to return to their normal activities may wish to consult their GP, practice nurse or occupational health service, or consider manual therapy (manipulative treatment) from a chartered physiotherapist, a registered chiropractor, or registered osteopath.

WARNING SIGNS

Severe pain which gets worse over several weeks instead of better, or being 'unwell' with backpain:

- difficulty passing or controlling urine
- numbness around back passage or genitals
- numbness, pins and needles or weakness in both legs
- unsteadiness on feet.

From Working Backs Scotland, with permission.

APPENDIX 15D PRELIMINARY DRAFT OF EUROPEAN GUIDELINES FOR THE MANAGEMENT OF ACUTE NON-SPECIFIC LOW BACK PAIN IN PRIMARY CARE

From COST ACTION B13, with permission.

Maurits van Tulder (chairman), Annette Becker, Trudy Bekkering, Alan Breen, Tim Carter, Maria Teresa Gil del Real, Allen Hutchinson, Bart Koes, Peter Kryger-Baggesen, Even Laerum, Antti Malmivaara, Alf Nachemson, Wolfgang Niehus, Etienne Roux, Sylvie Rozenberg

Note: This guideline was developed within the framework of the COST ACTION B13 "Low back pain: guidelines for its management", issued by the European Commission, Research Directorate-General, Department of Policy, Co-ordination and Strategy. The final version of this guideline and future guidelines on prevention and chronic low back pain will be on www.backpaineurope.org. Further information on the COST B13 project, the methodology, and dissemination and implementation is available on the website and in COST B13 Management Committee (2002).

Summary of recommendations for diagnosis of acute non-specific low back pain

- Undertake diagnostic triage at the first assessment to exclude red flag conditions and radicular syndrome (*level D*)
- Complete case history and brief examination should be carried out to identify possible "red flags" and radicular syndrome (*level A*)
- If history taking indicates "red flags" or radicular syndrome, carry out physical examination including neurological screening when appropriate (*level A*)
- Be aware of psychosocial factors, and review them in detail if there is no improvement (*level A*)
- Diagnostic imaging tests (including X-rays, CT and MRI) are not routinely indicated for non-specific low back pain (*level A*)
- Reassess patients who are not resolving within a few weeks after the first visit or who are following a worsening course (*level D*)

Summary of recommendations for treatment of acute non-specific low back pain

- Give adequate information and reassure the patient (*Level B*)
- Do not prescribe bed rest as a treatment (*Level A*)
- Advise patients to stay active and continue normal daily activities including work if possible (*Level A*)
- Prescribe medication, if necessary for pain relief; preferably to be taken at regular intervals; first choice paracetamol, second choice NSAIDs (*Level A*)
- Consider adding a short course of muscle relaxants on its own or added to NSAIDs, if paracetamol or NSAIDs have failed to reduce pain (*Level A*)
- Consider (referral for) spinal manipulation for patients who are failing to return to normal activities (*Level A*)
- Multidisciplinary treatment programs in occupational settings may be an option for workers with sub-acute low back pain and sick leave for more than 4–8 weeks (*Level B*)

OBJECTIVES

The primary objective of these European evidence-based guidelines is to provide a set of recommendations that can support existing and future national and international guidelines or future updates of existing guidelines.

These guidelines intend to improve the management of acute non-specific low back pain patients (adults) in primary care in Europe, by:

1. providing recommendations on the clinical management of acute non-specific low back pain in primary care
2. ensuring an evidence-based approach through the use of systematic reviews and existing clinical guidelines
3. providing recommendations that are generally acceptable by all health professions in all participating countries
4. enabling a multidisciplinary approach; stimulating collaboration between primary

health care providers and promoting consistency across providers and countries in Europe.

TARGET POPULATION

The target population of the guidelines consists of individuals or groups that are going to develop new guidelines or update existing guidelines, and their professional associations that will disseminate and implement these guidelines. Indirectly, these guidelines also aim to inform the general public, low back pain patients, health care providers (for example, general practitioners, physiotherapists, chiropractors, manual therapists, occupational physicians, orthopaedic surgeons, rheumatologists, rehabilitation physicians, neurologists, anesthesiologists and other health care providers dealing with acute nonspecific low back pain patients), and policy makers in Europe.

EVIDENCE

The strength of evidence was rated:

Level A: Generally consistent findings provided by (a systematic review of) multiple high quality studies.
Level B: Generally consistent findings provided by (a systematic review of) multiple low quality studies.
Level C: One study (either high or low quality) or inconsistent findings from (a systematic review of) multiple studies.
Level D: No relevant studies on prognosis, diagnosis or therapy.

INTRODUCTION

Definitions

Low back pain is defined as pain and discomfort, localised below the costal margin and above the inferior gluteal folds, with or without leg pain.

Acute low back pain is usually defined as the duration of an episode of low back pain persisting for less than 6 weeks; sub-acute low back pain as low back pain persisting between 6 and 12 weeks; chronic low back pain as low back pain persisting for 12 weeks or more. In this guideline,

recommendations are related to both acute and sub-acute low back pain unless specifically stated otherwise. Recurrent low back pain is defined as a new episode after a symptom-free period of 6 months, but not an exacerbation of chronic low back pain.

Non-specific low back pain is defined as low back pain not attributed to recognisable, known specific pathology (e.g., infection, tumour, osteoporosis, ankylosing spondylitis, fracture, inflammatory process, radicular syndrome or cauda equina syndrome).

Red flags

The initial clinical history taking should aim at identifying "red flags" of possible serious spinal pathology [41]. Red flags are risk factors detected in low back pain patients' past medical history and symptomatology and are associated with a higher risk of serious disorders causing low back pain compared to patients without these characteristics. If any of these are present, further investigation (according to the suspected underlying pathology) should be considered to exclude a serious underlying condition, e.g., infection, inflammatory rheumatic disease or cancer.

Red flags are [41]:

- Age of onset <20 or >55 years
- Violent trauma
- Constant progressive, non-mechanical pain (no relief with bed rest)
- Thoracic pain
- Past medical history of malignant tumour
- Prolonged use of corticosteroids
- Drug abuse, immunosuppression, HIV
- Systematically unwell
- Unexplained weight loss
- Widespread neurology (including cauda equina syndrome)
- Structural deformity
- Fever

Cauda equina syndrome is likely to be present when patients describe bladder dysfunction (usually urinary retention, occasionally overflow incontinence), sphincter disturbance, saddle anaesthesia, global or progressive weakness in the lower limbs or gait disturbance. This requires urgent referral.

Yellow flags

Psychosocial "yellow flags" are factors that increase the risk of developing, or perpetuating chronic pain and long-term disability (including) work-loss associated with low back pain [28]. Identification of "yellow flags" should lead to appropriate cognitive and behavioral management. However, there is no evidence on the effectiveness of psychosocial assessment or intervention in acute low back pain.

Examples of "yellow flags" are [28]:

1. Inappropriate attitudes and beliefs about back pain (for example, belief that back pain is harmful or potentially severely disabling or high expectation of passive treatments rather than a belief that active participation will help),

2. Inappropriate pain behavior (for example, fear-avoidance behavior and reduced activity levels),

3. Work related problems or compensation issues (for example, poor work satisfaction)

4. Emotional problems (such as depression, anxiety, stress, tendency to low mood and withdrawal from social interaction).

Epidemiology

The lifetime prevalence of low back pain is reported as over 70% in industrialised countries (one-year prevalence 15% to 45%, adult incidence 5% per year). Peak prevalence occurs between ages 35 and 55 [3].

Symptoms, pathology and radiological appearances are poorly correlated. Pain is not attributable to pathology or neurological encroachment in about 85% of people. About 4% of people seen with low back pain in primary care have compression fractures and about 1% has a neoplasm. Ankylosing spondylitis and spinal infections are rarer. The prevalence of prolapsed intervertebral disc is about 1% to 3% [13].

Risk factors are poorly understood. The most frequently reported are heavy physical work, frequent bending, twisting, lifting, pulling and pushing, repetitive work, static postures and vibrations [3]. Psychosocial risk factors include stress, distress, anxiety, depression, cognitive functioning, and pain behaviour, job dissatisfaction and mental stress at work [3,24,36].

Acute low back pain is usually self-limiting (recovery rate 90% within 6 weeks) but 2%–7% of people develop chronic pain. Recurrent and chronic pain accounts for 75% to 85% of total workers' absenteeism [18].

Outcomes

The aims of treatment for acute low back pain are to relieve pain, to improve functional ability, and to prevent recurrence and chronicity. Relevant outcomes for acute low back pain are pain intensity, overall improvement, back pain specific functional status, impact on employment, generic functional status, medication use, and physical parameters [14]. Intervention-specific outcomes (e.g., coping and pain behavior for behavioral treatment, strength and flexibility for exercise therapy, depression for antidepressants, and muscle spasm for muscle relaxants and EMG biofeedback) may also be relevant.

DIAGNOSIS OF ACUTE LOW BACK PAIN

For most patients with acute low back pain a thorough history taking and brief clinical examination is sufficient. The primary purpose of the initial examination is to attempt to identify any "red flags" and to make a specific diagnosis. It is, however, well-accepted that in most cases of acute low back pain it is not possible to arrive at a diagnosis based on detectable pathological changes. Because of that several systems of diagnosis have been suggested, in which low back pain is categorized based on pain distribution, pain behaviour, functional disability, clinical signs etc. However, none of these systems of classification have been critically validated.

A simple and practical classification, which has gained international acceptance, is by dividing acute low back pain into three categories – the so-called "diagnostic triage":

- Serious spinal pathology
- Nerve root pain/radicular pain
- Non-specific low back pain

The priority in the examination procedure follows this line of clinical reasoning. The first priority is to make sure that the problem is of musculoskeletal origin and to rule out non-spinal pathology. The next step is to exclude the presence of serious spinal pathology. Suspicion therefore is awakened by the history and/or the clinical examination and can be confirmed by further investigations. The next priority is to decide whether the patient has nerve root pain. The patient's pain distribution and pattern will indicate that, and the clinical examination will often support it. If that is not the case, the pain is classified as non-specific low back pain.

The initial examination serves other important purposes besides reaching a "diagnosis". Through a thorough history taking and physical examination, it is possible to evaluate the degree of pain and functional disability. This enables the health care professional to outline a management strategy that matches the magnitude of the problem. Finally, the careful initial examination serves as a basis for credible information to the patient regarding diagnosis, management and prognosis and may help reassuring the patient.

Recommendation D1

Undertake diagnostic triage at the first assessment to exclude serious spinal pathology and nerve root pain (level D).

Evidence D1

Although there is general consensus on the importance and basic principles of differential diagnosis, there is little empirical evidence on the diagnostic triage.

Clinical guidelines D1

All guidelines propose some form of diagnostic triage in which patients are classified as having (1) possible serious spinal pathology; "red flag" conditions such as tumor, infection, inflammatory disorder, fracture, cauda equina syndrome, (2) nerve root pain, or (3) non-specific low back pain.

Discussion/commentary D1

Individual red flags do not necessarily link to specific pathology but indicate a higher probability of a serious underlying condition that may require further investigation. Multiple red flags need further investigation.

Recommendation D2

Complete case history should be carried out to identify possible serious spinal pathology and nerve root pain (level A).

Evidence D2

One systematic review of 36 studies evaluated the accuracy of history, physical examination and erythrocyte sedimentation rate in diagnosing low back pain in general practice [45]. The review found that the diagnostic accuracy of these tests remains unclear to a substantial extent. Not one single test seemed to have a high sensitivity and high specificity for radiculopathy, ankylosing spondylitis and vertebral cancer.

Clinical guidelines D2

All guidelines are consistent in their recommendations that diagnostic procedures should focus on the identification of "red flags" and the exclusion of specific diseases (sometimes including radicular syndrome). "Red flags" include, for example, age of onset <20 or >55 years, significant trauma, thoracic pain, weight loss, widespread neurology.

Discussion/consensus D2

The group strongly agrees that history taking should be carried out by a health professional with competent skills. Competence will depend on appropriate training in different member states.

Recommendation D3

If history taking indicates serious spinal pathology or nerve root pain, carry out physical examination including neurological screening when appropriate (level A).

Evidence D3

One systematic review of 17 studies found that the pooled diagnostic odds ratio for straight leg raising was 3.74 (95% CI 1.2–11.4); sensitivity was high (1.0–0.88), but specificity was low (0.44–0.11) [12]. All included studies were surgical case-series at non-primary care level. Most studies evaluated the diagnostic value of SLR for disc prolapse. The pooled diagnostic odds ratio for the crossed straight leg raising test was 4.39 (95% CI 0.74–25.9); with low sensitivity (0.44–0.23) and high specificity (0.95–0.86). The authors concluded that the studies do not enable a valid evaluation of diagnostic accuracy of the straight leg raising test [12].

Clinical guidelines D3

The types of physical examination and physical tests that are recommended show some variation. Neurological screening, which is largely based on the straight leg raising test (SLR), plays an important role in most guidelines.

Discussion/consensus D3

The group agrees that extensive physical examination is not always necessary for patients without any indication of serious spinal pathology or nerve root pain, but considered a brief physical examination always an essential part of the management of acute low back pain. Straight leg raising test is the most accurate test to identify nerve root pain.

The group strongly agrees that physical examination should be carried out by a health professional with competent skills. Competence will depend on appropriate training in different member states.

Recommendation D4

Be aware of psychosocial factors (e.g., pain behavior, fear avoidance behavior, kinesophobia, distress), and review them in detail if there is no improvement (level A).

Evidence D4

One systematic review was found of 11 cohort and 2 case-control studies evaluating psychosocial risk factors for low back pain [24]. Strong evidence was found for low social support in the workplace and low job satisfaction as risk factors for low back pain. Insufficient evidence was found for an effect of a high work pace, high qualitative demands, low job content, low job control, and psychosocial factors in private life.

Another systematic review found that there is strong evidence that psychosocial factors play an important role in chronic low back pain and disability, and moderate evidence that they are important at a much earlier stage than previously believed [36].

Clinical guidelines D4

All guidelines, with varying emphasis, mention the importance of considering psychosocial factors as risk factors for the development of chronic disability. There is, however, considerable variation in the amount of detail given about how to assess psychosocial factors or the optimal timing of the assessment, and specific tools for identifying these factors are scarce. The UK guideline [41] gives a list describing four main groups of psychosocial risk factors, whilst the New Zealand guideline [2, 28] gives by far the most attention towards explicit screening of psychosocial factors, using a standardized questionnaire [35].

None of the guidelines (with the exception of some general principles in the New Zealand "Yellow Flags") give any specific advice on what to do about psychosocial risk factors that are identified, and there is no published scientific evidence on the effectiveness of psychosocial interventions for acute low back pain. However, there is some scientific support that behavioural treatment is effective in reducing disability in sub-acute low back pain [34].

Discussion/consensus D4

The group strongly agrees that there should be awareness of psychosocial factors from the first visit in primary care to identify patients with a high risk of chronic disability. The group suggests considering it useful information for later management. Explicit screening of psychosocial factors (for example by using specific questionnaires or instruments) may be performed when there are recurrent episodes or no improvement.

Recommendation D5

Diagnostic imaging tests (including X-rays, CT and MRI) are not routinely indicated for non-specific low back pain (level A).

Evidence D5

One systematic review was found that included 31 studies on the causal relationship between X-ray findings of the lumbar spine and non-specific low back pain [48]. The results showed that degeneration, defined by the presence of disc space narrowing, osteophytes and sclerosis, is consistently and positively associated with non-specific low back pain with odds ratios ranging from 1.2 (95% CI 0.7–2.2) to 3.3 (95% CI 1.8–6.0). Spondylolysis/listhesis, spina bifida, transitional vertebrae, spondylosis and Scheuermann's disease did not appear to be associated with low back pain.

A review of MRI literature concluded that there is no evidence that this technique has improved the treatment of common back syndromes [29]. MRI is associated with the detection of abnormalities in patients without pain or without nerve root pain.

Clinical guidelines D5

The guidelines are consistent in the recommendation that plain X-rays are not useful in acute non-specific low back pain and that X-rays should be restricted to cases suspected of specific underlying pathology (based on "red flags"). In some guidelines X-rays are suggested as optional in case of low back pain persisting for more than 4 to 6 weeks) [6, 7, 10, 41]. None of the guidelines recommend any form of radiological imaging for acute, non-specific low back pain while the US and UK guidelines overtly advise against [6, 41].

Discussion/consensus D5

Although there is some evidence for an association between severe degeneration and non-specific low back pain, the group agrees that it does not have any implications for further management. The risks of the high doses of radiation in X-rays of the lumbar spine do not justify routine use.

The group strongly agrees that diagnostic imaging tests should not be used if there are no clear indications of possible serious pathology or radicular syndrome. The type of imaging test that may be used in such cases is outside the scope of this guideline.

Recommendation D6

Reassess patients who are not resolving within a few weeks after the first visit or who are following a worsening course (level D).

Evidence D6

There is little empirical evidence on the reassessment of patients.

Clinical guidelines D6

Most guidelines do not specifically address reassessment. The New Zealand guidelines stated that "A reasonable approach for most patients is a review by the end of the first week, unless symptoms have completely resolved [2]. It may be appropriate to arrange an earlier review, to reinforce the message to keep active and avoid prolonged bed rest." The Dutch guidelines advise reassessment at follow-up visits after 1 week if severe pain does not subside, after 3 weeks if the symptoms are not diminishing, and after 6 weeks if there is still disability or if there is no progress in function, or if pain does not decline [17]. The Danish guidelines recommend re-evaluation after 2 and 4 weeks if low back pain is unchanged or worsened [10].

Discussion/consensus D6

The group feels that the thresholds for reassessment of 4–6 weeks used in most existing guidelines are arbitrary and suggests using them flexibly.

TREATMENT FOR ACUTE LOW BACK PAIN

Various health care providers may be involved in the treatment of acute low back pain in primary care. Although there may be some variations between European countries, general practitioners, physiotherapists, manual therapists, chiropractors, exercise therapists (e.g., Alexander, Feldenkrais, Mendendieck, Cesar therapists), McKenzie therapists, orthopaedic surgeons, rheumatologists, physiatrists (specialists in physical medicine and rehabilitation) and others, may all be involved in providing primary care for people with acute low back pain. It is important that information and treatment are consistent across professions, and that all health care providers closely collaborate with each other.

Treatment of acute low back pain in primary care aims at: 1) providing adequate information, reassuring the patient that low back pain is usually not a serious disease and that rapid recovery is expected in most patients; 2) providing adequate symptom control, if necessary; and 3) recommending the patient to stay as active as possible and to return early to normal activities, including work. An active approach is the best treatment option for acute low back pain. Passive treatment modalities (for example bed rest, massage, ultrasound, electrotherapy, laser and traction) should be avoided as monotherapy and not routinely be used, because they increase the risk of illness behaviour and chronicity.

Recommendations included in these guidelines relate mainly to pain causing activity limitations or to patients seeking care.

Referral to secondary health care should be limited to patients in whom there is a suspicion of serious spinal pathology or nerve root pain (see diagnostic triage).

Recommendations for treatment are only included if there is evidence from systematic reviews or RCTs on acute non-specific low back pain. No RCTs have been identified on various commonly used interventions for acute low back pain, for example acupuncture, heat/cold, electrotherapy, ultrasound, trigger point and facet joint injections, and physiotherapy (defined by a combination of information, exercise therapy and physical modalities (e.g., massage, ultrasound, electrotherapy).

Recommendation T1

Give adequate information and reassure the patient (level B).

Evidence T1

One review evaluated the effectiveness of educational interventions for back pain in primary care [44]. One study showed that an educational booklet decreased the number of visits to a general practitioner for back pain. Another study showed that a 15-minute session with a primary care nurse plus an educational booklet and a follow-up phone call resulted in greater short-term patient satisfaction and perceived knowledge compared with usual care, but symptoms, physical functioning and health care utilization were not different.

In another trial published after the review, patients were given either an experimental booklet (the "Back Book") or a traditional booklet [9]. Patients receiving the experimental booklet showed greater early improvement in beliefs and functional status. There was no effect on pain.

Guidelines T1

Most guidelines recommend reassuring patients. The UK, US, Swiss, Finnish and Dutch guidelines recommend providing reassurance by explaining that there is nothing dangerous and that a rapid recovery can be expected [6, 17, 26, 27, 37, 41]. The US guidelines also stated that patients who do not recover within a few weeks may need more extensive education about back problems and told that special studies may be considered if recovery is slow [6]. The Swiss guidelines added that it is important to reassure patients through adequate information instead of making them insecure by stating that "nothing was found" [26, 27]. The New Zealand guidelines stated that "it is important to let the patient know that, if a full history and examination have uncovered no suggestion of serious problems, no further investigations are needed" [2].

Discussion T1

The evidence shows that carefully selected and presented information and advice about back pain can have a positive effect on patients' beliefs and clinical outcomes. The group recommends reassuring the patient by acknowledging the pain of the patient, being supportive and avoiding negative messages. It is important to give a full explanation in terms that the patient understands, for example, back pain is very common; usually the outlook is very good; hurting does not mean harm; it could arise from various structures, such as muscles, disks, joints or ligaments, but nobody knows exactly which. Cover the points discussed elsewhere in this guideline as appropriate.

Core items of adequate information should be: good prognosis, no need for X-rays, no underlying serious pathology, and stay active. Consistency across professions is very important.

It has been proven that a booklet may be helpful. The "Back Book", which is available in several languages, might be used for this purpose.

Recommendation T2

Do not prescribe bed rest as a treatment (level A).

Evidence T2

Six systematic reviews (10 RCTs, no statistical pooling) evaluated the effect of bed rest for acute low back pain [6, 16, 21, 30, 47, 56]. Five RCTs ($n = 921$) compared bed rest to alternative treatments, e.g., exercises, physiotherapy, spinal manipulation, or NSAIDs. They found either no differences or that bed rest was worse (using outcomes of pain, recovery rate, time to return to daily activities and sick leave). Five RCTs ($n = 663$) found that bed rest was no different or worse than no treatment or placebo. Two RCTs ($n = 254$) found that seven days of bed rest was no different from 2 to 4 days' bed rest.

Adverse effects: Adverse effects of bed rest are joint stiffness, muscle wasting, loss of bone mineral density, and venous thrombo-embolism [6]. Prolonged bed rest may lead to chronic disability and may impair rehabilitation.

Clinical guidelines T2

There now appears to be broad consensus that bed rest should be discouraged as treatment for low back pain [26, 27, 37, 39, 55]. Some guidelines state that if bed rest is indicated (because of severity of pain), it should not be advised for more than 2 days [2, 7, 10, 17, 22]. The UK guideline suggests

that some patients may be confined to bed for a few days but that should be regarded as a consequence of their pain and should not be considered a treatment [41]. The US guidelines stated that the majority of back pain patients will not require bed rest, and that prolonged bed rest for more than 4 days may lead to debilitation and is not recommended [6].

Discussion/consensus T2

The group agrees that bed rest does not promote recovery.

Recommendation T3

Advise patients to stay active and continue normal daily activities including work if possible (level A).

Evidence T3

A systematic review of eight RCTs found that there is strong evidence that advice to stay active is associated with equivalent or faster symptomatic recovery, and leads to less chronic disability and less time off work than bed rest or usual care [56]. Advice to stay active was either provided as single treatment or in combination with other interventions such as back schools, a graded activity program or behavioral counseling. Two RCTs ($n = 228$) found faster rates of recovery, less pain and less disability in the group advised to stay active than in the bed rest group. Five RCTs ($n = 1500$) found that advice to stay active led to less sick leave and less chronic disability compared to traditional medical treatment (analgesics as required, advice to rest and "let pain be your guide"). Harms were not addressed.

Adverse effects: None reported.

Clinical guidelines T3

Guidelines in the Netherlands, New Zealand, Finland, United Kingdom, Australia, Germany, Switzerland and Sweden recommend advice to stay active [2, 5, 17, 22, 26, 27, 37, 39, 41, 55]. Other guidelines made no explicit statement regarding advice to stay active.

Discussion/consensus T3

The group feels that advice to stay at work or to return to work if possible is important. Observational studies indicate that a longer duration of work absenteeism is associated with poor recovery.

Recommendation T4

Do not advise specific exercises (for example strengthening, flexion, and extension exercises) for acute low back pain (level A).

Evidence T4

Five systematic reviews and 12 additional RCTs (39 RCTs in total, no statistical pooling) evaluated the effect of exercise therapy for low back pain [1, 6, 16, 47, 52]. Results for acute and chronic low back pain were not reported separately in three trials.

Twelve RCTs ($n = 1894$) reported on acute low back pain. Eight trials compared exercises with other conservative treatments (usual care by the general practitioner, continuation of ordinary activities, bed rest, manipulation, NSAIDs, mini back school or short-wave diathermy). Seven of these found no differences or even mildly worse outcomes (pain intensity and disability) for the exercise group. Only one trial reported better outcomes for the exercise therapy group on pain and return to work compared to a mini back school. Four trials ($n = 1234$) compared exercises with "inactive" treatment (i.e., bed rest, educational booklet, and placebo ultrasound) and found no differences in pain, global improvement or functional status. Two small studies ($n = 86$) compared flexion to extension exercises, and found a significantly larger decrease of pain and a better improvement in functional status with extension exercises.

Adverse effects: Most trials did not assess harms.

Clinical guidelines T4

Recommendations regarding exercise therapy also show some variation. In several guidelines, back-specific exercises (e.g., strengthening, flexion, extension, stretching) are considered not useful during the first weeks of an episode [5, 17, 37, 41]. Other guidelines state that low stress aerobic exercises are a therapeutic option in acute low back pain [6]. The Danish guidelines specifically mention McKenzie exercise therapy as a therapeutic option in some patients with acute low back pain [10]. The Australian guidelines state that therapeutic exercises are not indicated in acute low back pain, but that general exercises for maintaining mobility and avoiding sick role may be considered [55]. The Finnish guidelines recommend guided exercises as part of multidisciplinary rehabilitation for subacute low back pain [37]. Guidelines from Switzerland consider exercises (active therapy, mobilizing, relaxation, strengthening) optional in the first 4 weeks, and useful after 4 weeks as training programs within an activating approach [26, 27].

Discussion/consensus T4

The group agrees that advice to stay active or to get active should be promoted, and that increase in fitness will improve general health. However, the current scientific evidence does not support the use of specific strengthening or flexibility exercises as a treatment for acute non-specific low back pain.

Recommendation T5

Prescribe medication, if necessary, for pain relief. Preferably to be taken at regular intervals. First choice paracetamol, second choice NSAIDs (level A).

Evidence T5 paracetamol

Two systematic reviews found strong evidence that analgesics are not more effective than NSAIDs [6, 47]. There is strong evidence from a systematic review in other situations that analgesics provide short-term pain relief [11].

Six RCTs (total $n = 329$) reported on acute low back pain. Three compared analgesics with NSAIDs. Two of these ($n = 110$) found that meptazinol, paracetamol and diflunisal (a NSAID) reduced pain equally. The third trial found that mefenemic acid reduced pain more than paracetamol, but that aspirin and indometacin were equally effective. One small trial ($n = 40$) found that electroacupuncture reduced pain slightly more than paracetamol after 6 weeks. One RCT ($n = 73$) found that ultrasound treatment substantially increased the proportion of pain-free patients after four weeks compared to (unspecified) analgesics.

Adverse effects: Combinations of paracetamol and weak opioids slightly increase the risk of adverse effects with OR 1.1 (95% CI 0.8 to 1.5) for single dose studies and OR 2.5 (95% CI 1.5 to 4.2) for multiple dose studies [11].

Evidence T5 NSAIDs

Two systematic reviews found strong evidence that regular NSAIDs relieve pain but have no effect on return to work, natural history or chronicity [32, 51]. NSAIDs do not relieve radicular pain. Different NSAIDs are equally effective. Statistical pooling was only performed for NSAIDs v placebo in acute low back pain.

Versus placebo: Nine RCTs ($n = 1135$) found that NSAIDs increased the number of patients experiencing global improvement (pooled OR after 1 week 2.00, 95% CI 1.35 to 3.00) and reduced the number needing additional analgesic use (pooled OR 0.64, 95% CI 0.45 to 0.91). Four RCTs ($n = 313$) found that NSAIDs do not relieve radicular pain.

Versus paracetamol: Three trials ($n = 153$) found conflicting results. Two RCTs ($n = 93$) found no differences in recovery, and one RCT ($n = 60$) found more pain reduction with mefenamic acid than paracetamol.

Versus muscle relaxants and opioid analgesics: Five out of six RCTs ($n = 399$ out of 459) found no differences in pain and overall improvement. One RCT ($n = 60$) reported more pain reduction with mefenamic acid than with dextropropoxyphene plus paracetamol.

Versus non-drug treatments: Three trials ($n = 461$). One RCT ($n = 110$) found that NSAIDs improved range-of-motion more than bed rest and led to lesser need for treatment. One trial ($n = 241$) found no statistically significant difference. Two studies ($n = 354$) found no differences between NSAIDs and physiotherapy or spinal manipulation in pain and mobility.

Versus each other: 15 RCTs ($n = 1490$) found no difference in efficacy.

Adverse effects: Adverse effects (particularly at high doses and in the elderly) may be serious [6, 23]. Effects include gastritis and other gastrointestinal complaints (affect 10% of people). Ibuprofen and diclofenac have the lowest gastrointestinal complication rate, mainly due to the low doses used in practice (pooled OR for adverse effects compared to placebo 1.27, 95% CI 0.91 to 1.78) [23]. In two trials side-effects were more frequent in the NSAIDs with muscle relaxant combination groups.

Clinical guidelines T5

Guidelines of the USA, New Zealand, Switzerland, Denmark, Finland, the Netherlands, UK, Germany and Australia all recommend paracetamol and NSAIDs, in that order [2, 6, 10, 17, 22, 26, 27, 37, 41, 54]. The Israeli guidelines only recommend NSAIDs [7]. Guidelines of the Netherlands, UK and Sweden explicitly recommend a time-contingent prescription, while the other guidelines do not mention this [17, 39, 41].

Discussion/consensus T5

The group points out that there is no evidence for a time-contingent prescription of drugs, but that it reflects the way it has been used in RCTs and that it is consistent with advice to stay active and encouragement to continue ordinary activities.

There was consensus among the group that paracetamol is to be preferred as first choice medication for acute low back pain, because of the evidence of effectiveness from other studies outside the field of low back pain and because of the low risk of side-effects.

If the patient is already taking adequate doses of paracetamol, NSAIDs may be started. If the patient already takes an NSAID, a combination of NSAIDs and mild opiates, a combination of paracetamol and mild opiates or a combination of NSAIDs and muscle relaxants may be used.

Recommendation T6

Only consider adding a short course of muscle relaxants on its own or added to NSAIDs, if paracetamol or NSAIDs have failed to reduce pain (level A).

Evidence T6

Two systematic reviews (14 RCTs; no statistical pooling) found strong evidence that muscle relaxants reduce pain and that different types are equally effective [6, 45].

Fourteen RCTs were identified (total $n = 1160$). Nine trials ($n = 762$) compared a muscle relaxant (tizanidine, cyclobenzaprine, dantrolene, carisoprodol, baclofen, orphenadrine, diazepam) with placebo. Seven of these found that muscle relaxants reduced pain and muscle tension and increased mobility more than placebo between one and two weeks; two found no differences. Three trials (total $n = 236$) compared different types of muscle relaxants. Two of these found that carisoprodol provided more overall improvement than diazepam but not than cyclobenzaprine, and that there were no differences in pain intensity. One RCT also found no differences between methocarbamol and chlormezanone.

Adverse effects: Adverse effects include drowsiness and dizziness in up to about 70% of patients, and a risk of dependency even after one week of treatment [6, 47]. The trials found adverse effects more common with muscle relaxants than placebo; 68% of patients with baclofen experienced one or more adverse reactions compared to 30% with placebo. One RCT found more adverse effects (e.g., dyspepsia and drowsiness) with chlormezanone (14 out of 52 patients) compared with methocarbamol (6 out of 55 patients) [6, 47].

Clinical guidelines T6

The Danish, Dutch, New Zealand guidelines clearly state that muscle relaxants should not be used in the treatment of low back pain, because of the risk of physical and psychological dependency [2, 10, 17]. The German and Swiss guidelines state that muscle relaxants may be an option if muscle spasms play an important role [22, 26, 27]. The US guidelines state that muscle relaxants are an option in the treatment of acute low back pain, but that they have potential side-effects [6]. The UK guidelines recommend considering to add a short course (less than 1 week) if paracetamol, NSAIDs or paracetamol-weak opioid compounds failed to provide adequate pain control [41].

Discussion/consensus T6

The group acknowledges the disagreement that exists among the various guidelines and recommends very limited use of and only a short course of muscle relaxants, if any, due to the high risk of side-effects and the danger of habituation.

Recommendation T7

Epidural steroid injections are not recommended for acute non-specific low back pain (level C).

Evidence T7

Four systematic reviews included two small RCTs on acute low back pain [6, 33, 40, 47, 58]. One trial ($n = 57$, epidural steroids v subcutaneous lidocaine (lignocaine) injections in people with acute pain and sciatica) found no differences after 1 month, but more pain-free patients in the steroid group at 3 months. However, this was not presented for the subgroup of patients with non-specific low back pain. The second trial ($n = 63$, epidural steroids v epidural saline, epidural bupivacaine and dry needling) found no difference in number of patients improved or cured. We found conflicting evidence on the effectiveness of epidural steroids.

Adverse effects: Adverse effects are infrequent and include headache, fever, subdural penetration and more rarely epidural abscess and ventilatory depression [6].

Clinical guidelines T7

The German and US guidelines state that epidural steroid injections are an option for pain relief in patients with radicular symptoms, if previous conservative treatment was not successful [6, 22]. The Danish guidelines do not recommend epidural injections [10]. The other guidelines do not include any recommendations regarding epidural steroids for acute low back pain.

Discussion/consensus T7

General consensus. The group concludes that there is a lack of sufficient evidence on epidural steroid injections for acute non-specific low back pain.

Recommendation T8

Consider (referral for) spinal manipulation for patients who are failing to return to normal activities (level A).

Evidence T8

Five systematic reviews of 37 RCTs (16 RCTs in acute low back pain, 8 RCTs in chronic low back pain, no statistical pooling) were identified [6, 16, 31, 42, 47]. Thirteen RCTs included mixed populations of acute and chronic low back pain.

Five trials ($n = 383$) compared manipulation with placebo therapy and found conflicting results. Two trials found slightly more pain relief with manipulation up to three weeks, and two found no differences in pain relief. One trial found slightly faster recovery in the manipulation group. Twelve RCTs ($n = 899$) compared manipulation with other conservative treatments (e.g., short-wave diathermy, massage, exercises, back school, drug therapy). Three systematic reviews found that these RCTs were conflicting. One systematic review (7 RCTs, $n = 731$, manipulation v other conservative treatments) found that manipulation increased recovery at two to three weeks (NNT = 5*, 95% CI 3.6 to 14.3*) [42].

Adverse effects: Risk of serious complication is low (estimated risk: cauda equina syndrome <1 in 1 000 000) [4]. Current guidelines contraindicate manipulation in people with severe or progressive neurological deficit.

Clinical guidelines T8

Recommendations regarding spinal manipulation for acute low back pain show some variation. In most guidelines spinal manipulation is considered to be a therapeutic option in the first weeks of a low back pain episode. The US, UK, New Zealand and Danish guidelines consider spinal manipulation a useful treatment for acute low back pain [2, 6, 10, 41]. In the Dutch, Australian and Israeli guidelines spinal manipulation is not recommended for acute low back pain, although the Dutch advocate its consideration after 6 weeks [7, 17, 55].

Discussion/consensus T8

We do not know for which subgroup of patients spinal manipulation is most effective. Future studies should focus on identifying these subgroups.

Recommendation T9

We do not recommend back schools for treatment of acute low back pain (level B).

Evidence T9

A systematic review of three RCTs found conflicting evidence that back schools are effective [50].

Two RCTs ($n = 242$) compared back schools with other conservative treatments (McKenzie exercises and physical therapy). They found no difference in pain, recovery rate, and sick leave. One trial ($n = 100$, physical therapy (McKenzie exercises) v back school) found that exercises improved pain and reduced sick leave more than back school up to five years, but the back school in this study consisted of one 45 minute-session while exercises were ongoing. The other trial ($n = 145$) compared back schools with short-wave diathermy at lowest intensity, and found that back schools are better at aiding recovery and reducing sick leave in the short-term.

Adverse effects: Harms have not been reported.

Clinical guidelines T9

The US guidelines state that workplace back schools may be effective in addition to individual education efforts by a clinician [6]. The New Zealand guidelines state that there is insufficient evidence for back schools [2]. The Swiss and German guidelines recommend back schools for secondary prevention of chronicity and recurrences in patients with resolved acute low back pain [22, 26, 27]. The Danish guidelines recommended "modern" back schools (teaching focuses upon ignoring the pain as much as possible) for patients with low back pain if there is a clear need for rehabilitation, or when prevention at the workplace is being considered [10]. The other guidelines do not include recommendations on back schools for treatment of acute low back pain.

Discussion/consensus T9

The recommendations in favour of back schools in some of the national guidelines seem related to treatment of sub-acute low back pain or secondary prevention of chronic low back pain, but not to treatment of acute low back pain.

Recommendation T10

There is insufficient evidence to recommend behavioural therapy for treatment of acute low back pain (level C).

Evidence T10

Five systematic reviews were identified on behavioural therapy for low back pain [6, 16, 44, 47, 53]. There is limited evidence from one RCT ($n = 107$) that found that behavioural treatment reduced pain and perceived disability (at 9 to 12 months) more than traditional care (analgesics and exercise until pain had subsided).

Adverse effects: The trials did not assess harms.

Clinical guidelines T10

None of the international guidelines on acute low back pain included behavioural treatment.

Discussion/consensus T10

A behavioural approach may become more important in treatment of sub-acute low back pain or in the prevention of chronicity and recurrences. However, randomised trials evaluating a behavioural approach in primary care settings are still lacking.

Recommendation T11

Do not use traction (level B).

Evidence T11

Three systematic reviews (16 RCTs in total, no statistical pooling) found conflicting evidence [16, 46, 54].

Two RCTs reported on acute low back pain (total $n = 225$, traction v bed rest + corset, traction

v infrared). One small pilot-study found more overall improvement after one and three weeks, but the subsequent main study found no difference in overall improvement after two weeks.

Adverse effects: Harms were not reported in the RCTs.

Clinical guidelines T11

The UK guidelines state that traction does not appear to be effective for low back pain [41]. The New Zealand guidelines state that bed rest and traction should not be used for acute low back pain [2]. The Danish and US guidelines do not recommend traction [6, 10]. Other guidelines made no explicit statement regarding traction.

Discussion/consensus T11

General consensus.

Recommendation T12

There is insufficient evidence to recommend massage as a treatment for acute non-specific low back pain (level B).

Evidence T12

One systematic review found insufficient evidence to recommend massage as a stand-alone treatment for acute non-specific low back pain [19].

Two low quality RCTs investigated the use of manual massage as a treatment for acute non-specific low back pain. In both studies massage was the control intervention in evaluating spinal manipulation. There is limited evidence showing that massage is less effective than manipulation immediately after the first session. At the completion of treatment and at 3 weeks after discharge there is no difference between massage and manipulation.

Adverse effects: Not reported.

Clinical guidelines T12

The Danish guidelines do not generally recommend massage, but state that it may be considered for pain relief for localised muscle pain or for initial pain relief prior to using, for example, manipulation or exercise therapy [10]. The New Zealand, US and UK guidelines do not recommend massage due to insufficient evidence or due to lack of any effect on clinical outcomes [2, 6, 41]. Other guidelines made no explicit statement regarding massage.

Discussion/consensus T12

General consensus.

Recommendation T13

There is insufficient evidence to recommend transcutaneous electrical nerve stimulation (TENS) (level B).

Evidence T13

Two systematic reviews of two RCTs found insufficient evidence [6, 47].

One study ($n = 58$) compared a rehabilitation program with TENS to the rehabilitation program alone in an occupational setting and found no differences on pain and functional status. The other low quality study ($n = 40$) compared TENS with paracetamol and reported significantly better improvement in the TENS group after 6 weeks regarding pain and mobility.

Adverse effects: Harms were not reported.

Clinical guidelines T13

The US, Swiss and Danish guidelines do not recommend TENS [6, 10, 26, 27]. The New Zealand guidelines state that there is at least moderate evidence of no improvement in clinical outcomes with TENS [2]. The UK guidelines state that there is inconclusive evidence on the efficacy of TENS [41]. Other guidelines made no explicit statement regarding TENS.

Discussion/consensus T13

General consensus.

Recommendation T14

Multidisciplinary treatment programs in occupational settings may be an option for workers with sub-acute low back pain and sick leave for more than 4–8 weeks (level B).

Evidence T14

One systematic review of two RCTs ($n = 233$) found that multidisciplinary treatment leads to faster return to work and less sick leave than usual care [25]. In one study in patients who had been absent from work for 8 weeks the multidisciplinary "graded activity" program consisted of 1) measurement of functional capacity, 2) a workplace visit, 3) back school education, and 4) an individual, sub-maximal, gradually increased exercise program, with an operant-conditioning behavioral approach. In the other study in patients who had been absent from work for more than 4 weeks, the comprehensive multidisciplinary program consisted of a combination of clinical intervention (by a back pain specialist, back school, functional rehabilitation therapy, and therapeutic return to work), and occupational intervention (visit to an occupational physician and participatory ergonomics evaluation conducted by an ergonomist, including a work-site evaluation).

Adverse effects: Harms were not reported.

Clinical guidelines T14

The Finnish guidelines recommend active multidisciplinary rehabilitation after 6 weeks [37]. The Swiss, German and Dutch guidelines recommend multidisciplinary treatment for chronic low back pain only, not for acute or sub-acute low back pain [5, 17, 22, 26, 27]. The Swiss and German guidelines recommend back schools for secondary prevention of chronicity and recurrences in patients with resolved acute low back pain [22, 26, 27]. The Danish guidelines recommended "modern" back schools ("teaching focuses upon ignoring the pain as much as possible") for patients with low back pain if there is a clear need for rehabilitation, or when prevention at the workplace is being considered [10].

Discussion/consensus T14

Evidence from trials is related to multidisciplinary programs, which typically include a variety of interventions, such as exercises, back school education, workplace visit, ergonomic advice and behavioural treatment. It is unclear what the effectiveness of the various components of these programs is.

References

[Brackets indicate country of guidelines]

1. Abenhaim L, Rossignol M, Valat J P, Nordin M, Avouac B, Blotman F, Charlot J, Dreiser R L, Legrand E, Rozenberg S, Vautravers P. The role of activity in the therapeutic management of back pain. Report of the International Paris Task Force on Back Pain. Spine 2000; 25 (Suppl): 1S–33S.

2. ACC and the National Health Committee. New Zealand acute low back pain guide. Wellington, New Zealand, 1997. [New Zealand]

3. Andersson G B J. The epidemiology of spinal disorders. In: Frymoyer J W, ed. The adult spine: principles and practice. 2nd ed. New York: Raven Press, 1997: 93–141.

4. Assendelft W J J, Bouter L M, Knipschild P G. Complications of spinal manipulation: a comprehensive review of the literature. J Fam Pract 1996; 42: 475–80.

5. Bekkering G E, van Tulder M W, Hendriks H J M, Oostendorp R A B, Koes B W, Ostelo R W J G, Thomassen J. Dutch physiotherapy guideline for low back pain. (KNGF richtlijn lage rugpijn.) Ned Tijdschr Fysiother 2001; 111 (Suppl. 3): 1–24. [the Netherlands]

6. Bigos S, Bowyer O, Braen G et al Acute low back problems in adults. Clinical practice guideline no. 14. AHCPR publication no. 95-0642. Rockville, MD: Agency for Health Care Policy and Research, Public Health Service, US Department of Health and Human Services. December 1994. [USA]

7. Borkan J, Reis S, Werner S, Ribak J, Prath A. Guidelines for treating low back pain in primary care (Hebrew; available in English). The Israeli Low Back Pain Guideline Group. Harfuah 1996; 130: 145–151. [Israel]

8. Bronfort G. Spinal manipulation: current state of research and its indications. Neurol Clin 1999; 17: 91–111.

9. Burton A K, Waddell G, Tillotson K M, Summerton N. Information and advice to patients with back pain can have a positive effect. A randomized controlled trial of a novel educational booklet in primary care. Spine 1999; 24: 2484–91.

10. Danish Institute for Health Technology Assessment: Low back pain. Frequency, management and prevention from an HTA perspective. Danish Health Technology Assessment 1999. [Denmark]

11. De Craen A J M, Di Giulio G, Lampe-Schoenmaeckers A J E M, Kessels A G H, Kleijnen J. Analgesic efficacy and safety of paracetamol-codeine combinations vs paracetamol alone: a systematic review. Br Med J 1996; 313: 321–325.

12. Deville W L, van der Windt D A, Dzaferagic A, Bezemer P D, Bouter L M. The test of Lasegue: systematic review of the accuracy in diagnosing herniated discs. Spine 2000; 25: 1140–7.

13. Deyo R A, Rainville J, Kent D L. What can the history and physical examination tell us about low back pain? JAMA 1992; 268: 760–65.

14. Deyo R A, Battie M, Beurskens A J, Bombardier C, Croft P, Koes B, Malmivaara A, Roland M, Von Korff M, Waddell G. Outcome measures for low back pain research. A proposal for standardized use. Spine 1998; 23: 2003–13.

15. Ernst E, White A R. Acupuncture for back pain. A meta-analysis of randomized controlled trials. Arch Intern Med 1998; 158: 2235–41.

16. Evans G, Richards S. Low back pain: an evaluation of therapeutic interventions. Bristol: Health Care Evaluation Unit, University of Bristol, 1996.

17. Faas A, Chavannes A W, Koes B W, Van den Hoogen J M M, Mens J M A, Smeele I J M, Romeijnders A C M, Van der Laan J R. Clinical practice guidelines for low back pain. (Dutch, available in English.) Huisarts Wet 1996; 39: 18–31. [the Netherlands]

18. Frymoyer J W. Back pain and sciatica. N Engl J Med 1988; 318: 291–300.

19. Furlan A D, Brosseau L, Welch V, Wong J. Massage for low back pain (Cochrane Review). In: The Cochrane Library, Issue 4, 2000. Oxford: Update Software.

20. Gam A N, Johannsen F. Ultrasound therapy in musculoskeletal disorders: a meta-analysis. Pain 1995; 63: 85–91.

21. Hagen K B, Hilde G, Jamtvedt G, Winnem M. Bed rest for acute low back pain and sciatica (Cochrane Review). In: The Cochrane Library, Issue 4, 2000. Oxford: Update Software.

22. Handlungsleitlinie – Ruckenschmerzen. Empfehlungen zur Therapie von Rückenschmerzen, Artzneimittelkommission der deutschen Ärzteschaft. (Treatment guideline – backache. Drug Committee of the German Medical Society.) Zeitschrift fur Artzliche Fortbildung und Qualitatssicherung Aug 1997; 91(5): 457–460. [Germany]

23. Henry D, Lim L L Y, Rodriguez L A G et al Variability in risk of gastrointestinal complications with individual non-steroidal anti-inflammatory drugs: results of a collaborative meta-analysis. Br Med J 1996; 312: 1563–1566.

24. Hoogendoorn W E, van Poppel M N M, Bongers P M, Koes B W, Bouter L M. Systemic review of psychosocial factors at work and private life as risk factors for back pain. Spine 2000; 25: 2114–25.

25. Karjalainen K, Malmivaara A, van Tulder M, Roine R, Jauhiainen M, Hurri H, Koes B. Multidisciplinary biopsychosocial rehabilitation for subacute low back

pain among working age adults (Cochrane Review). In: The Cochrane Library, Issue 4, 2000. Oxford: Update Software.

26. Keel P, Perini Ch, Schutz-Petitjean D et al Chronicisation des douleurs du dos: problematique, issues. Rapport final du Programme National de Recherche No 26B. Bale: Editions EULAR 1996. [Switzerland]

27. Keel P, Weber M, Roux E et al Kreuzschmerzen: Hintergründe, Prävention, Behandlung. Basisdokumentation. Verbindung der Schweizer Ärzte (FMH), Bern, 1998. [Switzerland]

28. Kendall N A S, Linton S J, Main C J. Guide to assessing psychosocial yellow flags in acute low back pain: risk factors for long-term disability and work loss. Accident Rehabilitation & Compensation Insurance Corporation of New Zealand and the National Health Committee. Wellington, New Zealand, 1997. [New Zealand]

29. Kent D L, Larson E B. Disease, level of impact, and quality of research methods: three dimensions of clinical efficacy assessment applied to magnetic resonance imaging. Invest Radiol 1992; 27: 245–54.

30. Koes B W, van den Hoogen H M M. Efficacy of bed rest and orthoses of low back pain. A review of randomized clinical trials. Eur J Phys Med Rehabil 1994; 4: 86–93.

31. Koes B W, Assendelft W J J, van der Heijden G J M G, Bouter L M. Spinal manipulation for low back pain. An updated systematic review of randomized clinical trials. Spine 1996; 21: 2860–71.

32. Koes B W, Scholten R J P M, Mens J M A, Bouter L M. Efficacy of non-steroidal anti-inflammatory drugs for low back pain: a systematic review of randomised clinical trials. Ann Rheum Dis 1997; 56: 214–23.

33. Koes B W, Scholten R J P M, Mens J M A, Bouter L M. Epidural steroid injections for low back pain and sciatica: an updated systematic review of randomized clinical trials. Pain Digest 1999; 9: 241–47.

34. Lindstrom I, Ohlund C, Eek C, Wallin L, Peterson L E, Fordyce W E, Nachemson A L. The effect of graded activity on patients with subacute low back pain: a randomized prospective clinical study with an operant-conditioning behavioral approach. Phys Ther 1992; 72: 279–90.

35. Linton S J, Hallden K. Can we screen for problematic back pain? A screening questionnaire for predicting outcome in acute and subacute back pain. Clin J Pain 1998; 14: 209–15.

36. Linton S J. A review of psychological risk factors in back and neck pain. Spine 2000; 25: 1148–56.

37. Malmivaara A, Kotilainen E, Laasonen E, Poussa M, Rasmussen M. Clinical practice guidelines: diseases of the low back. (Finnish, available in English.) The Finnish Medical Association Duodecim 1999. [Finland]

38. Nachemson A, Vingard E. Assessment of patients with neck and back pain: a best-evidence synthesis. In: Nachemson A, Jonsson E, eds. Neck and back pain: the scientific evidence of causes, diagnosis, and treatment. Lippincott, Williams & Wilkins, Philadelphia 2000.

39. Nachemson A L, Jonsson E (Eds.) Neck and back pain: the scientific evidence of causes, diagnosis, and

treatment. Lippincott, Williams & Wilkins, Philadelphia, 2000. [Sweden]

40. Nelemans P J, de Bie R A, de Vet H C W, Sturmans F. Injection therapy for subacute and chronic benign low back pain. In: The Cochrane Library, Issue 4, 2001. Oxford: Update Software.

41. Royal College of General Practitioners. Clinical guidelines for the management of acute low back pain. London, Royal College of General Practitioners, 1996 and 1999. [UK]

42. Shekelle P G, Adams A H, Chassin M R, Hurwitz E L, Brook R H. Spinal manipulation for low back pain. Ann Intern Med 1992; 117: 590–8.

43. Turner J A, Denny M C. Do antidepressant medications relieve chronic low back pain? J Fam Pract 1993b; 37: 545–53.

44. Turner J A. Educational and behavioral interventions for back pain in primary care. Spine 1996; 21: 2851–9.

45. Van den Hoogen H M M, Koes B W, van Eijk J Th M, Bouter L M. On the accuracy of history, physical examination and erythrocyte sedimentation rate in diagnosing low back pain in general practice. A criteria-based review of the literature. Spine 1995; 20: 318–27.

46. Van der Heijden G J M G, Beurskens A J H M, Koes B W, de Vet H C W, Bouter L M. The efficacy of traction for back and neck pain: a systematic, blinded review of randomized clinical trial methods. Phys Ther 1996; 75: 93–103.

47. Van Tulder M W, Koes B W, Bouter L M. Conservative treatment of acute and chronic nonspecific low back pain: a systematic review of randomized controlled trials of the most common interventions. Spine 1997; 22: 2128–56.

48. Van Tulder M W, Assendelft W J J, Koes B W, Bouter L M. Spinal radiographic findings and nonspecific low back pain: a systematic review of observational studies. Spine 1997; 22: 427–34.

49. Van Tulder M W, Cherkin D C, Berman B, Lao L, Koes B W. The effectiveness of acupuncture in the treatment of low back pain (Cochrane Review). In: The Cochrane Library, Issue 4, 2000. Oxford: Update Software.

50. Van Tulder M W, Esmail R, Bombardier C, Koes B W. Back schools for non-specific low back pain (Cochrane Review). In: The Cochrane Library, Issue 4, 2000. Oxford: Update Software.

51. Van Tulder M W, Scholten R J P M, Koes B W, Deyo R A. Non-steroidal anti-inflammatory drugs (NSAIDs) for non-specific low back pain (Cochrane Review). In: The Cochrane Library, Issue 4, 2000. Oxford: Update Software.

52. Van Tulder M W, Malmivaara A, Esmail R, Koes B W. Exercise therapy for non-specific low back pain (Cochrane Review). In: The Cochrane Library, Issue 4, 2000. Oxford: Update Software.

53. Van Tulder M W, Ostelo R W J G, Vlaeyen J W S, Linton S J, Morley S J, Assendelft W J J. Behavioural treatment for chronic low back pain (Cochrane Review). In: The Cochrane Library, Issue 4, 2000. Oxford: Update Software.

54. Van Tulder M W, Jellema P, van Poppel M N M, Nachemson A L, Bouter L M. Lumbar supports for prevention and treatment of low back pain (Cochrane Review). In: The Cochrane Library, Issue 4, 2000. Oxford: Update Software.

55. Victorian Workcover Authority. Guidelines for the management of employees with compensable low back pain. Melbourne, Victorian Workcover Authority. 1993 and revised edition 1996. [Australia]

56. Waddell G, Feder G, Lewis M. Systematic reviews of bed rest and advice to stay active for acute low back pain. Br J Gen Pract 1997; 47: 647–52.

57. Waddell G, Feder G, McIntosh A, Lewis M, Hutchinson A. Low back pain evidence review. London: Royal College of General Practitioners, 1996. [UK]

58. Watts R W, Silagy C A. A meta-analysis on the efficacy of epidural corticosteroids in the treatment of sciatica. Anaesth Intensive Care 1995; 23: 564–9.

APPENDIX 15E: NEW ZEALAND *GUIDE TO ASSESSING PSYCHOSOCIAL YELLOW FLAGS IN ACUTE LOW BACK PAIN*

From Kendall et al (1997) with permission.

WHAT THIS GUIDE AIMS TO DO

This guide complements the *New Zealand Acute Low Back Pain Guide* and is intended for use in conjunction with it. This guide describes "yellow flags" – psychosocial factors that are likely to increase the risk of an individual with acute low back pain developing prolonged pain and disability causing work loss, and associated loss of quality of life. It aims to:

- provide a method of screening for psychosocial factors
- provide a systematic approach to assessing psychosocial factors
- suggest strategies for better management of those with acute low back pain who have "yellow flags" indicating increased risks of chronicity.

This guide is not intended to be a rigid prescription and will permit flexibility and choice, allowing the exercise of good clinical judgement according to the particular circumstances of the patient. The management suggestions outlined in this document are based on the best available evidence to date.

WHAT ARE PSYCHOSOCIAL YELLOW FLAGS?

"Yellow flags" are factors that increase the risk of developing, or perpetuating long-term disability and work loss associated with low back pain.

Psychosocial "yellow flags" are similar to the "red flags".

Yellow and red flags can be thought of in this way:

- yellow flags = psychosocial risk factors
- red flags = physical risk factors.

Identification of risk factors should lead to appropriate intervention. Red flags should lead to appropriate medical intervention; yellow flags to appropriate cognitive and behavioural management.

The significance of a particular factor is relative. Immediate notice should be taken if an important red flag is present, and consideration given to an appropriate response. The same is true for the yellow flags.

Assessing the presence of yellow flags should produce two key outcomes:

- a decision as to whether more detailed assessment is needed
- identification of any salient factors that can become the subject of specific intervention, thus saving time and helping to concentrate the use of resources.

Red and yellow flags are not mutually exclusive – an individual patient may require intervention in both areas concurrently.

WHY IS THERE A NEED FOR PSYCHOSOCIAL YELLOW FLAGS FOR BACK PAIN PROBLEMS?

Low back pain problems, especially when they are long-term or chronic, are common in our society and produce extensive human suffering. New Zealand has experienced a steady rise in the number of people who leave the work force with back pain. It is of concern that there is an increased proportion who do not recover normal function and activity for longer and longer periods.

The research literature on risk factors for long-term work disability is inconsistent or lacking for many chronic painful conditions, except low back pain, which has received a great deal of attention and empirical research over the last 5 years. Most of the known risk factors are psychosocial, which implies the possibility of appropriate intervention, especially where specific individuals are recognised as being "at risk".

Who is "at risk"?

An individual may be considered "at risk" if they have a clinical presentation that includes one or more very strong indicators of risk, or several less important factors that might be cumulative.

Definitions of primary, secondary and tertiary prevention

It has been concluded that efforts at every stage can be made towards prevention of long-term

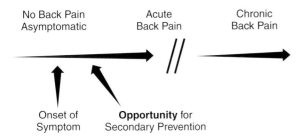

Figure 15E.1   Secondary prevention.

disability associated with low back pain, including work loss.

Primary prevention: elimination or minimisation of risks to health or well-being. It is an attempt to determine factors that cause disabling low back disability and then create programmes to prevent these situations from ever occurring.

Secondary prevention: alleviation of the symptoms of ill health or injury, minimising residual disability and eliminating, or at least minimising, factors that may cause recurrence (Figure 15E.1). It is an attempt to maximise recovery once the condition has occurred and then prevent its recurrence. Secondary prevention emphasises the prevention of excess pain behaviour, the sick role, inactivity syndromes, re-injury, recurrences, complications, psychosocial sequelae, long-term disability and work loss.

Tertiary prevention: rehabilitation of those with disabilities to as full function as possible and modification of the workplace to accommodate any residual disability. It is applied after the patient has become disabled. The goal is to return to function and patient acceptance of residual impairment(s); this may in some instances require work site modification.

The focus of this guide is on secondary prevention, which aims to prevent:

- excess pain behaviour, sick role, inactivity syndromes
- re-injury, recurrences
- complications, psychosocial sequelae, long-term disability, work loss.

DEFINITIONS

Before proceeding to assess yellow flags, treatment providers need to carefully differentiate between the presentations of acute, recurrent and chronic back pain, since the risk factors for developing long-term problems may differ even though there is considerable overlap.

Acute low back problems: activity intolerance due to lower back or back and leg symptoms lasting less than 3 months.

Recurrent low back problems: episodes of acute low back problems lasting less than 3 months but recurring after a period of time without low back symptoms sufficient to restrict activity or function.

Chronic low back problems: activity intolerance due to lower back or back and leg symptoms lasting more than 3 months.

GOALS OF ASSESSING PSYCHOSOCIAL YELLOW FLAGS

The three main consequences of back problems are:

- pain
- disability, limitation in function including activities of daily living
- reduced productive activity, including work loss.

Pain

Attempts to prevent the development of chronic pain through physiological or pharmacological interventions in the acute phase have been relatively ineffective. Research to date can be summarised by stating that inadequate control of acute (nociceptive) pain *may* increase the risk of chronic pain.

Disability

Preventing loss of function, reduced activity, distress and low mood is an important, yet distinct goal. These factors are critical to a person's quality of life and general well-being. It has been repeatedly demonstrated that these factors can be modified in patients with chronic back pain. It is therefore strongly suggested that treatment providers must prevent any tendency for significant withdrawal from activity being established in any acute episode.

Work loss

The probability of successfully returning to work in the early stages of an acute episode depends on the quality of management, as described in this guide. If the episode goes on longer, the probability of returning to work reduces. The likelihood of return to any work is even smaller if the person loses their employment, and has to re-enter the job market.

Prevention

Long-term disability and work loss are associated with profound suffering and negative effects on patients, their families and society. Once established they are difficult to undo. Current evidence indicates that to be effective, preventive strategies must be initiated at a much *earlier* stage than was previously thought. Enabling people to keep active in order to maintain work skills and relationships is an important outcome.

Most of the known risk factors for long-term disability, inactivity and work loss are psychosocial. Therefore, the key goal is to identify yellow flags that increase the risk of these problems developing. Health professionals can subsequently *target* effective early management to prevent onset of these problems.

Please note that it is important to avoid pejorative labelling of patients with yellow flags as this will have a negative impact on management. Their use is intended to encourage treatment providers to *prevent* the onset of long-term problems in "at risk" patients by interventions appropriate to the underlying cause.

HOW TO JUDGE IF A PERSON IS "AT RISK"

A person may be at risk if:

- there is a cluster of a few very salient factors
- there is a group of several less important factors that combine cumulatively.

There is good agreement that the following factors are important and consistently predict poor outcomes:

- presence of a belief that back pain is harmful or potentially severely disabling

- fear-avoidance behaviour (avoiding a movement or activity due to misplaced anticipation of pain) and reduced activity levels
- tendency to low mood and withdrawal from social interaction
- an expectation that passive treatments rather than active participation will help.

Suggested questions (to be phrased in treatment provider's own words):

- Have you had time off work in the past with back pain?
- What do you understand is the cause of your back pain?
- What are you expecting will help you?
- How is your employer responding to your back pain? Your co-workers? Your family?
- What are you doing to cope with back pain?
- Do you think that you will return to work? When?

HOW TO ASSESS PSYCHOSOCIAL YELLOW FLAGS

- If large numbers need to be screened quickly there is little choice but to use a questionnaire. Problems may arise with managing the potentially large number of "at risk" people identified. It is necessary to minimise the number of false positives (those the screening test identifies who are not actually at risk).
- If the goal is the most accurate identification of yellow flags prior to intervention, clinical assessment is preferred. Suitably skilled clinicians with adequate time must be available.
- The two-stage approach shown in Figure 15E.2 is recommended if the numbers are large and skilled assessment staff are in short supply. The questionnaire can be used to screen for those needing further assessment (Box 7.4, Ch. 7). In this instance, the number of false negatives (those who have risk factors, but are missed by the screening test) must be minimised.
- To use the screening questionnaire (Box 7.5, Ch. 7).
- To conduct a clinical assessment for acute back pain (Box 15E.1).

Clinical assessment of yellow flags involves judgements about the relative importance of factors for

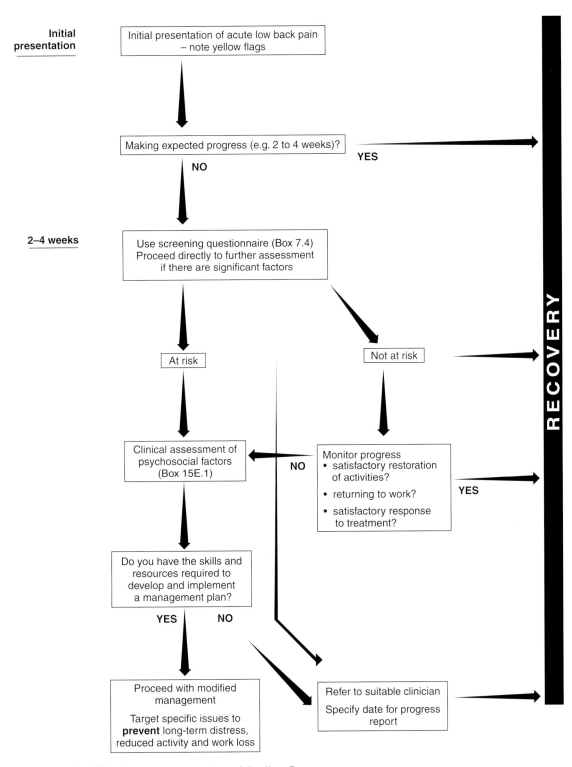

Figure 15E.2 Deciding how to assess psychosocial yellow flags.

Box 15E.1   Clinical assessment of psychosocial yellow flags

Attitudes and beliefs about back pain

- Belief that pain is harmful or disabling resulting in fear-avoidance behaviour, e.g. the development of guarding and fear of movement
- Belief that all pain must be abolished before attempting to return to work or normal activity
- Expectation of increased pain with activity or work, lack of ability to predict capability
- Catastrophising, thinking the worst, misinterpreting bodily symptoms
- Belief that pain is uncontrollable
- Passive attitude to rehabilitation

Behaviours

- Use of extended rest, disproportionate "downtime"
- Reduced activity level with significant withdrawal from activities of daily living
- Irregular participation or poor compliance with physical exercise, tendency for activities to be in a "boom–bust" cycle
- Avoidance of normal activity and progressive substitution of lifestyle away from productive activity
- Report of extremely high intensity of pain, e.g. above 10, on a 0–10 Visual Analogue Scale
- Excessive reliance on use of aids or appliances
- Sleep quality reduced since onset of back pain
- High intake of alcohol or other substances (possibly as self-medication), with an increase since onset of back pain
- Smoking

Compensation issues

- Lack of financial incentive to return to work
- Delay in accessing income support and treatment cost, disputes over eligibility
- History of claim(s) due to other injuries or pain problems
- History of extended time off work due to injury or other pain problem (e.g. more than 12 weeks)
- History of previous back pain, with a previous claim(s) and time off work
- Previous experience of ineffective case management (e.g. absence of interest, perception of being treated punitively)

Diagnosis and treatment

- Health professional sanctioning disability, not providing interventions that will improve function
- Experience of conflicting diagnoses or explanations for back pain, resulting in confusion
- Diagnostic language leading to catastrophising and fear (e.g. fear of ending up in a wheelchair)
- Dramatisation of back pain by health professional producing dependency on treatments, and continuation of passive treatment
- Number of times visited health professional in last year (excluding the present episode of back pain)
- Expectation of a "techno-fix", e.g. requests to treat as if body were a machine
- Lack of satisfaction with previous treatment for back pain
- Advice to withdraw from job

Emotions

- Fear of increased pain with activity or work
- Depression (especially long-term low mood), loss of sense of enjoyment
- More irritable than usual
- Anxiety about and heightened awareness of body sensations (includes sympathetic nervous system arousal)
- Feeling under stress and unable to maintain sense of control
- Presence of social anxiety or disinterested in social activity
- Feeling useless and not needed

Family

- Over-protective partner/spouse, emphasising fear of harm or encouraging catastrophising (usually well-intentioned)
- Solicitous behaviour from spouse (e.g. taking over tasks)
- Socially punitive responses from spouse (e.g. ignoring, expressing frustration)
- Extent to which family members support any attempt to return to work
- Lack of support person to talk to about problems

(Continued)

Box 15E.1   (Continued)

Work
- History of manual work, notably from the following occupational groups
  - fishing, forestry and farming workers
  - construction, including carpenters and builders
  - nurses
  - truck drivers
  - labourers
- Work history, including patterns of frequent job changes, experiencing stress at work, job dissatisfaction, poor relationships with peers or supervisors, lack of vocational direction
- Belief that work is harmful; that it will do damage or be dangerous
- Unsupportive or unhappy current work environment
- Low educational background, low socioeconomic status
- Job involves significant biomechanical demands, such as lifting, manual handling heavy items,

extended sitting, extended standing, driving, vibration, maintenance of constrained or sustained postures, inflexible work schedule preventing appropriate breaks
- Job involves shift work or working "unsociable hours"
- Minimal availability of selected duties and graduated return to work pathways, with unsatisfactory implementation of these
- Negative experience of workplace management of back pain (e.g. absence of a reporting system, discouragement to report, punitive response from supervisors and managers)
- Absence of interest from employer

Remember the key question to bear in mind while conducting these clinical assessments is *"What can be done to help this person experience less distress and disability?"*

the individual. Box 15E.1 lists factors under the headings of "attitudes and beliefs about back pain", "behaviours", "compensation issues", "diagnosis and treatment", "emotions", "family" and "work".

These headings have been used for convenience in an attempt to make the job easier. They are presented in alphabetical order since it is not possible to rank their importance. However, within each category the factors are listed with *the most important at the top*.

Please note, clinical assessment may be supplemented with the questionnaire method (i.e. the acute low back pain screening questionnaire – Box 7.4, Ch. 7) if that has not already been done. In addition, treatment providers familiar with the administration and interpretation of other pain-specific psychometric measures and assessment tools (such as the pain drawing, the multidimensional pain inventory, etc.) may choose to employ them. Become familiar with the potential disadvantages of each method to minimise any potential adverse effects.

The list of factors provided here is not exhaustive and for a particular individual the order of

importance may vary. *A word of caution*: some factors may appear to be mutually exclusive, but are not in fact. For example, partners can alternate from being socially punitive (ignoring the problem or expressing frustration about it) to being over-protective in a well intentioned way (and inadvertently encouraging extended rest and withdrawal from activity, or excessive treatment seeking). In other words, both factors may be pertinent.

WHAT CAN BE DONE TO HELP SOMEBODY WHO IS "AT RISK"?

These suggestions are not intended to be prescriptions, or encouragement to ignore individual needs. They are intended to assist in the prevention of long-term disability and work loss.

Suggested steps to better early behavioural management of low back pain problems

1. Provide a *positive expectation* that the individual will return to work and normal activity. Organise for a regular expression of interest from the

employer. If the problem persists beyond 2 to 4 weeks, provide a "reality based" warning of what is going to be the likely outcome (e.g. loss of job, having to start from square one, the need to begin reactivation from a point of reduced fitness, etc.).

2. Be directive in scheduling *regular reviews of progress*. When conducting these reviews shift the focus from the symptom (pain) to function (level of activity). Instead of asking "how much do you hurt?", ask "what have you been doing?" Maintain an interest in improvements, no matter how small. If another health professional is involved in treatment or management, specify a date for a progress report at the time of referral. Delays will be disabling.

3. *Keep the individual active and at work* if at all possible, even for a small part of the day. This will help to maintain work habits and work relationships. Consider reasonable requests for selected duties and modifications to the work place. After 4 to 6 weeks, if there has been little improvement, review vocational options, job satisfaction, any barriers to return to work, including psychosocial distress. Once barriers to return to work have been identified, these need to be targeted and managed appropriately. Job dissatisfaction and distress cannot be treated with a physical modality.

4. *Acknowledge difficulties* with activities of daily living, but avoid making the assumption that these indicate all activity or any work must be avoided.

5. Help to *maintain positive cooperation* between the individual, an employer, the compensation system and health professionals. Encourage collaboration wherever possible. Inadvertent support for a collusion between "them" and "us" can be damaging to progress.

6. *Make a concerted effort to communicate that having more time off work will reduce the likelihood of a successful return to work*. In fact, longer periods off work result in reduced probability of ever returning to work. At the 6 week point *consider suggesting vocational redirection, job changes*, the use of "knight's move" approaches to return to work (same employer, different job).

7. Be alert for the presence of individual beliefs that he/she should stay off work until treatment

has provided a "total cure"; watch out for expectations of *simple "techno-fixes"*.

8. Promote *self-management and self-responsibility*. Encourage the development of self-efficacy to return to work. Be aware that developing self-efficacy will depend on *incentives and feedback* from treatment providers and others. If recovery only requires development of a skill such as adopting a new posture, then it is not likely to be affected by incentives and feedback. However, if recovery requires the need to overcome an aversive stimulus such as fear of movement (kinesiophobia) then it will be readily affected by incentives and feedback.

9. Be prepared to ask for a second opinion, provided it does not result in a long and disabling delay. Use this option especially if it may help clarify that further diagnostic work-up is unnecessary. *Be prepared to say "I don't know"* rather than provide elaborate explanations based on speculation.

10. Avoid confusing the *report of symptoms* with the presence of emotional distress. Distressed people seek more help, and have been shown to be more likely to receive ongoing medical intervention. Exclusive focus on symptom control is not likely to be successful if emotional distress is not dealt with.

11. *Avoid suggesting* (even inadvertently) that the person from a regular job may be able to *work at home*, or in their own business because it will be under their own control. This message, in effect, is to allow pain to become the reinforcer for activity – producing a deactivation syndrome with all the negative consequences. Self-employment nearly always involves more hard work.

12. Encourage people to recognise, from the earliest point, that *pain can be controlled and managed* so that a normal, active or working life can be maintained. Provide *encouragement for all "well" behaviours* – including alternative ways of performing tasks, and focusing on transferable skills.

13. If barriers to return to work are identified and the problem is too complex to manage, referral to a multidisciplinary team is recommended.

WHAT ARE THE CONSEQUENCES OF MISSING PSYCHOSOCIAL YELLOW FLAGS?

Under-identifying "at risk" patients may result in inadvertently reinforcing factors that are disabling. Failure to note that specific patients strongly believe that movement will be harmful may result in them experiencing the negative effects of extended inactivity. These include withdrawal from social, vocational and recreational activities.

Cognitive and behavioural factors can produce important physiological consequences, the most common of which is muscle wasting.

Since the number of earlier treatments and length of the problem can themselves become risk factors, most people *should* be identified the second time they seek care. Consistently missing the presence of yellow flags can be harmful and usually contributes to the development of chronicity.

There may be significant adverse consequences if these factors are overlooked.

WHAT ARE THE CONSEQUENCES OF OVER–IDENTIFYING PSYCHOSOCIAL YELLOW FLAGS?

Over-identification has the potential to waste some resources. However, this is readily outweighed by the large benefit from helping to prevent even one person developing a long-term chronic back problem.

Some treatment providers may wonder if identifying psychosocial risk factors, and subsequently applying suitable cognitive and behavioural management can produce adverse effects. Certainly if the presence of psychosocial risk factors is misinterpreted to mean that the problem should be translated from a physical to a psychological one, there is a danger of the patient losing confidence in themselves and their treatment provider(s).

There are unlikely to be adverse consequences from the over-identification of yellow flags.

The presence of risk factors should alert the treatment provider to the possibility of long-term problems and the need to *prevent* their development. Specialised psychological referrals should only be required for those with psychopathology (such as depression, anxiety, substance abuse, etc), or for those who fail to respond to appropriate management.

QUICK REFERENCE GUIDE TO ASSESSING PSYCHOSOCIAL YELLOW FLAGS IN ACUTE LOW BACK PAIN

Differentiate acute, recurrent and chronic low back pain

Acute low back problems: activity intolerance due to lower back or back and leg symptoms lasting less than 3 months.

Chronic low back problems: activity intolerance due to lower back or back and leg symptoms lasting more than 3 months.

Recurrent low back problems: episodes of acute low back problems lasting less than 3 months' duration but recurring after a period of time without low back symptoms sufficient to restrict activity or function.

Key goal

To identify risk factors that increase the probability of long-term disability and work loss with the associated suffering and negative effects on patients, their families and society. This assessment can be used to target effective early management and prevent the onset of these problems.

The acute pain screening questionnaire

Useful for quickly screening large numbers. Interpret the results in conjunction with the history and clinical presentation. Be aware of, and take into account, reading difficulties and different cultural backgrounds.

Clinical assessment

There is good agreement that the following factors are important, and consistently predict poor outcomes:

- presence of a belief that back pain is harmful or potentially severely disabling
- fear-avoidance behaviour and reduced activity levels
- tendency to low mood and withdrawal from social interaction
- an expectation of passive treatment(s) rather than a belief that active participation will help.

Suggested questions (to be phrased in your own style)

- Have you had time off in the past with back pain?
- What do you understand is the cause of your back pain?
- What are you expecting will help you?
- How is your employer responding to your back pain? Your co-workers? Your family?
- What are you doing to cope with back pain?
- Do you think that you will return to work? When?

Chapter **16**

Information and advice for patients

Gordon Waddell   Kim Burton

Patients with back pain want information and advice about their problem. Indeed, once we exclude serious disease, that may be their main need. Deyo & Diehl (1986) showed that good communication and explanation lead to greater patient satisfaction with care.

All clinical guidelines recommend that we should give adequate information and reassure the patient. "There is no sign of anything serious and you should expect rapid recovery." The Swiss guidelines add that reassurance depends on providing *adequate* information. It can be hard to get the message right. For example, simply saying that "I can't find anything wrong" may imply that you are not sure and make patients worry more! The European guidelines (www.backpaineurope.org) suggest that reassurance depends on:

- acknowledging that the patient's pain is real
- providing empathy and support
- providing as much explanation as patients need, in terms they can understand
- providing positive messages; avoiding negative messages.

They recommend that the core items of adequate information should be:

- There is no underlying serious pathology.
- You do not need X-rays or other special investigations.
- The prognosis is good.
- You can stay active and get on with your life, despite the pain.

POSITIVE MESSAGES: "THE GOOD NEWS"

We have seen (Ch. 11) that patients get information from many sources, but health professionals are the most authoritative and potentially one of the most important. However, we must always remember that our impact can be positive or negative. We need to think carefully about what we say to patients and how we say it.

Certain key issues need further consideration.

Diagnostic labels

What's in a name? Labels are important (Cedraschi et al 1998, Bogduk 2000, Hamonet et al 2000). Diagnosis is "the process of determining the nature of a disorder." A good label shows that the doctor is taking the patient seriously and accepts the complaints are real. But names are also a kind of shorthand that encapsulate a set of ideas and beliefs. So the diagnoses we attach to back pain help to determine how we think about it and what we do about it. That is true for patients, for health professionals, and for society.

The dynasty of the disk was built on the diagnosis of "disk injury." It was so popular because the idea is so simple. "Arthritis," "degenerative disk disease," and "wear and tear" are equally seductive. These labels offer a simple, mechanical explanation that patients can understand. They can even see it on their own X-ray or scan, so that proves it! These beliefs may then become fixed and difficult to change. The fact that these diagnoses are irrelevant in most patients with non-specific back pain is a minor inconvenience. More important, they carry very negative messages (Abenhaim et al 1995, Deyo & Phillips 1996, Hamonet et al 2000) about permanent damage, fear of reinjury, and the need to rest or get fixed. They create beliefs and expectations about treatment that can be quite unrealistic. So the very diagnosis may become an obstacle to recovery.

We need an equally simple, plausible, and acceptable diagnosis that fits modern understanding of back pain and supports modern ideas of management. It should carry the messages that this is ordinary backache, it is not any serious disease, the outlook is good, and it is not disabling. We want a name that is medically accurate, but at the same time understandable and satisfactory to

patients. It must "legitimize" their pain (Borkan et al 1995, Stone et al 2002).

Non-specific or idiopathic low back pain are probably most honest and accurate. They certainly serve to remind health professionals of the limits to our knowledge. But they are really only diagnoses of exclusion. And these terms are meaningless and unsatisfactory to patients. Deyo & Phillips (1996) described it as "uncomplicated back pain" but that is not really much better. It only gives the negative side, and does not carry any positive messages. It is also somehow just a lay description rather than a medical diagnosis. We previously called it "simple" backache to reassure patients there was no damage to the nerves or any more serious spinal pathology. However, some critics felt that was too dismissive. They argued that it failed to acknowledge that backache can be very painful and disabling, and is not always "simple" to treat. In this edition we have described it as "ordinary backache" or "the kind of back pain that everyone gets." We mean that to include both everyday aches and pains and acute attacks or spells. Patients seem to understand that. Others have described it as "common" back pain.

We may try to dodge these difficulties by talking about "sprains and strains." This sounds medical. We mean, rather vaguely, that it is a simple soft-tissue problem and there is no serious damage. We realize that we cannot identify any precise anatomic damage, but we really do not face up to the common lack of evidence of any injury. If we redefine "strain" in terms of dysfunction (Ch. 9) this may be reasonably accurate. However, to our patients it still carries messages about injury and fear of reinjury.

Perhaps the old term lumbago met the need best. It was medically accurate, if only because of its lack of precision. It offered a respectable medical label, even if it really only translated as pain in the lower back. Everyone found it satisfactory and thought they knew what it meant, even if they all understood it differently and not always accurately. We need a modern equivalent of lumbago.

Our patients seem to accept the term "muscular" back pain. We agree there is rarely evidence of muscular *injury*, but musculoskeletal dysfunction appears the most likely explanation of non-specific back pain (Ch. 9). So "muscular" back pain may be reasonably accurate, even if it is an oversimplification. For those who wish a more technical term, we may use musculoskeletal dysfunction. For those who wish more detail, we may launch into the description of the cause and mechanism of back pain. This certainly carries the messages we want. It means there is no serious disease or damage, and reassures that this is a common problem that should resolve. It side-steps the question of injury. It is simple and understandable. It leads nicely into management by getting active and restoring function.

Stone et al (2002) provided support for this approach from a neurology clinic in Edinburgh. They asked patients how they understood various explanations for leg weakness with negative tests. These patients rejected labels that sounded "psychological." One of the most acceptable was "functional weakness." Doctors and therapists often use functional as a code-word for psychological or psychosomatic problems, but patients do not understand it that way. Patients do seem to understand the idea of disturbed function and dysfunction. The "number needed to offend" in this study was nine: eight out of nine patients found "functional" an acceptable label.

Along with red and yellow flags, perhaps we also need a "green flag" to reassure patients that it is safe to resume normal activities. Or perhaps we already have it. Nothing could convey the message more dramatically than the complete reversal of how we manage back pain. Traditional rest, bed rest, and even hospitalization carried very negative messages about a serious, disabling condition. Advice to stay active and continue ordinary activities as normally as possible because that is the way to get better, faster, carries a very different set of messages about the problem.

"The challenge remains to find a new term: one that is palatable to doctors, satisfying to patients, and which not only means there is nothing seriously wrong, but also conveys the message that the patient has no grounds for fear, and can expect recovery with straightforward, even minimal, management" (Bogduk 2000). That is still true today. We do not have a good, agreed label for back pain.

Moreover, words and usage vary in different places and settings. At the end of the day, you must use clinical judgment. You need an explanation that you are comfortable with and can deliver

with confidence. You must judge what your patients understand and accept, and adapt the message to suit each patient. But it should probably follow the above principles.

The cause of non-specific back pain

Patients want to understand their back pain, because that forms the basis for how they deal with it. This is more than just a diagnosis. Modern patients want to know something about the cause(s) and mechanism(s).

- What is causing my pain?
- Why is it not getting better? (Or, what is prolonging my pain?)
- (And the implication is – What can I do about it?)

Once again, we need an explanation that is simple, plausible, and acceptable to patients. It should fit modern understanding of the physical basis of back pain, and support modern ideas of management. We have already considered this in Chapter 9, the physical basis of back pain.

An explanation for patients

1. Back pain is a physical problem. (If required: psychosocial factors may influence how we react to pain and how it affects us, but they do not cause the pain. Back pain is *not* a psychological problem.) Back pain starts with a physical problem in the back. (This reinforces that you accept the pain is "real.")

2. Back pain is a mechanical problem. It is a movement disorder or an activity-related disorder of the musculoskeletal system. (This is the first step to explaining the problem. It is a disturbance of function rather than structural damage or disease. It generally affects the back as a whole rather than one anatomic site.)

3. Back pain is a common bodily symptom, like headache. We all get back aches and pains, and most of us get some more acute attacks or spells at some time in our lives. Back pain is not a disease. Most back pain is not a signal of any serious disease or damage to the back. (Further reassurance that there is nothing serious.)

4. Most back pain is simply a symptom of physical dysfunction or malfunction. Pain and (dys)function are intimately related to each other. Your back is "not working properly" or as it should. It is "out of condition," like a car engine that is out of tune. Your posture may be poor. (This does not imply that poor posture is the cause of back pain; pain may cause poor posture.) Your back is not moving as it should, but may be stiff or "seized up." Your muscles are not working as they should, but may be weak and wasted and tire easily. There may be loss of strength and endurance and coordination. This leads to fear and guarded movements. The small joints and other working parts "seize up." Changes in the nervous system and psychological changes can lead to increased sensitivity to pain. Loss of fitness makes it harder to rehabilitate. This all leads to a vicious circle. The whole pattern of painful dysfunction is the core of the problem and becomes self-perpetuating. It is much more important than any original, long-gone, trigger for the pain. (This is the core of the explanation. It explains why the pain does not get better.)

5. This has obvious implications for management. The original cause or site of the pain really does not matter much any more. Whatever the original trigger, pain will continue as long as there is dysfunction. Recovery and relief of pain depend on getting your back working again and restoring normal function. The answer is to get moving and get fit again. This leads to a sports medicine analogy, and sports medicine principles of rehabilitation. It also depends very much on you taking responsibility for what you do, rather than depending on a doctor or therapist to "fix it." (The practical implications.)

You may also use the examples and analogies in Chapter 9.

The outlook is good

Von Korff (1999) asked primary care patients in a US health maintenance organization about their goals when they saw the doctor. He found that patients wanted to understand:

- the likely course of their back pain and associated activity limitations
- how to manage their back pain
- how to return to usual activities quickly
- how to minimize the frequency and severity of recurrences.

Patients ranked these concerns even higher than seeking a cause for their back pain or a diagnosis.

Here, we need to strike a balance between honesty and optimism. The harsh reality is that back pain is often a recurrent or fluctuating problem over long periods of our lives (Ch. 5). And there is no magic answer. It is dishonest to pretend anything else, and false reassurance may come back to haunt you.

But the epidemiology is not all doom and gloom. We should present its bright side. Back pain is very common, and most people manage to cope with it pretty well most of the time. Most acute attacks settle quite quickly, at least enough to get back to most ordinary activities and get on with your life. The risk of chronic, intractable pain and long-term incapacity is very low: a few percent. So *your* odds are very good. Even if there is no magic cure, there are a lot of treatments that can help to relieve or control the pain. And there is a lot you can do to help yourself. So even if you might continue to have some back pain at times, the good news is that you should be able to deal with it, with a little bit of help when you need it.

EDUCATIONAL MATERIAL

One-to-one communication between doctor or therapist and patient is the most important method of providing information and advice. However, we can supplement this with printed material. Leaflets and booklets on their own have a limited effect. They are simply an aid to reinforce information and advice from the doctor and therapist. The message is more likely to get through if patients get consistent information and advice from all members of the health care team. Any educational material must reinforce that.

There is a profusion of material for patients with back pain: hundreds of leaflets and pamphlets and booklets, and dozens of books. And there is now an enormous range of websites (Li et al 2001, Butler & Foster 2003). Potentially, this could play a useful role in helping patients to learn about their condition and how best they can manage it. Unfortunately, the content is of very variable quality. It often comes from vested interests, which are not always obvious. A lot of it is blatant or disguised advertising. Even professional society sites are often promotional. Much of the information and advice is not evidence-based and does not conform to current guidelines. Some of it is downright wrong and harmful – for example, about bed rest and exercise. You may wish to search the internet yourself to see what is currently available. The National Institutes of Health (NIH) guideline website (www.guide line.gov) now lists about 40 sites about back pain (www.nlm.nih.gov/medlineplus/ backpain.html). These have been screened by NIH though they do not say what criteria they used. Yet these sites still offer the same mish-mash of information. You are probably better to advise patients not to use the internet, unless you can direct them to a site that you have checked and know it conforms to your management. And remember that internet sites and material can change very rapidly. That is why we do not recommend any sites, because they might soon become outdated.

This chapter will focus on printed leaflets and booklets. There are two completely different types of educational material: traditional biomedical education and modern biopsychosocial information and advice (Burton & Waddell 2002). These have very different content and goals (Table 16.1). The traditional approach was factual education. It imparted biomedical information and provided instructions about physical activities and treatment. From a psychosocial perspective, it often gave negative messages with damaging effects on patients'

beliefs and behaviors (Deyo & Phillips 1996, Hamonet et al 2000). The modern approach tries to prevent the development of chronic pain and disability by addressing these very issues. Its main focus is on beliefs and behavior. It promotes self-help, builds confidence, and reduces unnecessary worry (Burton & Main 2000). Turner (1996) was one of the first to make this distinction. She reviewed earlier studies and suggested that traditional back schools had little long-term effect. However, she suggested that educational and behavioral interventions that activated patients and encouraged active management were more promising.

Traditional biomedical education

The vast majority of the available material is based on traditional ideas about spinal disorders and medical treatment or physical therapy. More recent material usually gives some modern, evidence-based information, e.g., the lack of serious damage; no indication for X-rays; avoid bed rest and stay active; good prognosis. However, that is often buried in the overwhelming biomedical thrust. The possible impact on patients' beliefs or behavior is often ignored.

There is very little evidence on the effectiveness of that kind of material (Turner 1996, Van Tulder et al 2000, Burton & Waddell 2002).

Cherkin et al (1996) compared different methods of giving information to patients with back pain in a US health maintenance organization. Patients received a booklet alone, or a 15-minute session and follow-up phone call from a primary care nurse (plus the booklet), or usual care. They wrote a new

Table 16.1   A comparison of traditional and biopsychosocial information and advice

Traditional biomedical education	Modern biopsychosocial information and advice
Focus on pain	Focus on disability *and* pain
Impart knowledge	Change beliefs and behavior
Provide medical information about anatomy, pathology, diagnosis, indications, and methods of treatment	Provide information about epidemiology, natural history, prognosis. How people react and cope with back pain
Instruction on ergonomics, lifting, and back-specific exercises	Focus on staying active, continuing ordinary activities as normally as possible, and activities of daily living
Facilitate patient cooperation with treatment. Patient remains the passive recipient of professional treatment	Enable individual to share or take over responsibility for his or her own continued management

booklet for the trial: *Back in Action – a guide to under-standing your low back pain and learning what you can do about it.* It was based on current scientific knowledge and guidelines. It addressed patients' concerns about the cause, the good prognosis, actions to aid recovery, and the value of return to normal activities as soon as possible. However, the presentation and content still followed a conventional biomedical pattern. The booklet started with two pages of anatomy. Then there was information about pathology, investigation and referral, therapy options, and back exercises. The nurse-led information gave greater short-term patient satisfaction and perceived knowledge. Those who received the booklet alone showed no effect. There was no difference between the three groups in worry, symptoms, physical function, or health care use.

Cherkin et al (1998) used the same booklet for the control group in a randomized controlled trial (RCT) of McKenzie physical therapy and chiropractic. Both physical therapy and chiropractic produced marginally greater improvement in self-reported symptoms and disability, compared with the booklet alone. There was no difference in sickness absence. Although the therapies were effective, the magnitude of the effect was quite small. Cherkin et al questioned their cost-effectiveness compared with a cheap booklet.

Little et al (2001) carried out an RCT in UK patients attending their family doctor with back pain. Four groups received the leaflet alone, verbal advice on exercise from the doctor, both, or neither. All patients got advice to keep as mobile as possible, to minimize bed rest, and take simple painkillers. The leaflet gave rather mixed messages. There was traditional biomedical information on anatomy and the physical causes of back pain. (Though that was not all evidence-based, e.g., sitting was given as "a major cause of back pain.") Modern messages included the strength of the spine, the limited role of X-rays, and the good prognosis. The major focus was on practical hints about how to perform activities of daily living. There was advice to minimize bed rest, keep mobile, and progressively increase activity. However, there was also advice to take "great care" with bending, sitting, and lifting. There was mild encouragement to return to work even with some symptoms. Roberts et al (2002) showed that patients did learn and use some of the practical hints. Little et al (2001) showed that either the leaflet or advice from the doctor gave modest improvement in self-reported pain and function at 1 week, though that disappeared by 3 weeks. The combination of both verbal advice and the leaflet was *less* effective. This suggests that verbal and written advice must be closely matched, or patients are likely to become confused.

Biopsychosocial information and advice

As traditional clinical management of back pain failed, it is hardly surprising that traditional educational material was also ineffective. If we are going to change clinical management, we must also change patient information and advice. It must be in line with modern understanding of back pain and disability. It should be evidence-based and fit modern clinical guidelines (Box 16.1). Even more

---

Box 16.1   Information and advice from health professionals

It is important that all doctors, therapists, and any other health professionals give consistent advice, in line with clinical guidelines and other information material.

- *Reassure* that there is no serious damage or disease
- *Explain* back pain as a symptom that the back is "not working properly"
- *Avoid* labeling as injury, disk trouble, degeneration, or wear and tear
- *Reassure* about good natural history, providing you stay active, but with accurate information about recurrent symptoms and how to deal with them
- *Advise* to use simple, safe treatments to control symptoms
- *Encourage* staying active, continuing daily activities as normally as possible, and staying at work. This gives the most rapid and complete recovery and less risk of recurrent problems
- *Avoid* "let pain be your guide"
- *Encourage* patients to take responsibility for their own continued management

Backache should not cripple you unless you let it.

important, we believe that it should be directed to psychosocial just as much as biologic issues. The impact on patients' beliefs and behavior is crucial. Indeed, that appears to be more important than any likely therapeutic benefit from the advice given.

Roland & Dixon (1989) wrote the first *Back Book*. This was arguably the first psychosocial booklet for patients, even if what it tried to do was limited and the approach quite primitive. Not surprising, it could not escape completely from the conventional biomedical format of the time. There was a brief account of the anatomy of back pain, advice to rest, practical advice on daily activities, and back-specific exercises. However, in some ways it was quite innovative. It presented the information in a very simple and reader-friendly way. It stressed that back pain is rarely due to any serious disease. More important, the whole emphasis of the booklet was on self-care, with the subliminal message to stay away from doctors. The conscious intent of the booklet to change patients' thinking and behavior was quite different from any previous material. Roland & Dixon tested this booklet in a small RCT of primary care patients with acute or chronic low back pain. Patients who received the booklet made fewer visits to the general practitioner during the next year. There was no difference in sickness absence.

Symonds et al (1995) developed the first true psychosocial leaflet: *Back Pain – don't suffer needlessly*. It was based on the fear-avoidance model and aimed to shift passive beliefs and attitudes. It used blunt, positive messages written in simple language: "Back pain is not usually a serious problem. Continued back pain is not inevitable. Most people can take care of it themselves." It gave reassurance that activity and work do not hinder recovery and encouraged early return to ordinary activities. It used a dramatic contrast between the "coper" and the "avoider." Copers take a positive approach, cope with the pain, and get on with their lives. Avoiders take a negative approach, rest a lot, and wait for the pain to get better or someone to fix it for them. Symonds et al gave this leaflet to workers in one factory, and a traditional biomedical leaflet to those in another factory. Workers who got the new leaflet showed a positive shift in beliefs about the inevitability of consequences

from back pain. Those who got the traditional leaflet showed a negative shift. The factory that got the new leaflet had a marked fall in days of sickness absence and spells of extended absence.

The back book

We wrote *The Back Book* (Roland et al 1996) to accompany the UK RCGP (1996) guidelines. At the time, it was innovative and challenged traditional teaching and advice about how to deal with back pain. We had difficulty getting any publisher to produce it, and released it with some trepidation. It is now the established market leader and has been translated into many languages. Building on that success, in the second edition (Roland et al 2002) we have been more confident about some of the contentious issues. It spells out the risks of chronic pain and disability, and tries to get the patient to address obstacles to recovery. It also deals with work issues. We have recently published an American edition (Bigos et al 2002). We have also made a video *Get Back Active* that has even won a film award! This supplements *The Back Book* or offers an alternative presentation for those who wish it. It is suitable for use in a class, in occupational health, or in a clinic.

We developed *The Back Book* from the original *Back Book* by Roland & Dixon (1989) and the industrial leaflet by Symonds et al (1995). It is strictly evidence-based and in line with current concepts and guidelines. We made a conscious decision to reduce the biomedical content, and to focus on shifting beliefs and behavior. We put a great deal of effort into making it easy to read. The messages are sharply focused and uncompromising: the spine is strong; back pain is not a disease; the natural history is benign; rest is bad, activity is good; self-coping is the answer, doctors are not. We deliberately tried to "de-medicalize" the problem.

The end product is deceptively simple, but do not imagine you can improve it one evening with a few mates over a bottle of your favorite hooch! It took six of us nearly a year to write about a dozen drafts, peer review, rewrite, pilot at various stages on patients, rewrite again and again, format, and illustrate some 3000 words. Of course someone will do it better some day: but be prepared for a lot of hard work. And no matter how good you think your writing is, always test it on the end-users. You will always get surprises, and some of them are instructive.

Burton et al (1996) made a pilot study of *The Back Book* in 124 patients attending an osteopath or a community physical therapy department. Almost all the patients found the booklet very easy to read, interesting, believable, and helpful. They said they would recommend it to family or friends (Table 16.2). Despite concern from some health professionals, neither workers nor primary care patients took offense at the idea of copers and avoiders. They got the main messages (Table 16.3).

Burton et al (1999) then tested *The Back Book* in an RCT in primary care. Patients received either *The Back Book* or a traditional biomedical booklet (Table 16.4) in a sealed envelope at the end of the consultation. There was no other intervention, and apart from that, all patients received "usual care." Patients who received *The Back Book* showed a substantial improvement in beliefs about the inevitability of back problems at 2 weeks, and this was maintained at 1 year (Fig. 16.1). Patients with high fear-avoidance beliefs showed improvement in their beliefs about physical activity at 2 weeks, and this was followed by improvement in self-reported disability at 3 months. There was no effect on pain. There were insufficient patients off work to show any effect on return to work.

The video *Get Back Active* has not been formally tested yet.

Table 16.2 Patients' acceptance of *The Back Book*

Very easy to read	88%
Information clear and interesting	100%
Gives new and helpful information[a]	90%
Believe most of what it says	90%
Would tell a friend or family to read it	100%
Length is about right	86%
Think it will help people	100%

[a]Only 4 patients said they "knew most of the information anyway".

Table 16.3 The most important messages that patients took from *The Back Book*

Message	Percentage of readers
Exercise is good	63
Normal activity is good	41
Too much rest is bad	31
Positive attitudes are helpful	22

Table 16.4 Comparison of the main messages given in the *The Back Book* and the traditional biomedical booklet in the randomized control trial

The Back Book	Handy Hints
• There is no sign of any serious disease • The spine is strong. There is no permanent damage. Even when it is very painful, that does not mean there is any serious damage to your back. Hurt does not mean harm • Back pain is a symptom that your back is simply not moving and working as it should. It is unfit or out of condition • There are a number of treatments that can help to control the pain, but lasting relief then depends on your own efforts • Recovery depends on getting your back moving and working again and restoring normal function and fitness. The sooner you get active, the sooner your back will feel better • Positive attitudes are important. Do not let your back take over your life. "Copers" suffer less at the time, get better quicker, and have less trouble in the long term	• Traditional biomedical concepts of spinal anatomy, injury, and damage. (Implicit messages that the spine is easily damaged, you need health professionals to diagnose and treat the problem, but there is often permanent damage) • "Let pain be your guide" to limit activity when in pain; your doctor may advise bed rest • Describes further investigations and surgery. (This reinforces the message that back pain is a medical problem, and there is little the patient can do) • Concentrates on pain rather than function. (Implicit message that restoring function must await relief of pain) • Encourages patient to be passive recipient of health care

Adapted from Burton et al (1999).

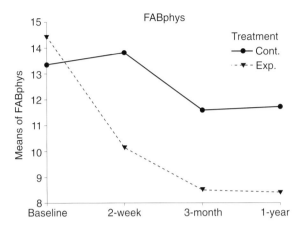

Figure 16.1 Shift in fear-avoidance beliefs about physical activity (FABphys) produced by *The Back Book*. Cont, control group; Exp, experimental group. Reproduced with permission from Burton et al (1999).

Other biopsychosocial material

Several other educational programs have used similar psychosocial messages but presented them in different ways.

Linton & Andersson (2000) in Sweden carried out an RCT of three forms of information. Their aim was to prevent long-term disability in patients with acute or subacute low back pain. The main intervention was a cognitive-behavioral program (Ch. 18) of six 2-hour group sessions. The goals were to reassure and activate patients, correct dysfunctional beliefs, and promote coping. Patients in the two control groups received either a Swedish translation of the Symonds leaflet, or a package of more conventional biomedical material. All patients received usual care. All three groups showed improvement in pain, fear avoidance, and catastrophizing. The cognitive-behavioral group had a ninefold reduction in the risk of > 30 days' sickness absence in the next 6 months. They also used less health care. Clearly, the cognitive-behavioral intervention was by far the most effective. However, suitable pamphlets might be a cheap and cost-effective alternative for some patients at lower risk.

There is one other RCT of a biopsychosocial leaflet that is instructive because it had negative results. Hazard et al (2000) wrote and tested a leaflet *Good News About Low Back Pain*. They included ideas from various recent guidelines and educational materials. The main aim was to encourage self-care, staying active, and early return to work. This was an A4-size leaflet similar in style to Symonds et al (1995), with bullet points and "danger" signs. It was a biopsychosocial leaflet and the advice and messages were to some extent comparable to *The Back Book*. However, there was less overt attempt to challenge and change dysfunctional beliefs. The leaflet was mailed to workers who filed claims for back injuries: they and the controls otherwise received usual care. Unfortunately, workers perceived this coming from the Workers' Compensation Authority, and 56% either did not reply or refused to take part in the trial. The pamphlet made no difference to days lost from work over the next 6 months. Most such educational material is designed for use in primary health care. The results of this trial suggest that the presentation and setting are also important.

Von Korff et al (1998) reported an RCT of self-management, group education for US primary care patients with subacute back pain. Each group met for four sessions and was led by a lay person. It applied problem-solving techniques to the self-management of back pain. This was supplemented by a book and video giving similar messages to *The Back Book* but in much greater detail. The educational program reduced worry and improved confidence. These patients also had more improvement in self-reported disability on the Roland score at 6 and 12 months.

The same group carried out a second RCT of a similar intervention led by a clinical psychologist (Moore et al 2000). Patients had two group sessions supplemented by a book and videos. It was designed to provide accurate information about back pain, reduce fears and worries, promote self-care, develop personal action plans, and improve functional outcomes. This reduced back-related worries and fear-avoidance beliefs. It also produced modest but significant improvements in pain and functional outcomes at 3–12 months. Overall, the results were similar to the earlier study but tended to occur faster.

Buchbinder et al (2001a, b) described the first public education program for back pain in Victoria, Australia. Neighboring New South Wales acted as a control. The Victorian Workcover Authority ran a multimedia public education campaign called *Back Pain: Don't Take it Lying Down*. It lasted about 2 years.

It was based on the messages of *The Back Book*, and promoted the benefits of staying active, avoiding prolonged rest, and staying at work. Prime-time TV adverts featured medical experts, and national sporting and television personalities. Radio and printed advertisements, billboards, posters, seminars, workplace visits, and publicity articles supported the messages. *The Back Book* was translated into 11 languages and distributed widely. All doctors in Victoria received evidence-based guidelines giving the same messages. Surveys of doctor and population samples over 2 years measured the impact in Victoria and New South Wales. The education campaign produced a positive shift in population beliefs about back pain. Doctors also showed a shift to more active management. The number of workers' compensation claims, days lost, and medical costs all fell slightly. There was no change in any of these outcomes in New South Wales over the same period. These effects were relatively modest, but no one had ever managed to produce such a shift at a population level. And in view of the massive impact of back pain, even modest improvements were well worthwhile. The whole campaign was cost-effective.

Working Backs Scotland is a national educational campaign that has been running since October 2000. It is a true national partnership, involving all the health professions who treat back pain, national organizations, employers, unions, and patients. It is led by the Health Education Board for Scotland (HEBS), which is an international leader in the field. It is "badged" to HEBS and the Health and Safety Executive, both of whom enjoy wide public recognition and trust. Its aims are:

- to share new understanding about the management of back pain
- to make sure everyone gets consistent advice
- to get employers, employees, and health practitioners to work together.

We did not try to reinvent the wheel, but built on the RCGP (1999) and the UK occupational health guidelines (Carter & Birrell 2000) and *The Back Book*. We then devoted our efforts to presenting the main messages in a simple, user-friendly way:

- Stay active.
- Try simple pain relief.
- And, if you need it, get advice.

Table 16.5 Change in advice from family doctors

	Sept–Oct 2000	Nov 2000–June 2001	Sept 2001–May 2002	Sept–Dec 2002
Stay active	13%	24%	25%	31%
Rest/restrict activity	21%	15%	11%	11%

Unpublished data from Working Backs Scotland.

We developed slogans, single-page leaflets for each user, and posters. We put together an information pack containing all our material and background resources (see Appendices 15B, 16B, 16C and 17D. You can download everything from www.workingbacksscotland.com). The core of the campaign was commercial radio adverts – played 1777 times on 15 stations in the first 4 weeks, and reaching 60% of adults. We got extensive (free!) press and TV news cover. We distributed 35 000 packs to every health professional treating back pain in Scotland. We got 120 000 hits on our website in the first few months. Since that time we have had periodic "booster" campaigns. And we have developed additional resources for family doctors, occupational health, and orthopedic surgeons. We are still struggling to develop material and to get through to small and medium-sized enterprises, but that is a common problem for any such campaign.

We carried out population surveys of 1000 adults per month (like the standard political polls) for 2 months before the launch and ever since. These show high awareness of the campaign. Table 16.5 shows the shift in the advice patients receive from family doctors. This is all the more impressive because it is what patients report they were actually told, not what GPs say they advise.

Figure 16.2 shows the shift in beliefs about how to manage back pain. This is a massive 20% reversal from a majority in favor of rest to a majority in favor of staying active. It occurred within a month or two of the launch and has been maintained for more than 2 years. This is almost unbelievable. Most health education – like an antismoking campaign – does well if it achieves a 3–5% shift at population level. And the effect usually decays over months. Obviously the Working Backs Scotland campaign did not occur in isolation. It is possible

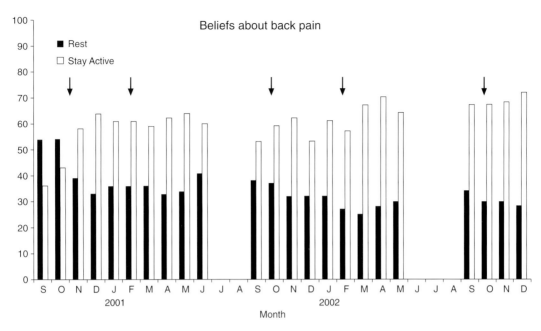

Figure 16.2 Population shift in beliefs about the management of acute low back pain. Unpublished data from Working Backs Scotland, with thanks.

that we were lucky in our timing and boosted a change in opinion that was occurring anyway. Alternatively, Bogduk (personal communication) suggests that most health education campaigns tell people to stop doing things they enjoy – like smoking, eating, or sex! Our message was emotionally neutral. Indeed, we have some feedback that it was telling people what they already knew or wanted to hear. We have some tentative hints that there is a fall in self-reported disability and time of work. However, we will need to wait a year or two before we have the statistics to tell if we have had any impact on sickness absence or long-term incapacity.

CONCLUSIONS

- Information and advice from doctors and therapists can have a powerful *positive or negative* impact on patients' beliefs, behaviors, clinical outcomes, and sickness absence.
- Carefully selected educational material *can* produce a positive shift in beliefs and potentially improve clinical outcomes and sickness absence.
- The material should be evidence-based and in line with modern guidelines.
- A focus on shifting beliefs and behavior appears to be more effective than attempts to impart biomedical knowledge.
- The format, presentation, and setting are important.
- Printed material on its own is likely to have modest impact. It is designed to supplement information and advice from doctors and therapists. All health professionals and any educational material should provide consistent messages. Ideally, this should be integrated into a cohesive educational package.

References

Abenhaim L, Rossignol M, Gobeille D et al 1995 The prognostic consequences in the making of the initial medical diagnosis of work-related injuries. Spine 20: 791–795

Bigos S, Roland M, Waddell G, Moffett J K, Burton K, Main C 2002 The back book, American edition. The Stationery Office, London

Bogduk N 2000 Editorial: what's in a name? The labelling of back pain. Medical Journal of Australia 173: 400–401

Borkan J M, Reis S, Hermoni D, Biderman A 1995 Talking about the pain: a patient-centered study of low back pain in primary care. Social Science and Medicine 40: 977–988

Buchbinder R, Jolley D, Wyatt M 2001a Population based intervention to change back pain beliefs and disability: three part evaluation. British Medical Journal 322: 1516–1520

Buchbinder R, Jolley D J, Wyatt M 2001b Effects of a media campaign on back pain beliefs and its potential influence on the management of low back pain in general practice. Spine 26: 2535–2542

Burton A K, Main C J 2000 Obstacles to return to work from work-related musculoskeletal disorders. In: Karwowski W (ed.) International encyclopedia of ergonomics and human factors. Taylor & Francis, London, pp. 1542–1544

Burton A K, Waddell G 2002 Educational and informational approaches. In: Linton S J (ed.) New avenues for the prevention of chronic musculoskeletal pain and disability. Elsevier Science, Amsterdam, pp 245–258

Burton A K, Waddell G, Burtt R, Blair S 1996 Patient educational material in the management of low back pain in primary care. Bulletin of the Hospital for Joint Diseases 55: 138–146

Burton A K, Waddell G, Tillotson K M, Summerton N 1999 Information and advice to patients with back pain can have a positive effect: a randomized controlled trial of a novel educational booklet in primary care. Spine 24: 2484–2491

Butler L, Foster N E 2003 Back pain online: a cross-sectional survey of the quality of web-based information on low back pain. Spine 28: 395–401

Carter J T, Birrell L N (eds) 2000 Occupational health guidelines for the management of low back pain at work. Faculty of Occupational Medicine, London. Available online at: www.facoccmed.ac.uk

Cedraschi C, Nordin M, Nachemson A L, Vischer T L 1998 Health care providers should use a common language in relation to low back pain patients. In: Nordin M, Cedraschi C, Vischer T L (eds) New approaches to the low back pain patient. Baillière's clinical rheumatology vol. 12. Baillière Tindall, London, pp 1–15

Cherkin D C, Deyo R A, Street J H, Hunt M, Barlow W 1996 Pitfalls of patient education: limited success of a program for back pain in primary care. Spine 21: 345–355

Cherkin D C, Deyo R A, Battie M, Street J, Barlow W 1998 A comparison of physical therapy, chiropractic manipulation, and provision of an educational booklet for the treatment of patients with low back pain. New England Journal of Medicine 339: 1021–1029

Deyo R A, Diehl A K 1986 Patient satisfaction with medical care for low back pain. Spine 11: 28–30

Deyo R A, Phillips W R 1996 Low back pain: a primary care challenge. Spine 21: 2826–2832

Hamonet C, Boulay C, Heiat A et al 2000 Les mots qui font mal. Douleurs 2: 29–33

Hazard R G, Reid S, Haugh L D, McFarlane G 2000, A controlled trial of an educational pamphlet to prevent disability after occupational low back injury, Spine 25: 1419–1423

Li L, Irwin E, Guzman J, Bombardier C 2001 Surfing for back pain patients: the nature and quality of back pain information on the internet. Spine 26: 545–557

Linton S J, Andersson T 2000 Can chronic disability be prevented? A randomized trial of a cognitive-behavior intervention and two forms of information for patients with spinal pain. Spine 25: 2825–2831

Little P, Somerville J, Williamson I et al 2001 Randomised controlled trial of self management leaflets and booklets for minor illness provided by post. British Medical Journal 322: 1214–1216

Moore J E, Von Korff M, Cherkin D, Saunders K, Lorig K 2000 A randomised trial of a cognitive-behavioral program for enhancing back pain self-care in a primary care setting. Pain 88: 145–153

RCGP 1996, 1999 Clinical guidelines for the management of acute low back pain. Royal College of General Practitioners, London. Available online at: www.rcgp.org.uk

Roberts L, Little P, Chapman J et al 2002 The Back Home trial: general practitioner-supported leaflets may change back pain behavior. Spine 27: E1821–1828

Roland M, Dixon M 1989 Randomized controlled trial of an educational booklet for patients presenting with back pain in general practice. Journal of the Royal College of General Practitioners 39: 244–246

Roland M, Waddell G, Klaber-Moffett J, Burton K, Main C, Cantrell T 1996 The back book. Stationery Office, Norwich. Available online at: www.clicktso.com

Roland M, Waddell G, Klaber-Moffett J, Burton K, Main C, 2002 The back book, 2nd edn. Stationery Office, Norwich. Available online at: www.clicktso.com

Stone J, Wojcik W, Durrance D et al 2002 What should we say to patients with symptoms unexplained by disease? The "number needed to offend". British Medical Journal 325: 1449–1450

Symonds T L, Burton A K, Tillotson K M, Main C J 1995 Absence resulting from low back trouble can be reduced by psychosocial intervention at the work place. Spine 20: 2738–2745

Turner J A 1996 Educational and behavioral interventions for back pain in primary care. Spine 21: 2851–2859

Van Tulder M W, Esmail R, Bombardier C, Koes B W 2000 Back schools for non-specific low back pain (Cochrane review). In: The Cochrane Library, issue 4. Update Software, Oxford

Van Tulder M W, Becker A, Bekkering T et al 2002 European guidelines for the management of acute nonspecific low back pain in primary care. COST action B13, Brussels. Available online at: www.backpaineurope.org

Von Korff M 1999 Pain management in primary care: an individualized stepped-care approach. In: Gatchel R J, Turk D C (eds) Psychosocial factors in pain: clinical perspectives. Guildford Press, New York, pp 360–373

Von Korff M, Moore J E, Lorig K et al 1998 A randomized trial of a lay person-led self-management group intervention for back pain patients in primary care. Spine 23: 2608–2615

APPENDIX 16A *THE BACK BOOK*

The best way to deal with back pain
Based on the latest research

THE NEW APPROACH TO BACK PAIN

Back pain is very common and causes a great deal of misery but, fortunately, serious or permanent damage is rare. There has been a revolution in thinking about back care and we now deal with it in a different way. This booklet sets out the facts and shows you how to get better as quickly as possible. It's based on the latest research.

What you do about back pain yourself is usually more important than the exact diagnosis or treatment.

An attack of back pain can be alarming. Even a minor back strain can be very painful and it's natural to think that something dreadful might have happened. But stop and look at the facts:

Serious or permanent damage is rare.
There are lots of things you can do to help yourself.

BACK FACTS

- Most back pain is not due to any serious disease.

- The acute pain usually improves within days or a few weeks, at least enough to get on with your life. The long-term outlook is good.

- Sometimes aches and pains can last for quite a long time. But that doesn't mean it's serious. It does usually settle eventually – even though it's frustrating that no one can predict exactly when! Most people can get going quite quickly, even while they still have some pain.

- About half the people who get backache will get it again within a couple of years. But that still does not mean it's serious. Between attacks most people return to normal activities with little, if any, pain.

- What you do in the early stages is very important. Rest for more than a day or two usually does not help and may actually prolong pain and disability.

- Your back is designed for movement: it needs movement – a lot of movement. The sooner you get moving and doing your ordinary activities as normally as possible, the sooner you will feel better.

- The people who cope best with back pain are those who stay active and get on with life despite the pain.

Back pain need not cripple you, so don't let it!
The sooner you get on with your life, the sooner you will feel better.

CAUSES OF BACK PAIN

Your spine is one of the strongest parts of your body. It is made of solid bony blocks joined by discs to give it strength and flexibility. It is reinforced by strong ligaments, and surrounded by large and powerful muscles that protect it. Most simple back strains do not cause any lasting damage.

It is surprisingly difficult to damage your spine.

Despite what you might have heard:

- Only a few people with back pain have a slipped disc or a trapped nerve. Even then, a slipped disc usually gets better by itself. Very few back problems ever need surgery.

- X-rays and MRI scans can detect serious spinal injuries, but they don't usually help in ordinary back pain. They may even be misleading. Doctors sometimes mention "degeneration", which sounds frightening, but it's not damage or arthritis. These are the normal changes with age – just like grey hair.

- Your doctor or therapist will often not be able to pinpoint the source of the pain. Again, it's frustrating not to know exactly what is wrong. Actually, in another way it's good news – you do not have any serious damage to your spine.

Most back pain comes from the working parts of your back – the muscles, ligaments and small joints. Your back is simply not moving and working as it should. You can think of it being "out of condition". So what you should do is get your back moving and working properly again. This stimulates its natural ability to recover.

REST OR STAY ACTIVE?

The old-fashioned treatment for back pain was rest. Some people with back pain were sent to bed for weeks or even months on end, just waiting for the pain to disappear. We now know that bed rest for more than a day or two is the worst possible treatment, because in the long term it actually prolongs the pain:

- Your bones get weaker.
- You get stiff.
- Your muscles get weak.
- You lose physical fitness.
- You get depressed.
- The pain feels worse.
- It is harder and harder to get going again.

Bed rest is bad for backs.

No wonder it didn't work! We no longer use bed rest to treat any other common condition and it's time to stop bed rest for back pain.

You may be limited in how much you can do when the pain is bad. You might even be forced to stay in bed at the start. But only for a day or two. Bed rest is not a treatment – it's simply a short-term consequence of the pain. The most important thing is to get moving again as soon as you can.

ACTIVITY IS GOOD

Your whole body must keep active to stay healthy. It thrives on use.

Regular physical activity:

- gives you stronger bones
- develops your muscles
- keeps you supple
- makes you fit
- makes you feel good
- releases natural chemicals that reduce the pain.

Use it or lose it.

Even when your back is painful, you can make a start without putting too much stress on it:

- walking
- swimming
- exercise bike
- dancing/yoga/keep fit
- In fact, most daily activities and hobbies.

Exercise gets your back moving again by stretching tight muscles and joints, and stops the working parts seizing up. It also makes your heart and lungs work and improves physical fitness.

Different things suit different people. Experiment – find what works best for you and your back. Your goal is to get moving and steadily increase your level of activity. Do a little bit more each day.

Getting stiff joints and muscles working *can* be painful. Athletes accept that when they start training, their muscles can hurt and they have to work through the pain barrier. But that does not mean they are doing any damage. So don't worry if exercise makes you a bit sore at first – that's usually a sign you are actually making progress! As you get fully fit the pain should ease off.

No one pretends it's easy. Painkillers and other treatments can help to control the pain to let you get started, but you still have to do the work. There is no other way. You have a straight choice: rest and get worse, or get active and recover.

Do not fall into the trap of thinking it will be easier in a week or two, next month, next year. It won't! The longer you put it off, the harder it will be to get going again. The faster you get back to normal activities and back to work the better – even if you still have some restrictions.

The sooner you get active, the sooner your back will feel better.

DEALING WITH AN ATTACK OF BACK PAIN

Most people manage to deal with most attacks themselves. What you do depends on how bad your back feels. However, because there's no serious damage, you can usually:

- use something to control the pain
- modify your activities for a time, if necessary
- stay active and get on with your life.

Some people have more persistent pain – but the same principles apply.

Control of pain

There are many treatments which can help – even if there is no miracle cure. They may not remove the pain completely, but they should control it enough to let you get active and so make yourself better.

Painkillers

You should not hesitate to use painkillers if you need them. You can safely mask the pain to get active: your body will not let you do any harm. Paracetamol is the simplest and safest painkiller. Or you can use anti-inflammatory tablets like ibuprofen.

It may surprise you, but these simple over-the-counter painkillers are often the most effective for back pain. The problem is that many people do not use them properly. You should take the full recommended dose and take them regularly every 4–6 hours – do not wait till your pain is out of control. You should usually take the painkillers for a few days, but you may need to take them for a week or two. Few people require anything stronger.

Do not take ibuprofen or aspirin if you are pregnant or if you have asthma, indigestion or an ulcer.

Heat and cold

Heat or cold can be used for short-term relief of pain and to relax muscle spasm. In the first 48 hours you can try a cold pack on the sore area for 5–10 minutes at a time – a bag of frozen peas wrapped in a damp towel. Other people prefer heat – a hot water bottle, a bath or a shower.

Massage

Massage is one of the oldest treatments for back pain. Many people find gentle rubbing eases the pain and relaxes muscle spasm.

Manipulation

Most doctors now agree that manipulation can help back pain. It is safe if done by a qualified professional: osteopaths, chiropractors, some physiotherapists and a few doctors with special training. You should begin to feel the benefit within a few sessions and it's not a good idea to have treatment for months on end.

Other treatments

Many other treatments such as electrotherapy machines, acupuncture or alternative medicine are used for back pain and some people feel they help.

But be realistic. Despite the claims, these treatments rarely provide a quick fix. Once again, you should feel any benefit quite quickly and there is no value in treatment for months on end. What really matters is whether they help you get active.

Anxiety, stress and muscle tension

Anxiety and stress can increase the amount of pain we feel. Tension can cause muscle spasm and the muscles themselves can become painful.

Many people get anxious about back pain, especially if it doesn't get better as fast as they expect. You may get conflicting advice – from your family and friends or even from doctors and therapists – which may make you uncertain what best to do. Trust the advice in this booklet – it comes from the latest research. Remember, serious damage is rare and the long-term outlook is good. So do not let fear and worry hold back your recovery.

Stress can aggravate or prolong pain. If stress is a problem you need to recognise it at an early stage and try to do something about it. You cannot always avoid stress, but you can learn to reduce its effects by controlled breathing, muscle relaxation and mental calming techniques. One of the best ways of reducing stress and tension is exercise.

The Swedish relaxation exercise

1. Don't try too hard to relax.
2. Find a comfortable position, sitting or lying down – somewhere quiet.
3. Take deep breaths "slow and steady"; hold for about 15–20 seconds and exhale.
4. Focus your mind on something calm and repetitive.
5. "Let go" when exhaling. Imagine and concentrate on breathing – not on relaxing.

The "relaxation response" can sometimes be achieved quite quickly, but deep relaxation may take 10–15 minutes.

The risk of chronic pain

There has been a lot of research in recent years to identify people at risk of long-term pain and disability. What may surprise you is that most of the warning signs are about what people feel and do, rather than medical findings.

Signs of people at risk of long-term pain:

- believing that you have a serious injury or damage; being unable to accept reassurance
- believing that hurt means harm and that you will become disabled
- avoiding movement or activity due to fear of doing damage
- continued rest and inactivity instead of getting on with your life
- waiting for someone to fix it rather than believing that you can help yourself recover
- becoming withdrawn and depressed.

This all develops gradually and you may not even notice. That's why it is so important to get going as soon as possible *before* you develop chronic pain. If you – or your family and friends – spot some of these early warning signs, you need to do something about it. Now, before it is too late. Use the advice in this booklet to work out what you can do to change direction and get on with your life. If you need extra help to get going, you should ask your doctor or therapist.

You may meet a practical problem here. Doctors and therapists deal best with clear-cut diseases and injuries for which they have a cure. We are often not so good at dealing with more ordinary symptoms like back pain. For example, it's no good staying off work and doing nothing for weeks on end to attend therapy. Or waiting months for a surgeon to tell you that you don't need an operation. That simply delays your recovery! Which is why it really does depend on what you do yourself. You have to make it clear to your doctor or therapist that you realise all this, and what you want is help to get on with your life.

If you are still off work after about a month, you are at risk of developing long-term problems. There is then a 10% risk you will still be off work in a year's time. You could even lose your job. Long before you get to that stage you really need to face up to the problem and take urgent action.

HOW TO STAY ACTIVE

As we've explained, the sooner you start getting mobile and active again the better. Only if the pain is particularly severe do you need to rest up or be off work. But even then you can still do most daily activities if you think about them first. Work out a plan. What are the problems and how can you get around them? Can you do things in a different way?

Try to strike a balance between being as active as you can and not putting too much strain on your back. The basic rules are simple:

- Keep moving.
- Do not stay in one position for too long.
- Move about before you stiffen up.
- Move a little further and faster each day.
- Don't stop doing things – just change the way you do them.

Sitting

Choose a chair and position that is comfortable for you – experiment. Try some support in the small of your back. Get up and stretch regularly – take advantage of TV adverts!

Desk work

Adjust the height of your chair to suit your desk. Arrange your keyboard and VDU so that you are comfortable and not strained. Get up and stretch regularly.

Driving

Adjust your seat from time to time. Try some support in the small of your back.

Stop regularly for a few minutes' break. Get out of the car, walk about and stretch.

Lifting

Think before you lift. Do not lift more than you need to. Keep the load close to your body. Don't twist while you are lifting but turn with your feet.

Carrying and shopping

Think if you need to carry at all. Carry things hugged to your body or split the load between both hands. Don't carry further than you need to. Use wheels!

Daily activities/hobbies

Don't do one thing for too long. Keep changing activities.

Sports

Continuing with your normal sport is fine, but you may need to reduce the intensity.

Swimming: try to vary your stroke – backstroke, side stroke, crawl.

Sleeping

Some people find a firmer mattress helps – or you can try a sheet of chipboard beneath the mattress. Experiment.

Try painkillers an hour before you go to bed.

Sex

Fine! – but you may need to try different positions.

Getting on with your life

You will have good days and bad days. That's normal.

It is important to maintain the momentum of your life – and that includes staying at work if you possibly can. Doing things will distract you from the pain, and your back will usually not get any worse at work than it will at home. If you have a heavy job, you may need some help from your work mates. Simple changes may make your job easier.

If you are seeing a doctor or therapist, tell them about your work. Talk to your supervisor or boss if you need to. Tell them about any parts of your job that may be difficult to begin with, but stress that you want to be at work. Offer your own suggestions about how to overcome these problems – you might even show them this booklet.

If you do have to stay off work, it helps to get back as soon as possible – usually within days or a couple of weeks – and even if you still have some pain. The longer you are inactive and off work the more likely you are to develop long-term pain and disability.

If you are not at work within about a month you should be planning with your doctor, therapist and employer how and when you can get back. Your occupational health department or health and safety rep may be able to assist. Temporary modification to your job or pattern of work may help you get back sooner.

What doctors can and can't do

Although we have stressed that you can deal with most back pain yourself, there may be times you are uncertain and feel the need to check. That's quite reasonable. But remember there is no quick fix for back pain. So you should be realistic about what you expect from a doctor or therapist.

They can:

- make sure you don't have any serious disease and reassure you
- suggest various treatments to help control your pain
- advise you on how you can best deal with the pain and get on with your life.

Try to accept that reassurance and don't let needless worry delay your recovery. You have to share responsibility for your own progress. Some doctors and therapists may be hesitant about handing over and letting you take control. You may have to tell them straight out this really is what you want.

Doctors and therapists can help to ease the pain but only you can get your back going!

Warning signs

If you have severe pain which gets worse over several weeks instead of better, or if you are unwell with back pain, you should see your doctor.

Here are a few symptoms, which are all very rare, but if you do have back pain and suddenly develop any of these you should see a doctor straight away:

- difficulty passing or controlling urine
- numbness around your back passage or genitals
- numbness, pins and needles or weakness in both legs
- unsteadiness on your feet.

Don't let that list worry you too much.

Remember that back pain is rarely due to any serious disease

IT'S YOUR BACK

We've shown you that back pain is rarely due to anything serious and it should not cripple you unless you let it. You've got the facts and the most up-to-date advice about how to deal with back pain. The important thing now is for you to get on with your life. How your back affects you depends on how you react to the pain and what you do about it yourself.

There is no instant answer. You will have your ups and downs for a while – that's normal. But look at it this way:

There are two types of sufferer

One who avoids activity ☹ *and one who copes* ☺

☹ The avoider gets frightened by the pain and worries about the future.

- The avoider is afraid that hurting always means further damage – it doesn't.
- The avoider rests a lot, and just waits for the pain to get better.

☺ The coper knows that the pain will get better and does not fear the future.

- The coper carries on as normally as possible.
- The coper deals with the pain by being positive, staying active and getting on with life.

Who suffers most?

☹ Avoiders suffer the most. They have pain for longer, they have more time off work and they can become disabled.
☺ Copers get better faster, enjoy life more and have less trouble in the long run.

So how do I become a coper and prevent unnecessary suffering?

Follow these guidelines – you really can help yourself

☺ Live life as normally as possible. This is much better than giving in to the pain.

- Keep up daily activities – they will not cause damage. Just avoid really heavy things.
- Try to stay fit – walking, cycling or swimming will exercise your back and should make you feel better. And continue even after your back feels better.
- Start gradually and do a little more each day so you can see the progress you are making.
- Either stay at work or go back to work as soon as possible. If necessary, ask if you can get lighter or modified duties for a week or two.

- Be patient. It's normal to get aches or twinges for a time.

☹ Don't rely on painkillers alone. Stay positive and take control of the pain yourself.

- Don't stay at home or give up doing things you enjoy.
- Don't get frightened. Continuing pain does not mean you are going to become an invalid.
- Don't listen to other people's horror stories.
- Don't get gloomy on the down days.

Get on with life – you'll get better quicker and have less trouble later.

Remember

- Back pain is common but it is rarely due to any serious disease. The long-term outlook is good.
- Even when it is very painful, that doesn't usually mean there's any serious damage to your back. Hurt does not mean harm.
- Bed rest for more than a day or two is usually bad for you.
- Staying active will help you get better faster and prevent more back trouble.
- The sooner you get going, the faster you will get better.
- If you don't manage to get back to most normal activities quite quickly, you should seek additional help.
- Regular exercise and staying fit help your general health and your back.
- You have to get on with your life. Don't let your back take over.

That's the message from the latest research – you really can help yourself.

Availability

The Back Book is available from the Stationery Office, PO Box 29, Norwich NR3 1GN www.tso.co.uk or bookshops (ISBN 011 702949 1, price £1.25, Prices for bulk orders, call 0870-600-5522).

The American edition is available in the US from Balogh International Inc., 1911 N. Duncan Road, Champaign, Illinois 61822 www.balogh.com (ISBN 011-702950-5).

The video *Get Back Active* is also available from the Stationery Office: mail, telephone and fax orders only (ISBN 011-702940-8).

APPENDIX 16B WORKING BACKS SCOTLAND SHEETS FOR PEOPLE WITH BACK PAIN AND ON STAYING ACTIVE

If you have back pain..

follow these simple steps
to stay in control

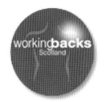

(www.workingbacksscotland.com)

Back pain affects nearly everyone at some point in his or her life but is rarely serious.

If you have severe pain which gets worse over several weeks instead of better, or if you are unwell with back pain, you should see your doctor. You should see a doctor straightaway if you have:

- difficulty passing or controlling urine
- numbness around your back passage or genitals
- numbness, pins and needles or weakness in both legs
- unsteadiness on your feet.

But remember that back pain is rarely due to any serious disease.

Simple painkillers can be used to help manage your pain (follow the instructions).

A cold pack or local heat can be used for short-term symptomatic relief.

It is important to stay active and continue as normally as possible.

Try to remain at work or get back as soon as possible even if you still have some low back pain. The longer you stay off work the more likely you are to develop chronic pain and disability.

Manual therapy (manipulative treatment) may help with pain relief. You can go to a chartered physiotherapist, a registered chiropractor or a registered osteopath, or ask you GP, practice nurse, or occupational health service to refer you.

Traction and lumbar corsets may be used for pain relief to help you to get ot active but do not provide lasting benefit.

Tell your doctor, nurse or therapist about you work duties. You may also wish to discuss the problem with your employer.

Most people are back to normal activites by about six weeks. If not you should be getting help to get fully active.

If you have not returned to work by about six weeks you should be talking with your GP, therapist and your employer about how and when you will. Your occupational health department or health and safety representative may be able to assist. Temporary adapation of the job or pattern of work may help.

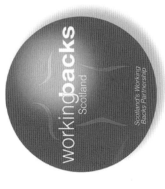

Staying active

Keep it moving

Keeping your back moving stops the working parts from seizing up. It may hurt a bit at first, but it does not do any damage—**hurt is not the same as harm**. It's worth working through any initial discomfort —because you'll get **back to normal** that much quicker.

You don't have to do special exercises. Simply continue to do your ordinary activities as normally as possible. Being fit and active will help you get better faster and prevent more back trouble later.

Strike a balance

Of course, you may need to take it a little easier or move a bit more carefully at first. But don't stop altogether. You can still do most normal activities without putting too much strain on your back—just use common sense!

- Don't sit or stand in one position for too long—change position often.
- Get up and walk about to avoid stiffening up.
- Take breaks when driving.
- Some things may take a little longer or you may need to change how you do them.
- Pain killers may help you get going.
- Walking and swimming are good forms of regular exercise.

What about work?

Some tasks may be more difficult when your back is sore, but back pain is not usually caused by work. Work is good for physical and mental health. So staying active and **getting on with your life** means staying at work or returning to work as soon as possible. You don't have to wait till the pain is 100% gone. In fact, getting back to work can help you recover faster. And don't be afraid to ask colleagues for help if you need to.

Get on with your life

You know that activity is good for your health—it's just the same for your back. The most important thing is for you to get on with your life. You really can help yourself.

Chapter 17

Occupational health guidelines

Gordon Waddell   Kim Burton

CHAPTER CONTENTS

Most of us think that our job is to treat our patients' symptoms. Most of the time, we simply assume they will recover and return to work. For more than 90% of patients who do recover rapidly and uneventfully, that may be a reasonable approach. For those who fail to do so, it is a dangerous false assumption. Treatment might still help symptoms, but symptomatic treatment alone is then quite ineffective at returning people to work (Scheer et al 1997, van der Weide et al 1997, van Tulder et al 2000).

Clinical guidelines (Ch. 15) focus on clinical management and outcomes and pay little attention to work issues. From one point of view that is understandable, because that is what clinical guidelines are about. But in view of the importance of work-related issues in back pain it is unfortunate. Recent occupational health guidelines fill that gap and address the management of the worker with low back pain. Although they are primarily for occupational health professionals, they have important messages for all clinicians.

Occupational health is about "health at work." It is not only about work injuries and occupational diseases. Nor is it just about sickness absence. Much more broadly, it deals with the two-way relationship between work and health. That includes the effects of work on health and how the worker's health may influence his or her work. The World Health Organization (WHO) defined occupational health as "the promotion and maintenance of the highest degree of physical, mental and social well-being of workers" (Harrington et al 1998). Ideally, it should prevent ill health rather than simply deal with it after it occurs. So helping workers remain at work with back pain is just as important as helping them to return to work after sickness absence. (See Harrington et al (1998) for an introduction to occupational health.)

Thus, for management, it really does not matter whether or not back pain was *caused* by work. Any back pain, whatever its cause, may *affect* work and is the concern of occupational health. Occupational health physicians, nurses, and therapists have a particular responsibility to apply modern concepts of management in the work setting. But none of us can limit our management to clinical issues alone. All doctors and therapists dealing with back pain should be aware of and deal with work-related issues (Box 17.1). Health care is not an end in itself and we must all share responsibility for what happens to our patients in the real world.

Even though questions about back pain and work and the relation between them are so important, many doctors and therapists remain ignorant of these issues. We are often barely aware of our patient's job, never mind what it involves. How often do you ask a patient about his or her job tasks or demands (both physical and mental)? Even if they tell you, do you really understand? Have you ever been in a factory and seen what some of these jobs are like? Do you discuss how back pain affects doing their job – or vice versa? Or if there is anything they can do about it?

There is a general lack of communication between health care and the workplace. Apart from official forms, when did you last speak or write to a patient's employer or supervisor or occupational health department? Any improvement will depend on whether we actually communicate. Because of confidentiality, this requires the patient's consent. But it is almost always in the patient's own interests for doctor or therapist, patient and employer to communicate and work together to achieve what should be our common aim.

INFORMATION AND ADVICE

The information and advice we give to patients are so important that we devoted Chapter 16 to it. But in no area is information and advice more important than about work.

Unfortunately, traditional biomedical information and advice carried a lot of very negative messages about back pain and work. There are many occupational myths about back pain (Table 17.1) shared by patients, therapists, and doctors alike. These myths convey inaccurate and harmful messages, and may act as obstacles to work retention or return to work.

Many authors comment on such issues, but Anema et al (2002) made one of the few actual studies. They looked at 300 Dutch patients who were still off work for an average of 4.5 months with low back pain. They questioned occupational health physicians about how these patients' clinical care might act as obstacles to return to work (Table 17.2). In fairness, the same health care system treated most people successfully and this study only looked at the failures. Nevertheless, the results are sobering. Even worse, they felt these "iatrogenic" obstacles were more common than any individual psychosocial factors in the workers. Despite these concerns, in only 19% of these patients was there *any* communication between treating

---

Box 17.1   Occupational issues in clinical practice

- Be aware of your patient's job
- What are the physical and mental demands of that job?
- Do any of these demands affect their back pain – or vice versa? Which? How?
- Can they/you identify any obstacles to them returning to work?
- *But* – think very carefully before you give any advice about work. How will the patient understand what you say? What are the short-and long-term implications? Is your advice realistic?
- What can the patient/the employer/you do to help overcome any obstacles to return to work?
- Aim for better communication and cooperation between health care, the workplace, and rehabilitation
- The ultimate outcome measure of your management is whether and how quickly your patient gets back to work

and occupational health physicians. And that was in a country with good occupational health systems, so in many countries it must be much worse.

A recent UK government study found that 40% of people who gave up work because of sickness or disability had been advised to do so by a health professional.

Table 17.1 Occupational myths about back pain

Myths	What the evidence says
Your back pain is due to wear and tear	X-ray changes are largely a normal, age-related finding
Wear and tear is caused by heavy work	Physical demands of work and occupational loading are not a major cause of degeneration
Your back pain is caused by your work	Back pain may be work-related but most back pain is not *caused* by work
You must have some time off work	Most people with back pain do not (need to) take sick leave
You should stay off work till you are free from pain	It is not necessary to remain off work till completely symptom-free
Your job is too heavy – you should change to a lighter job	Most people can and do return to their previous job. That is always the easiest option
Giving up that work would be good for your back	In practice, that may mean unnecessary early retirement

Table 17.2 Ineffective disability management as an obstacle to return to work

Duration of symptomatic medical treatment	43%[a]
Waiting periods for treatment	41%
Worker passive or uncooperative	33%
Views of treating doctor	25%

[a] Percentage of patients.
Adapted from Anema et al (2002).

Too often, we offer advice about work quite casually. We do not really think about what we are saying, or about its impact on our patients and their families. Just imagine if someone told you that your job was bad for you and implied that you should give it up. Just write off years of training and experience and all your skills. Never mind what else you might do, or how (or even if) you would get another job. Or the financial impact on you and your dependants. How would you react? Education, knowledge, and insight would probably allow you to discount such advice. Your patients may not be so lucky – they may trust you.

Fundamental to these myths and to better management of occupational issues is how we think about the relationship between back pain and work. It may help if we distinguish the underlying back problem from the symptom of back pain. As we saw in Chapter 6, only a modest proportion of back problems are actually *caused* by work. Back trouble is common in adults of working age. Physical demands at work may precipitate or aggravate back pain. And back pain, whatever its cause, can affect capacity to work. So back pain is certainly "occupational" in the sense that it is "work-related," but most of the time we cannot actually attribute back problems to work. This has important implications for return to work. Back pain may make it difficult to return to some work tasks or limit initial return to modified duties. But if the back problem is not attributable to work, then any restriction is simply an *effect* of the pain. There is no medical reason why back pain per se (as opposed to any associated restriction of function) should preclude work. Work may produce some temporary increase in symptoms, but there is no reason to fear further damage or reinjury. We must certainly acknowledge that some patients are presently unable to do some job tasks because of their back pain. But many patients are able to work despite their back pain and there is then no medical reason to advise them to stay off work. Nor do we not need to wait till the pain is 100% "cured" before returning to work. Epidemiology shows that most people do continue working most of the time despite back pain (Ch. 5). All the evidence is that remaining at work or returning to work as early as possible is the best possible treatment for back pain. It does not aggravate the problem or cause reinjury but actually leads to faster recovery and less trouble in the long term (Waddell & Burton 2000). That is why all occupational guidelines agree that we should encourage and support workers with back pain to stay at work or return to work as early as possible (Staal et al 2003).

We recognize this may not be easy. Many doctors, therapists, and patients have deeply entrenched ideas about back pain being caused by work and work injuries. These ideas are difficult to overcome. Yet the scientific evidence is clear. Clinical guidelines about advice to stay active are clear. Occupational health guidelines about staying at work or return to work as early as possible are clear. There is strong evidence that advice produces faster recovery and fewer long-term problems. We must try to dispel these irrational fears and we must not allow them to cloud our professional judgment or advice.

OUTCOMES

Traditionally, doctors and therapists judge the success of treatment by clinical ratings such as "improvement." The problem is that these may not reflect the patient's perspective, so there is now increasing use of patient-centered outcomes such as pain and self-reported disability and satisfaction with care (Deyo et al 1998). These are certainly more valid and important than professional ratings of the technical success of treatment. The strength of these measures is that they are subjective and depend on qualitative judgments by the patient. But that is also their major limitation, because they are open to problems of reliability and bias. Thus, there is a powerful argument that these clinical measures should be supplemented by an occupational outcome. The single most crucial impact of back pain for the individual of working age, and for society, is on ability to work. Return to work is the most important social and economic measure of the success of treatment. At the same time it is the most objective outcome measure that is hardest to manipulate or fudge, even if it is most subject to widely varying influences.

Using (sustained) return to work as the ultimate outcome measure changes our whole view of clinical management. It is no longer a question of whether we regard our treatment as "successful."

It is no longer enough that our patients feel better or say they are satisfied with our care. Now we must face up to whether we really have managed to help our patients get on with their lives. That is a much more brutal test. It demands a whole new perspective on what health care is all about.

OCCUPATIONAL GUIDANCE

Staal et al (2003) have reviewed the international occupational health guidelines, and Box 17.2 gives some of the common elements. All of these guidelines recognize the complexities of the issues and the limitations of the evidence. But they all emphasize that the starting point is to get all the players – patient, health professional(s), and employer – on side (Frank et al 1998). Regrettably, the players who should be most open to evidence-based education – health professionals – may be hardest to change. Instead of helping, doctors and therapists sometimes form an obstacle for return to work (Table 17.2). Clearly, we must make sure that our management does actually produce the outcomes we want, and that we *do no harm*.

Box 17.2 summarizes some of the important occupational issues that can supplement usual clinical care. This approach is not easy, and for most of us it goes against our traditional teaching – but it is what the evidence suggests. Of course, we all have a professional duty to support and care for the worker with back pain. This new approach is not inconsistent with that duty. In fact, it will enhance it, because the interests of the worker take priority over the pain.

SAMPLE GUIDELINES

We have included:

- Appendix 17A: UK *Occupational Health Guidelines for the Management of Low Back Pain at Work* (Carter & Birrell 2000). These are the first truly evidence-based occupational health guidelines for back pain. Brief and full versions of the guidelines and the accompanying evidence tables are available on www.facoccmed.ac.uk. The full bibliography is available on the website or in Waddell & Burton (2001).

Box 17.2 Improving clinical management for occupational outcomes

- Ask patients about their job and any difficulties – do this during routine clinical assessment, not as a last-minute afterthought
- Consider the "yellow flags" for risk of chronicity (Ch. 7)
- Do not actually suggest sick leave unless there is a strong clinical reason (which is rare)
- Educate the patient:
  - Avoid diagnostic labeling, especially those that may link symptoms to work
  - Explain that continuing work, though possibly somewhat difficult or uncomfortable, will speed recovery and reduce recurrences
- Say that you are there to help and support
- Offer to discuss any problems and the benefits of work retention with the employer
  - Do not recommend work modifications too readily, and do not recommend belts and corsets
- If sick leave is unavoidable, make it short-term and review the patient regularly
  - Encourage return to normal duties as soon as possible – do not wait till symptom-free
  - Only if necessary suggest *temporary* use of modified work, and then only to facilitate early return to work

- Offer to discuss modified duties with the employer or occupational health department
- Build up liaisons with local employers, and encourage them to contact you
- Advise the employer of the benefits of sympathetic yet positive contact during sick leave
- If early return to work proves difficult, make sure the patient (and employer) appreciate the disadvantages of long-term absence
  - If you have the expertise, offer to discuss job demands more closely and advise the employer on suitable temporary modifications to facilitate return. Or refer to an occupational health professional who can supply this advice
  - Reassess and address psychosocial obstacles to work return
  - If these steps are clearly failing, explain the importance of shifting from symptomatic treatment to an active rehabilitation program. Try to refer the patient to such a program, preferably linked to the workplace with input from the employer (Ch. 18)

- Appendix 17B: COST European guidelines: *Back Pain and Work*. You may also want to look at Staal et al (2003) for an international review of occupational health guidelines.

- Appendix 17C: *Active and Working!* Managing acute low back pain in the workplace: an employer's guide (Kendall 2000). This is designed to accompany the New Zealand guidelines and

is available on www.acc.org.nz. We consider this to be by far the best and most readable guide for employers.

- Appendix 17D: Working Backs Scotland summary sheet for employers. All of the Working Backs Scotland material is available on www.workingbacksscotland.com.

References

Anema J R, van der Giezen A M, Buijs P C, van Mechelen W 2002 Ineffective disability management by doctors is an obstacle for return-to-work: a cohort study on low back pain patients sicklisted for 3–4 months. Occupational and Environmental Medicine 59: 729–733

Carter J T, Birrell L N (eds) 2000 Occupational health guidelines for the management of low back pain at work – principal recommendations. Faculty of Occupational Medicine, London. Available online at: www.facoccmed.ac.uk

Deyo R A, Battie M, Beurkens A J H M et al 1998 Outcome measures for low back pain research: a proposal for standardized use. Spine 23: 2003–2013

Frank J, Sinclair S, Hogg-Johnson S et al 1998 Preventing disability from work-related low-back pain. New evidence gives new hope – if we can just get all the players onside. Canadian Medical Association Journal 158: 1625–1631

Harrington J M, Gill F S, Aw T C, Gardiner K 1998 Occupational health, 4th edn. Pocket consultant series. Blackwell Science, London

Kendall N A S 2000 Active and working! Managing acute low back pain in the workplace: an employer's guide. Accident Rehabilitation and Compensation Insurance Corporation of New Zealand and the National Health Committee, Wellington, New Zealand. Available online at: www.acc.org.nz

RCGP 1999 Clinical guidelines for the management of acute low back pain. Royal College of General Practitioners, London. Available online at: www.rcgp.org.uk

Scheer S J, Watanabe T K, Radack K L 1997 Randomized controlled trials in industrial low back pain. Part 3 Subacute/chronic interventions. Archives of Physical Medicine and Rehabilitation 78: 414–423

Staal J B, Hlobil H, van Tulder M W et al 2003 Occupational health guidelines for the management of low back pain:

an international comparison. Occupational and Environmental Medicine (in press)

van der Weide W E, Verbeek J H A M, van Tulder M W 1997 Vocational outcome of intervention for low back pain. Scandinavian Journal of Work and Environmental Health 23: 165–178

van Tulder M W, Goossens M, Waddell G, Nachemson A 2000 Conservative treatment of chronic low back pain. In: A Nachemson, E Jonsson (eds) Neck and back pain: the scientific evidence of causes, diagnosis and treatment. Lippincott, Williams & Wilkins, Philadelphia, pp. 271–304

Waddell G, Burton A K 2000 Occupational health guidelines for the management of low back pain at work – evidence review. Faculty of Occupational Medicine, London. Available online at: www.facoccmed.ac.uk

Waddell G, Burton A K 2001 Occupational health guidelines for the management of low back pain at work: evidence review. Occupational Medicine 51: 124–135

APPENDIX 17A *UK OCCUPATIONAL HEALTH GUIDELINES FOR THE MANAGEMENT OF LOW BACK PAIN AT WORK*

These guidelines represent the main recommendations and evidence statements derived from a detailed Evidence Review and developed by a multidisciplinary group of practitioners. They concern the occupational health management of workers with non-specific low back pain. They focus on actions to be taken to assist the individual and do not specifically cover legal issues, health and safety management, job design and ergonomics. They assume that a risk assessment has been conducted and used to define the control measures required, including the need for occupational health advice.

These guidelines complement and should be used in conjunction with the RCGP (1999) *Clinical Guidelines for the Management of Acute Low Back Pain* (Ch. 15).

The evidence and guidance is presented under a logical sequence of occupational health situations:

A. Background
B. Pre-placement assessment
C. Prevention
D. Assessment of the worker presenting with back pain
E. Management principles for the worker presenting with back pain
F. Management of the worker having difficulty returning to normal occupational duties at approximately 4–12 weeks

Summary

The evidence is weighted as follows:
*** Strong evidence – generally consistent findings in multiple, high quality scientific studies
** Moderate evidence – generally consistent findings in fewer, smaller or lower quality scientific studies
* Limited or contradictory evidence – one scientific study or inconsistent findings in multiple scientific studies
– No scientific evidence – based on clinical studies, theoretical considerations and/or clinical consensus

Notes

1. "LBP" within these guidelines means non-specific low back pain, unless stated otherwise.
2. "Worker" is used to describe all those in employment (including the self-employed, trainees and apprentices).
3. "Employer" is used as a collective term for all those with managerial responsibilities, including all types of employers, line managers, supervisors and their representatives.

Evidence statements for each situation are preceded by an introduction to the relevant issues and some important areas are given additional discussion. Full evidence tables and bibliography are available on www.facoccmed.ac.uk or in Waddell & Burton (2001).

A BACKGROUND

Non-specific low back pain (LBP) can be occupational in the sense that it is common in adults of working age, frequently affects capacity for work, and often presents for occupational health care. It is commonly assumed this means that LBP is *caused* by work but the relationship between the physical demands of work and LBP is complex and inconsistent. A clear distinction should be made between the presence of symptoms, the reporting of LBP, attributing symptoms to work, reporting "injury", seeking health care, loss of time from work and long term damage. LBP in the occupational setting must be seen against the high background prevalence and recurrence rates of low back symptoms, and to a lesser extent disability, among the adult population. Workers in heavy manual jobs do report rather more low back symptoms, but most people in lighter jobs or even those who are not working have similar symptoms. Jobs with greater physical demands commonly have a higher rate of reported low back injuries, but most of these "injuries" are related to normal everyday activities such as bending and lifting, there is usually little if any objective evidence of tissue damage (though clinical examination and current in vivo investigations may be insensitive tools to detect this), and the relationship between job demands and symptoms or injury rates is inconsistent. Physical stressors may overload certain structures in individual

A Background

Recommendation	Evidence

You, as an occupational health practitioner, have a professional duty to support the worker with LBP and should do so whether or not occupational factors play any role in causation.

Recommendation	Evidence
Make employers and workers aware that: ● LBP is common and frequently recurrent but acute attacks are usually brief and self-limiting ● Physical demands at work are one factor influencing LBP but are often not the most important ● Prevention and case management need to be directed at both physical and psychosocial factors	*** Most adults (60–80%) experience LBP at some time and it is often persistent or recurrent. It is one of the most common reasons for seeking health care and it is now one of the commonest health reasons given for work loss *** Physical demands of work (manual materials handling, lifting, bending, twisting, and whole body vibration) can be associated with increased reports of back symptoms, aggravation of symptoms and "injuries" * There is limited and contradictory evidence that the length of exposure to physical stressors at work (cumulative risk) increases reports of back symptoms or of persistent symptoms *** Physical demands of work (manual materials handling, lifting, bending, twisting, and whole body vibration) are a risk factor for the incidence (onset) of LBP, but overall it appears that the size of the effect is less than that of other individual, non-occupational and unidentified factors ** Physical demands of work play only a minor role in the development of disc degeneration *** Care-seeking and disability due to LBP depend more on complex individual and work-related psychosocial factors than on clinical features or physical demands of work
Establish a partnership, involving workers, employers and health professionals in the workplace and the community, with a common consistent approach to agreed goals, to manage back pain and prevent unnecessary disability	

cases but, in general, there is little evidence that physical loading in modern work causes permanent damage. Whether low back symptoms are attributed to work, are reported as "injuries", lead to health care seeking and/or result in time off work depends on complex individual psychosocial and work organisational factors. The development of chronic pain and disability depends more on individual and work-related psychosocial issues than on physical or clinical features. People with physically or psychologically demanding jobs may have more difficulty working when they have LBP, and so lose more time from work, but that can be the effect rather than the cause of their LBP.

In summary, physical demands of work can precipitate individual attacks of LBP, certain individuals may be more susceptible and certain jobs may be higher risk but, viewed overall, physical demands of work only account for a modest proportion of the total impact of LBP occurring in workers.

B PRE-PLACEMENT ASSESSMENT

Individual health, fitness and strength can affect the ability to perform tasks. Pre-placement assessment aims to identify those who may be at higher risk for LBP in a given occupational setting. The main factors that have been investigated include clinical and historical features, physical strength parameters and psychosocial factors. The recurrent nature of LBP means that previous history is the best predictor of future LBP, and all other

B Pre-placement assessment

Recommendation	Evidence
LBP is common and recurrent and is not a reason for denying employment in most circumstances. However care should be taken when placing individuals with a strong history of LBP in physically demanding jobs	
Enquire about previous history of LBP as part of the pre-placement assessment, in particular the frequency and duration of attacks, time since last attack, radiating leg pain, previous surgery and sickness absence due to LBP	*** The single, most consistent predictor of future LBP and work loss is a previous history of LBP, including in particular the frequency and duration of attacks, time since last attack, radiating leg pain, previous surgery and sickness absence due to LBP
Do not routinely include clinical examination of the back, lumbar X-rays, back function testing, general fitness or psychosocial factors in the pre-placement assessment	** Examination findings, including in particular height, weight, lumbar flexibility and straight leg raising (SLR), have little predictive value for future LBP or disability ** The level of general (cardiorespiratory) fitness has no predictive value for future LBP * There is limited and contradictory evidence that attempting to match physical capability to job demands may reduce future LBP and work loss *** X-ray and MRI findings have no predictive value for future LBP or disability *** Back-function testing machines (isometric, isokinetic or isoinertial measurements) have no predictive value for future LBP or disability *** For symptom-free people, individual psychosocial findings are a risk factor for the incidence (onset) of LBP, but overall the size of the effect is small
Placement should take account of the risk assessment and requirements under the Disability Discrimination Act 1995 to provide "suitable and reasonable" adjustments, but it is ultimately a question of professional judgement	

pre-placement measures have no predictive value at all, or only a weak and unreliable predictive value.

High risk patients/physically demanding jobs

There is a pragmatic argument that individuals at highest risk of LBP should not be placed in jobs that impose the greatest physical demands. The basic concern is that workers with physically (or psychologically) demanding work report rather more low back symptoms, have more work-related back "injuries" and lose more time off work with LBP. Even if physical demands of work may be a relatively modest factor in the primary *causation* of LBP (see Background above), people who have

LBP (for whatever cause) do have more difficulty managing physically demanding work. It may be argued, therefore, that avoiding putting people at highest risk of recurrent LBP and sickness absence into more physically demanding work would be in the interests of the individual worker, the employer and the total societal burden of LBP.

The problem is, a previous history of LBP simply identifies people who are more likely to have recurrent problems, but that has little to do with the job: they are probably likely to have such problems irrespective of which job they are recruited for – and even if they are not recruited. Indeed, those who remain unemployed may be at highest risk of all for chronic LBP and disability. Because a previous history of LBP is so common, it could exclude many people who are medically fit for most work. At the same time, all pre-placement assessment methods miss many people who may later develop LBP. There is no clear evidence for a threshold of what constitutes a strong history of LBP or excessive job demands. Most of the evidence is from a population-based perspective whilst pre-placement assessment must try to predict future risks for the individual, which is a different matter. It may be concluded that the present evidence base is insufficient for reliable selection of individuals for particular types of work. Attempts to match individual susceptibility for LBP against a risk assessment of the job (and reduction of the risk of injury to the lowest level "reasonably practicable") are therefore very much a question of judgement, and there is limited empirical evidence on their effectiveness. Refusal of employment on the basis of such judgements carries substantial personal, societal, legal and political implications, and may

need to take into account the requirement under the Dis-ability Discrimination Act 1995 to provide "suitable and reasonable" adjustments.

C   PREVENTION

Employers have a statutory and moral responsibility to safeguard the health, safety and welfare of workers, and to take reasonably practicable steps to prevent avoidable injuries. Over the last 50 years, there have been considerable reductions in the physical demands of most work and much effort has gone into ergonomic improvements: that has reduced many serious occupational health risks, but there is inconsistent evidence on whether or to what extent it has reduced occupational LBP. Low back symptoms are common and non-specific, physical demands of work are only one causal factor, and non-occupational and psychosocial issues are important, so it may be questionable to what extent

C Prevention

Recommendation	Evidence
Advise on current good working practices such as specified in the Manual Handling Regulations and associated guidance	
Do not recommend lumbar belts and supports or traditional biomedical education as methods of preventing LBP. There is insufficient evidence to advocate general exercise or physical fitness programmes	* There is contradictory evidence that various general exercise/physical fitness programmes may reduce future LBP and work loss; any effect size appears to be modest *** Traditional biomedical education based on an injury model does not reduce future LBP and work loss − There is preliminary evidence that educational interventions which specifically address beliefs and attitudes may reduce future work loss due to LBP *** Lumbar belts or supports do not reduce work-related LBP and work loss
Advise employers that high job satisfaction and good industrial relations are the most important organisational characteristics associated with low disability and sickness absence rates attributed to LBP	*** Low job satisfaction and unsatisfactory psychosocial aspects of work are risk factors for reported LBP, health care use and work loss, but the size of that association is modest
Encourage employers to: ● consider joint employer–worker initiatives to identify and control occupational risk factors ● monitor back problems and sickness absence due to LBP ● improve safety and develop a "safety culture"	* There is limited evidence but general consensus that joint employer–worker initiatives (generally involving organisational culture and high stakeholder commitment to identify and control occupational risk factors and improve safety, surveillance measures and "safety culture") can reduce the number of reported back "injuries" and sickness absences, but there is no clear evidence on the optimum strategies and inconsistent evidence on the effect size

occupational interventions can realistically be expected to reduce the societal impact of LBP. It seems reasonable in principle to attempt to reduce the incidence and prevalence of LBP by interventions designed to reduce known occupational "risk factors", but the fundamental limitation of this approach may be the lack of any clear causal link (see Background). Much depends on whether the target is reduction of symptoms, "injuries", sickness absence or long term disability: different interventions may well have differing effects. There is a lack of convincing evidence that it is possible substantially to reduce the incidence or prevalence of the symptom of LBP. Interventions to reduce physical workload have generally had an inconsistent impact on occupational LBP – when there has been an effect

it remains unclear if the interventions actually reduced "symptoms" or "injuries", or simply modified reporting patterns and altered what workers do about their LBP. Organisational change interventions, directed to improving job satisfaction and psychosocial aspects of work, are difficult to implement and there is conflicting evidence that they have any significant effect on health outcomes (though little of that evidence is specifically about LBP).

D   ASSESSMENT OF THE WORKER PRESENTING WITH BACK PAIN

There is general consensus that a simple clinical interview and examination can distinguish between simple back pain manageable at the primary care

D Assessment of the worker presenting with back pain

Recommendation	Evidence
Screen for serious spinal diseases and nerve root problems (see "Diagnostic Triage", Algorithm 15B.1)	** Screening for "red flags" and diagnostic triage is important to exclude serious spinal diseases and nerve root problems
Clinical examination may aid clinical management (RCGP 1999), but is of limited value in planning occupational health management or in predicting the vocational outcome	** Examination findings, including in particular height, weight, lumbar flexibility and SLR are of limited value in planning occupational health management or in predicting the prognosis of non-specific LBP.
Take a clinical, disability and occupational history, concentrating on the impact of symptoms on activity and work, and any obstacles to recovery and return to work	** Patients who are older (particularly > 50 years), have more prolonged and severe symptoms, have radiating leg pain, whose symptoms impact more on activity and work, and who have responded less well to previous therapy are likely to have slower clinical progress, poorer response to treatment and rehabilitation, and more risk of long term disability
Consider psychosocial "yellow flags" to identify workers at particular risk of developing chronic pain and disability (Ch. 15E). Use this assessment to instigate active case management at an early stage	*** Individual and work-related psychosocial factors play an important role in persisting symptoms and disability, and influence response to treatment and rehabilitation. Screening for "yellow flags" can help to identify those workers with LBP who are at risk of developing chronic pain and disability. Workers' own beliefs that their LBP was caused by their work and their own expectations about inability to return to work are particularly important
X-rays and scans are not indicated for the occupational health management of the patient with LBP	*** In patients with non-specific LBP, X-ray and MRI findings do not correlate with clinical symptoms or work capacity
Ensure that any incident of LBP which may be work-related is investigated and advice given on remedial action. If appropriate, review the risk assessment	

level and those pathological conditions requiring specialist referral ("red flags"). However, conventional clinical tests of spinal and neurological function are of limited value in determining appropriate clinical or occupational management of non-specific LBP. Furthermore, "diagnostic labelling" may have detrimental effects on outcome. X-rays and MRI are primarily directed to the investigation of nerve root problems and serious spinal pathology. Much more relevant to occupational health management is the identification of individual and work-related psychosocial issues which form risk factors for chronicity ("yellow flags"). General disaffection with the work situation, attribution of blame, beliefs and attitudes about the relationship between work and symptoms, job dissatisfaction and poor employer–employee relationships may also constitute "obstacles to recovery".

E　MANAGEMENT PRINCIPLES FOR THE WORKER PRESENTING WITH BACK PAIN

Clinical aspects of management should follow the RCGP (1999) clinical guidelines. Occupational health management should focus on supporting the worker with LBP and facilitating remaining at work or returning to work as rapidly as possible, and should deal with any occupational issues that may form obstacles to achieving these goals. Occupational health practitioners should liaise closely with primary care. All stakeholders (i.e., the worker with LBP, supervisor(s) and management, union and health and safety representatives, the occupational health team and other health professionals undertaking clinical management) need to work closely together with a common, consistent approach to agreed goals.

Return to work with back pain

Concern about return to work with residual symptoms is often expressed by workers themselves, their representatives, primary care health professionals, and occupational health professionals as well as supervisors and management, particularly if the LBP is attributed to work and if there is thought to be a risk of "reinjury". This concern is natural but illogical. A recent study has highlighted the variability in physician advice on return to work and that recommendations often reflect personal attitudes of the physicians and their perception of the severity of symptoms. Studies of the natural history show that LBP is commonly a persistent or recurrent problem, and most workers do continue working or return to work while symptoms are still present: if nobody returned to work till they were 100% symptom free only a minority would ever return to work. Epidemiological and clinical follow-up studies show that early return to work (or continuing to work) with some persisting symptoms does not increase the risk of "re-injury" but actually reduces recurrences and sickness absence over the following year. Conversely, the longer someone is off work the *lower* the chance of recovery. Undue caution will form an obstacle to return to work and lead to protracted sickness absence, which then aggravates and perpetuates chronic pain and disability, and actually increases the risk of a poor long term outcome: this clearly is not in the interest of either the worker or the employer. Concerns are also sometimes expressed about legal liability for "re-injury" if the worker returns to work before they are completely "cured" which is also illogical. Again, the natural history shows that LBP is commonly a persistent or recurrent problem, so expectations of "cure" are unrealistic and recurrences are likely irrespective of work status. Refusing to allow a worker to return to work because they still have some LBP increases the likelihood of a break-down in worker–employer relationships and of the worker making a claim; and the longer the sickness absence the higher the cost of any claim. Helping and supporting the worker to remain at work, or in early return to work, is in principle the most promising means of reducing future symptoms, sickness absence and claims. Reducing any legal liability is best achieved not by forcing the worker into protracted sickness absence and possibly an adversarial situation, but by addressing the issues of job reassessment ("newly assessed duties"), the provision of modified work with adequate support, and good worker–employer relationships. All of these goals may best be achieved by the proposed active rehabilitation programme and organisational interventions. That is also more in keeping with the spirit and the requirements of the Disability Discrimination Act.

E Management principles for the worker presenting with back pain

Recommendation	Evidence
Clinical Clinical management should follow the RCGP (1999) guidelines. Discuss expected recovery times, and the importance of continuing ordinary activities as normally as possible despite pain	*** Advice to continue ordinary activities of daily living as normally as possible despite the pain can give equivalent or faster symptomatic recovery from the acute symptoms, and leads to shorter periods of work loss, fewer recurrences and less work loss over the following year than "traditional" medical treatment (advice to rest and "let pain be your guide" for return to normal activity)
Ensure that workers with LBP receive the key information in a form they understand	** The above advice can be usefully supplemented by simple educational interventions specifically designed to overcome fear avoidance beliefs and encourage patients to take responsibility for their own self-care
Occupational Encourage the worker to remain in his or her job, or to return at an early stage, even if there is still some LBP – do not wait until they are completely pain-free. Consider the following steps to facilitate this: ● Initiate communication with their primary health care professional early in treatment and rehabilitation ● Advise the worker to continue as normally as possible and provide support to achieve this ● Advise employers on the actions required, which may include maintaining sympathetic contact with the absent worker ● Consider temporary adaptations of the job or pattern of work	** Communication, co-operation and common agreed goals between the worker with LBP, the occupational health team, supervisors, management and primary health care professionals is fundamental for improvement in clinical and occupational health management and outcomes *** Most workers with LBP are able to continue working or to return to work within a few days or weeks, even if they still have some residual or recurrent symptoms, and they do not need to wait till they are completely pain free * Advice to continue ordinary activities as normally as possible, in principle, applies equally to work. The scientific evidence confirms that this general approach leads to shorter periods of work loss, fewer recurrences and less work loss over the following year, although most of the evidence comes from intervention packages and the clinical evidence focusing solely on advice about work is limited * There is general consensus but limited scientific evidence that workplace organisational and/or management strategies (generally involving organisational culture and high stakeholder commitment to improve safety, provide optimum case management and encourage and support early return to work) may reduce absenteeism and duration of work loss

F MANAGEMENT OF THE WORKER HAVING DIFFICULTY RETURNING TO NORMAL OCCUPATIONAL DUTIES AT APPROXIMATELY 4–12 WEEKS

In general, the longer a worker is off work with LBP the more disabling the condition becomes, the less successful any form of treatment, and the greater the probability of long term sickness absence. This could be explained to some extent by selection bias in that those who are off work longer are simply those with a more severe problem. However, the clinical evidence suggests that there is little if any physical difference in their backs and intervention studies show that there is usually no insurmountable physical barrier to rehabilitation. There are strong logical and humanitarian arguments, and strong empirical evidence, that treatment at the sub-acute stage (approximately 4–12 weeks) is more effective at preventing chronic pain and disability

F Management of the worker having difficulty returning to normal occupational duties at approximately 4–12 weeks

Recommendation	Evidence
Ensure that workers, employers and primary care health professionals understand that the longer anyone is off work with LBP, the greater the risk of chronic pain and disability, and the lower their chances of ever returning to work Address the common misconception among workers and employers of the need to be pain-free before return to work. Some pain is to be expected and the early resumption of work activity improves the prognosis	*** The longer a worker is off work with LBP, the lower their chances of ever returning to work. Once a worker is off work for 4–12 weeks they have a 10–40% risk (depending on the setting) of still being off work at one year; after 1–2 years absence it is unlikely they will return to any form of work in the foreseeable future, irrespective of further treatment
Encourage the employer to establish a surveillance system to identify those off work with LBP for over 4 weeks so that appropriate action can be taken. Intervention at this stage is more effective than delaying and having to deal with established intractable chronic pain and disability	*** Various treatments for chronic LBP may produce some clinical improvement, but most clinical interventions are quite ineffective at returning people to work once they have been off work for a protracted period with LBP
Advise employers on ways in which the physical demands of the job can be temporarily modified to facilitate return to work	** From an organisational perspective, the temporary provision of lighter or modified duties facilitates return to work and reduces time off work — Conversely, there is some suggestion that clinical advice to return only to restricted duties may act as a barrier to return to normal work, particularly if no lighter or modified duties are available.
If medical treatment fails to produce recovery and return to work by 4–12 weeks, communicate and collaborate with primary health care professionals to shift the emphasis from dependence on symptomatic treatment to rehabilitation and self-management strategies	** Changing the focus from purely symptomatic treatment to an "active rehabilitation programme" can produce faster return to work, less chronic disability and less sickness absence. There is no clear evidence on the optimum content or intensity of such packages, but there is generally consistent evidence on certain basic elements. Such interventions are more effective in an occupational setting than in a health care setting
Where practicable, refer the worker who is having difficulty returning to normal occupational duties at 4–12 weeks to an active rehabilitation programme. Such a rehabilitation programme needs to be carefully designed to fit local circumstances and should consist of a multidisciplinary "package" of interventions	** A combination of optimum clinical management, a rehabilitation programme, and organisational interventions designed to assist the worker with LBP return to work, is more effective than single elements alone

than attempts to treat chronic, intractable pain and disability once it is established. There is strong evidence that intervention packages at the sub-acute stage *can* produce desirable occupational outcomes, and these efforts are likely to be more cost-effective (though there is only limited empirical evidence on costs and cost-effectiveness). There is therefore a convincing argument for intense efforts to get workers with LBP back to work before disability and sickness absence become protracted.

Rehabilitation programmes

Most of the above principles could be combined in an active rehabilitation programme, although there is wide variation, lack of clear definition and considerable confusion about exactly what constitutes an effective rehabilitation programme. Some forms of "back school" or "multidisciplinary rehabilitation" at the sub-acute stage have produced faster recovery of pain and disability, faster return to work and fewer recurrences over the following year than other treatments to which they have been compared. However, the results are inconsistent, probably because most studies are of packages of interventions of widely varying content and intensity. There is no clear evidence on the optimum content or intensity of such packages, although there is generally consistent evidence on certain basic elements.

Education alone is a relatively weak intervention. Traditional biomedical information and advice based on spinal anatomy, biomechanics and an injury model is largely ineffective but completely different information and advice, designed to overcome fear avoidance beliefs and promote self-responsibility and self-care, can produce positive shifts in beliefs and reduce disability.

All of the effective rehabilitation programmes have included a progressive active exercise and physical fitness element. Such exercise programmes can produce short-term improvement in pain and disability for sub-acute and chronic LBP, although there is no clear evidence that any specific type of exercise has any specific physical effect.

There are theoretical considerations and empirical evidence that most of the effective programmes are based on behavioural principles of pain management, but there are few studies which look at this approach in isolation. There is moderate evidence that these programmes are more effective in an occupational setting.

The interventions, resources and costs should be strictly controlled. There is insufficient evidence to justify intensive and expensive programmes and they are likely to be less cost effective. The rehabilitation programme should be closely audited and evaluated to check that it is effective and not having any unplanned adverse effects.

EVIDENCE GAPS IN OCCUPATIONAL HEALTH MANAGEMENT OF LBP

This review has found considerably more scientific evidence on the occupational health management of LBP than originally anticipated, despite the methodological problems in a workplace setting. There is sufficient evidence to permit a number of strong and moderate evidence statements and recommendations for occupational health management. However, this review has also identified inadequacies in the evidence in some important areas.

There is a need for further rigorously designed and carefully controlled studies (where appropriate by RCTs and with sub-categorisation of patients) on:

- Pre-placement assessment, particularly matching (strong) previous history of LBP, physical capabilities and job demands.
- "Innovative" education approaches to prevention and management specifically designed to overcome psychosocial issues (e.g. fear avoidance beliefs) and encourage patients to take responsibility for their own self-care.
- Company policies on accident prevention, "safety culture", surveillance and monitoring to reduce reported back "injuries" and claims.
- The relative benefits and costs of prescribing sick certification for LBP.
- Early interventions to overcome obstacles to recovery (e.g., focused clinical interventions targeting individual "yellow flags" for chronicity).
- The optimum combination and relative importance of individual components in an active rehabilitation programme.
- The optimum organisation, content and combination of case management, active rehabilitation and return to work programmes.

APPENDIX 17B PRELIMINARY DRAFT OF EUROPEAN COST B13 GUIDELINES FOR THE MANAGEMENT OF ACUTE NON-SPECIFIC LOW BACK PAIN IN PRIMARY CARE: APPENDIX ON BACK PAIN AND WORK

Maurits van Tulder (chairman), Annette Becker, Trudy Bekkering, Alan Breen, Tim Carter, Maria Teresa Gil del Real, Allen Hutchinson, Bart Koes, Peter Kryger-Baggesen, Even Laerum, Antti Malmivaara, Alf Nachemson, Wolfgang Niehus, Etienne Roux, Sylvie Rozenberg

These guidelines are directed at the management of back pain in primary health care settings. Effective collaboration with those providing occupational health services, managers responsible for defining the tasks undertaken at work and social security administrations may be required whenever back pain occurs in people of working age. This appendix outlines the contributions which good occupational health practice can make to back pain management and identifies where the evidence base for such practice can be found. Detailed guidelines are not presented as these will vary considerably between member states depending on the provisions for occupational health and social security.

Low back pain is a very common problem in people of working age. The physical demands of work can precipitate individual attacks of low back pain and the risks are higher in jobs where there is:

- heavy manual labour
- manual material handling
- awkward postures
- whole body vibration.

The demands of work may also influence the ease of return after an episode of pain (1).

However although work may be a contributory cause, it is not responsible for a large proportion of episodes of pain. Back pain is common in all occupations and is a major cause of absence from work and one of the leading reasons for long term incapacity and medical retirement. Thus employers and social security administrations should have a strong incentive to ensure that disability from back pain is minimised and to collaborate with primary care providers to secure effective case management.

Good occupational health practice for back pain management has been addressed in guidelines produced in the Netherlands (2), UK (3, 4, 5), Australia (6, 7), Japan (8), and USA (9).

The key evidence based principles for back pain management in the occupational health setting are:

- Recognising that selection at recruitment will not reduce incidence significantly. There is no evidence that clinical examination or diagnostic tests such as X-rays are valid predictors of future risk. Hence they have no place in routine pre-placement screening or selection.

- Understanding that while ergonomic measures will bring some benefits there are no well-validated preventative techniques. This means that some incidents of back pain in any workforce are inevitable.

- Ensuring that the need for an active approach to case management is understood by employees and employers and planning for this in anticipation of future incidents. The educational element in this would include a shared understanding that active management reduces pain and disability and that return to work before the person is pain free will often be the best way of speeding resolution of the discomfort.

- Securing a collaborative approach to case management with primary care providers as soon as possible after an incident of back pain in order to plan an early and effective return to work, with temporary modification to tasks or working arrangements if this is likely to hasten recovery.

- Arranging access to rehabilitation for anyone who has been away from work for more than four weeks.

IMPLICATIONS FOR PRIMARY CARE PROVIDERS

1. Giving a patient entitlement to absence from work because of non-specific back pain may be essential in severe cases but should be avoided where possible as it is likely to delay rather than hasten recovery.

2. Where there is occupational health provision led by a clinical health professional the provider of primary care is recommended to secure consent from the patient for an early discussion with the occupational health practitioner to agree a shared plan for case management. This should include arrangements for referral for rehabilitation if the pain persists and for prevention of return to work within four weeks.

3. Where there is no clinical occupational health service the primary care provider is recommended to review the options for collaboration on occupational aspects with the patient and liaise as appropriate to ensure that the principles outlined above are followed, if pain persists and prevents return to work.

4. If the patient is of working age but not in employment liaison with the social security, administration as specified in national regulations will be required. It will often be to the benefit of the patient to propose a treatment plan to the administration and obtain their support for it, especially in relation to access to rehabilitation services and retraining should this be needed.

References

1. Research on work related low back disorders. Luxembourg Office for Official Publications of the European Union (2000), ISBN 92 95007 02 6

2. Nederlandse Vereniging voor Arbeids- en Bedrijfsgeneeskunde. Handelen van de bedrijfsarts bij werknemers met lage rugklachten. Geautoriseerde richtlijn, 2 april 1999./Dutch Association for Occupational Medicine. Management by the occupational physician of employees with low back pain. Authorised Guidelines, April 2, 1999, ISBN 90 76721 01 7 [the Netherlands]

3. Carter J T, Birrell L N. Occupational Health Guidelines for the Management of Low Back Pain at Work: recommendations. Faculty of Occupational Medicine, London 2000, ISBN 1 86016 131 6 (also on www.facoccmed.ac.uk) [UK]

4. Waddell G, Burton A K. Occupational Health Guidelines for the Management of Low Back Pain at Work: evidence review. Faculty of Occupational Medicine, London 2000, ISBN 1 86016 131 6 (also on www.facoccmed.ac.uk) [UK]

5. Waddell G, Burton A K. Occupational Health Guidelines for the Management of Low Back Pain at Work: evidence review. Occup Med 2001; 51: 124–35 [UK]

6. Steven ID (ed.) Guidelines for the management of back-injured employees. Adelaide: South Australia Workcover Corporation 1993 [Australia]

7. Victorian Workcover Authority. Guidelines for the management of employees with compensable low back pain. Melbourne, Victorian Workcover Authority. 1993 and revised Edition 1996 [Australia]

8. Yamamoto S. Guidelines on Worksite Prevention of Low Back Pain Labour Standards Bureau Notification No. 57. Industrial Health 1997; 35: 143–172 [Japan]

9. Fordyce WE (ed.) Back Pain in the Workplace: Management of Disability in Non-specific Conditions. Seattle, IASP Press. 1995 [US – International]

APPENDIX 17C NEW ZEALAND ACC EMPLOYER'S GUIDE: *ACTIVE AND WORKING!*

AN OVERVIEW

These are the key steps to helping employees with acute low back pain stay in work. These simple strategies, explained in this guide, can help you minimise work loss and prevent ongoing problems.

FOREWORD

Nearly all adults experience back pain during their working lives. This common problem has become one of the leading causes of work loss in industrialised countries. It is clearly an expensive problem for our society, resulting in lost productivity and individual suffering.

The effective management of back pain has undergone one of the most radical changes

	Your employee can	As the employer, you can	The treatment provider can
Before a problem occurs		• Set up your systems • Identify advisors you can use • Prepare functional job descriptions	
Onset of pain (up to 1 week)	• Use self-help approach • Take simple pain relief • Stay active and modify activities if necessary	• Encourage early reporting of pain	
Report pain (up to 1 week)	• Report pain if tasks or safety affected • Tell work about difficult tasks	• Activate your systems • Respond quickly with modified tasks/hours • Review any worksite factors involved • Make recommended changes • Be aware of "flags" and serious symptoms • Keep records	
Seek treatment (if no improvement)	• Stay active and at work • Follow treatment advice about work tasks and hours, activities, pain relief	• Foster "stay in work" approach • Identify suitable tasks and hours • Assign someone to keep in touch	• Check for Red Flags • Encourage to "stay in work" • Reassure and explain • Advise on work tasks and hours, activities, pain relief
If off work	• Keep in touch with work • Attend work meetings and social events • Stay active	• Set return to work plan • Get occupational advice if needed • Keep in touch – weekly • Liaise with treatment providers – advise of available tasks	• Set return to work plan • Encourage activity • Refer for expert treatment • Identify and address Yellow Flags
Return to work	• Gradually increase hours and tasks • Continue as many usual activities as possible	• Start graded return to work plan • Get occupational advice if needed	• Review regularly • Encourage activity • Address ongoing Yellow Flags
Ongoing symptoms (4–12 weeks)	• Tell work about tasks that are still difficult • Stop unhelpful treatment • Consider work options	• Suggest all parties meet to discuss employment options	• Intensify return to work efforts • Stop unhelpful treatments • Use people with expertise in workplace rehabilitation • Liaise with Case Manager

witnessed in the history of modern health care. Traditional concepts emphasising bed rest and passive treatment have been demonstrated as ineffective by high quality scientific research. Instead it has been shown that keeping a person as active as possible in their normal life is the most effective method of managing the problem. The role of the workplace in facilitating rapid rehabilitation has therefore become a principal focus.

It is now inappropriate to think of work merely as a place to return to once a person is fully recovered. We know that the workplace is integral to the rehabilitation process. Employers (through managers and supervisors) have a critical role in providing the opportunity for a person with back pain to maintain their work habits and daily routine through the temporary provision of a safe and accommodating workplace.

Dr Nicholas Kendall
Chairman – Acute Low Back Pain Expert Panel

In this guide …

- What is acute low back pain about?
- Employers are key players
- You can help speed recovery
- When should you get involved?
- An update on current treatment
- Everyone has a role to play
- Workplace checklist

Low backs can be a pain

Acute low back pain is very common and causes significant costs in terms of suffering, lost work time and profitability, treatment and compensation. But the latest findings from around the world show that acute low back pain can be effectively managed. And one of the most important key players is you – the employer.

This guide brings you up to date information, and outlines strategies you can use in your workplace to minimise the impact on both your business and your employees. You might find some of it quite surprising – ideas on how to manage acute low back pain have undergone a radical reversal.

We have focused entirely on the management of acute low back pain – rather than covering prevention. Why? Quite simply because, unlike with

serious injuries, acute low back pain is common and it's almost impossible to prevent. And unfortunately it often results in lost work time – even when the pain didn't start at work.

The good news is that quick action and proper management works – and in most cases improvement is relatively quick. It doesn't have to become an ongoing problem for you and your employee.

The prevention and management of serious back injuries remains an important issue for employers. However, a full discussion of serious back injuries is beyond the scope of this guide.

Active and working helps backs best! We now know that staying active and at work, even if tasks have to be modified for a time, helps people recover better and more quickly. And of course faster recovery means less work time lost – so everyone benefits.

WHAT IS ACUTE LOW BACK PAIN ABOUT?

Acute low back pain is common (nine out of ten people will feel it at some time) but it's not usually serious. Where once the advice given was to lie down and rest, it is now clear that staying active and at work, if possible, is extremely important – it helps speed the recovery process. Scientific views on acute low back pain and its management have changed dramatically. Here's a quick overview.

How does it happen?

The reasons are not clear, although there are some known risk factors. People may associate the onset of acute low back pain with work, sport or home activities – or it can occur for no particular reason. It often starts during an everyday activity that has not caused pain before. A small proportion of acute low back pain begins due to an accident such as slipping or falling.

What are the risk factors?

There have been many studies and there is a lot of debate over risk factors. All that we can confidently state is that there can be a range of causes and often there is no definable event at all.

There is some evidence that heavy work, lots of lifting and forceful movements, bending and twisting, and a lot of driving are risk factors. Heredity, gender and build make little difference. Keeping fit, not smoking and avoiding excess weight may help prevent acute low back pain – but are more likely to have a greater impact on recovery than prevention.

Is it serious?

In most cases it's not possible to give a specific diagnosis – and the term "non-specific" is often used to describe the condition. In fact, exact diagnosis isn't necessary for effective management in most cases. Serious back injuries or disease are not common. Serious conditions are easily detected and usually require specialist treatment. This guide only covers non-specific acute low back pain.

What is the impact?

Non-specific acute low back pain can cause quite high levels of pain and difficulty with daily tasks. But the presence of pain doesn't mean that work and activity are harmful (research shows the opposite). The pain is usually self-limiting, so your employee may not be able to do some tasks for a short time. But severe symptoms won't last long and usually improve in a few days, or a few weeks at most. During this time the way you assist your employee can have a marked effect on their recovery.

What can I do?

As an employer you have a key role in helping staff to recover quickly. In the severe stages most people benefit from advice and strategies to help them

- report their pain appropriately
- seek suitable treatment
- modify or continue their work.

Someone with acute low back pain also needs support and reassurance – they may be worried about their job. If they do need time off work, it's important to keep in touch.

Of course how acute low back pain is managed in the workplace depends on the tasks the person usually does, what they can cope with and their treatment provider's advice.[1] The most important thing is that it is managed. This has benefits for both your staff and your business.

Taking control benefits everyone. As an employer you have a key role. Managing acute low back pain in the workplace benefits your staff and your business. It can cut the cost of lost work time and productivity and helps reduce extra costs such as recruitment, retraining and compensation.

EMPLOYERS ARE KEY PLAYERS

As an employer you have a key role in helping staff recover quickly from acute low back pain. Assisting staff to stay at work – or to return as soon as they can – helps the recovery process and reduces the cost to your business.

How does work help?

Research shows that people who are off work for long periods are less likely to return to work than those who are only off work for a short time, or who stay at work doing modified tasks.

Work is important to recovery for many reasons. For instance it can provide purpose, a sense of identity, social contacts, the opportunity to develop skills and financial security. So the best thing you can do is to help your employee stay at work – or to return as early as possible if they need time off.

But does it help me?

Keeping people at work, or speeding their return, is good for business – and it can help reduce costs. The cost of lost work time and compensation can be easily measured, but there are also hidden costs such as recruitment, retraining and lost productivity to consider. And of course ongoing lost work time can affect the risk assessment for your workplace or industry – and your premium.

What do I need to do?

The workplace is extremely important in ensuring an early and safe return to work. You can't just leave it up to the employee or their treatment provider – everyone needs to work closely together.

---

[1] By treatment provider we mean a doctor, nurse, physiotherapist, chiropractor, osteopath or Maori healer.

The workplace environment is vital. You need to

- have good management systems in place before the problem occurs
- show a commitment and interest in helping staff stay at work, or return early
- provide options for modified work tasks[2] and a gradual return to work[3]
- foster co-operation between the treatment provider, workplace and employee.

Identifying and managing the factors that can delay or stop people returning to work are also important. Once slow recovery was put down to the physical demands of work. Now there is a lot of information to show that psychosocial factors are also influential.

Studies show that people have less time off work – for any reason – when the workplace is friendly and supportive, when tasks are varied, demands are reasonable and there is a good level of job satisfaction.

What can I do now?

Having good systems in place will help you manage the situation better when a problem does occur – whether it's acute low back pain or another injury or illness.

Here are some steps you can take now:

- Create a work environment that enables staff to ask for help. Make sure they know that you are willing to provide modified work tasks so they can stay at work

- Set up systems for reporting and recording cases – and for communication between all parties. Everyone needs to be clear about when and how to report a problem – and what their roles are

- Nominate someone to manage cases. This could be someone like a human resources or health and safety professional, or someone external like a case manager or occupational therapist

- Identify a treatment provider who can act in an advisory role – someone who knows the issues in your workplace and who can provide staff with workplace-based guidance

- Prepare functional job descriptions with lists of alternative tasks that can be given to treatment providers as needed. You may want to seek professional help with this.

Can I prevent back pain occurring?

Injury prevention programmes that focus on reducing employees' exposure to very heavy loads, extreme bending and twisting, excessive whole-body vibration, and falls from a height can help prevent serious back injuries. However, studies show it's almost impossible to prevent the more common "acute low back pain" because there are many factors involved. But the condition can be managed to help stop it becoming an ongoing problem for you and your employee.

It's also essential to investigate any workplace situation that may have contributed to the problem – so the person can do their job and to help prevent things getting worse. When problems do arise there is usually a chain of events, such as stressful deadlines, increased work loads and other workplace hazards – so you may need to address more than one factor to make your workplace safe.

The management of low back pain at work is most likely to be successful in a workplace where priority is given to health and safety at all levels of the organisation.

---

[2] A modified work task could mean a change in the task itself – or how long it is done for – but the change is made with the intention that it is not permanent and the person will return to full duties.

Other terms commonly used to mean the same include alternative, transitional, or light duties.

[3] A gradual or graded return to work could mean gradually increasing the hours at work each day – or attending for normal hours but working intermittently, say every second hour, for a while.

YOU CAN HELP SPEED RECOVERY

Here is a summary of the most important things you can do to promote recovery once acute low back pain has occurred. There may be non-work factors you can't control that will slow recovery – but you can make up for this by intensifying efforts in the areas you do have control over.

Identify and modify "difficult" tasks

Pain may make some tasks too difficult to do for a while. Not everyone is affected the same, so you'll need to consider what your employee tells you they can do and what their treatment provider recommends. Generally the most difficult tasks involve heavy work, lots of lifting and forceful movements, bending and twisting, or a lot of driving.

Encourage graded return to work

If your employee needs time off, a graded return can help them get back to work sooner. You may need professional help to work out a plan. A good plan usually sets out hours and tasks as well as what progress can be expected. Some people insist on working even if they are getting worse. Modified tasks may help in these cases. Discuss this with them and enlist the help of their treatment provider if necessary.

Modify the plan if necessary

If progress is slower than expected you may need to modify the plan. The treatment provider or case manager may be able to help.

Address workplace factors

It's important to address workplace factors that may have been involved in the onset of pain:

- Investigate accidents or injuries immediately
- Make changes to minimise future problems – expert advice may help
- Have clear health and safety policies – and follow them.

Keep in touch

Assign someone to keep in weekly contact with your employee (maybe their manager or the person your company has nominated to look after cases). If they're off work ask co-workers to also call them each week. Let them know their work is valued and you're looking forward to their return. Invite them to staff training, meetings, morning tea and social events. Encourage them to return.

Can you see the progress? Reducing pain is one measure of improvement. But changes you are more likely to see first include ability to work longer and do more tasks, more periods of comfort, better morale, and a feeling of improved strength and fitness. An action plan can help make progress more visible to the person with low back pain. It should include simple goals (like being able to do the dishes or go to a movie) and activities which can bring relief (like listening to music and walking).

Talk with the treatment provider

Contact with the person treating your employee is important, especially if recovery is delayed. Let them know what work tasks are available and seek their advice on suitable tasks and a return to work plan. This is where having a pre-prepared functional job description comes in handy. You can expect the treatment provider to carry out regular reviews, especially if someone is off work. If you're concerned about how long someone is off work (two weeks could be too long) call the treatment provider. If you're concerned about your employee's progress, suggest they visit their treatment provider again, or call them yourself.

Create the right environment

Studies show that people are less likely to have time off (for any reason) when

- their job content is well defined, demands are reasonable, tasks are varied and there is a good level of job satisfaction
- the workplace is friendly, there is good support from co-workers and there are no conflicts with other staff or supervisors.

Watch for those who need extra support

There are some people who find it harder to get back to work. They may have had back pain before, think work will harm their back, do heavy work or not always enjoy their job. It's important to keep a special eye out for these people – and it may help to call in a treatment provider early if you think the person needs extra support.

If improvement is much slower than expected, ask for a meeting between yourself, your employee, their case manager and treatment provider to help sort out any underlying issues. Around four weeks is a good time to do this if your employee is still off work.

Some points to remember

- Acute low back pain is common
- The exact causes are unclear, although there are some known risk factors
- The best treatment is to stay active and at work – with temporary modifications if needed
- There are many factors, physical and non-physical, that can affect returning to work
- The workplace has a key role to play in helping people stay at work or return early.

Making contact with treatment providers can be tricky. It's good to contact the treatment provider and show your support by explaining the options at your workplace. If you want to discuss the employee you'll need to involve them in the process, and you'll need consent to share health or personal information. If there's a problem it's best to contact the case manager (if one has been assigned) so they can work with everyone to try and resolve things.

Take an active role. Support and encouragement to work can speed recovery. Just waiting until your employee is pain-free, or leaving it all up to the treatment provider can slow it down.

WHEN SHOULD YOU GET INVOLVED?

Early intervention is the key to successfully managing acute low back pain. There are many simple strategies that can be used to help recovery and prevent a claim. It's also important to know when seeking treatment and making a claim is the best course of action.

When do you need to know?

You need a system in place to encourage your employees to report acute low back pain early. Early reporting and management can help prevent problems and claims. As a simple guide, staff should report their pain as soon as they can't complete work tasks or carry them out safely – or if their pain is getting worse. This is important even if the pain started outside work. Although non-work related pain won't affect your premiums, it can still affect your employees' safety and productivity at work. Staff should be clear about when and how to let you know there is a problem.

What do you need to do next?

Most people will try some form of self-management first (such as taking pain medication). So reporting their pain means that they are telling you they need help. Quick action at this stage can speed the recovery process and prevent problems. The most important early steps you can take include

- modifying tasks that are difficult to do
- addressing workplace factors involved
- encouraging the employee to stay in work.

You may require specialised help with rehabilitation advice and workplace assessments. Large companies often have on-site occupational health nurses or doctors who can provide these services. Other businesses may need to seek advice from treatment providers.

When should treatment advice be sought?

If you have taken steps to modify tasks or hours and this doesn't bring improvements you need to encourage your employee to seek treatment advice. Remember some people will continue on regardless and this puts them at risk of an ongoing problem – so you need to take an active role.

We're not suggesting you should make decisions related to someone seeking treatment – but it's important that you know what to look out for. Your employee definitely needs to seek advice from a treatment provider if they mention the following symptoms:

- Severe, worsening low back pain despite efforts to relieve it
- Generally feeling unwell
- Difficulty with bowel or bladder control
- Numbness in the groin
- Unsteadiness when walking
- Pins and needles or pain in the leg.

How can the treatment provider help?

Unfortunately there is no "quick fix" for acute low back pain. The treatment provider can provide reassurance and encouragement to continue normal activities. And they can advise on pain relief, treatment, appropriate exercise and modifying activities (your functional job description will help them make decisions about suitable work tasks). They'll also check for any serious problems.

There are also treatment providers who specialise in occupational or workplace advice. They can help by assessing the physical tasks your employee can do and matching them to your worksite – and with "work hardening" programmes to help the employee regain their strength.

If your employee is off work or not recovering well you need to liaise with them and their treatment provider. Everyone needs to work together closely to monitor progress and deal with problems quickly.

Here's a couple of tricky issues…

What if recovery is delayed?

Sometimes, despite everyone's efforts, your employee may not be able to return to their old job. You need to arrange a case meeting to identify what they can and can't do. You may need a treatment provider with specialist skills to help with this. It may be a good idea for the employee to have a support person or a union representative present. The outcome might be that you can offer your employee an alternative job. If not, you can still help them on the road to recovery by liaising with the case manager and helping your employee to find a new job.

Should you employ someone with back pain?

Some employers are concerned about taking on people who have had back pain in the past. But low back pain is very common and not usually serious. And whilst many people have more than one episode of pain it is usually short-lived. With good health and safety procedures in your workplace a recurrence, if any, should have a minimal effect. So it makes better sense to employ the best person for the job than to be overly concerned about whether back pain will recur.

Is it a claim? There can be many factors involved in acute low back pain – it's not always due to injury. The treatment provider must decide if their patient should make a claim by considering all the circumstances surrounding the onset of pain and taking a fair view.

AN UPDATE ON CURRENT TREATMENT

Treatment is only one aspect of managing acute low back pain – but it can be an important one. Here we explain the current "state of the art" treatment for acute low back pain. This information can help you support your employee. If their treatment seems markedly different or things are not improving it's important to ask how you can help – and to take an active role. A co-operative approach between you, your employee and their treatment provider will provide the best results.

The first visit – what happens?

The treatment provider will examine your employee and take their history. They will try and identify the circumstances relating to the onset of pain.

If there are indicators of a serious problem (Red Flags), the treatment provider may investigate further with blood tests or X-rays for example – or refer your employee to a specialist. There's no need for X-rays or scans in the first four weeks unless there are Red Flags.

If the acute low back pain is not due to a serious problem the best treatment will be

- assurance and explanation
- advice to continue usual activities at home
- advice to continue work if appropriate
- simple pain relief (paracetamol and anti-inflammatories)
- manipulation (in the first four to six weeks only).

Work activities or hours may need to be modified. Some home activities may also need to be modified but should be continued where possible. Bed rest for more than two days is not recommended.

What are Red and Yellow Flags?

Red Flags help identify potentially serious conditions. Yellow Flags indicate psychosocial barriers to recovery.

Red Flags include...	Yellow Flags include...
• Severe worsening pain, especially at night • Significant trauma (such as a fall from height) • Problems controlling legs, bladder, bowel • Numbness in the groin • Weight loss, history of cancer, fever • Use of intravenous drugs or prescribed steroids (for example asthma drugs)	• Belief that pain and activity are harmful • "Sickness behaviours" (like extended rest) • Low or negative moods, social withdrawal • Treatment that doesn't fit "best practice" • Problems with claim and compensation • History of back pain, time off, other claims • Problems at work, poor job satisfaction • Heavy work, unsociable hours • Overprotective family – or lack of support

What about ongoing treatment?

The treatment provider, you and the employee should work together to ensure that things improve as expected. Regular review is important, particularly if the symptoms are severe, activity is severely limited, there is a history of recurrent pain or there are barriers to recovery.

If the symptoms persist and don't reduce in intensity after four weeks, a full reassessment is needed. This should include a history and examination, screening for Red and Yellow Flags, appropriate investigations, ongoing treatment and X-rays. Scans and surgery are usually not required unless there are Red Flags.

What if the pain recurs?

Many people have more than one episode of acute low back pain. This doesn't mean that it's serious, although the pain may be severe and limit activity. There is strong evidence that the symptoms will pass quickly and that staying in work, with modified tasks if necessary, is the best treatment.

Once the presence of Red Flags has been eliminated it's okay to take simple pain medication and keep going – it won't cause harm. But it's still important to try and improve workplace factors that aggravate pain.

EVERYONE HAS A ROLE TO PLAY

Acute low back pain impacts on a number of life areas. Most people will need support from a variety of sources during their recovery.

What can the employee do?

Your employee can help themselves by

- taking control of the problem
- staying as active as possible
- reporting their low back pain early
- identifying the tasks and hours they can do
- seeking treatment if they need it
- following the advice in the Patient Guide to Acute Low Back Pain Management
- keeping in touch if they are off work.

What can you do as the employer?

You need to be proactive in ensuring your employee gets the best available help, gets back to work as soon as possible and has a safe work environment to come back to.

This means that you need to

- set up clear reporting and recording systems
- address circumstances that lead to low back pain
- make "staying in work" part of your health and safety policy
- assign someone to keep in touch with your employee and their treatment provider
- tell the treatment provider about available work tasks
- know where to get advice on rehabilitation and return to work plans.

What is the role of treatment providers?

Treatment providers can help people stay in work by

- giving "best practice" advice based on the evidence

- assessing work tasks and encouraging people to stay at work
- liaising with employers and case managers
- reviewing their patient's progress regularly
- referring patients for expert treatment if they don't improve.

Who else can help?

Case managers usually get involved if someone is off work. They can help with queries about claims and payments, tell you who can help with rehabilitation and return to work plans, and liaise between everyone involved in supporting the person with the back pain.

Your employee's partner and family can provide support and encouragement to keep your employee active and at work, and ensure they stick to their treatment programme.

Co-workers and colleagues have an important role. Studies show that support from co-workers can help people return to work faster. Encourage your staff to stay in touch with people who are off work.

WORKPLACE CHECKLIST

Are you committed to health and safety at all levels of your organisation?

Is there anything you can do to improve the work environment?

Do you have clear reporting and recording procedures for accidents, injury, illness?

Is supporting staying in work/early return a company policy?

Do you know who can help with workplace assessment and return to work plans?

When an employee reports acute low back pain...

Do you review the circumstances leading up to the acute low back pain?

Do you implement recommended changes to job tasks, content or worksite?

Could the employee stay in work doing normal tasks – or with modified tasks or hours if necessary?

Have you let the treatment provider know about the range of tasks available?

Have you assigned someone to keep in touch?

Has the "Action plan" in the *Patient Guide to Acute Low Back Pain Management* been completed?

If your employee is off work...

Can you implement a graded return to work plan?

Do you keep in regular contact?

Is the treatment provider doing regular reviews?

Have you sought expert advice on workplace-based rehabilitation?

If return to work is proving difficult have you suggested a meeting with everyone involved?

Has the "Return to work plan" in the *Patient Guide to Acute Low Back Pain Management* been completed?

APPENDIX 17D WORKING BACKS SCOTLAND SHEET FOR EMPLOYERS

Low back pain evidence-based recommendations

Employers

(www.workingbacksscotland.com)

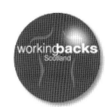

Take back pain seriously whatever its cause; it is the largest reported reason for sickness absence but it need not be.

Help the back pain sufferer to stay at work. Consider temporarily adapting job demands if necessary.

If sickness absence occurs, keep in touch and discuss how you can help the worker with back pain return to work as soon as possible.

Make sure you are not contributing to the problem; revise your risk assessments and take appropriate action.

Encourage early reporting of back pain and monitor sickness absences to help identify and deal with workplace issues.

Talk with the worker with back pain and those providing treatment to discuss how you can help.

Ensure you comply with health and safety legislation. Review your risk identification and assessment systems.

Establish partnerships with local GP's, nurses, therapists and occupational health services to provide quick access to advice and support.

Involve your employees and their health and safety representatives to help you develop better plans to manage back pain and reduce its effect in the workplace. Consider initiatives to identify workplace factors and devise and review strategies for return to work.

From Working Backs Scotland, with permission.

Chapter **18**

Rehabilitation

Gordon Waddell   Paul J. Watson

Rehabilitation is now flavor of the month, and everyone wants to jump on the bandwagon. But what exactly is "rehabilitation"? Despite what many doctors and therapists assume, it is not just health care. Nor better health care. Nor even earlier and more efficient delivery of health care. There is a strong argument for better, more timely, and more effective health care for back pain, but that is a separate issue. Health care and rehabilitation share some common goals, but there are differences in emphasis and in the means of reaching these goals (Table 18.1).

At the simplest level, the goal of health care is to make people better; the goal of rehabilitation is to enable them to return to normal activities. These goals overlap. Most patients with back pain do get better and return to their normal activities and work. So we can argue that routine clinical care does "rehabilitate" many patients, especially those who get better quickly. But the link is weak, especially for those who do not recover rapidly. For them, clinical improvement is not the same as recovery. Some patients get relief and even stop health care, but do not return to work. So "successful" clinical management may fall short of rehabilitation. Other people remain at work or return to work despite con- tinued symptoms and even if health care fails to give relief. So rehabilitation does not always depend on health care.

Thus, disability and rehabilitation are not just medical matters. The new *International Classification of Functioning* (ICF) is based on the biopsychosocial model of illness (WHO 2000). It helps to explain the

Table 18.1   The different emphasis of health care and rehabilitation

Health care	Rehabilitation
● Back pain is a symptom	● Disability is restricted activity
● Health care aims to make people better	● Rehabilitation aims to restore normal function
● Therapy is directed to relief of symptoms	● Rehabilitation usually requires a combination of
● Clinical management is directed to symptoms *and* disability	clinical, psychosocial, and work-related interventions
● Everyone expects that relief of symptoms will let	● Restoration of function is addressed directly
patients return to normal activities	● The most important outcome measure of rehabilitation
● The main clinical outcome measures are pain,	for back pain is sustained return to regular work
self-reported disability, and satisfaction with care	

origins and effects of disability. It acknowledges that disease influences the level of physical activity and social participation. But it also sets the rehabilitation agenda firmly in a social setting (Wade & de Jong 2000):

● Maximize the patient's participation in his or her social setting.
● Minimize the patient's pain and distress.
● Minimize the stress on the patient's family and work.

Trade unions define rehabilitation as *"any method by which people with a sickness or injury (that interferes with their ability to work to their normal or full capacity) can be returned to work"* (TUC 2000). They stress that no profession has a monopoly on rehabilitation and a multidisciplinary approach is almost always best. "This can involve medical or other treatment, vocational rehabilitation or retraining, adaptations to the work environment or working patterns".

Rehabilitation is now well established for conditions like stroke. Neurologists accept their responsibility to extend clinical care into rehabilitation. However, such "clinical" rehabilitation is mainly at the level of self-care and independent living. It is more difficult to apply this approach to a problem like back pain and to vocational outcomes. Nevertheless, there does seem to be an emerging consensus (adapted from Nocon & Baldwin 1998):

● The general aim of rehabilitation is to restore (to the maximum degree possible) function (physical or mental) and role participation (within the family, social network, or workforce).

● Back pain is most of a problem in adults of working age. The major impact for the individual and his or her family, for society, and economically is on capacity for work. (Chronic intractable pain that interferes with self-care is less common and is really a different problem.) Thus, in back pain, the most important goal and outcome measure of rehabilitation is capacity for work.

● Rehabilitation usually requires a combination of therapeutic, psychosocial, and work-related interventions that address the clinical problem *and* issues in the individual's physical and social environment.

● Rehabilitation services need to: be responsive to users' needs and wishes; be goal-directed; involve a number of agencies and disciplines; and be available when required.

● Rehabilitation is often a function of services: it is not necessarily a separate service.

This leads to a very different way of thinking (Table 18.2). In "old think," rehabilitation was a mechanistic process of "physical medicine." In "new think," it is a comprehensive social process. Patients used to be the recipients of a professional intervention. They were taken out of normal social life, rehabilitated, and then returned to work. Now, patients should be in the lead role, being enabled to get on with their lives. Employers used to contract out rehabilitation to health professional(s) and hand over responsibility. Now, rehabilitation is an occupational health issue. It is goal-directed, it is sited in or linked to the workplace, and the employer retains responsibility.

Table 18.2   Models of vocational rehabilitation

Old think	New think
Form of medical care	Partnership of patient, employer, and health professional(s)
Delivered by health professional(s)	Combined approach and responsibility of patient, employer, and health professional(s)
Delivered in a health care setting (usually secondary or tertiary care)	Delivered in or linked to the workplace
Focus on progressive exercise	Focus on increasing physical activity and overcoming obstacles to return to work
Discharged when package of care completed	Graded return to work and may need some continued support

TIMING

In the bad old days, rehabilitation was a separate, second stage after "proper" treatment was complete. Rehabilitation dealt with any residual "permanent impairment." In other words, rehabilitation was for when clinical management had failed. When we finally admitted there was "nothing more we could do," we got rid of these patients by referring them for rehabilitation. Too many clinicians still think this way, but it is no longer acceptable. Clinical management and rehabilitation go together. *Every doctor and therapist who treats back pain must be interested in rehabilitation. Failure to do so amounts to professional negligence.*

Throughout this book, we have emphasized the importance of timing. Clinical and psychosocial status changes over time. The passage of time is fundamental to the development of chronic disability and long-term incapacity. It involves biopsychosocial changes that may all influence further clinical progress and response to treatment. They may form obstacles to recovery, and these obstacles change over time. So when we provide rehabilitation is critical. And we must tailor the rehab intervention to suit the point in the time-course of sickness absence.

At the acute stage, most patients will recover rapidly and uneventfully with minimal intervention.

All they require is good clinical management and good information and advice on restoring function. Provided you check that your patients are managing to return to their ordinary activities and to work, there is no need for formal rehabilitation. The time to start thinking of rehabilitation is at about 3–6 weeks' sickness absence. Please note – weeks, not months or years. All patients who still have difficulty returning to ordinary activities at 3–6 weeks are at risk of chronic incapacity. That is when they need rehabilitation. It is also when it is likely to be easiest, most effective, and cost-effective (Frank et al 1996, 1998, Waddell & Burton 2000, Staal et al 2002). Once patients are on long-term incapacity and have lost their jobs, rehabilitation becomes much more difficult (Waddell et al 2002). In principle, rehabilitation should still be possible and worthwhile. However, the obstacles to return to work are much greater and harder to overcome. For all these reasons, rehabilitation at 1–6 months is likely to be most effective.

Von Korff (1999) and Von Korff & Moore (2001) described a "stepped-care approach" based on functional progress (Table 18.3). It starts with simple, low-intensity, low-cost measures and "steps up" the intensity of intervention till the patient does manage to return to normal activities.

It is clearly logical to direct more intensive resources to those patients who need it most, but there is little hard evidence. One study by Haldorsen et al (2002) confirms the value of this approach in patients with musculoskeletal pain who were sicklisted for at least 8 weeks. They divided the patients into three groups with good, medium, or poor prognosis for return to work. They then randomized them to usual medical care, a light multidisciplinary program, or an intensive multidisciplinary program. Those with a good prognosis returned to work as well with usual care as with a rehab program. Those with medium prognosis returned to work equally well with either light or intensive rehab. Those with poor prognosis returned to work better with the intensive rehab program.

MANAGING SYMPTOMS

The focus of rehabilitation is, rightly, to restore function. That is sometimes taken to mean ignore the pain or focus on function *despite* pain, but we

Table 18.3   A stepped-care approach (adapted from Von Korff & Moore 2001)

Step 1	Most patients at the acute stage	Identify and address the common worries of patients with back pain Simple, symptomatic measures Information and advice to encourage the resumption of ordinary activities
Step 2	The substantial minority of patients who do not resume ordinary activities by 3–6 weeks with simple advice	Brief, structured interventions that help patient to identify obstacles to recovery, set functional goals, and develop plans to achieve them. Provide support for physical exercise and return to ordinary activities
Step 3	The small minority of patients who have persisting disability in work or family life and who require more intensive intervention	Address dysfunctional beliefs and behavior A progressive exercise or graded-activity program Enable and support patients to return to ordinary activities

believe that is wrong. Pain and function are *both* important. When patients seek health care for back pain, their main desire is relief of pain. Relief of pain is the primary goal of clinical management. Pain is also one of the main limits on performance. Patients are unlikely to engage in rehabilitation if they feel the doctor or therapist is making light of their symptoms or suggesting they should be ignored. That may make patients angry or lose confidence in the clinician. So control of pain is the essential first step to engage the patient in rehabilitation and in raising activity levels.

This is actually a similar approach to pain management programs (Spanswick & Million 2000), which focus on function but make sure the analgesic regime has been optimized first.

It really does not matter how we achieve control of pain – whether by better analgesia, manual therapy, or more invasive procedures – so long as they are evidence-based. But it is very important how we present it to the patient. It must be clear that control of symptoms is not the final solution. It is only the means to an end – restoring normal function. Too often, patients get the impression that pain relief is the "clever" part of their treatment, particularly if it involves technical and invasive procedures. Too often, patients remain the passive recipients of treatment. That destroys the whole philosophy of rehabilitation. As we have already discussed, patients only reach this stage because purely symptomatic treatment has failed. So, by this stage, pain relief is no longer sufficient *in itself*, and should not be used in isolation. The aim of adequate pain control is to create a window of opportunity for

rehabilitation. Everyone – doctor, therapist, and patient – must agree a clear rehabilitation plan beforehand. That plan must not get derailed by repeated symptomatic interventions, which only divert patient and health professionals from the real goal of rehabilitation.

Many studies show that successful rehabilitation and improved physical function are strongly associated with *improvement* in pain. One of the best is by Mannion et al (1999, 2001a, b), which we have already looked at in Chapter 9. The strongest link they found over the course of treatment was between reduction in pain and improvement in disability. This was equally true for physiotherapy, aerobic training, or muscle reconditioning. Improvement in pain was by far the strongest factor they could identify in successful rehabilitation. Strand et al (2001) showed that rehabilitation could influence this relationship. In patients who had "usual care," return to work depended only on improvement in pain. In those who had a multidisciplinary rehab program, it depended on improvement in both pain and in physical function.

What is not clear is whether this is all cause or effect. First clinical impression might suggest that relief of pain produces or permits improved function. But overcoming dysfunction might also reduce pain (Ch. 9). The links between pain and disability are intimate and complex. Psychological factors affect perception of pain, and disability. As Mannion emphasized, it is ultimately a matter of performance. In practice, perhaps what matters is to address *both* pain and function, simultaneously. We can't treat one without the other.

OBSTACLES TO RECOVERY

The biopsychosocial model and ICF analysis provide a framework for a problem-oriented approach to rehabilitation. Medical, psychological, and social obstacles to recovery are all important. Perhaps we should also look more specifically at obstacles to return to work.

The first requirement is that the physical capacity of the worker must match the physical demands of his or her job. However, this often leads to negative thinking about limitations and restrictions and incapacity. A few patients with back pain have severe physical restrictions and a few jobs have very heavy physical demands. But most people with back pain do not have any absolute physical limitation for most jobs in modern society. For many patients, that way of thinking may actually create an obstacle to return to work. Do you remember the discussion about ability and performance in Chapter 9? It may be more helpful to think about the patient's current activity level compared with the physical requirements of the job. We might overcome any imbalance either by improving the patient's activity level or reducing the demands by modified work, or sometimes both. But for most patients this should not be an insurmountable obstacle. This may be a much more positive approach that leads directly to rehabilitation.

More often, the issue is pain. I have too much pain to manage my job. Or, trying to do my job would make my pain worse, so I cannot or should not do it or even attempt it. The first step is adequate pain control. The second step is to restore activity levels and give patients confidence that they can achieve them within acceptable pain limits. Ultimately, this is largely about beliefs.

Psychological obstacles are perceptions, beliefs, and expectations (Main & Burton 2000, Burton & Main 2000). Those about back pain and work and the relationship between them are probably most important. Some patients attribute their back pain to work, whether an accident or simply the physical demands. They may attribute blame to their work or employer, which may create an adversarial situation and undermine any cooperation about return to work. They may believe they have damaged something. They may have fear of pain, of activity, or of reinjury. They may believe that the best treatment for back pain is rest rather than staying active.

They are avoiders. They may believe it is not up to them and there is nothing they can do about it, but they are waiting for someone to "fix it." They may be convinced that they cannot and should not attempt to return to work till they are completely painfree. Some patients catastrophize, and this may influence their thinking about work. They may have little confidence, low expectations, and poor self-efficacy. They may not like their job, and have low job satisfaction. They may have problems with more specific psychosocial aspects of work. They may have other non-health reasons that discourage them from work or encourage sickness absence.

These are all likely to be obstacles to the patient feeling able or ready to return to work. Rehabilitation depends on identifying and overcoming such dysfunctional beliefs. We must reduce fears, restore confidence, and promote the patient's own ability to cope. We must create positive expectations about return to work. We have already talked about the physical need to increase activity levels, but it is also important psychologically. Rehabilitation is a matter of improving performance, and we know that is both physical and psychological. Rehabilitation depends on changing behavior.

Marhold et al (2002) tried to develop a questionnaire to measure obstacles to return to work. We do not think this is ready for general use, but they did have some interesting findings. In their study, the main obstacles they identified were:

- intensity of pain
- perceptions of work being too heavy and likely to cause harm
- lack of social support at work
- low expectations about return to work
- depression.

The most important social obstacles to return to work concern employment. We will use "employer" to cover all levels, but line managers and supervisors are probably most important. The most common and most important obstacle is lack of contact and communication between patient and employer during sickness absence. We must establish contact before we can achieve anything else. The employer may lack understanding of back pain and its modern management. Some employers believe that back pain and its treatment automatically mean sickness absence. Many employers still believe that pain must be 100% "cured" before they can "risk" return to work, for fear of reinjury and liability. There are often organizational barriers. Many employers insist that workers must be able to do everything, and do not even consider modified work. The rules of work and duties and sick pay may be rigid and unable to accommodate the worker with back pain. The whole work culture may be unhelpful or even adversarial. Return to work depends on overcoming these occupational barriers. That is why involvement of the employer in rehabilitation is vital.

Clinical management, rehabilitation, and return to work take place within a broader social framework. Health care itself may create obstacles to rehabilitation and return to work (BSRM 2000):

- waiting times, long gaps between appointments
- medical focus on impairment
- inadequate provision of rehabilitation
- lack of vocational aspects to rehabilitation
- lack of case management and appropriate advice.

Thornton (1998) considered some of the system obstacles to rehabilitation:

- assessment for rehabilitation is still dominated by medical issues. Most clinicians lack knowledge, awareness, or even interest about occupational and rehabilitation issues
- long delays of months for assessment or decisions
- limited facilities and waiting lists for rehabilitation
- often, workers have lost their jobs before they actually receive any active rehabilitation
- lack of funding for rehabilitation
- rehabilitation facilities fragmented and uncoordinated. Multiple providers. Competing philosophies and policy aims.

There may be financial obstacles, with lack of incentive or even frank disincentive to return to work. The social security or compensation system may create "benefit traps". Gardiner (1997) listed some of the obstacles that patients may face in coming off compensation or social security benefits and returning to work:

- personal characteristics such as (lack of) skills and work experience
- the (local) labor market
- disincentives for spouses to work created by the benefits system

- loss of certain benefits on moving into work
- anxiety about whether return to work will be successful, and if they can reclaim benefits in the future
- lack of access or facilities for retraining
- lack of information on the options available.

There may be little that health professionals or a rehab program can do about some of these system obstacles. But we should at least be aware of them. We should make sure that patients who need it get advice to find their way through the system.

Once a patient has lost his or her job and is on long-term incapacity, that may open a whole different can of worms (Waddell et al 2002). They may be physically unfit to return to a job with very heavy physical demands, particularly if they are getting older. They may have chronic pain. At the very least, they face a new and more difficult set of social obstacles to getting any alternative employment. There may be early retirement issues. They may require retraining, though that really goes beyond what we normally think of as rehabilitation.

Against that background of obstacles to recovery, let us now look at the physical, psychological, and social elements of rehabilitation.

EXERCISE

Van Tulder & Koes (2002) reviewed the current evidence on exercise for chronic low back pain. There are now 37 randomized controlled trials (RCTs). They concluded that there is strong evidence that exercise therapy improves self-reported pain and disability, compared with other treatments and "usual care". They found no clear evidence in favor of any one kind of back-specific exercises. There is limited evidence that exercise alone has much effect on return to work.

The physiologic effect of exercise

How does exercise work? Physiotherapists are experts in therapeutic exercise and different schools argue the merits of each type of exercise. These have different physiologic goals:

- mobilization
- strengthening
- endurance
- aerobic conditioning

- coordination
- stabilization.

The theory is that back pain and disability are due to specific dysfunctions, which can be corrected by corresponding exercises. Many studies have shown that each kind of exercise can produce improvement in the corresponding physiologic and physical measures. Strength exercises can increase muscle size and force. Stabilizing exercise can improve multifidus function. Aerobic conditioning can improve cardiorespiratory fitness. However, these are specific physiologic effects. There is rarely any close relationship to change in disability or return to work. Mannion et al (2001a) found that some physiologic and performance measures did occur with each of the three types of exercise. Changes in pain and disability were non-specific and similar in all three groups. Direct comparisons of different exercises have failed to show that one is any more effective than another (Oldervoll et al 2001, Petersen 2002).

Research into intensity has often been confounded by comparing different types and duration of exercise. However, several careful analyses have found no evidence of a dose–response relationship between the physical intensity of exercise and clinical outcomes (Faas 1996, Vuori 2001, Van Tulder & Koes 2002). One reason may be that patients do not adhere to the exercise program or fail to continue exercising after treatment finishes. A more likely explanation is that the specific exercises are not as important as physical activity.

So specific back exercises can produce specific physiologic effects, both in healthy subjects and in patients with back pain. But physiologic change is not the same as improved function or physical performance or rehabilitation. There does not seem to be any clear relationship between the type or intensity of exercise, physical performance, or improvements in pain and disability. That is also true of rehabilitation and return to work.

Exercise vs rehabilitation

Exercise is not the same as rehabilitation. Active rehabilitation uses exercise, but concentrates on function. Exercise is the means to achieve the rehab goals of restoring full function and regaining

physical fitness. Rehabilitation is also more intensive and structured. It is the difference between prescribing quadriceps exercises for an elderly woman with a fractured femur and teaching her to walk again (Fig. 18.1).

Physical therapy is the rehabilitation specialty *par excellence*. This is what therapy is all about in most musculoskeletal disorders. The 84-year-old woman in Figure 18.1 fractured the neck of her femur 36 hours before that photograph was taken, and had a major life-threatening operation. That morning, two bright young therapists came to her bedside: "Right, Granny, we're here to get you walking again." She looked at them in astonishment: "But I can't walk, I've broken my hip." "We know," they replied, "but you've had your operation, and you've got a pin to hold the bone in place." "But I can't walk," she repeated. "We know, but we're here to help you." "But it's still painful," she made a final protest. "Of course it is, you'd expect that at this stage. But your

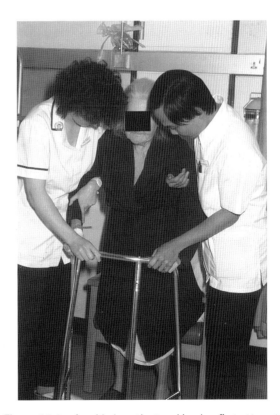

Figure 18.1   An elderly patient making her first attempt to walk, 24 hours after major surgery for a fractured neck of femur.

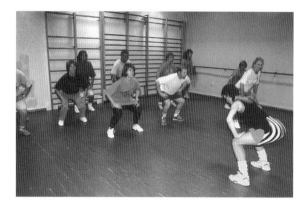

Figure 18.2   A back training class in Norway. From H B Finckenhagen, with thanks.

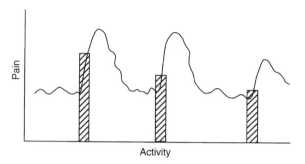

Figure 18.3   The problem of overenthusiastic bursts of activity and the need for pacing. After Hazard, personal communication.

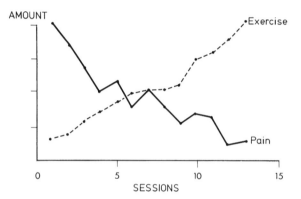

Figure 18.4   The importance of incremented increases in activity levels. Contrary to common belief, increased exercise does not cause increased pain, but actually leads to progressive reduction in pain levels. From Fordyce et al (1981, with permission).

painkillers should be working soon, and that won't stop you walking." These therapists concentrate on getting her walking again. And, if she survives, this gives her the best chance of getting mobile, independent, and back to her own home. What a contrast with back pain! Our argument is simply that therapists should apply the same rehabilitation principles and professional skills to back pain that they use in every other musculoskeletal condition (Fig. 18.2).

People with back pain require: a rationale for returning to activity; a safe environment to engage in *physical exercise* to restore confidence in movement; and the opportunity and encouragement to return to normal *physical activity*. It is the latter, where treatment becomes rehabilitation, that is the key to why physical exercise works. When patients ask: "What are the best exercises for back pain?" the answer is "The one(s) that you actually do!" It's not *what* you do that matters, it's the fact that you do it.

Increasing activity levels

Activity levels should increase by planned, fixed increments over time. It may be reasonable to set the starting point according to the patient's present symptoms and capacity. From this point on, there should be steadily increasing increments of activity level and exercise quotas. These are time-dependent, not symptom-dependent (Fordyce et al 1981): do what you plan, not what you feel. However, the rate of increase must be realistic. It is no use trying to do too much, too fast, provoking a pain crisis, and abandoning the effort (Fig. 18.3).

Many patients need to pace themselves, particularly at first. The rate and size of the increments will depend on the severity and duration of the patient's symptoms. It is a question of judgment and experiment to find a balance between what is realistically possible and achieving the goal within a reasonable time-scale. For most acute patients, this may be a matter of days or a few weeks. Even for chronic patients, it should usually be over a period of weeks or a few months at most if it is to have any chance of success. The most important message is that, contrary to common belief, progressive, incremented exercise levels lead to progressive decrease in pain (Fig. 18.4). But we must accept, and warn our patients, that there may be some temporary exacerbations of pain along the way. That is normal, and must be accepted and overcome. And even after, they must live with and be prepared to cope with the long-term natural history of recurrences and exacerbations.

Exercise and beliefs

Most doctors, therapists, and patients think the purpose of exercise is to restore physical and physiologic function. However, improved performance may be as much a matter of changing beliefs and behavior as any physiologic change.

Fixed beliefs and dysfunctional coping strategies are likely to be resistant to simple information and advice. Personal experience that challenges existing misconceptions and forces patients to rethink their whole approach to the problem is a much more powerful agent for change. Actions speak louder than words. Perhaps we need to redesign our therapy and rehabilitation for back pain to meet these goals, rather than thinking it is all about muscle physiology.

We found an unexpected effect of exercise on fear-avoidance beliefs during reliability studies of isokinetic assessment (Newton et al 1993). We got 20 patients to repeat the test four times over 7–10 days. Before we tested them we carried out a complete clinical assessment, including self-report of disability, and they told us all the things they could not do. We then put them on the isokinetic equipment (Fig. 18.5). From the outside this equipment looks rather frightening, but it actually gives patients a feeling of support and security. We put them through a test protocol and at the end of it, several patients turned to us in amazement: "I never thought I could do that!" So we tested their fear-avoidance beliefs over the series of four assessments (Table 18.4).

Remember, this was only a test protocol. These patients did not exercise enough to have any physiologic effect. We had also explained the study honestly. The patients knew it was only an assessment, and we did not pretend it was treatment. Yet their experience of what they could do in a single assessment session produced a significant shift in their fear-avoidance beliefs about physical activity. The series of four tests over 7–10 days gave a further shift in fear-avoidance beliefs, which in turn led to improvement in their pain and disability. The amount of exercise was too small, and the change too rapid, for this to be a physiologic effect.

Many other studies show that exercise and increased activity can change beliefs and behavior.

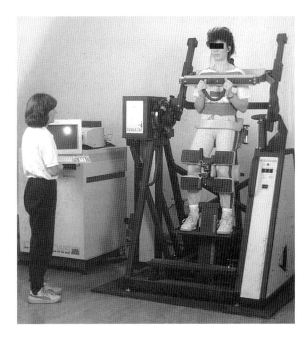

Figure 18.5 Isokinetic assessment on the Cybex II trunk flexion–extension device.

Table 18.4 Change in fear-avoidance beliefs (FABs) with isokinetic assessment

Baseline		After one assessment	After four assessments
FAB activity beliefs	17.2	14.0*	10.3**
Pain	48.7	45.9	36.5**
Disability	9.4	8.9	7.1*

*$P < 0.05$; ** $P < 0.001$.
Unpublished data from Dr. M Newton, with thanks.

Dolce et al (1986a, b) showed that exercise quotas increase exercise performance and expectancies of exercise capability while reducing anxiety about exercise. Rainville et al (1992) found that a functional restoration program could improve the physical performance of patients with chronic low back pain, despite lack of consistent improvement in pain. They suggested that experience of successful physical performance during rehabilitation modifies patients' ability to control and cope with their pain. Jensen et al (1994b) studied the mechanisms by which a pain management program worked. Clinical improvement depended most on reducing

Table 18.5   Changes in beliefs and coping strategies that relate to improvement in disability

Change	Correlation with improvement in disability
Reduce guarding	0.52
Reduce use of rest for pain	0.41
Reduce catastrophizing	0.36
Increased feelings of control	0.31

I Jensen, personal communication.

catastrophizing, guarding, and resting (Table 18.5). They suggested that exercise may be a powerful method of changing patients' beliefs in their own abilities, which can lead in turn to changes in behavior.

Vlaeyen et al (2002a, b) described an experimental approach to fear-avoidance beliefs. The basic idea is that systematic *exposure* to physical activity reduces fear. At first sight, this appears similar to a graded-activity program in that it gradually increases activity levels despite pain. Conceptually and in practice, however, it is quite different. Graded-activity programs focus on shaping behavior by positive reinforcement when predefined exercise quotas are met. Exposure deliberately confronts and overcomes fear. Individual fears are identified and arranged in a hierarchy. These activities are then tackled in ascending order of difficulty. Vlaeyen's studies showed that personal experience can reduce fear of movement and reinjury, expectancy of pain, and catastrophizing. Such mechanisms may be fundamental to rehabilitation.

Vowles & Gross (2003) tested this in an interdisciplinary treatment program for chronic pain. They found that improvement in specific fears about work-related injury was the best predictor of improved functional capacity for work.

Conclusion

- Rehabilitation can reduce pain and increase activity levels, regardless of the type of exercise used to engage the patient in the rehabilitation process.
- Specific physical exercises can produce specific physical and physiologic effects.

- Improvements in specific physical performance measures do not predict improvement in disability and return to work.
- Programs involving intense physical exercise are no more effective than those that involve moderate exercise.
- Exercise programs that also address psychosocial issues are likely to be more effective.

PSYCHOLOGICAL APPROACHES TO PAIN MANAGEMENT

Pain management programs deal mainly with patients who have chronic, intractable pain and have exhausted medical care. At least 50% have back pain. Pain management is too large a subject to cover here, and if you wish to read more we would recommend Main & Spanswick (2000). However, all doctors and therapists should be aware of certain principles, because they also apply to clinical care and rehabilitation (Linton 2002, Gatchel & Turk 2002).

The basic idea is that if psychological and behavioral factors can aggravate and perpetuate pain and disability, then it may help to address these issues. We will look at two main psychological approaches relevant to rehabilitation:

- behavioral approaches
- cognitive and cognitive-behavioral approaches.

Behavioral approaches focus on changing patients' pain behavior. Cognitive approaches focus on mental events – changing how patients think about and cope with their pain. However, there is no such thing as a purely cognitive approach. Most pain management now uses a combined cognitive-behavioral approach.

Behavioral management

Behavioral psychologists focus on pain behavior rather than the subjective experience of pain (Fordyce 1976). They concentrate on actions and behaviors that they can observe, and are less interested in reports of pain, because these are subjective and difficult to measure. They argue that behavior is governed mainly by its consequences. Positive or negative social reinforcement determines whether pain behavior continues, whatever the original cause of the pain. The effects depend partly on the strength of the reinforcement and are often temporary, so reinforcement must be repeated. Reinforcement tends to be specific to the situation, so patterns of behavior learned in one setting may not continue in a different situation.

Assessment focuses on pain behaviors by which other people know that the patient is in pain, such as limping, resting in bed, or taking medication. It looks for direct positive reinforcement such as encouragement and support of these behaviors by family or health professionals. It looks for avoidance behavior, and for negative reinforcement or blocks to well behavior. Interview of the patient and his or her partner may show how they interact. We should always ask about the information and advice patients have had from health professionals, because that often reinforces pain behavior.

Behavioral therapy tries to shape and change pain behavior by manipulating the social context. It tries to extinguish pain behavior by withdrawal of its reinforcements. At the same time, it develops healthy behavior by positive reinforcement. This is operant-conditioning. It usually sets specific goals:

- increase mobility and social activity
- reduce medication use
- reduce health care use.

It removes positive reinforcement such as medication, sympathetic attention, bed rest, and release from daily activities and duties. Staff and families are taught to ignore pain behavior. It encourages and reinforces well behavior. It usually involves increasing daily activities. Patients receive analgesics at regular fixed times, not in response to pain or on demand. Rest and attention are used to reinforce meeting exercise targets, but are withheld for failure to meet the quota. Patients get feedback on their progress.

Training involves the patient's partner and family so that they continue the same management at home. Family members become aware of how they have reinforced pain behaviors, and how they should reinforce well behaviors instead. All health professionals involved in the patient's continuing care must take the same approach. Otherwise, those who reinforced pain behavior in the first place may continue to sabotage progress!

Critics argue that a purely behavioral approach ignores more subjective issues. What about mental, emotional, and psychological factors and the complex interactions between them? It defines successful outcomes in terms of reduced pain behavior, but does that really mean less pain or disability?

Cognitive and cognitive–behavioral approaches

Partly in response to these criticisms of the behavioral approach, cognitive approaches focus more on patients' thoughts and feelings about their pain (Turk et al 1983):

- the meaning of the pain to the patient, their fears and beliefs
- beliefs about how to deal with the pain
- expectations of treatment
- coping skills and strategies.

There are several stages to cognitive therapy (Turk et al 1983):

- Help patients to rethink their beliefs about the pain, and what they do about it. This also depends on building confidence in their own ability and skills.
- Teach patients to use mental techniques to reduce pain
  — stop unhelpful thoughts
  — change the focus of attention
  — redefine pain as a different sensation.
- Teach patients to manage stress more effectively, and to use these skills to help cope with their pain and exacerbations.
- Patients practice and consolidate these skills, with special attention to situations that can lead to relapse (Turk & Rudy 1991).

The behavioral and cognitive approaches are conceptually different, but in practice they are two sides of the same coin. Cognitive therapy tries to change mental approaches to pain, but uses that to change behavior. Even if there could be such a thing as a purely cognitive program, it would still use behavior change as the main outcome. We may caricature the behavioral approach as social manipulation to produce a reflex response, but that is not completely true either. Active involvement, learning, and self-help are fundamental. Changing pain behavior also changes and reinforces the patient's thinking about the pain.

Cognitive-behavioral approaches combine these ideas (Turk et al 1983, Gatchel & Turk 2002).

They help patients to restructure the way they think about their pain and at the same time change their pattern of behavior. The goal is to address all the psychological aspects of the pain experience. Cognitive-behavioral programs:

- develop a new understanding of pain and disability
- help patients to identify and change unhelpful thoughts, feelings, and behavior
- help patients to acquire better coping skills, and the ability and confidence to use them on their own
- use behavioral methods to promote change; however, they also use changed behavior to provide feedback on the patient's fears and beliefs – "learning by doing"
- are active, time-limited, and structured
- use a wide range of treatment strategies and techniques, either individually or in groups
- help patients to take over management of their pain and daily activities.

Linton (2002) has applied these cognitive-behavioral principles to early interventions for back pain. His present program consists of six group sessions led by a clinical psychologist (Linton & Andersson 2000, Marhold et al 2001). This is a structured program with a manual (Table 18.6). Each session lasts 2 hours and starts with no more than 15 minutes of information. The rest of the time is spent developing and practicing coping skills. Individual homework is assigned and reviewed each week. This is a pure cognitive-behavioral program aimed at the secondary prevention of chronic pain and disability. There is no active exercise and no work intervention or focus. This group has performed three recent RCTs. Linton & Andersson (2000) studied patients with average 3–5 days' sickness absence in the past 6 months who saw themselves at risk of long-term problems. The program reduced the risk of long-term sickness absence (>30 days in the next 6 months) ninefold. Linton & Ryberg (2001) studied subjects from the general population who had recurrent back pain but very little sickness absence.

Table 18.6   Early cognitive-behavior program

Session	Focus	Skills
1	Causes of pain and prevention of chronic problems	Problem-solving Applied relaxation Learning about pain
2	Managing your pain	Activities; maintaining daily routines Activity scheduling Relaxation training
3	Promoting good health; controlling stress at home and at work	Warning signals Cognitive appraisal Beliefs
4	Adapting for leisure and work	Communication skills Assertiveness Risk situations Applying relaxation
5	Controlling flare-ups	Plan for coping with flare-ups Coping skills review Applied relaxation
6	Maintaining and improving results	Risk analysis Plan for adherence

Reproduced with permission from Linton & Andersson (2000).

The program produced a slight but significant reduction in sickness absence. Only 5% had more than 14 days' sickness over the next 6 months compared with 15% of the control group. Marhold et al (2001) studied patients from the National Insurance register with either about 3 months' or >12 months' sickness absence. The program reduced further days off by more than one-third in those with short-term sickness absence. It had no effect on those with long-term sickness absence.

Results of pain management

Morley et al (1999) reviewed RCTs of behavioral and cognitive-behavioral therapy for chronic pain. They found improvement in various measures of pain, positive coping measures, and pain behavior. There was no effect on depression, catastrophizing, or social role functioning. A more recent review by Van Tulder & Koes (2002) found similar results compared with no treatment, placebo, or waiting-list controls. There were conflicting results when compared with other forms of treatment. There was no clear difference between different types of behavioral therapy. There is no evidence of any significant effect on return to work (Scheer et al 1997, Morley et al 1999, Peat et al 2001, Van Tulder & Koes 2002). However, in fairness, that is not the goal of most chronic pain management programs or their patients.

This makes Linton's results even more impressive. It is not clear how he got such good sick-leave outcomes with a pure cognitive-behavioral program with no physical rehabilitation and no occupational intervention or focus. It may have something to do with timing or patient selection. Most of his studies were in people with a previous history of sick leave, but they were currently working. The goal was prevention rather than rehabilitation. However, it is possible there is something else about his program or patients or Swedish setting that we are missing. Whatever, his work does show very clearly the potential power of shifting beliefs and behavior.

OCCUPATIONAL INTERVENTIONS

Return to work has at least as much to do with the workplace as with health care. So it is no surprise that work-related interventions may be among the most effective ways of helping workers to remain at work or to return as early as possible.

Krause et al (1998) reviewed 29 studies of modified work. There were limitations to many of the studies, but the evidence was consistent. Providing modified work can double the number of injured workers who return to work and halve their time off work. Most modified work consisted of lighter duties, though there were also some trials of graded work exposure and work trial periods. In most of these studies, modified work was part of a broader occupational program.

However, doctors and therapists must be careful with the idea of modified work. These trials showed that *when the employer provides the opportunity for modified work*, that facilitates return to work. We must always remember this is a workplace intervention, and depends on the employer. Doctors or therapists are often tempted to recommend return to "light duties," but we often do this just to "play safe." The trap is that many employers do not provide modified work. Our recommendation may then become a prescription *only* to return to light duties and actually be an obstacle to return to regular work (Hall et al 1994). Imposing restrictions may continue to medicalize the problem. It may create an adversarial situation with some employers. We must also be realistic. Most workers return quickly to their usual job and do not need modified work, so there is no need to raise the question. Employers can only provide a limited number of modified posts, and usually only for a limited period. We cannot expect them to give every worker with back pain open-ended light duties. As always, our aim is to assist recovery and we must make sure that our advice does not create obstacles instead.

We must also remember that the ultimate goal is not simply return to work, but sustained return to regular work (Evanoff et al 2002). Reduced activities or modified work is not a long-term solution. It is always a temporary and unstable situation. The worker remains at risk of further injury, further sickness absence, and even long-term incapacity. The goal must always be to progress through this stage and to return to ordinary activities and regular work.

Modified duties are usually only part of a broader occupational program. This often includes accident prevention and health promotion, accident and sickness monitoring, and clinical or occupational health management protocols. The Paris Task Force (Abenhaim et al 2000) recommended that return to work interventions might include:

- evaluation of the worker's physical capacity
- work station assessment and, if necessary, ergonomic modification
- management of the return to work process by occupational health and human resources
- communication between the worker and supervisor
- regular clinical follow-up during the adaptation period.

Return to work must involve the employer, and that depends on communication. Wood (1987) is the classic study on the value of good communication. When workers were off work their supervisor phoned to say: "How are you? We are thinking about you. You are a vital part of the team. Your work is important and your job is waiting for you." That simple message, and the culture it reflected, cut the number of workers with back injuries staying off long-term from 7.1% to 1.7%. Frank et al (1996, 1998) looked at the broader issue of "getting all the players on side." Table 18.7 shows how health care and workplace interventions interact. The Canadian Medical Association Policy Statement (Kazimirski 1997) gives further guidance on how physicians might assist the return to work process. It highlights:

- communication between patient and employer for early treatment and return to work
- the importance of addressing obstacles to recovery
- developing a modified work plan
- recognizing workers' family and workplace roles
- the importance of the employer–employee relationship in return to work.

KEY STUDIES

We have tried to review the scientific trials of rehabilitation for back pain (Table 18.8). We had to decide which studies to include, and that meant we had to define what does and what does not count as rehabilitation (Staal et al 2002). This was an instructive exercise (Box 18.1) – especially deciding what is *not* really rehabilitation. This is not to deny the value of some of these other interventions. But it does help to focus our minds on what rehabilitation is really about.

Rehabilitation is a "program," which has several components. Some reviews define it as multidisciplinary, but that puts too much emphasis on the

Table 18.7　The role of health care and occupational interventions in return to work

Factors contributing to chronic incapacity	Intervention	Stakeholders
Acute		
Clinical: iatrogenic disability, obstacles to return to work	Health care according to clinical guidelines	Patients, health professionals, payers
Workplace: lack of communication, inappropriate organization	Prompt management according to occupational health guidelines Modified work if necessary	Patients/workers, employers, occupational health professionals, labor unions, payers
Subacute		
Biopsychosocial factors leading to chronic pain and incapacity	Intensive work-related case management: 　Comprehensive case review 　Graded-activity program 　Ergonomic assessment and modified work	Workers, employers, health professionals, occupational health professionals, labor unions, payers

After Frank et al (1998).

Table 18.8 Scientific studies of rehabilitation for low back pain

Study	Intervention	Outcomes	
Acute and recurrent			
Lindequist et al (1984)	(Early) back school	Rate of recovery	NS
RCT *n* = 56	Physical therapy training program	Days off work	NS
Family practice, Sweden	Encourage physical activity	Satisfaction	Better
	despite pain	Recurrences	Fewer and shorter
		1 year sick leave	Less (NS)
		Chronic disability	NS
Fordyce et al (1986)	Time-contingent analgesics	6 weeks	NS
RCT *n* = 107	Programmed restoration of activity	1 year: Disability	NS
Family practice, emergency room	Strong behavioral principles	Chronic sickness	Less
or orthopedic clinic, US		Futher health care	Less
Van Doorn (1995)	Early intervention	Reduced mean time off work from	
Cohort study. Time controls	Time-dependent approach	136 to 98 days	
Insurance company study	Evaluation of medical, psychosocial,	Number of claimants off work at	
Self-employed doctors,	and ergonomic factors	1 year reduced by 56%	
therapists, dentists, and vets	Progressive activity and gradual RTW		
The Netherlands	Good communication between		
	insurance physician, patient, and		
	treating physician		
Ryan et al (1995)	Early injury reporting and intervention	Fewer back injury claims	
Prospective study in a new	Workforce education – changing	Median time off work 10 days	
mine, with control site	perceptions	No worker off work >60 days	
Occupational health,	Encouragement and support for		
Australia	early return to work		
	Management and employee involvement		
	(No active exercise program)		
Yassi et al (1995),	Early intervention focusing on reducing	23% decrease back injury rate	
Cooper et al (1996),	perception of disability	44% decrease lost-time back injuries	
Tate et al (1999)	Comprehensive physiotherapy rehab	29% decrease sickness absence	
Controlled trial: high-risk wards	Occupational therapy assessment		
vs other wards	Return to modified work (No explicit		
Occupational health, nurses	cognitive-behavioral program)		
with work-related injuries, Canada			
Subacute – chronic			
Aberg (1984)	6-week inpatient rehab program	No significant effect on	
RCT *n* = 353	Education – ergonomics	vocational outcomes	
Chronic LBP, Sweden	"complete physiotherapy service"		
	(limited data provided)		
Sachs et al (1990)	4-week rehab program:	73% of rehab group employed at	
Controlled trial (not RCT) *n* = 78	biomedical education	6-month follow-up compared with	
Average 11 months off work	Graded exercise and work hardening	38% of control group *but*, selected	
with LBP	Functional capacity evaluation	groups and high loss to follow-up	
Rehab Unit, US	Behavioral modification and psychosocial		
	counseling		

(Continued)

Table 18.8   (Continued)

Study	Intervention	Outcomes
Altmaier et al (1992) RCT $n = 45$ 3–30 months off work with LBP Orthopedic Dept, USA	Standard 3-week inpatient rehab program: education, support, and physical reconditioning ± psychological component: relaxation, coping skills, and behavioral reinforcement	57% returned to original work and 81% to some form of work or retraining. No difference between standard rehab program and addition of psychological component
Lindstrom et al (1992a, b, 1995) RCT $n = 103$ Industrial blue-collar workers Sick-listed 8–12 weeks Sweden	Graded-activity program Operant conditioning Workplace assessment and modifications Swedish back school	Males: Return to work Faster 1 year sick leave Less Chronic disability Less (NS) No effect in females
Jarvikoski et al (1993) Quasiexperimental comparison of two groups (not RCT) $n = 309$ Average 133 days off work in past year (but 50% working at present) Rehab center, Finland	Two intensive inpatient rehab programs (a) Physiotherapy exercises "guided by pain," modified Swedish back school, congnitive-behavioral group therapy (b) More intensive physical training, overcome fear-avoidance beliefs: "no pain – no gain" (no vocational intervention)	Both programs produced improvement in pain and functional capacity over next 12 months, though slightly greater in (b) Both reduced sickness absence, but no significant difference
Jensen et al (1994a) Cohort study with matched controls (not RCT) $n = 35 + 88$ Patients with >3 months spinal pain Sweden	Cognitive-behavioral package Standardized physical training module Education Education of supervisors	Trend to less pain, disability, depression, and absenteeism. But lack of comparable absenteeism data for controls
Indahl et al (1995, 1998) RCT $n = 975$ Sick-listed 8–12 weeks Population-based (NI claims) Norway	Intense personal advice Reduce fear Increase activity, normal walking Reduce sick behavior Set goals	Days off work Less Return to work More Chronic disability Less
Hagen et al (2000) RCT $n = 457$ Sick-listed 8–12 weeks Population-based, Norway	Modified Indahl program Information and advice to stay active Individual advice on exercise from physiotherapist Light mobilization	Returned to work: Intervention Control 3 months 52% 36% 6 months 61% 45% 12 months 68% 56% Men: fewer days' sickness absence
Loisel et al (1997, 2002) RCT $n = 130$ Sick-listed > 4 weeks Occupational health, Canada	Back school Fitness, work hardening Cognitive-behavioral approach Site visit, ergonomic assessment Modified work and progressive return to work	Full intervention gave 2.4 × faster return to work Occupational intervention accounted for most of this Sickness absence reduced by 70% over next 6 years

(Continued)

Table 18.8   (Continued)

Study	Intervention	Outcomes	
Friedrich et al (1998) RCT $n = 93$ Chronic LBP (duration of sickness absence unclear) Orthopedic physical therapy, Austria	Individual exercise program (10 sessions with physical therapist) Motivation program – five interventions, including counseling, record-keeping, and reinforcement	Pain Self-reported disability 20% of the compliance group returned to their previous level of work by 4 months compared with none of the physio therapy group	Less Less (NS)
Bendix et al (1998) (a) RCT $n = 106$ Chronic LBP >6 months "threatening work situation" (but 30% still working) Tertiary referrals, Denmark	Intensive 6-week program: intensive physical training Psychological pain management including relaxation and biofeedback Biomedical education (no vocational component)	Fit for work Sick leave over next 2 years Disability pensions Median sick leave 15 days cf. 123 days in control group of "usual care"	NS Less NS
Bendix et al (1998) (b) RCT $n = 132$ Chronic LBP >6 months "threatening work situation" (but 30% still working) Tertiary referrals, Denmark	Intensive program as above Compared with less intensive physical program ± psychological pain management	Fit for work Sick leave over next 2 years Disability pensions Results maintained at 5 years	More Less Fewer
Moffett et al 1999 Moffett & Frost (2000) RCT $n = 187$ Family practice UK	Progressive exercise program Cognitive-behavioral approach (no occupational component)	Self-reported disability Sickness absence reduced by 37%	Less (NS)
Haldorsen et al (1998) Strand et al (2001) RCT $n = 117$ Sick-listed >8 weeks, Norway	4 weeks, 5 days/week, 6 hours/day Individual and group physical training Education Cognitive and behavioral modification Some communication with workplace Sick certification and RTW left to primary care physician	50% returned to work at 1-year, cf. 58% of control group	
Haldorsen et al (2002) Skouen et al (2002) RCT $n = 195$ Sick-listed average 3 months, Norway	Light vs extensive rehab program Individual graded-exercise program Address fear-avoidenace beliefs Reduce illness behavior and increase activity levels Some workplace visits	Both programs increased RTW by 6 months for men (70% cf. controls 42%). This was sustained beyond 1 year for the light program but not for the extensive program. Neither program had any effect in women.	
Jensen et al (2001) RCT $n = 214$ Sick-listed 1–6 months (average > 4 months) Sweden	Detailed medical assessment, education on psychology of chronic pain, ergonomic advice, and worksite visits (1) Behavior-oriented physical therapy (2) Cognitive-behavioral therapy (3) Both combined (4) Treatment as usual	(1) and (2) produced similar results to (3) Overall, no significant effect on sick-listing. Some gender differences in early retirement	

(Continued)

Table 18.8 (Continued)

Study	Intervention	Outcomes
Chronic pain and long-term incapacity		
Richardson et al (1994) Cohort study $n = 109$ Chronic pain patients, 74% unemployed for average 4.3 years, UK	Cognitive-behavioral pain management program Progressive exercise program One session on work issues	30% of unemployed patients returned to work during 1 year follow-up, though employment status fluctuated greatly
Kendall & Thompson (1998) Quasiexperimental waiting list controls (not RCT) $n = 81$ Patients with chronic pain and long-term unemployment referred to pain management center, New Zealand	Cognitive-behavioral pain management program Vocational rehabilitation	10% of intervention group returned to full-time work and 10% to part-time work. No return to work in waiting-list control group
Watson (2001) Pilot study $n = 84$ Long-term social security benefit recipients, UK	Cross-agency rehab program: physical rehabilitation Psychological support and pain management principles Vocational counseling	40% working at 6 months

Outcomes are significant ($P < 0.05$), unless otherwise stated.
RCT, randomized controlled trial; NS, not significant; RTW, return to work; LBP, low back pain; NI, National Insurance.

professionals. We believe it is more important to focus on the components of the program. The biopsychosocial model and the ICF analysis offer the best explanation of disability, so we used that as our starting point. Biopsychosocial issues may all be obstacles to recovery, either singly or in combination. So, to address disability and overcome obstacles to recovery, a rehab program should cover all three of these areas. First, almost all programs include some form of active exercise or graded-activity component. This may correct physiologic dysfunction in the back and improve physical fitness, but it is not just about "treating" the back with back-specific exercises. The goal is to reactivate the patient and restore normal activity levels. This is not to deny the importance of pain, which requires symptomatic treatment. We have already argued that adequate pain control is essential to the early stages of rehabilitation. But restoration of function is the best route to recovery and long-term relief, and that is the goal of rehabilitation. Second, we have

seen that beliefs drive behavior, so there should be some attempt to correct dysfunctional beliefs and behavior. This may be modern information and advice or some form of cognitive-behavioral component and/or principles. Third, there should be explicit social goal(s): to restore normal social function, most commonly capacity for work. From a preliminary review, the social component appears to be least clear. It may be a work-related intervention or the program may be in an occupational setting. The minimum is probably that everyone agrees that return to work is what the program is all about.

Table 18.8 shows the trials we included as "rehabilitation." We will look at functional restoration programs separately, so we have not put its trials into this table.

These studies all look at different rehab packages, and it can be difficult to see the exact components of each program. They often deal with different patients. Some of the findings may only apply in particular settings. Many of the studies are quite

<table>
<tr><td>

Box 18.1   Inclusion and exclusion criteria for what counts as a rehabilitation program

Minimum content
- Physical: progressive exercise or graded-activity component
- Psychological: explicit attempt to address beliefs and behavior
- Social: explicit functional and/or vocational goals and outcome measures

Exclusion criteria
- Prevention (aim to reduce future sick leave. Working at present)
- Information and advice (education) alone
- Exercise "therapy" alone
- Traditional "back school" with biomedical and ergonomic education, exercises, and relaxation
- Pure pain management program with no exercise/activity component or occupational focus
- Guideline implementation or case management (i.e., earlier and/or more efficient delivery of health care)
- Ergonomic or modified work initiatives alone
- Organizational/administrative/incentive and control interventions alone
- Postsurgical rehabilitation (this is a specialized area)

</td></tr>
</table>

- The health professionals generally thought they had done a good job. Workers were generally satisfied with the services. Employers' reactions were more mixed. Some were satisfied and supportive but others were more skeptical.

- There is no evidence that any of the pilot schemes had any real impact on back pain, sickness absence, or long-term incapacity.

The message seems to be that it is not enough just to re-badge health care as "rehabilitation".

Lindstrom et al (1992a, b, 1995) in Sweden carried out the first RCT of a modern rehab program for subacute back pain. It had all three of our key components. It had an individual graded-activity program for mobility, strength, and fitness, aimed at improving functional capacity. It used an operant-conditioning, behavioral approach, after Fordyce. It was in an occupational health setting, had a workplace visit with the physiotherapist, and the clear goal of return to work. The median time to return to work was 5 weeks, compared with 9 weeks for those treated "as usual". Average sick leave due to back pain in the second follow-up year was 12 weeks, compared with nearly 20 weeks for the control group. The number of patients going on to permanent disability pensions was reduced by three-quarters (though these were small numbers). But why did it only work for males, and not for females?

Indahl et al (1995, 1998) took a much more clinical approach. They probably had a more difficult group of all social security recipients who were sick-listed for 8+ weeks; Lindstrom studied a single, blue-collar work force in the Volvo company. Indahl gave patients a detailed assessment and reassured them there was no serious damage. They then got a "mini-back school" lasting 2 hours. This was reinforced by a further 1-hour, one-to-one session with the doctor 2 weeks later and follow-up at 3 months and 1 year. The explanation of "injury" and what was happening in the back was rather idiosyncratic, but bore some similarities to that in Chapters 9 and 16. There was strong advice and rationale for "light mobilization," but no formal exercise program. The main recommendation was to walk as normally and with as much flexibility as possible. Patients got some ergonomic advice about activities of daily living. The whole package was

small. Despite these problems, there is a wealth of information here and it is worth looking more closely at a few key studies.

The UK Back in Work initiative funded 18 small pilot studies to tackle back pain in the workplace. Thirteen dealt with prevention, 12 more efficient delivery of various forms of treatment, 12 "rehabilitation," 14 manual handling, and 11 general working practices and policies. The results (Brown 2002) suggest that:

- These were usually small groups of health professionals "doing their own thing." There were some interesting new collaborations, e.g., between emp- loyer, union, and occupational health to address manual handling. There were no really innovative approaches.

designed to reduce fear and uncertainty, and to promote activity. "Do not worry about your back. There is no need to be cautious. Stay active." However, there was no more formal cognitive-behavioral intervention. This was really a cross between traditional biomedical education and modern information and advice to shift beliefs and behavior (Ch. 16). There was no specific advice about return to work, no vocational intervention, and no contact with the employer. Indeed, the research design deliberately left sick certification and return to work to the primary care physician.

After 200 days, 70% had stopped sick leave compared with 40% of the control group treated as usual. At 5 years, 81% were working compared with 65% of the control group. This intervention may be good health care rather than rehabilitation, but the results are remarkable.

How does it work? Indahl is a charismatic doctor and when I first met him I thought this might be a personal effect. However, there was no difference between the patients who saw him or another doctor (A Indahl, personal communication). His nurse and physiotherapist also did a great job. However, an independent study by Hagen et al (2000) has now given similar results. Hagen could not identify which elements achieve the effect and suggested the complete package is important. "The advice is given by experts; the examination is thorough; and the team at the clinic is enthusiastic and optimistic about treatment results." The problem is that many unsuccessful programs could claim the same. No one has replicated this outside Norway, and perhaps there is something unique about the setting. Or perhaps the message is simply that we should not discount the value of good clinical management.

Jensen et al (1994a, 2001) and Haldorsen et al (1998, 2002) used the same behavioral medicine approach that appears to have all our key components. The first study by Jensen et al (1994a) showed a trend only to improvement in sickness absence, and only in women. Jensen et al (2001) showed that, if anything, those who received the full cognitive-behavioral rehab program had *more* sickness absence over the next 18 months. The first study by Haldorsen et al (1998) had no effect on return to work. The second study by Haldorsen et al (2002) did improve return to work in men, but not in women. Both the light and extensive

programs had the same initial effect, but why did the more intensive program paradoxically lose its effect beyond 9 months? Why do these various studies have such inconsistent results, when the programs seem to have the same basic components? Is this really multidisciplinary rehabilitation or is it more of a cognitive-behavioral pain management program? Jensen et al (2001) themselves raised the possibility that the full program might be too "psychological." How much occupational intervention was there in practice? In Haldorsen's studies it is not clear just how much link there was with the workplace. The rehab team deliberately did not give any advice about when to stop sick certification or return to work. However, Jensen et al (2001) did include ergonomic advice and worksite visits. Is it something about the social security setting in Sweden and Norway, where 20–50% go on to ill health retirement? Yet Indahl appears to have had largely similar patients in the same setting.

Loisel et al (1997) in Canada tested the relative impact of health care vs occupational interventions. This was a highly organized system of occupational health care. There was close cooperation between the injured worker, health care, the supervisor, and labor and management representatives. The clinical intervention started with an early visit to a back specialist, and a back school. The occupational intervention started with assessments by an occupational health physician and an ergonomist. The ergonomist, worker, and supervisor then visited the work site together. They observed the worker's tasks, reached an "ergonomic diagnosis", and recommended any changes in work tasks to assist stable return to work. Workers who were still off work at 12 weeks had a multidisciplinary functional restoration program.

Patients were randomized to usual care, the clinical intervention alone, the occupational intervention, or both. The clinical intervention alone did not give any faster return to work. Those who received the combined intervention returned to work fastest, but those who received the occupational intervention alone did nearly as well. This clinical intervention did little to promote return to work, either on its own or when added to the occupational intervention. Perhaps that reflects the weakness of back school and functional restoration programs. Or the failure to address beliefs and behavior specifically.

Or it shows that the occupational intervention is most important. Or the importance of the whole package and "getting all the players on side."

The ISSA study looked at *Who Returns to Work and Why?* (Bloch & Prins 2001, Hansson & Hansson 2001). This was an observational study, comparing what happened in Denmark, Germany, Israel, the Netherlands, Sweden, and the US. It looked at social security benefit recipients who were still off work at 3 months with back pain, who were all at high risk of long-term incapacity. None of the medical interventions had any effect on return to work at 1 or 2 years. Non-medical and vocational interventions were difficult to assess. Only workplace accommodations and therapeutic work resumption seemed to have a consistent effect in various countries. Disability assessment had a negative effect, which might reflect moves towards termination of employment or disability pension. Case management also seemed to have a negative effect, though that might reflect case selection.

Watson (2001) carried out one of the most promising pilot studies. This was part of the UK government's New Deal for Disabled People (www.newdeal.gov.uk). He studied 84 social security benefit recipients who had chronic low back pain and had not worked for a mean of 38 months. Most social security studies round the world suggest these patients nearly all remain on long-term incapacity and nothing can change that (Waddell et al 2002). This study formed a partnership between employment, health, and vocational training agencies. They developed a work-focused program of physical rehabilitation, psychological support, and vocational counseling. It was based on pain management principles. The initial study was in Salford and it was then replicated in Bristol.

- 56% of those who were referred joined the program
- 97% of those who started, completed the program
- 39.5% were employed at 6 months (Salford 43%, Bristol 36%)
- a further 26% were in job training, education, or voluntary work.

One of the most interesting findings was the effect of return to work (Fig. 18.6). Pain and disability improved in most patients after the program. There

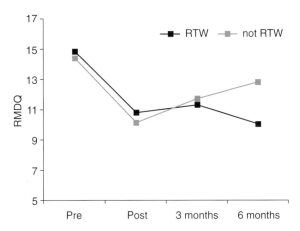

Figure 18.6 Continued improvement in disability following return to work (RTW) after a rehabilitation program (based on data from Watson 2001). RMDQ, Roland Morris Disability Questionnaire.

was little difference between those who did and those who did not return to work. In those who did return to work, pain and disability continued to improve over the next 6 months. In those who did not return to work, disability deteriorated again. This was a small, selected, and uncontrolled study, but the results are impressive. They show that at least some of these apparently intractable patients can be helped back into work if they get suitable cross-agency support. A proper RCT is now underway.

FUNCTIONAL RESTORATION

Mayer developed the first functional restoration program for chronic back pain in Dallas (Mayer et al 1985, 1987, Mayer & Gatchel 1988). The focus "was no longer on diagnosis or treatment but on promoting and maximizing functional abilities in the face of on-going pain" (Teasell & Harth 1996). The general view is that these programs "essentially ignore the complaint of pain," though Mayer argues that is not entirely true. Improved function often leads to less pain. In contrast, subjective expressions of pain usually do not improve unless there is improved function. Despite that argument, any impact on pain is clearly secondary.

One of the hallmarks of Mayer's approach was the use of objective measures of function, such as range of movement, strength, endurance, and aerobic capacity. The most novel element, however, was dynamic measurement of trunk strength using the new iso-machines (Fig. 18.5). This showed the importance of deconditioning. It also gave a tool to monitor progress and provide very graphic feedback to the patient. There have been two main claims about these machines. First, that they measure "real" physical impairment associated with low back pain and that this measure is objective, reliable, and valid. Second, that only maximal effort can produce a consistent recording and so these machines can assess "effort." Critical review casts doubt on these claims (Newton & Waddell 1993). These machines do produce objective, reliable measures but they are measures of performance, not strength or capacity. There is also no good evidence that these machines can assess "effort." It is clear that we should not overinterpret the results of isokinetic assessment.

Functional restoration programs are usually full-time for 3–4 weeks. The core is an intensive program of incremented physical activity. The goal is physical reconditioning based on sports medicine principles. Subjective reports of symptoms are ignored, and there are no passive treatment modalities. Assessment of progress and the continued program depend on objective measures of function instead of subjective reports of pain. The entire program is based on behavioral principles.

A complete functional restoration program needs an interdisciplinary team of health professionals. A physician leads the team, to address medical concerns and provide clinical direction. Physical therapists guide the reconditioning program. Occupational therapists provide training in task performance and advise patients on socioeconomic problems of disability and return to work. Psychologists help patients and other team members to understand and deal with barriers to recovery.

The main outcome measure is return to work.

The results of functional restoration

The first two studies by Mayer et al (1985, 1987) and Hazard et al (1989) gave return to work rates of 85% and 81%. A review by Cutler et al (1994) concluded that functional restoration was effective.

However, it is worth looking at these studies in some detail (Teasell & Harth 1996). The key thing is that they were not RCTs. Mayer et al (1985, 1987) studied 199 patients with chronic low back pain who had been off work an average of 13 months. These were selected patients in a workers' compensation setting. The 85% success was for 116 patients who completed the program. The treatment comparison group was 72 patients who were refused third-party funding. There was a separate group of 11 drop-outs from the program. Only 39% of those who were refused treatment and 13% of the drop-outs returned to work. But these groups were not comparable. They were preselected groups of different patients and the drop-outs were really treatment failures. Hazard et al (1989) analyzed their results in the same way, with the same criticisms.

Oland & Tveiten (1991) tried to replicate a functional restoration program in Norway but only 32% returned to work by 6 months. As you might expect, this generated a heated debate. It also led to two proper RCTs (Alaranta et al 1994, Mitchell & Carmen 1994).

Alaranta in Finland studied 293 patients, aged 30–47 years, with low back pain for more than 6 months. Most had been off work for several months. Their 3-week, inpatient program included an intensive fitness, muscle-strengthening, and endurance exercise program. Patients then continued an exercise program on their own. They had intensive psychosocial training but no specific vocational intervention. The approach and goals of this program were very similar to those of Mayer, even if the detail varied. The control group had the same length of treatment, which was mainly physical therapy, and the authors estimated that the intensity of exercise was about 40–50%. The control group had no psychosocial training.

This study had 98% follow-up at 1 year. At 3 months, the functional restoration patients improved their range of movement, muscle strength, and endurance. However, the gains were greater in men than in women and fell off by 12 months. Self-reports of physical performance and disability improved in males and females and were maintained at 12 months. These improvements in physical performance were similar to those reported by Mayer. Both the treatment and control groups showed variable improvements in their psychological status. However, there was *no* difference in the amount of sick leave over the following year.

Initial results of functional restoration in the Workers' Compensation Board (WCB) of Ontario suggested that more than 80% returned to work compared with about 70% of matched controls (Mitchell & Carmen 1990). Mitchell & Carmen (1994) then carried out an RCT on 542 injured workers in Toronto. There was no preselection of patients, and none were refused funding. All patients were working full-time before their injury and had been off work for 3–6 months before starting treatment. All had "components of inappropriate illness behavior with continued pain." This extensive functional restoration program lasted 8–12 weeks, with 40 treatment days lasting 7 hours/day:

- an active exercise routine using a sports medicine approach
- an individualized goal-oriented program
- intensive psychological support.

Patients in the control group were sent back to their primary care provider for routine management in the community. This study had 100% follow-up. At 1 year, 79% of the treatment group was working full-time, compared with 78% of the control group.

Sinclair et al (1997) studied the subsequent performance of these Ontario WCB rehab clinics. They followed a further group of over 1500 injured workers for 1 year. The rehab program made no difference to any subjective measures such as pain, disability, or quality of life. However, patients who got the rehabilitation program were off work an average of 7 days *longer*, presumably while they were attending the program. Average treatment costs were almost double. Sinclair & Hogg-Johnson (2002) offered two possible explanations. Over the years there was a change in when workers reached the program. Many now came within the first 4 weeks, when they were more likely to get better quickly, with or without treatment. For political reasons, the WCB also stopped any contact between the rehabilitation physician and employers. Decisions about return to work were also left to the patients' routine physician. This meant there was no effective occupational intervention or partnership.

Why have functional restoration programs not lived up to their initial promise? Why are these results so different? The first and most important explanation is trial design. The first two reports were controlled trials, but they were not randomized. The controls were selected, with built-in bias. That is why proper RCTs are so important. The actual RCTs showed conflicting effects on pain, self-reported disability, and physical performance. The most striking difference was the lack of effect on sick leave or return to work. However, there were also differences in the patients, the exact content of the programs, and the settings.

Conclusion

Functional restoration is an important rehabilitation principle. It is a well-established and successful approach for conditions such as stroke and spinal cord injury. It is probably the best and most powerful *physical* approach ever devised for the rehabilitation of back pain. Yet, on critical examination, the evidence is that it does not achieve the goal of getting patients back to work (Teasell & Harth 1996, Guzman et al 2001). Why, then, does it not work?

Perhaps part of the problem is that it is such a hard, physical approach. To some patients, it may deny the legitimacy of their primary complaint – pain. The emphasis on "objective" measures may make it difficult to address more subjective issues. The program is based on psychological principles, but it is a behavioral approach based on operant-conditioning principles. In practice, it does not appear to address perceptions and beliefs, which are vital. An occupational therapist provides occupational assessment and advice, but there is no actual vocational intervention. There is little or no direct contact with the workplace or any attempt to get "all the players on side."

It may be useful at this point to compare different approaches to chronic pain (Main & Benjamin 1995). Traditional medical care tries to diagnose and treat the cause of pain. Pain management tries to improve quality of life, with a focus on pain, distress, and quality of life. Functional restoration tries to "normalize" back function, with a focus on physical performance and return to work. Pain management is subjective and "internalized". Functional restoration is more objective and "externalized". Pain management sometimes seems to have forgotten return to work issues. Functional restoration sometimes seems to have forgotten the more personal and human aspects of pain.

None of these approaches are successful at getting patients back to work. Perhaps that is because each only deals with part of the problem. Medicine treats symptoms. Pain management addresses beliefs and behavior. Functional restoration restores physical performance. They all fail to address other obstacles to return to work.

PRINCIPLES OF REHABILITATION

Can we pull this all together and extract some basic principles (Staal et al 2002)? A biopsychosocial framework lets us relate the components of a rehab program to the obstacles to recovery they aim to overcome (Table 18.9).

We must never forget the fundamental importance of good clinical management, with appropriate information and advice. Rehabilitation is no substitute, after bad, failed treatment.

The primary goal for patients and health care is relief of pain. Many patients will then rehabilitate themselves. For those patients who do not manage to return to ordinary activities and work by 4–6 weeks, further symptomatic treatment *on its own* is not enough. Continued or improved pain control should then be used to create a window of opportunity for rehabilitation.

This review suggests that there are three key ingredients to rehabilitation (Table 18.9).

Rehabilitation is reactivation. The goal is progressive increase in activity levels and restoration of function. Exercise has direct physiologic benefits, but that is really only the means to an end. It may help to focus on graded activity rather than progressive exercise, because that is the goal. We must translate gains from the health care setting into everyday life and work. We must address the inevitable relapses and recurrences.

Table 18.9   Components of a rehabilitation program: overcoming obstacles to recovery

	Obstacles to recovery	Components of rehab program
Bio-	Activity level vs job demands	Graded activity
Psycho-Social	Beliefs and behavior	Cognitive-behavioral
	Employment (system)	Occupational intervention; communication (policy)

Recovery and return to work require change in behavior. Behavior is driven by beliefs and fears about back pain, about how we should deal with it, and about back pain and work. Successful rehabilitation depends on changing beliefs and behavior. This is quite different from traditional medical education about back pain, and more than accurate information and advice. It must focus on and address those dysfunctional beliefs and behavior that may be obstacles to recovery. The evidence suggests this component should be cognitive-behavioral and not just behavioral alone.

The most important goal of rehabilitation for back pain is to maintain or restore capacity for work, and to minimize sickness absence. Everyone – patient, health professionals, and employer – must recognize and agree with this occupational goal. All the players must be on side. Many successful rehab programs include a specific occupational intervention. Many are in an occupational rather than a health care setting, which may have an important influence on beliefs and behavior. Some of the best evidence is for modified return to work. The main outcome measure is sustained return to regular work.

Now that we have a clearer idea of the three main components, let us look again at the key studies from Table 18.8. We have only included RCTs. We defined success in terms of work outcomes. (We left out Moffett et al (1999) because their results were unclear. They did reduce sickness absence by about one-third, but the numbers were small and did not reach significance.) Which rehab programs met these stricter criteria for each component

Table 18.10   Key components of successful and unsuccessful rehab programs

Components	Graded activity	Cognitive-behavioral	Occupational
Successful occupational outcomes			
Fordyce et al (1986)	+	+	−
Lindstrom et al (1992a, b)	+	+	+
Indahl et al (1995)	? (self)	? (information and advice)	−
Hagen et al (2000)	? (self)	? (information and advice)	−
Loisel et al (1997)	+	+	+
Bendix et al (1998)	+	+	−
Haldorsen et al (2002)	+	+	? (occasional)
Unsuccessful occupational outcomes			
Lindequist et al (1984)	+	−	−
Altmaier et al (1992)	+	+	−
Aberg (1994)	?	−	−
Friedrich et al (1998)	+	−	−
Haldorsen et al (1998)	+	+	? (occasional)
Jensen et al (2001)	+	+	+

+ component present in that study; ? present but inadequate or wrong type; − component missing in that study.

(Table 18.10)? It seems clear that graded activity alone is not enough. Most successful programs address beliefs in one way or another, and some of them also include an occupational intervention. Most of the programs that do not explicitly address these two issues are unsuccessful.

Two rehab programs do not seem to fit the pattern. Indahl's seems to be a clinical program with few of our key components, yet it was highly successful. Jensen's and Haldorsen's programs seem to have all our key components, yet did not have any consistent impact on sick leave. We really don't know why.

In addition to the three key components, there appear to be several other important conditions for a successful rehab program.

Timing is everything. Any intervention must be appropriate to the point in the time-course of sickness absence. The studies in Table 18.10 provide strong evidence that rehab programs can be effective at the subacute or early chronic stage, between about 6 weeks and 6 months. Very few studies focus on patients who have lost their jobs and are on long-term incapacity benefits. And none of them are RCTs. Clinical experience suggests that rehab

programs at this stage need to be more complex, intensive, and costly in time and resources. The social security literature shows that the success rate is also likely to be much lower (Waddell et al 2002).

Rehabilitation does not occur in a vacuum, but in a particular setting. It depends on a delivery system. Moffett & Frost (2000) discuss some of the practical issues and problems. It takes place within a particular organizational and policy framework. Ideally, patient, health professional(s), and employer should all work together in partnership, with a common, consistent approach to achieve agreed goals. This depends on communication: we cannot work together if we do not talk to each other! All the evidence is that the success of rehabilitation depends on the situation and setting. So we must design each rehab program to suit its particular situation. Changing beliefs and behavior and successful rehabilitation must also take account of the background culture surrounding back pain, disability, and work (Waddell et al 2002).

There are still many unanswered questions about rehabilitation (Carter & Birrell 2000). We need more research into the basic scientific principles.

We also need to develop more effective delivery systems.

- better screening for the early identification of patients at high risk of long-term incapacity
- better understanding of obstacles to return to work and specific interventions to address them
- more effective exercise, fitness, or graded-activity programs
- more effective methods of overcoming dysfunctional beliefs and behaviors
- more effective occupational interventions
- the best and minimal combination of these components into a rehabilitation program
- improved communication and partnership between all the players
- more timely, efficient, and effective delivery of rehabilitation.

We are well aware that many of the ideas in this chapter are speculative. This is not a systematic review. We have been selective and have chosen the material that we judge to be important. We have tried to develop some basic principles (Box 18.2). We have tried to generate ideas to explore with further research. But rehabilitation involves complex and difficult issues, many of which we do not fully understand. These ideas must be tested and we need further proof of what does or does not work. Hopefully, in another 5 years, this chapter will stand on much firmer ground.

Box 18.2   Principles of rehabilitation

Key principles
- Good clinical management is fundamental
- The primary goal of patients and health care is pain relief but
- For patients who do not recover quickly, health care alone is not enough

The three key components of rehabilitation
- Reactivation and progressive increase in activity levels
- Address dysfunctional beliefs and behavior
- An occupational component and/or setting

In addition
- Patient, health professional(s), and employer must communicate and work together to common, agreed goals
- Identify and address obstacles to return to work
- The main goal is job retention and (early) return to work

Delivery
- Timing
- Setting
- Organizational/policy framework
- Culture of rehabilitation and return to work

Outcome
- The measure of successful rehabilitation is sustained return to regular work

---

References

Abenhaim L, Rossignol M, Valat J-P et al 2000 The role of activity in the therapeutic management of back pain. Report of the International Paris Task Force on back pain. Spine 25 (suppl. 4S): 1S–35S

Aberg J 1984 Evaluation of an advanced back pain rehabilitation program. Spine 9: 317–318

Alaranta H, Rytokoski U, Rissanen A et al 1994 Intensive physical and psychosocial training program for patients with chronic low back pain. A controlled clinical trial. Spine 19: 1339–1349

Altmaier E M, Lehmann T R, Russell D W, Weinstein J N, Kao C F 1992 The effectiveness of psychological interventions for the rehabilitation of low back pain: a randomized controlled trial evaluation. Pain 49: 329–335

Bendix A F, Bendix T, Labriola M, Boekgaard P 1998 Functional restoration for chronic low back pain: two-year follow-up of two randomized clinical trials. Spine 23: 717–725

Bloch F S, Prins R (eds) 2001 Who returns to work and why? International Social Security Series (ISSA). Transaction, New Brunswick

Brown D 2002 Initiative evaluation report: back in work. HSE contract research report 441/2002. HSE books 01787-881165. Health & Safety Executive, London

BSRM 2000 Vocational rehabilitation: the way forward. British Society of Rehabilitation Medicine. London

Burton A K, Main C J 2000 Obstacles to recovery from work-related musculoskeletal disorders. In: Karwowski W (ed.) International encyclopedia of ergonomics and human factors. Taylor & Francis, London, pp 1542–1544

Carter J T, Birrell L N (eds) 2000 Occupational health guidelines for the management of low back pain at work – principal recommendations. Faculty of Occupational Medicine, London

Cooper J E, Tate R B, Yassi A, Khokhar J 1996 Effect of an early intervention program on the relationship between subjective pain and disability measures in nurses with low back injury. Spine 21: 2329–2336

Cutler R B, Fishbain D A, Rosomoff H L et al 1994 Does non-surgical pain center treatment of chronic pain return patients to work? A review and meta-analysis of the literature. Spine 19: 643–652

Dolce J J, Crocker M F, Moletteire C, Doleys D M 1986a Exercise quotas, anticipatory concern and self-efficacy expectancies in chronic pain: a preliminary report. Pain 24: 365–372

Dolce J J, Doleys D M, Raczynski J M, Lossie J, Poole L, Smith M 1986b The role of self-efficacy expectancies in the prediction of pain tolerance. Pain 27: 261–272

Evanoff B, Abedin S, Gayson D, Dale A M, Wolf L, Bohr P 2002 Is disability under-reported following work injury? Journal of Occupational Rehabilitation 12: 139–150

Faas A 1996 Exercises: which ones are worth trying, for which patients, and when? Spine 21: 2874–2879

Fordyce W E 1976 Behavioural methods for chronic pain and illness. Mosby, St Louis

Fordyce W E, McMahon R, Rainwater G et al 1981 Pain complaint–exercise performance relationship in chronic pain. Pain 10: 311–321

Fordyce W E, Brockway J A, Bergman J A, Spengler D 1986 Acute back pain: a control group comparison of behavioural vs traditional management methods. Journal of Behavioral Medicine 9: 127–140

Frank J W, Brooker A-S, DeMaio S E et al 1996 Disability resulting from occupational low back pain. Part II: What do we know about secondary prevention? A review of the scientific evidence on prevention after disability begins. Spine 21: 2918–2929.

Frank L, Sinclair S, Hogg-Johnson S et al 1998 Preventing disability from work-related low-back pain. New evidence gives new hope – if we can just get all the players on side. Canadian Medical Association Journal 158: 1625–1631

Friedrich M, Gittler G, Halberstadt Y, Cermak T, Heiller I 1998 Combined exercise and motivation program: effect on the compliance and level of disability of patients with chronic low back pain: a randomized controlled trial. Archives of Physical Medicine and Rehabilitation 79: 475–487

Gardiner J 1997 Bridges from benefit to work: a review. Joseph Rowantree Foundation, York

Gatchel R J, Turk D C 2002 Psychological approaches to pain management, 2nd edn. Guilford Publications, New York

Guzman J, Esmail R, Karjalainen K, Malmivaara A, Irvin E, Bombardier C 2001 Multi-disciplinary rehabilitation for chronic low back pain: systematic review. British Medical Journal 322: 1511–1516

Hagen E M, Eriksen H R, Ursin H 2000 Does early intervention with a light mobilization program reduce long-term sick leave for low back pain? Spine 25: 1973–1976

Haldorsen E M H, Kronholm K, Skouen J S, Ursin H 1998 Multimodal cognitive behavioral treatment of patients sicklisted for musculoskeletal pain. Scandinavian Journal of Rheumatology 27: 16–25

Haldorsen E M H, Grasdal A L, Skouen J S, Risa A E, Kronholm K, Ursin H 2002 Is there a right treatment for a particular patient group? Comparison of ordinary treatment, light multidisciplinary treatment, and extensive multidisciplinary treatment for long-term sick-listed employees with musculoskeletal pain. Pain 95: 49–63.

Hall H, McIntosh G, Melles T, Holowachuk B, Wai E 1994 Effect of discharge recommendations on outcome. Spine 19: 2033–2037

Hansson T H, Hansson E K 2001 The effects of common medical interventions on pain, back function and work resumption in patients with chronic low back pain. A prospective 2-year cohort study in six countries. Spine 25: 3055–3064

Hazard R G, Fenwick J W, Kalisch S M et al 1989 Functional restoration with behavioural support: a one year prospective study of patients with chronic low back pain. Spine 14: 157–161

Indahl A, Velund L, Reikeraas O 1995 Good prognosis for low back pain when left untampered. A randomized clinical trial. Spine 20: 473–477

Indahl A, Haldorsen E H, Holm S, Reikeras O, Ursin H 1998 Five-year follow-up study of a controlled clinical trial using light mobilization and an informative approach to low back pain. Spine 23: 2625–2630

Jarvikoski A, Mellin G, Estlander A et al 1993. Outcome of two multimodal back treatment programs with and without intensive physical training. Journal of Spinal Disorders 6: 93–98

Jensen I B, Nygren A, Lundin A 1994a Cognitive-behavioral treatment for workers with chronic spinal pain: a matched and controlled cohort study in Sweden. Occupational and Environmental Medicine 51: 145–151

Jensen M P, Turner J A, Romano J M 1994b Correlates of improvement in multidisciplinary treatment of chronic pain. Journal of Consulting and Clinical Psychology 62: 172–179

Jensen I B, Bergstrom G, Ljungquist T, Bodin L, Nygren A L 2001 A randomized controlled component analysis of a behavioral medicine rehabilitation program for chronic spinal pain: are the effects dependent on gender? Pain 91: 65–78

Kazimirski J C 1997 Canadian Medical Association policy statement. The physician's role in helping patients return to work after an illness or injury. Canadian Medical Association Journal 156: 680A–680C

Kendall N A S, Thompson B F 1998 A pilot program for dealing with the co-morbidity of chronic pain and long-term unemployment. Journal of Occupational Rehabilitation 8: 5–26

Krause N, Dasinger L K, Neuhauser F 1998 Modified work and return to work: a review of the literature. Journal of Occupational Rehabilitation 8: 113–139

Lindequist S, Lundberg B, Wikmark R et al 1984 Information and regime at low back pain. Scandinavian Journal of Rehabilitation Medicine 16: 113–116

Lindstrom I, Ohlund C, Eek C et al 1992a The effect of graded activity on patient with subacute low back pain: a randomized prospective clinical study with an operant conditioning behavioral approach. Physical Therapy 72: 279–291

Lindstrom I, Ohlund C, Eek C, Wallin L, Peterson L-E, Nachemson A 1992b Mobility, strength and fitness after a graded activity program for patients with subacute low back pain. Spine 17: 641–652

Lindstrom I, Ohlund C, Nachemson A 1995 Physical performance, pain, pain behavior and subjective disability in patients with subacute low back pain. Scandinavian Journal of Rehabilitation Medicine 27: 153–160

Linton S J (ed.) 2002 New avenues for the prevention of chronic musculoskeletal pain and disability. Pain research and clinical management, vol. 12. Elsevier, Amsterdam

Linton S J, Andersson T 2000 Can chronic disability be prevented? A randomized trial of a cognitive-behavior intervention and two forms of information for patents with spinal pain. Spine 25: 2855–2831

Linton S J, Ryberg M 2001 A cognitive-behavioral group intervention as prevention for persistent neck and back pain in a non-patient population: a randomized controlled trial. Pain 90: 83–90

Loisel P, Abenhaim L, Durand P et al 1997 A population-based, randomized clinical trial on back pain management. Spine 22: 2911–2918

Loisel P, Lemaire J, Poitras S et al 2002 Cost-benefit and cost-effectiveness analysis of a disability prevention model for back pain management: a six year follow-up study. Occupational and Environmental Medicine 59: 807–815

Main C J, Benjamin S 1995 Psychological treatment and the health care system; the chaotic case of back pain. Is there a need for a paradigm shift? In: Mayou R, Bass C, Sharpe M (eds) Treatment of functional somatic symptoms. Oxford University Press, Oxford, pp 214–230

Main C J, Burton A K 2000 Economic and occupational influences on pain and disability. In: Main C J, Spanswick C C (eds) Pain management. An interdisciplinary approach. Churchill Livingstone, Edinburgh, pp 63–87.

Main C J, Spanswick C C (eds) 2000 Pain management: an interdisciplinary approach. Churchill Livingstone, Edinburgh

Mannion A F, Muntener M, Taimela S, Dvorak J 1999 A randomized clinical trial of three active therapies for chronic low back pain. Spine 24: 2435–2448

Mannion A F, Taimela S, Muntener M, Dvorak J 2001a Active therapy for chronic low back pain: part 1. Effects on back muscle activation, fatigability and strength. Spine 26: 897–908

Mannion A F, Junge A, Taqimela S et al 2001b Active therapy for chronic low back pain: part 3. Factors influencing self-rated disability and its change following therapy. Spine 26: 920–929

Marhold C, Linton S J, Melin L 2001 A cognitive-behavioral return-to-work program: effects on pain patients with a history of long-term versus short-term sick leave. Pain 91: 155–163

Marhold C, Linton S J, Melin L 2002 Identification of obstacles for chronic pain patients to return to work: evaluation of a questionnaire. Journal of Occupational Rehabilitation 12: 65–75

Mayer T G, Gatchel R J 1988 Functional restoration for spinal disorders: the sports medicine approach. Lea & Febiger, Philadelphia, pp 1–321

Mayer T, Gatchel R, Kishino N et al 1985 Objective assessment of spine function following industrial injury. A prospective study with comparison group and one-year follow-up. Spine 10: 482–493

Mayer T G, Gatchel R J, Mayer H, Kishino N D, Keeley J, Mooney V 1987 A prospective two-year study of functional restoration in industrial low back injury. Journal of the American Medical Association 258: 1763–1767

Mitchell R I, Carmen G M 1990 Results of a multicenter trial using an intensive active exercise program for the treatment of acute soft tissue and back injuries. Spine 15: 514–521

Mitchell R I, Carmen G M 1994 The functional restoration approach to the treatment of chronic pain in patients with soft tissue and back injuries. Spine 19: 633–642

Moffett J K, Frost H 2000 Back to fitness programme: the manual for physiotherapists to set up the classes. Physiotherapy 86: 295–305

Moffett J K, Torgerson D, Bell-Syer S et al 1999 Randomised controlled trial of exercise for low back pain: clinical outcomes, costs and preferences. British Medical Journal 319: 279–283

Morley S, Eccleston C, Williams A 1999 Systematic review and meta-analysis of randomized controlled trials of cognitive behaviour therapy and behaviour therapy for chronic pain in adults, excluding headache. Pain 80: 1–13

Newton M, Waddell G 1993 Trunk strength testing with iso-machines. Part I: review of a decade of clinical evidence. Spine 18: 801–811

Newton M, Thow M, Somerville D, Henderson I, Waddell G 1993 Trunk strength testing with iso-machines. Part II. Experimental evaluation of the Cybex II back testing system in normal subjects and patients with chronic low back pain. Spine 18: 812–824

Nocon A, Baldwin S 1998 Trends in rehabilitation policy. King's Fund, London

Oland G, Tveiten G 1991 A trial of modern rehabilitation for chronic low-back pain and disability: vocational outcome and effect on pain modulation. Spine 16: 457–459

Oldervoll L M, Ro M, Zwart J-A, Svebak S 2001 Comparison of two physical exercise programs for the early intervention of pain in the lower back in female hospital staff. Journal of Rehabilitation Medicine 33: 156–161

Peat G M, Moores L, Goldingay S, Hunter M 2001 Pain management program follow-ups. A national survey of current practice in the United Kingdom. Journal of Pain and Symptom Management 21: 218–226

Petersen T, Kryger P, Ekdahl C, Olsen S, Jacobsen S 2002 The effect of McKenzie therapy as compared with that of intensive strengthening training for the treatment of patients with subacute or chronic low back pain: a randomized controlled trial. Spine. 27: 1702–1708

Rainville J, Ahern D K, Phalen L, Childs L A, Sutherland R 1992 The association of pain with physical activities in chronic low back pain. Spine 17: 1060–1064

Richardson I H, Richardson P H, Williams A C deC, Featherstone J, Harding V R 1994 The effects of a cognitive-behavioural pain management programme on the quality of work and employment status of severely impaired chronic pain patients. Disability and Rehabilitation 16: 26–34

Ryan W E, Krishna M K, Swanson C E 1995 A prospective study evaluating early rehabilitation in preventing back pain chronicity in mine workers. Spine 20: 489–491

Sachs B, David J-O F, Olimpio D, Scala A D, Lacroix M 1990 Spinal rehabilitation by a work tolerance based on objective physical capacity assessment of dysfunction: a prospective study with control subjects and twelve-month review. Spine 15: 1325–1332

Scheer S J, Watanabe T K, Radack K L 1997 Randomized controlled trials in industrial low back pain. Part 3. Subacute/chronic pain interventions. Archives of Physical Medicine and Rehabilitation 78: 414–423

Sinclair S J, Hogg-Johnson S 2002 Early rehabilitation: the Ontario experience. In: Linton S J (ed.) New avenues for the prevention of chronic musculoskeletal pain and disability. Pain research and clinical management, vol. 12. Elsevier, Amsterdam, pp 259–268

Sinclair S, Hogg-Johnson S, Mondloch M V, Shields S A 1997 Evaluation of effectiveness of an early, active intervention program for workers with soft tissue injuries. Spine 22: 2919–2931

Skouen J S, Grasdal A L, Haldorsen E M H, Ursin H 2002 Relative cost-effectiveness of extensive and light multidisciplinary treatment programs versus treatment as usual for patients with chronic low back pain on long-term sick leave. Spine 27: 901–910

Spanswick C C, Million R 2000 Medical assessment. In: Main C J, Spanswick C C (eds) Pain management: an interdisciplinary approach. Churchill Livingstone, Edinburgh, pp 139–157

Staal J B, Hlobil H, van Tulder M W, Köke A J A, Smid T, van Mechelen W 2002 Return to work interventions for low back pain: a descriptive review of contents and concepts of working mechanisms. Sports Medicine 32: 251–267

Strand L I, Ljunggren A E, Haldorsen E M H, Espehaug B 2001 The impact of physical function and pain on work status at 1-year follow-up in patients with back pain. Spine 26: 800–808

Tate R B, Yassi A, Cooper J 1999 Predictors of time loss after back injury in nurses. Spine 24: 1930–1936

Teasell R W, Harth M 1996 Functional restoration: returning patients with chronic low back pain to work – revolution or fad? Spine 21: 844–847

Thornton P 1998 International research project on job retention and return to work strategies for disabled workers. International Labour Office, Geneva

TUC 2000 Consultation document on rehabilitation: getting better at betting back. Trades Union Congress, London

Turk D C, Rudy T E 1991 Neglected topics in the treatment of chronic pain patients: relapse, noncompliance and treatment adherence. Pain 44: 5–28

Turk D C, Meichenbaum D H, Genest M 1983 Pain and behavioural medicine. A cognitive-behavioural perspective. Guilford Press, New York

Van Doorn J W 1995 Low back disability among self-employed dentists, veterinarians, physicians and physical therapists in the Netherlands. Acta Orthopaedica Scandinavica 66 (suppl. 263): 1–64

Van Tulder M W, Koes B W 2002 Low back pain and sciatica: chronic. Clinical Evidence 8: 1171–1187. Available online at: www.clinicalevidence.com

Vlaeyen J W S, de Jong J, Geilen M, Heuts P H T G, van Breukelen G 2002a The treatment of fear of movement/(re)injury in chronic low back pain: further evidence on the effectiveness of exposure in vivo. Clinical Journal of Pain 18: 251–261

Vlaeyen J W S, de Jong J, Sieben J M, Crombez G 2002b Graded exposure in vivo for pain-related fear. In: Gatchel R, Turk D C (eds) Psychological approaches to pain management. Guildford Press, New York

Von Korff M 1999 Pain management in primary care: an individualized stepped-care approach. In: Gatchel R J, Turk D C (eds) Psychosocial factors in pain: clinical perspectives. Guilford Press, New York, pp 360–373

Von Korff M, Moore J C 2001 Stepped care for back pain: activating approaches for primary care. Annals of Internal Medicine 134: 911–917

Vowles K E, Gross R T 2003 Work-related fears about injury and physical capability for work in individuals with chronic pain. Pain 101: 291–298

Vuori I M 2001 Dose–response of physical activity and low back pain, osteoarthritis, and osteoporosis. Medicine and Science in Sports and Exercise 33(suppl. 6): S551–S586

Waddell G, Burton A K 2000 Occupational health guidelines for the management of low back pain at work – evidence review. Faculty of Occupational Medicine, London

Waddell G, Aylward M, Sawney P 2002 Back pain, incapacity for work and social security benefits: an international literature review and analysis. Royal Society of Medicine Press, London

Wade D T, de Jong B A 2000 Recent advances in rehabilitation. British Medical Journal 32: 1385–1388

Watson P J 2001 Back to work: report to the Department of Employment on the efficacy of integrated vocational rehabilitation for social security benefits recipients with low back pain. National Disability Development initiative. Department for Education and Employment, Bristol

WHO 2000 International classification of functioning, disability and health (ICF). World Health Organization, Geneva

Wood D J 1987 Design and evaluation of a back injury prevention program within a geriatric hospital. Spine 12: 77–82

Yassi A, Tate R, Cooper J E et al 1995 Early intervention for back-injured nurses at a large Canadian tertiary care hospital: an evaluation of the effectiveness and cost benefits of a two-year poilot project. Occupational Medicine 45: 209–214

Chapter 19

UK health care for back pain

We all spend our working lives treating individual patients, and it is difficult to see the broad picture of health care. Let us now try to look at it from a different perspective. What health care services and resources are devoted to back pain? Let us look first at the UK, where the National Health Service (NHS) makes it easier to see the whole picture.

Remember the background of need (Ch. 5). There are now 55 million people in the UK, but back trouble mainly affects adults, and the number of people aged 16 or over is 44 million. Roughly 27 million are employed: 15 million men and 12 million women, although many women only work part-time. Thirty-seven percent of adults have back pain lasting at least 24 hours each year – that is about 16 million people. Three to four percent of those aged 16–44 years, and 5–7% of those aged 45–64 years, say their back trouble is a "chronic illness."

So, who gets health care for back pain in the UK? Who do they see? And what happens to them?

THE NATIONAL HEALTH SERVICE

The health care system in the UK is very different from that in the US. The NHS provides 97–98% of all health care in the UK. The NHS was started in 1948 with the basic principle that care should be free at the time of need and should be funded from taxation. UK expenditure on sickness and health care is now about 7% of gross domestic product, which despite recent increases is still lower than the European average. It is not possible to meet unrestrained demand with limited resources and the result is waiting lists. You often wait several days for an appointment to see a family doctor. It takes weeks or even months to see a therapist. It takes months – sometimes many months – to see a specialist. You can wait weeks or months for a scan. You then join another waiting list for surgery and in some places that will take more than a year. Despite many political attempts at reform over the past 20 years, waiting lists are still a major problem. On the whole, the NHS is quite good at seeing urgent and emergency cases. The problem is how to provide an adequate service for the large numbers of "routine" patients – and most back pain is regarded as routine.

Access to NHS service is through your family doctor or general practitioner (GP). Everyone in the UK has a GP and many people stay with the same GP for years. In principle, and often in practice, GPs know their patients. They know their medical histories and their social and family background. The GP is the "gate keeper" who controls referral to a specialist and the choice of specialist, although patients can request referral and a second opinion. Access to physiotherapy – the British term for physical therapy – is also through the GP. Osteopathy and chiropractic are rarely available on the NHS. The only way to bypass your GP for NHS treatment is through a hospital Accident and Emergency (A&E) department. Each year nearly half a million people attend A&E departments with back pain. These departments are really meant for medical emergencies but patients can walk in off the street. This may sometimes give a more direct route to hospital services, but at other times that attempt is rebuffed.

All NHS staff, therapists and MDs alike, are salaried. So there is no direct financial incentive to NHS investigation or treatment.

Private medicine only provides 2–3% of all health care in the UK. It includes medical specialists (MDs), who usually work mainly in the NHS and part-time in private practice, some physiotherapists, and all chiropractors and osteopaths. Private medical specialists in the UK function very much as in the US. In the UK, however, patients usually get their GP to refer them to a private medical specialist and do not self-refer. Physiotherapy practice in the UK is very similar to physical therapy in the US. Chiropractors in the UK have very similar training, professional status, and practice as in the US, but they are still fewer. Osteopaths, however, are very different. In the US, a DO is more or less the

same as an MD and functions very much as any other physician, whether in family practice or as a medical specialist. In the UK, however, osteopaths function much more like chiropractors. Most patients go directly to an osteopath or chiropractor, though more GPs are now advising patients to seek such care. Access to private therapy is usually within a matter of days, which is one of its major advantages over the NHS. Many private health care insurance schemes cover osteopathy or chiropractic, but only if authorized by a GP or medical specialist. So, in practice, most patients consult and pay for an osteopath or chiropractor themselves.

Patients also attend their GP for sick certificates. Employers, private insurance, and state benefits all demand sick certificates from an MD. Registered osteopaths and chiropractors can legally issue sick certificates, but they rarely do. Since 1982, patients sign their own sick certificates for up to 7 days.

Health care statistics

We can get information about health care from patients or from medical records, but these sources are very different. They ask different questions and get different results. They have different problems and errors.

Population surveys depend on patients' memory of the health care they receive. The answers are subjective and there is no cross-check. The answers vary with the exact wording of the questions. The questions usually define a time period, often of 1 year, but the longer the period, the less accurate the answers. If a patient has had a lot of trouble, he or she is more likely to answer "yes," even if that treatment was actually before the time period of the question. Many questions simply ask "Have you seen …?" or "Have you had …?" but perhaps back pain was not the main reason for consulting. Patient and doctor may have different ideas of what the consultation was about. The patient may indeed have back pain, but the doctor may not think that was the main reason for consulting. For all these reasons, population surveys probably overestimate health care for back pain. Or they may overestimate serious health problems but underestimate minor problems because people forget.

Medical records have other problems. They focus on medical diagnosis or at least the clinical problem, but this does not always reflect the patient's concerns or reason for consulting. They record the main problem but may not include all secondary symptoms or problems. Patients with back pain often have other problems and the doctor must judge which to record as the main problem. Medical records are often sparse and the coding of data is crude. For example, it is often difficult to separate low back problems from neck problems in official UK statistics. These statistics depend on large numbers of clerical staff collecting and sorting data. With all these potential problems, it is not surprising that most NHS statistics have an error of at least 15% and sometimes more. Data also come from different sources and methods and may not be comparable. The data reflect official interest and do not give a complete picture. Social security records, for example, are about benefits paid, which is not the same as work loss or sickness. NHS figures omit all private health care. For all these reasons, official statistics probably underestimate health care for back pain.

The true figure probably lies between these two estimates. Or they may tell us different things. Medical records may give a better estimate of health care resources used mainly for back pain. Population surveys may give a better estimate of total perceived need for health care for back pain.

Official UK statistics are now quite up-to-date, but that was not always so in the past. Most health care use for back pain increased up to the 1990s, so we must place all data in its correct time frame.

WHO CONSULTS?

No health worker who treats back pain should ever forget that most people deal with it themselves most of the time. The Consumers' Association (1985) found that, of those British people who had ever had back pain, about one-third had sought care in the previous year; one-third had treatment at some time in the past but not in the previous year; and one-third had never seen anyone about it. Current Working Backs Scotland surveys still show that only about one-third of those with back pain in the previous year sought health care.

There is no imperative about health care for back pain. It is not life-threatening and no one has to get treatment. Nor is it only a question of severity of pain. People with more severe and more prolonged

pain are more likely to seek help, while those with less severe and shorter periods of pain are more likely to deal with it themselves (Tables 19.1 and 19.2). But a surprising number of people who say that their pain is very severe and present all or most of the year do not seek any health care. Eighteen percent of those who say they have "unbearable pain" have never seen a doctor.

The South Manchester Study (Croft et al 1994) also found little difference in the back pain described by people who saw their GP and those who dealt with it on their own (Table 19.3). The greatest difference was that more of those who were off work saw their doctor, but that may just reflect the need to see a doctor for a sick certificate.

What people do about back pain depends as much on the person as on the medical condition. *The Nuprin Pain Report* (Taylor & Curran 1985)

Table 19.1 How severity of pain affects consulting in the UK

	Seen GP in the past year	No health care in the past year
Duration of back pain in the past year		
None	12	211
Part of the year	132	310
All or most of the year	126	79
Severity of back pain on a scale 0–10		
0–4	48	190
4–7	111	141
7–10	99	59

Based on data from Consumers' Association (1985).

Table 19.2 How severity of pain affects consulting in the US

Severity of back pain on a scale 0–10	Percentage who have ever consulted a doctor
Slight 0–3	39
Moderate 4–6	51
Severe 7–9	74
Unbearable 10	82

Based on data from *The Nuprin Pain Report* (Taylor & Curran 1985).

Table 19.3 Nature of low back pain and disability in adults who have had pain in the past year

	Adults with back pain who have not consulted[a] (%)	Adults who have consulted their GP[a] (%)
Continuous pain	18	31
Pain down leg	46	36
More than 3 months of pain in the past year	37	38
Restricted activity	44	55
Needed bed rest	18	20
Off work due to low back pain	8	23

[a]Percentages of those with back pain.
From the South Manchester Study, with permission.

found that people with more stress are more likely to seek medical help. It is a matter of how they view the problem, how they react, and how they try to deal with it. Many factors affect whether they seek health care (Mechanic 1968):

- severity of symptoms
- effect on quality of life
- fear and anxiety
- attitudes and beliefs about backache and what they should do about it
- family and fellow workers' attitudes and beliefs
- expectations and experience of health care for backache
- availability, social costs, and benefits of health care
- need for sick certification to stay off work.

Waxman et al (1998) studied influences on GP consultations for back pain in UK. The single most important factor was the belief that pain management was a matter for professionals rather than a personal responsibility. The influences varied at different stages. In the first 2 weeks, consultation depended on severity of pain. After 2 weeks, it depended more on disability. After 3 months, it was associated with depression.

There are many steps in health care utilization:

- recognize symptoms
- self-treatment
- communication with family and fellow workers

- assess symptoms
- express concern
- assume sick role
- assess treatment options
- choice of treatment
- consultation
- investigation and treatment
- assess how treatment affects symptoms
- recovery and rehabilitation.

Patients with chronic pain may recycle through some of these steps again and again. Different patients may have very different reasons for consulting. The same patient may have different reasons at different times. Recognizing and meeting their needs may be the key to a successful consultation and patient satisfaction.

Summary

Most people deal with back pain themselves most of the time
- Only about a third of people who have back pain each year consult a doctor
- There is little difference in the back pain described by those who consult a doctor and those who deal with it themselves
- Many factors influence the decision to seek health care for back pain

GP consultation

Earlier surveys showed that about 85% of people who sought any health care for back pain in the UK saw their GP. Recent Working Backs Scotland surveys show the same. Most of the others attend some kind of therapist.

Altogether, 78% of the UK population consult their GP each year: 43 million people see their GPs some 130 million times. Although back pain is one of the two or three most common bodily symptoms, overall it is only the fifth most common reason for seeing a doctor in the UK (Scottish Health Service statistics 2000). Respiratory conditions are by far the most common reason: 19% of men and 30% of women consult for these reasons each year. Genitourinary problems are nearly as common in women. Next come mental health problems and

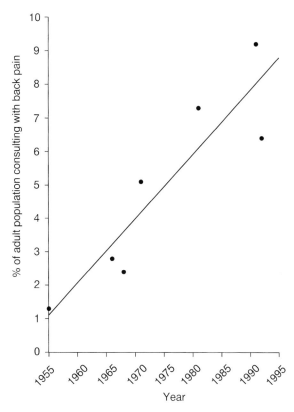

Figure 19.1   The rising trend in GP consultations for back pain up to the early 1990s. Has it now plateaued?

Table 19.4   GP consulting rates for back pain per annum as a percentage of the population

Age (years)	Male	Female
5–15	1.1	1.3
16–24	4.7	6.0
25–44	8.2	9.6
45–64	10.5	12.6
65–74	8.7	10.6
75–84	8.2	9.9
All ages	6.7	8.1

Based on data from the Fourth National Morbidity Study (McCormick et al 1995).

then hypertension and skin conditions. Back pain is the most common reason for consulting in men aged 25–44 years and the second most common in men aged 45–64. There is no age group of women in whom it is higher than fourth. It is a much less common reason for consulting in the young and the elderly.

Up to the early 1990s, there was a steady increase in the number of people who saw their GP with back pain (Fig. 19.1). The Fourth National Morbidity Study (McCormick et al 1995) recorded that 9.2% of adults saw their GP with back pain in 1991–1992. The most recent Working Backs Scotland surveys in 2002 give a comparable figure of 8.5%. That is roughly 4 million people in the UK each year. Each patient who saw their GP with back pain attended an average of 1.6 times (McCormick et al 1995). It varied from 1.4 times for sprains and strains of the back to 2.0 times for disk disorders. In the South Manchester Study, 40% of those who

attended with back pain saw their GP again within 3 months. However, only 25% came again with back pain and the other 15% with some other complaint. If 4 million people attend their GP an average of 1.6 times, there are about 6.5 million GP consultations for back pain each year in the UK. So, just over 4% of all GP consultations in the UK are for back pain.

At least up to the early 1990s, GPs visited about 10% of these 4 million people at home because the pain was so "acute." Compare that with the rarity of domiciliary visits in the US!

Consulting rates vary with gender and age (Table 19.4). Women consult slightly more than men, with back pain as for all health reasons. Consulting rates for back pain increase from early adult life, with a peak in late middle life and a slight fall in older age.

A recent survey in Glasgow (Furniss et al 2002) found that one-third of patients attended their GP within 1 week of onset of back pain and 72% within 4 weeks. Forty-six percent received an appointment within 48 hours and 83% within 5 days.

Table 19.5 shows GP diagnoses of back problems in the UK. Remember that medical diagnosis of non-specific low back pain follows fads and fashions and has little to do with pathology. There is some variation in diagnosis with age. Sprains and strains are most common in the young. Osteoarthritis of the spine increases with age. Intervertebral disk disorders peak at 45–64 years. This may to some extent reflect the age range of different pathologies, but it probably also depends on diagnostic beliefs and customs.

Table 19.5   GP diagnosis of back disorders

Diagnosis	Percentage of population consulting	Average number of consultations
Ankylosing spondylitis and related disorders	0.10	1.8
Spondylosis and allied disorders (or osteoarthritis of the spine)	1.19	1.7
Intervertebral disk disorders	0.39	2.0
Other disorders of cervical region	0.91	1.3
Sciatica	1.20	
Backache and lumbago[a]	2.52	
Sprains and strains	2.12	1.4

[a]Together these are "other and unspecified disorders of the back." Based on data from the Fourth National Morbidity Study (McCormick et al 1995).

Perhaps more important is how GPs perceive patients with back pain and how that influences their management. Skelton et al (1995) interviewed GPs in 12 practices in Nottingham. They found six main ways that they differentiated these patients:

1. Psychological status. Most patients were "normal" but a small minority had some form of "psychological disturbance."
2. Clinical condition. "Acute" patients had a short episode of severe pain, which usually resolved quickly. "Chronic" patients had a longer duration of pain, did not respond to treatment, and were difficult and frustrating.
3. Patients' approach to management – whether they were motivated, took advice and took responsibility for self-management. (Most did not.)
4. Whether the patient was "genuine," i.e., if they were "obviously" in severe pain and stoical.
5. Social class. This was often stereotyped.
6. Gender and occupation. This was again often stereotyped.

The "ideal" patient was easy to treat, and would cooperate, respond, and be satisfied. These GPs had no good answer for the "difficult" patient. You can guess which was which!

TREATMENT

GP treatment

Table 19.6 shows the treatment patients receive from their GPs. There has been a dramatic shift since the early 1990s.

In all the earlier studies, most medical treatment for back pain was passive. The most common treatment was analgesics and anti-inflammatory agents. More than half of those who saw their GP were prescribed bed rest. GPs issued sick certificates to stay off work for almost a quarter of those who came to see them. If they continued to attend with back pain over several months, they would probably get an X-ray and be referred for physiotherapy. About 20% were referred to a hospital specialist, but most later rather than sooner. They were then often referred again and again.

Our recent surveys show that treatment is now much more active. This particular data may be partly due to the Working Backs Scotland education campaign (Ch. 16) and it will be interesting to compare this with up-to-date data from England. There appears to be little or no change in the use of analgesics. Most patients now get advice to stay active instead of to restrict their activities. Bed rest is now rare. Only about 5% now receive a sick certificate. There has possibly been a slight increase in

Table 19.6   Treatment received from GPs (as a percentage of those who consult)

What the GP did	Early 1990s[a]	2002[b]
Advised analgesics	64	64
Gave advice to restrict activities	80	10
Gave advice to stay active	10–20	31
Prescribed bed rest	>50	3
X-ray	20	20
Refer to specialist	17	17
Refer to physiotherapy	11	15
Sick certification	22	5

[a]Based on data from an unpublished survey of Scottish GPs (1985), Mason (1994), Croft et al (1994).
[b]Based on unpublished data from Working Backs Scotland 2002.

the number referred for physiotherapy. Croft et al (1994) found that only 2% got physiotherapy within 3 months of their first visit to their GP. They do now seem to be getting it earlier. There has been little change in the use of X-ray. Nor is there any obvious change in the pattern of referral to specialists. That may simply reflect availability, which has not changed in the last decade.

Therapy

About 2.3 million people in the UK get some form of physical therapy for back pain each year. The average course of physiotherapy, osteopathy, or chiropractic is about six to seven sessions. However, a few patients continue to attend for months or even years. Table 19.7 details UK statistics for these three forms of therapy for back pain. To some extent these figures simply reflect the numbers of the three kinds of therapists. Remember that only physiotherapy is available free to NHS patients. It is striking that private practitioners now provide more than half of all physical therapy for back pain in the UK. No other condition approaches this. And few NHS staff are aware of it.

Foster et al (1999) and Gracey et al (2002) surveyed UK physiotherapy for back pain in 1994–1997. The most common treatments were practical advice (90%), Maitland (60–90%) or McKenzie (50–70%) treatments, and interferential electrotherapy (30–40%). Therapy at that time was still largely passive. There was little agreement on the best kind of exercise. Despite the scientific evidence, there was very little manipulation, fitness or multidisciplinary programs, or use of cognitive-behavioral principles. There is no doubt that physiotherapy for back pain in UK is now changing. There is growing interest in a biopsychosocial approach (Gifford 2000). There is much less use of passive modalities. There are more, and more active "back classes" (Fig. 18.2, Ch. 18). The NHS Modernisation Agency has set up a National Back Pain Collaborative (www.modern.nhs.uk/orthopaedics) which provides a forum to exchange ideas and experience. Fifteen teams covering 30 health communities around the UK have already joined. Let me give one example of a local, physiotherapy-led Back Service in Glasgow (Furniss et al 2002). The pilot scheme was funded by the Primary Care Development Fund. It was set up as a dedicated service with two and a half specialist physiotherapists. The goal was to implement the RCGP (1999) guidelines. The practical aims were to:

- establish an algorithm for patients with acute or recurrent low back pain (<8 weeks)
- provide evidence-based practice using appropriate assessment and treatment methods
- identify and provide educational material for patients
- develop lines of communication and referral with GPs
- set up fast-track links with orthopedics
- monitor uptake, delivery, and satisfaction with the service
- identify areas of potential development for the service, in order to provide the best possible patient care
- educate physiotherapy colleagues.

Patients who presented with "red flags" went direct to the appropriate specialty. As far as we can tell, none were missed. All other patients with back pain went to the Back Service. After assessment, those with acute nerve root problems were "fast-tracked" to orthopedics. Treatment for those with non-specific back pain and non-surgical root pain included information and advice, symptomatic measures (to facilitate exercise and rehabilitation), manual therapy (Maitland or McKenzie),

Table 19.7 UK staffing and workload of various forms of therapy for back pain

Type of therapy	Number of therapists[a]	Percentage of time spent on back pain	Number of patients treated for back pain each year[b]
NHS			
Physiotherapy	12 000	10	1.0 million
Private			
Physiotherapy	2200	?	0.3 million
Osteopathy	2500	67	0.7 million
Chiropractic	1000	50	0.3 million
Total private			1.3 million

[a]Estimated number working, in full-time equivalents.
[b]Based on 1993 data, before the CSAG (1994) report.

individual exercises and fitness, and training in self-management.

A total of 1281 patients were referred to the service in the first 12 months, 65% of them from their first GP visit. Eighty-nine percent were seen within 2 weeks. Sixty-two percent were appropriate referrals and the patients attended their first appointment. There was some initial problem of GPs trying to refer patients with more chronic problems, and 16% of patients failed to keep their first appointment. Patients then had an average of one assessment session and six treatment sessions over 5 weeks. Only 5 patients with acute nerve root problems needed to be fast-tracked to orthopedics. Over the course of treatment, mean pain intensity fell from 5.3 to 1.4 and the Roland & Morris disability score fell from 8 to 1. Thirty-three percent were off work at initial assessment, and only 5% at discharge. Eighty-eight percent of all patients felt the treatment was very good and met all their needs. Only 5% sought any further treatment.

We should not overinterpret these results. This was a pilot service run by enthusiasts. It was a selected group of patients whose natural history was to get better anyway. It was uncontrolled. Yet it does show that it is possible to deliver a much more efficient and satisfactory service even with limited NHS resources. There are a growing number of such services in UK, though there are also many gaps. There are no up-to-date national data on therapy services for back pain.

Hospital outpatient clinics

In the UK, NHS patients see medical specialists in hospital outpatient clinics. Various sets of data suggest that about 1.6 million people attend an NHS specialist with back pain each year. Back pain is the reason for about 5% of all new outpatient visits in all adult specialties in NHS hospitals.

The South Manchester Study gave the most detailed information, and there is no evidence this has changed. They found that the four "back pain specialties" were orthopedics, rheumatology, pain clinics, and neurosurgery. Every patient whose back pain was due to a spinal problem or a mechanical problem in his or her back went to one of these departments. Small numbers of patients going to other specialties had "back pain at least in part the

reason for referral." In all of these patients, however, the symptom of back pain was a minor part of some other condition. GP triage between primary back disorders and other non-spinal disease does seem to be reasonably accurate.

Of the four back pain specialties, orthopedics has by far the largest clinics and about half the patients with back trouble attend there (Table 19.8). That is where patients with back pain go. Looking at it from another perspective, back pain is a large part of the outpatient workload of each of the four back pain specialties (Table 19.9).

In the South Manchester Study, 28% of new patients with back disorders were seen within 3 months, and 83% within 6 months. In a national survey, 29% of all routine orthopedic outpatients were seen within 4 months. NHS reforms in the 1990s

Table 19.8 Percentage of patients with back pain seen in each specialty clinic

Clinic	Hope Hospital	Stockport hospitals
Orthopedic	48	61
Rheumatology	22	14
Pain	7	8
Neurosurgery	6	
General medicine	8	6
Urology and gynecology	8	10
General surgery	2	
Psychiatry		2
Total patients with any back pain	100%	100%

From the South Manchester Study, with permission.

Table 19.9 Back pain as a proportion of the total workload of specialty clinics: proportion of new patients at each clinic who present with back pain

Clinic	Hope Hospital	Stockport hospitals
General orthopedic (excluding knee and hand clinics)	45%	28%
Rheumatology	36%	27%
Pain	41%	52%
Neurosurgery	21%	

From the South Manchester Study, with permission.

seemed at first to be reducing waiting lists, but more recent data show they are longer than ever.

The South Manchester Study also obtained clinical detail on these patients referred to hospital. Their back pain was severe and long-standing. Ninety-one percent had back pain for more than 3 months in total in the past year; 73% had continuous rather than recurrent pain; 62% had other medical problems as well as back pain. Despite being "new" referrals, 36% had seen a specialist before with back problems. Only 10% were in full-time work outside the home. Half said they had lost or changed their job because of their back, and 63% were "not working because of ill health or disability."

At the clinic, 35% had X-rays and 34% were given blood tests. The most common treatments were physiotherapy for 38% and further medication for 25%. Thirty-one percent got a return appointment to the same clinic and 15% were referred on to another hospital specialist.

What do specialist consultations achieve?

Coulter et al (1989, 1991) studied GP referrals to NHS outpatient clinics. Table 19.10 shows the reasons GPs gave for referring patients with back pain. In my practice, reassuring the patient or GP was a more common reason than these GPs admit. But the striking thing is that GPs do seem to have realistic expectations and do not often refer these patients looking for a magic cure.

The GPs referred 20% of these patients within 6 months of their first visit with back pain. But they treated 59% of them for at least 2 years before their

first specialist referral. So it seems that GPs use specialist referral as a last rather than a first resort. However, 46% of these GP referrals had already seen a specialist before with back trouble, and for 8% this was at least their fourth specialist referral. So when GPs do refer patients with back pain to a specialist, they then often refer them again and again.

Coulter et al (1989) also looked at the outcome of these referrals. What actually happened was very different from what the GP was looking for. Sixty-nine percent of patients sent for reassurance or advice only actually got some form of treatment. Many of these patients then had multiple clinic appointments and 33% were still attending their GP 5 years later with back pain.

The South Manchester Study interviewed patients 3 months after their outpatient visit. Most said they had no change in their condition and 91% still had backache. Almost half had been a little (29%) or very disappointed (19%) with their clinic visit. That was a regional center with many problem patients who would respond poorly to treatment, so these figures probably do not reflect the national pattern. But it is still a depressing picture.

X-rays and imaging

There are now about 1.5 million plain X-rays of the lumbar spine in UK each year, which is little changed since 1993. GPs arrange about 0.6 million of these and specialists about 0.9 million. That is 3% of all medical and dental X-rays, but because of the high dose of lumbar X-rays it is about 12% of total medical radiation (National Radiation Protection Board data).

There are now about 63 000 computed tomography (CT) scans of the lumbar spine in the UK each year, compared with 54 000 in 1989.

There are now something like 200 000 magnetic resonance imaging (MRI) scans of the lumbar spine in the UK each year, which is about a quarter of all MRIs.

General X-ray rates in the UK are comparable to the Netherlands and about half those in the US, Germany, and Japan.

Historically, most spinal imaging in the UK was carried out at the request of a specialist. Some experts still argue that we should only image patients with back pain after a surgeon has made a

Table 19.10 Reasons GPs gave for referring patients with back pain to a specialist

Reason	Percentage
For advice on management	29
To establish diagnosis	25
For treatment	18
To take over management	14
For specific investigation	3
To reassure patient	3
To reassure GP	3
Other	5

Based on data from Coulter et al (1989).

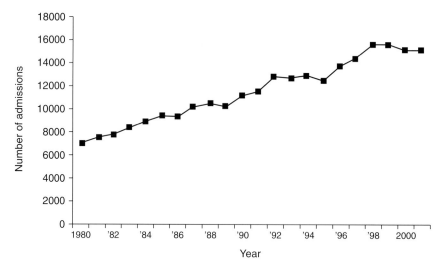

Figure 19.2 Trends in number of patients admitted to hospital with spinal disorders in Scotland (based on data from the Scottish Health Services, Information and Statistics Division).

clinical decision that they may require surgery. In practice, however, imaging is now often used as part of assessment and diagnosis. A few centers provide direct GP access to spinal imaging, though that is still a matter of debate. And some patients now arrive at specialists with their MRI scan in their hand looking for an operation. Britain may be heading down the same slippery slope as the US, although I hope it is not yet too late to stop this.

Hospitalization

There were about 100 000 hospital admissions for back problems in the UK in 1993, occupying 770 000 bed-days. There were another 30 000 day-case admissions. By 2001–2002 the number who received some form of inpatient treatment had risen to about 200 000. However, the average stay had fallen, so the number of bed-days fell to about 560 000. Figure 19.2 shows the rising trend of admissions over the past 20 years. Political pressure to reduce bed occupancy appears to have had more impact on the length of stay in hospital rather than on the number of admissions.

Table 19.11 shows where they go. About half are in the surgical specialties of orthopedics and neurosurgery, but only about a third of these patients have some form of procedure. A large proportion of NHS bed occupancy for back problems is still for assessment, investigation, or non-surgical treatment.

Table 19.11 Hospital inpatients for spinal disorders in Scotland

Specialty	Discharges	Bed–days	Average stay
Orthopedics	4012	30 550	7.6
Neurosurgery	1364	7683	5.6
Other specialties	4932	44 452	9.0
Total	10 308	82 685	8.0

Based on data from the Scottish Health Services, Information and Statistics Division.

Surgery

In 1982 there were about 9000 disk operations and another 2000 spinal fusions in England and Wales (OHE 1985). By 1990 this had risen to about 17 000 operations (Table 19.12). The number of low back operations has stayed more or less constant since that time, even though cervical, deformity, and fracture surgery rates have doubled. There are another 27 000 "other procedures" – mainly epidural and facet injections.

Regional variation

There is not much regional variation in low back pain or disability across the UK, but there is a lot of difference in health care. Porter & Hibbert (1986)

Table 19.12   Surgical operations for back disorders in England

Operation	Number	
	1989–1990	2001–2002
Cervical disk operations	1869	3387
Fusion	503	243
Thoracic spine	532	532
Lumbosacral disk operations	12 040	12 698
Fusion	1164	1179
Deformity	857	1333
Fracture–dislocation	258	777
Total	17 223	20 149

Based on NHS inpatient statistics: www.doh.gov.uk.hes.

Table 19.13   GP consulting rates for back pain by social class

Social class	Standardized ratios all ages	
	Male	Female
I and II (professional and managerial)	72	85
IIINM (skilled non-manual)	92	92
IIIM (skilled manual)	110	115
IV and V (partly skilled and unskilled)	134	110
Average (all social classes)	100	100

Based on data from the Third National Morbidity Survey 1981–1982 (RCGP 1986).

looked at patients with back pain in four GP practices in different parts of the UK. The number who had ever had an X-ray varied from 23 to 44%, those who had ever seen an orthopedic surgeon varied from 13 to 55%, and those who had ever been off work varied from 46 to 90% – and that was in a very small sample of four practices! Some GPs and practices must vary much more, either way.

Most earlier studies showed a higher GP consulting rate for back pain in the north of England and Scotland, where the GP is also more likely to prescribe medication. People with back pain in the south-east and south-west are more likely to feel that their GP cannot do anything for back pain and are less likely to receive NHS physiotherapy. Those in London, the south-east, and the south-west are more likely to attend an osteopath. Those in the south-east and the south-west are more likely to attend a chiropractor.

CSAG (1994) found wide variation in access to NHS specialists in different parts of the UK. Numbers of orthopedic surgeons, rheumatologists, neurosurgeons, and pain clinics vary greatly in different areas. Routine waiting times for a specialist appointment vary from about 6 weeks to more than 1 year. Patients in London, the Midlands, and the south-east are more likely to see a private specialist. Those in the north of England and Scotland are more likely to receive hospital inpatient treatment. Referral patterns depend on the individual specialists in the area, local custom, and waiting times. Who you see and how long you

wait depends on your post code. This in turn determines the treatment you receive and the waiting times may decide your outcome.

All these patterns probably simply reflect the availability of NHS and private services for back pain. The greatest differences however, as in the US, seem to be between individual GP practices and hospitals. These differences depend partly on socioeconomic factors, but they probably depend most of all on how individual GPs and specialists practice.

There is also some variation in health care for back pain with social class (Table 19.13). Mason (1994) showed the same pattern, but gave more clinical detail. Social classes IIIM–V have more GP visits, specialist referrals, X-rays, and physiotherapy. Social classes I–II are more likely to deal with the problem on their own, but if they do seek professional health care they are more likely to see an osteopath or chiropractor privately.

TOTAL HEALTH CARE USE

Benn & Wood (1975) made one of the first attempts to estimate the size of the problem of back pain in the UK, using data from the 1950s and 1960s. At that time they found that about 2.7% of people consulted their GP with back disorders each year. Of these, 1 in 2.3 would see a hospital specialist, 1 in 4 would get a spinal support, 1 in 30 would be admitted to hospital, and 1 in 200 would have a disk operation. They pointed out that this pattern of health care looks very different to people with

1985

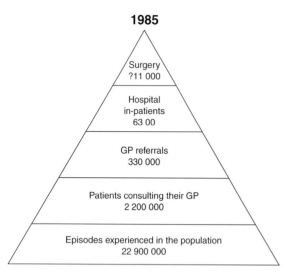

Figure 19.3   Estimated health care for back pain in the UK in 1985. From OHE (1985), with permission.

1993

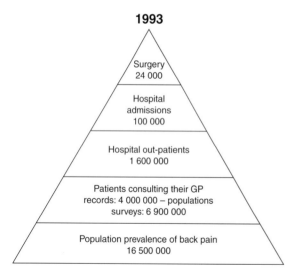

Figure 19.4   Estimated NHS care for back pain in the UK in 1993. Based on CSAG (1994).

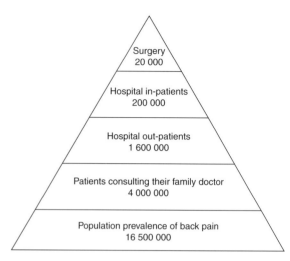

Figure 19.5   Estimated NHS care for back pain in the UK in 2002.

back pain in 1993 (Fig. 19.4). Fig. 19.5 gives the latest update for 2001–2002.

Some of the figures for 1985 are not directly comparable to the more recent figures. The data were from different sources, the definitions were different, and some of the estimates were of variable quality. Many of the OHE estimates were little more than guesses. The 1993 and 2001–2002 figures are based on much better population surveys and NHS data. Through 1955–1990, there was a steady rise in the number of people who visit their GP with back pain. The rise in the number going to specialists came later in the 1980s. Since 1993, the number of consultations seems to have plateaued. The number of patients treated in hospital has continued to rise, but the average length of stay has fallen so total bed occupancy has also fallen. The number of spinal operations rose up to 1993, but since then has plateaued.

We can now summarize health care for back pain in the UK. Most people with back pain in the UK deal with it themselves most of the time. If they seek medical care, most go first to the NHS. About 4 million people consult their GP for back pain each year, which is 9% of the adult population. 1.6 million of these patients attend a hospital specialist. 1.5 million have X-rays and more than 100 000 have a CT or MRI of the lumbar spine. 1.0 million have NHS physiotherapy. About 200 000 receive some form of hospital inpatient treatment and 20 000 have spinal surgery.

back pain and to health professionals. Few people with back pain in the UK received any specialist treatment, but the specialist only saw a select few of those with back pain.

The Office of Health Economics (OHE) (1985) tried to estimate total health care for back pain in the UK in the mid-1980s (Fig. 19.3). CSAG (1994) made a similar summary of NHS health care for

But many people with back pain in the UK seek private health care. Each year about 0.5 million people see a private medical specialist for back pain. 0.3 million attend a private physiotherapist, 0.7 million an osteopath, and 0.3 million a chiropractor. Fifteen percent of patients who seek health care for back pain stay away from the NHS altogether and depend entirely on the private sector. More than half of all therapy for back pain is private. As far as I know, back pain is the only common condition where this is true. Access to and satisfaction with NHS services for back pain are so bad that many patients vote with their feet and their wallets.

Summary

In the UK, back pain accounts for:

- 4% of all family doctor consultations
- 5% of elective referrals to medical specialists
- 13.5% of state incapacity benefit

Table 19.14   Estimated costs of back pain in UK in 1998

Resource	Best estimate (£ millions)
GP consultations	134
Prescribed drugs	94
Outpatient consultations	159
Physiotherapy	126
X-rays	106
Inpatient bed-days (including surgery)	200
A&E attendances	26
Total NHS costs	**845**
Private medical consultations	50
Private therapy	227
Over-the-counter analgesics	24
Private health care costs	**301**
Social security benefits	3600
Sickness absence[a]	1350–3500
Total	**£6–8.2 billion**

[a]Depending on how lost production costs are calculated.

THE COST OF BACK PAIN

It is difficult to get accurate figures on the cost of back pain in the UK. Different authors give widely varying figures (Coyle & Richardson 1994, Moffett et al 1995, Maniadakis & Gray 2000). There are the problems of estimating health care use for back pain that we have seen throughout this chapter. Costs within the state-funded NHS are somewhat artificial. Most previous calculations of social security costs used the basic benefit rate and did not allow for the actual level of benefit paid. Some authors have confused social security benefits with sickness absence (Ch. 5). Economists have great difficulty deciding how to calculate the employment-related costs of sickness absence. Days lost × average wages is probably an overestimate of lost production. The "friction method" is probably conservative.

Table 19.14 gives my best estimate for the cost of back pain in the UK. Total NHS costs are now about £0.8 billion. Private health care is another £0.3 billion. But these health care costs are swamped by the social costs of £5–7 billion. Because of changes in the methods of calculation, it is difficult to compare this with earlier estimates. CSAG (1994) estimated at that time the total cost of back pain was rising by £0.5 billion every year. Since then, health care costs have continued to rise, but the social costs have probably plateaued. Any such estimates have a considerable range of error. But depending on how you look at it, this is either a great deal of money or not nearly enough to meet the need.

THE STATE OF NHS SERVICES FOR BACK PAIN IN 1994

CSAG (1994) was a major Department of Health report on NHS services for back pain in the UK. We visited eight districts in different parts of the country. At each visit we met GPs and hospital specialists and heard about their experience. We looked at standards of care and compared them with clinical guidelines. Guidelines were new in the UK, but most people at the meetings welcomed them. However, few districts felt that they met these standards in 1994. We heard many common criticisms of services at that time:

- Everyone agreed that diagnostic triage is fundamental to referral. But family doctors could not put this into practice because there were no different NHS services for patients with different kinds of back trouble. The main problem was that, in practice, we did not separate patients with serious spinal disease and nerve root problems from those with ordinary backache.

- Most specialist services were designed to investigate and treat patients with serious spinal disease, nerve root problems, and those who might require surgery. Emergency and urgent referrals of these patients were usually dealt with satisfactorily. Routine referrals of these patients suffered long delays due to waiting lists caused by large numbers of patients with ordinary backache.

- These specialty services were usually inappropriate for patients with ordinary backache. They provided them with a very poor service. And they were ineffective.

- There were no NHS services specifically designed for patients with ordinary backache, apart from a few isolated examples.

- Only half the districts felt that spinal X-rays for back pain followed the Royal College of Radiology guidelines. Too many patients still had repeat X-rays because previous X-rays or reports were not available due to simple clerical inefficiency. Some GPs wanted direct access to spinal imaging, but it seemed that they often used this simply as a mechanism to bypass specialist waiting lists. Most agreed that was not the ideal way to run a service.

- There was very variable access to physiotherapy. Some districts had direct GP access, while others set criteria for referral or used specialist clinics and their waiting lists as a filter to control demand. Waiting times for physiotherapy varied greatly. Very few NHS patients with back pain actually received any form of physical therapy at the acute stage.

- Many health professionals felt that the system created the chronic pain patient. It was still common practice to give analgesics and send patients home for bed rest without information or advice about their problem. There were too many delays before patients got any active treatment. They were then sent to the wrong specialist, often with unrealistic expectations of a cure. Delayed access

might lead to chronic pain and by that time they might also have lost their job.

- We heard frequent comment about the "revolving door" of specialist care for chronic back pain. Patients waited months to see a specialist and then found that he had nothing to offer. A typical example was waiting to see a surgeon with ordinary backache that was not a surgical problem. Then they had to wait all over again to see another specialist, with the same result. Or they were passed from one specialist to another.

- Pain services in the UK were usually the last resort for patients with chronic intractable pain. They often had long waiting lists. Anesthesiologists ran most NHS pain clinics and the main treatment they offered was medication and regional anesthesia. Many GPs and other specialists felt that NHS pain services were of limited value for patients with back problems.

- GPs were under a lot of pressure to give sick certificates. Sometimes this was for social rather than health reasons, to get social security benefits. Many GPs felt this was a particular problem with back pain where they found it difficult to assess fitness for work. Some felt it would be better to separate sick certification from health care.

Summary: NHS services 1994

- Most patients attending hospital specialists have chronic low back pain and disability
- Many of them are not working
- They have often seen other specialists before
- Specialist treatment achieves little and leaves many patients dissatisfied
- There is lack of triage between possible spinal pathology, nerve root problems, and ordinary backache
- Most specialist services are designed for the investigation and treatment of patients with serious spinal pathology, nerve root problems, and those who require consideration of surgery
- These specialist services provide an inappropriate and ineffective service for patients with ordinary backache
- There are very few services designed to meet the needs of patients with ordinary backache

Many GPs and specialists were dissatisfied with 1994 specialist services for back pain. Patients also were disillusioned. There was wide agreement on what was wrong with NHS services for back pain, and on the need for change. Up till then, there had been little will to do anything about it.

RECENT ADVANCES 1994–2003

There has been such a radical shift in thinking about back pain, that it is difficult to remember what it used to be like and how much has changed in such a short time. Let me try to pick out some key elements:

- a biopsychosocial model in place of a purely medical model
- diagnostic triage
- a positive strategy of advising and supporting patients to stay active instead of a negative strategy of rest
- the scientific evidence base for treatment
- active therapy instead of passive modalities

Table 19.15   UK initiatives on clinical management and health services for back pain

Date	Source	Product	Reference
May 1994	Clinical Standards Advisory Group (CSAG)	Report on NHS services for LBP. Appendix: Management guidelines for LBP	CSAG (1994)
Jan 1996	Health Care Evaluation Unit	*Low Back Pain: An Evaluation of Therapeutic Interventions.*	Evans & Richards (1996)
Sept 1996	Royal College of General Practitioners (RCGP: multidisciplinary)	Clinical guidelines for the management of acute LBP	
Sept 1996	The Stationery Office	*The Back Book* (a booklet for patients)	Roland et al (1996)
Feb 1999	Royal College of General Practitioners (multidisciplinary)	*Clinical Guidelines for the Management of Acute LBP*, 2nd edn	RCGP (1999) www.rcgp.org.uk
1999–2001	Joint Dept of Health (DoH)/Health and Safety Executive (HSE)	Back in Work pilot initiatives	DoH/HSE (2001)
Mar 2000	Faculty of Occupational Medicine	*Occupational Health Guidelines for the Management of Low Back Pain*	Carter & Birrell (2000), www.facoccmed.ac.uk
August 2000	Institute for Musculoskeletal Research and Clinical Implementation	Audit toolkit for acute back pain	Breen et al (2000) www.imrci.ac.uk
Oct 2000	HSE	European Week for Health and Safety at Work: Turn your back on musculoskeletal disorders	
		Back in work: managing back pain in the workplace: a leaflet for employers and workers	HSE (2000): www.hse.gov.uk
	HSE/Health Education Board of Scotland	Launch of Working Backs Scotland campaign	www.workingbacksscotland.com
2002	National Institute for Clinical Excellence	Piloting guide on referral practice, based on RCGP guidelines	www.nice.org.uk
2002	RCGP Scottish Programme of Improving Clinical Effectiveness in primary care	GP quality improvement programme. Desk-top memo, recording, and audit system	www.ceppc.org/spice
2002	NHS Modernisation Agency	National Back Pain Collaborative	www.modern.nhs.uk/orthopaedics
2003	Dept for Work and Pensions (formerly Dept of Social Security)	Job retention and rehabilitation pilot schemes	

NHS, National Health Services; LBP, Low back pain.

- the importance of psychosocial issues
- clinical guidelines
- changes in clinical practice
- occupational health issues
- changed public perceptions.

The question is, how much has changed in practice? Most countries now have clinical guidelines and agree how back pain should be managed. Yet most have put much less effort into implementing the guidelines or looking at the implications for health care delivery. That is where the UK may differ (Waddell 2002). Table 19.15 lists the main UK initiatives since 1994.

Little et al (1996) had doubts about whether family doctors' management at that time matched guidelines. Two surveys in 1996–1997 questioned whether there was any real change in NHS services for back pain (Underwood et al 1997, Barnett et al 1999). However, more recent surveys show that GPs are now much more aware of guidelines (Deane & Crick 1998, Frankel et al 1999, Schers et al 2000). We have already seen the radical shift in GP advice (Table 16.5, Ch. 16) and the shift in public perceptions about back pain and its management (Fig. 16.2, Ch. 16). We finally have evidence that there has been a massive shift in primary care management of back pain, even if it is still not universal.

Physiotherapy also seems to be changing, at least in places. There is no evidence yet of much shift in hospital specialist services for back pain.

CONCLUSION

Back pain in the UK accounts for:

- 4% of all GP consultations
- 5% of all NHS specialist referrals
- 13.5% of UK incapacity benefits.

Yet back disorders get less than 1.8% of total NHS spending. Even worse, we spend that money in the wrong way. We still fail to provide the best possible care and waste limited and expensive resources. There is wide agreement that many traditional specialist services are inappropriate and ineffective for non-specific back pain. Patients, GPs, and specialists alike remain dissatisfied with much of the present service.

There is now wider agreement on the need for change and what direction this should take. The situation is improving, at least in places. But there is still a long way to go to provide a satisfactory service across the country. And there is still a lot of resistance to change, especially when it involves changing established professional practice or spending money.

References

Barnett A G, Underwood M R, Vickers M R 1999 Effect of UK national guidelines on services to treat patients with acute low back pain: a follow up questionnaire survey. British Medical Journal 318: 919–920

Benn R T, Wood P H N 1975 Pain in the back: an attempt to estimate the size of the problem. Rheumatology and Rehabilitation 14: 121–128

Breen A C, Langworthy J, Vogel S et al 2000 Primary care audit tool kit: acute back pain. Institute for Musculoskeletal Research and Clinical Implementation, Bournemouth. Available online at: www.imrci.ac.uk

Carter J T, Birrell L N (eds) 2000 Occupational health guidelines for the management of low back pain. Faculty of Occupational Medicine, London. Available online at: www.facoccmed.ac.uk

Consumers' Association 1985 Back pain survey. Consumers' Association, London

Coulter A, Noone A, Goldacre M 1989 General practitioners' referrals to specialist outpatient clinics. British Medical Journal 299: 304–306

Coulter A, Bradlow J, Martin-Bates C 1991 Outcome of general practitioner referrals to specialist out-patient clinics for back pain. British Journal of General Practice 41: 450–453

Coyle D, Richardson G 1994 The cost of back pain. In: The epidemiology of back pain. Annex to the Clinical Standards Advisory Group's report on back pain. HMSO, London, pp 65–72

Croft P, Joseph S, Cosgrove S et al 1994 Low back pain in the community and in hospitals. A report to the Clinical Standards Advisory Group of the Department of Health. Prepared by the Arthritis and Rheumatism Council, Epidemiology Research Unit, University of Manchester

CSAG 1994 Report on back pain. Clinical Standards Advisory Group. HMSO, London, pp 1–89

Deane M, Crick D 1998 Outcome of low back pain in general practice: evidence based practice can improve outcome. British Medical Journal 317: 1083

DoH/HSE 2001 UK Department of Health/Health and Safety Executive. Back in work pilot initiatives: final conference. DoH/HSE, London

Evans G, Richards S 1996 Low back pain: an evaluation of therapeutic interventions. Health Care Evaluation Unit, Bristol

Foster N E, Thompson K A, Baxter G D, Allen J M 1999 Management of nonspecific low back pain by physiotherapists in Britain and Ireland. Spine 24: 1332–1342

Frankel B S M, Moffett J K, Keen S, Jackson D 1999 Guidelines for low back pain: changes in general practice. Family Practice 16: 216–222

Furniss J, Johnstone R, Shand L 2002 A service development in North East Glasgow. Report to Greater Glasgow Health Board

Gifford L (ed.) 2000 Physiotherapy pain association yearbook. Topical issues in pain 2: Biopsychosocial assessment and management. CNS Press, Cornwall

Gracey J H, McDonough S M, Baxter G D 2002 Physiotherapy management of low back pain: a survey of current practice in Northern Ireland. Spine 27: 406–411

HSE 2000 Back in work: managing back pain in the workplace. A leaflet for employers and workers in small businesses. Health and Safety Executive, London. Available online at: www.hse.gov.uk

Little P, Smith L, Cantrell T, Chapman J, Langridge J, Pickering R 1996 General practitioners' management of acute back pain: a survey of reported practice compared with clinical guidelines. British Medical Journal 312: 485–488

Maniadakis N, Gray A 2000 The economic burden of back pain in the UK. Pain 84: 95–103

Mason V 1994 The prevalence of back pain in Great Britain. Office of Population Censuses and Surveys Social Survey Division. HMSO, London, pp 1–24

McCormick A, Fleming D, Charlton J 1995 Morbidity statistics from general practice. Fourth national study 1991–1992. Office of Population Censuses and Surveys series MB5 no. 3. HMSO, London, pp 1–366

Mechanic D 1968 Medical sociology. Free Press, New York

Moffett J K, Richardson G, Sheldon T A, Maynard A 1995 Back pain: its management and cost to society. Discussion paper 129. Centre for Health Economics, York, pp 1–67

OHE 1985 Back pain. Office of Health Economics, London

Porter R W, Hibbert C S 1986 Back pain and neck pain in four general practices. Clinical Biomechanics 1: 7–10

RCGP 1986 Morbidity statistics from general practice; third national morbidity survey 1981/1982. Royal College of General Practitioners/HMSO, London

RCGP 1999 Clinical guidelines for the management of acute low back pain. London, Royal College of General Practitioners. Available online at: www.rcgp.org.uk

Roland M, Waddell G, Moffett J K et al 1996 The back book. Stationery Office, Norwich. Available online at: www.tsonline.co.uk

Schers H, Braspenning J, Drijver R, Wensing M, Grol R 2000 Low back pain in general practice: reported management and reasons for not adhering to the guidelines in the Netherlands. British Journal of General Practice 50: 640–644

Skelton A M, Murphy E A, Murphy R J L, O'Dowd T C O 1995 General practitioner perceptions of low back pain patients. Family Practice 12: 44–48

Taylor H, Curran N M 1985 The Nuprin pain report. Louis Harris, New York, pp 1–233

Underwood M R, Vickers M R, Barnett A G 1997 Availability of services to treat patients with acute low back pain. British Journal of General Practice 47: 501–502

Waddell G 2002 Recent developments in low back pain: UK 1994–2001. IASP refresher course. IASP Press, Seattle

Waxman R, Tennant A, Helliwell P 1998 Community survey of factors associated with consultation for low back pain. British Medical Journal 317: 1564–1567

Chapter 20

US health care for back pain

The health care system in the US is very different from the UK and that affects the treatment Americans receive for back pain.

There is no universal, federal health service in the US. Most treatment is provided in a competitive health care market, paid on an item of service basis. Funding is from many sources: private health insurance, workers' compensation and government programs, and some from patients themselves. But about 15% of Americans have little or no health insurance. This system produces wide variations in treatment for a problem like back pain where any health care is a matter of choice.

We must also see health care for back pain in its US context. Americans are very health-conscious and pain is a prominent concern. They live in a drug culture and consume large quantities of all kinds of medication. They have more faith in medical technology than Europeans. So, even with a symptom like ordinary backache, they want to know every detail of their medical condition and all the treatment options. They expect to get fixed (Box 20.1). Unfortunately, this kind of approach may not be helpful for a problem like back pain.

BACK PAIN AND DISABILITY IN THE US

The population of the US is 288 million: about 142 million men and 146 million women. Clinical back pain mainly affects the 212 million adults aged 18 and over.

About 70–85% of Americans have back pain at some time in their life. About a third of adults have some back pain each year: about 70 million people.

Box 20.1   Popular US myths about health care for back problems (adapted from Deyo 1998)

- Everyone with back pain should have a spine X-ray
- X-rays, CT, and MRI scans can identify the cause of the pain
- If you have a slipped disk, you need surgery
- High-tech medicine should be able to fix the problem

In population surveys, some 7–14% of US adults say they have had some restriction of their daily activities due to back pain in the past year. The number who say they are chronically disabled by back pain rose from about 1 million in 1987 to 1.5 million in 1993 and then fell between 1993 and 1996 (E Volinn, personal communication). Remember, however, that is all about self-reported symptoms.

The number of all workers' compensation claims fell from 2.5 million in 1987 to 1.7 million in 1998. Back injuries make up a steady two-fifths of these. There are now about 700 000 workers' compensation claims for work-related back injuries each year (Waddell et al 2002).

About 8.5 million Americans now receive social security benefits for some form of permanent disability. They increased by 3 million in the 1990s, much more than workers' compensation claims fell. About 1.5 million receive these benefits for musculoskeletal conditions, of which about half are back conditions. That is roughly three-quarters of a million people. However, there are no good US data on social security trends for back pain (Waddell et al 2002).

INFORMATION AVAILABLE ON HEALTH CARE

Deyo et al (1994) reviewed official sources of data on US health care for back pain. The National Center for Health Statistics (NCHS) now provides more information online at www.cdc.gov/nchs.

NCHS carries out regular federal surveys on samples of many thousands of adults covering the entire US. The National Health and Nutrition Examination Surveys (NHANES) obtain health histories and include physical examinations. The National Health Interview Surveys ask questions about health status and health care use but do not include any examinations. The National Ambulatory Medical Care Surveys give record-based data on visits to office-based physicians. The National Hospital Discharge Surveys give record-based data on hospital discharges. Health insurance data such as workers' compensation, Medicare and Medicaid cover selected groups of patients. By their nature, all of these surveys collect general information about all conditions, so they give limited information about back pain. What they do is set back pain in the broader health care picture.

The problem is finding your way through this labyrinth. In the past few years, more of the data is available online, but it is still often 2–5 years old. Earlier data were never readily available. Much of the data is only published in summary form or under the main diagnostic groups. It takes a major effort to learn each system and to make sure you extract and interpret the data correctly. So, in practice, we depend on experts. NCHS does publish good summaries, but they are usually broad and do not give much detail on back pain. It is particularly difficult to get data on longer-term trends. Beware of attempts to estimate trends from two isolated figures, often only a few years apart and perhaps not directly comparable. Fortunately, various research groups have analyzed back pain data from the various surveys and have published papers that provide this information in user-friendly form.

Even then, we must recognize the limitations of this data. It is always dated. Some scientific papers published in 2002 were still based on data from before 1994! So we must always set findings in their time frame. Most of the surveys are for administrative purposes and we must be careful using the data to answer questions for which it was not designed. Often, the information we want is simply not there. The data are also open to error and bias. There may be selection of subjects, the questions, and the way of presenting the data. There is a major problem with missing data and that may produce further bias. More detailed studies that focus on back pain can obtain more clinical detail. By their nature, these studies involve more resources and effort, so they cannot be on a national scale.

They usually provide data on a local area such as Washington state or North Carolina. We must then be careful trying to extrapolate the findings to the whole country. They are again often years out of date by the time they are published.

Despite these caveats, we should not be too pessimistic. Provided we are cautious, we can build a reasonable picture of health care for back pain in the US.

WHO SEEKS HEALTH CARE AND WHO DO THEY SEE?

We must always remember that there are two separate systems of health care for back pain in the US. Conventional medicine and alternative medicine are completely independent and competing. Conventional medicine offers a wide range of specialties. But alternative medicine also offers a wide range of choices, of which chiropractic is simply the largest and most powerful. There are fundamental differences in philosophy and practice between the different health care systems, even though they share some therapies in common.

However, that may be a very professional view. Patients do not make such a sharp distinction. For them, the type of clinician seems to be less important than whether they feel the care meets their needs. The most common pattern of back care in the US now is probably to see more than one provider, and to mix conventional and alternative care and self-treatment (Druss et al 2003, Wolsko et al 2003).

The number of visits

The Nuprin Pain Report (Taylor & Curran 1985) found that about 70% of people with "more than occasional" back pain said they had seen a medical doctor at some time. That would suggest about 25% of US adults seek medical care for back pain at some time in their lives. Half of them had sought medical care for back pain in the previous year. However, as we saw in the last chapter, such survey data is likely to overestimate the true picture.

Using health records from 1974 to 1982, Shekelle et al (1995a, b) estimated that about 6% of US adults sought some form of health care for back pain each year. That would mean about 12 million people. At that time, medical doctors were the main providers

Table 20.1 Common reasons for physician office visits in 1995–1998

Reason for visit	Percentage of all visits
Routine and special examinations for various conditions	21.8
Diagnostic testing	4.1
Coughs	3.5
Upper respiratory infections	2.6
Back pain	2.4

Based on data from the National Ambulatory Medical Care Survey.

of care for 7.2 million people, and chiropractic doctors were the main providers for the other 4.8 million. A number of earlier studies supported Shekelle's estimates.

Many authors still state that back pain is the second most common reason for all physician office visits in the US. This has been repeated ad nauseam in the introduction to papers about back pain till it has become a kind of creed. It comes from an old paper by Cypress (1983), using data from 1977–1978, and questionable diagnostic coding. It gives a very false impression. The National Ambulatory Medical Care Surveys from 1995–1998 show that back pain was the fifth most common reason for an office visit to a physician (Table 20.1). It was the primary diagnosis in a meager 2.4% of all office visits, compared with 2.8% in the 1980s.

Physician visits for back pain rose from 12 million in 1980–1981 to 15 million in 1989–1990, which was the same increase as for all conditions (Hart et al 1995). Through the 1990s, at least up to 1998, it remained fairly constant at just over 16 million (Table 20.2). (Note that these figures are for numbers of visits, while Shekelle's figures were for numbers of patients. That fits with each patient having an average of about 1.5 visits.)

Shekelle et al (1995a) looked at "episodes of health care." Of those who sought any health care for back pain, 71% had only a single episode of care over 3–5 years. Sixteen percent had two episodes, 9% had three episodes, and 4% had four or more episodes. Half of all episodes of health care for back pain lasted 1 week or less; two-thirds lasted 1 month

Table 20.2 Physician visits for back conditions in 1998 (millions)

	Male	Female	Total
Back injury	2.0	1.5	3.5
Disk disorders	1.4	1.2	2.6
Other back conditions	4.5	5.8	10.3
Total	7.8	8.5	16.4

Based on data from the National Ambulatory Medical Care Survey.

Table 20.3 Who patients visited for health care visits for back pain

	1987 (%)	1997 (%)
MD (or DO) only	38	35
Non-MD only	14	6
Both	49	59

As a percentage of those with back pain who sought any professional care.
Based on data from Druss et al (2003).

or less; and only 8% lasted more than 6 months. The average patient had 1.5 visits during an episode. (Note again, this is not about duration of symptoms but duration of episodes of health care.)

Eisenberg et al (1993, 1998) carried out national surveys of alternative medicine use for all conditions in 1990 and again in 1997. In 1990, 34% of adults said they used alternative medicine and by 1997 this had risen to 42%. By 1997, total visits to alternative medicine practitioners exceeded total visits to all primary care physicians. The number who attended chiropractors rose from 10% in 1990 to 11% in 1997. There was also an increase in the use of massage from 7% in 1990 to 11% in 1997.

Hurwitz et al (1998) reviewed a national sample of patients who received chiropractic treatment in the US and Canada in 1985–1991. Coulter et al (2002) carried out a more detailed prospective national survey of chiropractic patients in 1992–1994. Cherkin et al (2002) made the most recent survey of complementary and alternative medicine in 1998–1999. About 40% of chiropractic visits were for back pain and another quarter for neck pain.

Coulter et al estimated that use of chiropractic in the US has doubled in the past 15 years.

This fails to allow for overlap between conventional and alternative care. Druss et al (2003) analyzed National Ambulatory Care Survey data from 1987 and 1997 (Table 20.3).

Wolsko et al (2003) surveyed 2055 US adults in 1997. Sixty-six percent of those with back or neck pain said they had used some form of health care in the past year. This is high compared with other surveys and seems to include self-care. Thirty-seven percent of those with back pain sought some form of conventional medical care. Fifty-eight percent used complementary therapy, but again some of this was self-administered. There was a lot of overlap. Of those who sought any care in the past year, 18% used conventional care alone, 44% used complementary care alone, and 38% used both. Chiropractic was still the most common form of complementary medicine, but it no longer dominated the picture. Of those who used alternative therapy, 20% attended a chiropractor, 14% used massage, and 12% used relaxation techniques (though again some of these were self-care). Despite its earlier popularity, less than 1% of people with back pain now used acupuncture.

It is not clear whether most patients attend different professionals at different times, move back and forth, or attend more than one professional at the same time. Some 85% of chiropractic patients self-refer and only about 5% are referred from a medical doctor (Cherkin et al 2002). When they attend, it emerges that about a sixth are receiving care from an MD, and the chiropractor then communicates with the MD in about two-thirds of these cases. This is probably the best example of communication between alternative and conventional providers. It seems likely that most conventional and many alternative providers are unaware if their patients are getting care elsewhere.

Conventional medicine

The pattern of medical care for back pain seems to have stayed constant over many years (Cypress 1983, Deyo & Tsui-Wu 1987, Hart et al 1995, Shekelle et al 1995a, b). About two-thirds of medical care for back pain is in the primary care specialties of family practice, osteopathic medicine, and general internal

Table 20.4 Specialty market share and workload of back pain in 1989–1990

Specialty	Percentage market share of all back pain visits	Back pain as a percentage of specialty office visit caseload
General/family physician		
MD	30	2.6
DO	11	5.4
Internal medicine	14	2.4
Orthopedic surgery	25	11
Neurosurgery	7	35
Neurology	4	10

Based on data from Hart et al (1995).

Table 20.5 Back diagnosis by specialty in 1989–1990

	General/ family practice (%)	Orthopedic surgery (%)	Neuro- surgery (%)
Non-specific low back pain	76	40	19
Herniated disk	3	20	46
Degenerative changes	10	19	6

Based on data from Hart et al (1995).

medicine. One-third is provided by medical specialists, particularly orthopedic surgeons.

Table 20.4 shows the specialty market share of back pain visits and the proportion that back pain forms of each specialty's caseload. Most patients go directly to family doctors, DOs, and internists. Some patients are then referred to a specialist. But in the US, unlike in the UK, many patients go directly to a specialist of their choice without any screening. That applies to 55% of those who go to orthopedic surgeons, 27% to neurosurgeons, and 26% to neurologists.

Table 20.5 shows back pain diagnosis by specialty. The case mix may vary between specialties and that reflects both referral patterns and pathology. We should interpret these figures with caution. In most non-specific back pain, it is not possible to make any firm diagnosis. Physicians often simply provide a label, which may reflect their specialty leaning more than actual pathology. Moreover, that only reflects the broad differences between the specialties. Even more important, each doctor may have an individual *diagnostic signature*. That may produce much greater variation between doctors within each profession, and may be quite idiosyncratic.

Medical vs chiropractic care

There is some uncertainty about whether patients who go to a chiropractor are comparable to those who go to a physician (Carey et al 1995b, Nyiendo et al 1996, Hurwitz et al 1998, Cherkin et al 2002, Coulter et al 2002). Some studies suggest they may have less pain and disability, but others suggest they have about the same. Most patients who attend a chiropractor have recurrent pain and anything from 30 to 80% have seen a chiropractor before. Forty to 50% attend within 3 weeks of onset of their back pain, but 20–25% have had pain for more than 6 months. Carey et al (1995b) found that those seeking chiropractic care were in better general health, were more likely to have good health insurance, and had less severe pain. Coulter et al (2002) found that chiropractic patients had comparable levels of low back disability but poorer mental health.

Coulter et al (2002) also found that chiropractors and their patients share similar beliefs about health care. Saunders et al (1999), meantime, found that physician office visits were influenced by patient beliefs that pain required "medical" treatment and prescription analgesics. Such contrasting beliefs are likely to influence each patient's choice of care. Use of chiropractic varies most with region of the country and availability of practitioners. Cherkin et al (2002) found that 80% of chiropractic patients are young and middle-aged adults. Two-thirds are women. Whites are more likely to attend a DC or DO. The poorly educated are more likely to attend a family doctor (MD).

Hart et al (1995) and Shekelle et al (1995b) both gave information on average numbers of visits (Table 20.6). Family doctors (MDs) have the lowest number of return visits, while DOs and surgeons have more, and chiropractors have by far the highest number. Shekelle et al (1995b) also considered costs (Table 20.6). Health care costs per episode depend on the number of visits, cost per visit, drug costs, investigations, and hospitalization. Surgeons are by far the most expensive, mainly because of high-tech investigations, and hospitalization. Perhaps surprisingly, chiropractic care may not be cheaper than medical care. In Shekelle's study, low chiropractic cost per visit, low investigation costs, and lack of hospital costs were balanced by the large number of chiropractic visits per episode. However, some chiropractors dispute these figures, and argue they do not compare like with like.

Family practice and chiropractic should potentially be the cheapest and most cost-effective types of health care for an episode of non-specific low back pain. Most of the high costs of medical care are due to investigations and hospitalization, much of which may be unnecessary. If family practice could reduce these, it might be by far the cheapest. On the other hand, many chiropractic visits may be unnecessary. If chiropractic could control the number of visits per episode, it might be the cheapest.

Baldwin et al (2001) reviewed the evidence on the relative effectiveness and cost-effectiveness of medical and chiropractic care for back pain. There are now four randomized controlled trials (RCTs: Meade et al 1990, Cherkin et al 1998, Skargren et al 1998, Hurwitz et al 2002) and two cohort studies that show chiropractic and physiotherapy are equally effective in reducing symptoms and improving function. One RCT (Hurwitz et al 2002) and four cohort studies give conflicting evidence on the effectiveness of medical vs chiropractic care. Most studies find that chiropractic patients are more satisfied with their care. Baldwin et al (2001) found five cohort studies comparing costs and cost-effectiveness, but they all suffered methodologic problems. They concluded that, on the current evidence, it is not possible to say whether medical or chiropractic care is more cost-effective. (References to the cohort studies can be found in Baldwin et al 2001.)

WHAT HAPPENS TO THEM?

The average medical consultation for back pain in US primary care lasts 15 minutes. The average first chiropractic visit is about 30 minutes and each return visit is about 15 minutes. Some other forms of alternative therapy last up to 60 minutes.

Table 20.7 shows what happens to patients with back pain when they visit different providers. Once again, we must allow for case mix.

MDs and DOs are very alike in US family practice, but there are some differences with back pain. MDs take more X-rays and prescribe more drugs for back pain. DOs order more physical therapy, and more than 50% recommend manipulation for back pain compared with less than 7% of MDs.

Table 20.6   Number and relative costs of visits to each specialty in 1982

Specialty	Mean number of visits/episode	Cost/episode (relative to family doctor)
Chiropractor	10.4	1.41
Family doctor		
MD	2.3	1.00
DO	5.3	1.95
Internist	3.4	1.67
Orthopedic surgeon	5.0	2.67

Based on data from Shekelle et al (1995a, b).

Table 20.7   Percentage of visits at which each treatment ordered in 1989–1990

Specialty	X-ray	Drugs	Physical therapy
General/family medicine			
MD	13	60	16
DO	6	45	30
General/internal medicine	18	57	32
Orthopedic surgery	28	35	23
Neurosurgery	21	26	13[a]
Chiropractic	50	?	

[a] 27% admitted to hospital after initial visit; all other specialties, 0–2%.

Based on data from Hart et al (1995).

Shekelle et al (1995b) found that chiropractors are more likely to give patients a specific diagnosis such as "sacroiliac injury," "disk displacement," and "disk dislocation." MDs are more likely to give a vague diagnosis such as "pain in the back" and "back injury."

In contrast to medical care, chiropractic is entirely outpatient, non-surgical and "drug-free." Shekelle et al (1995b) confirmed that no patient under chiropractic care had hospitalization or surgery during the 3–5-year period of their study. Surprisingly, however, drug costs of chiropractic patients were *not* any lower. In fairness, it was not clear to what extent these drugs were prescribed by the chiropractor or a primary care doctor or were over-the-counter. Chiropractors also now order as many X-rays and scans for back pain as primary care physicians.

Cherkin et al (1994a) carried out a fascinating study of how different medical specialists would investigate and treat back pain in 1991. They described three case scenarios of acute back pain, acute back pain with sciatica, and chronic low back pain. There was little agreement on the use of diagnostic tests. Rheumatologists were more likely to order blood tests. Neurosurgeons and neurologists were more likely to order imaging. Neurologists and physiatrists were more likely to order electromyograms. Physiatrists were also more likely to order psychological evaluation. Investigations seemed to vary more with the specialty of the doctor than with the clinical condition of the patient. Cherkin et al concluded that "who you see is what you get." Once again, the *diagnostic signature* may produce much greater individual variation.

In the second part of their study, Cherkin et al (1995) looked at treatment for these three patients. In 1991, bed rest, back exercises, and physical therapy were most frequent for all three patients. Patients with acute back pain or sciatica were more likely to be prescribed bed rest. Patients with chronic pain were more likely to be prescribed back exercises and physical therapy. At that time, 59% of physicians prescribed more than 3 days' bed rest for acute sciatica, 30% for acute back pain, and 17% for chronic back pain. The mean duration of bed rest was 5.8 days for acute sciatica, 4.5 days for acute back pain, and 5 days for chronic back pain. Neurologists and neurosurgeons were no

more likely to prescribe bed rest, but if they did, they gave longer periods of 7.5 days for all three patients. Emergency medicine physicians were most likely to order bed rest, imaging, and surgical referral (Table 20.8). They used high-tech and costly interventions too early, without clear clinical indications. At the same time, 10% would refer the patient with acute back pain and 28% would refer the patient with chronic back pain to a rehabilitation specialist.

There is much anecdotal evidence but little direct evidence that the *treatment signature* of individual doctors may produce the greatest variation of all.

What physicians say they would do in a questionnaire may not be quite the same as what they actually do in practice. So it is worth looking also at patients' reports about the treatment they receive.

Tacci et al (1998, 1999) studied the management of acute (<30 days), uncomplicated, work-related back injuries. This was in 1995, a year after the AHCPR (1994) guidelines. The treating physicians were still quite aggressive in their management. Sixty-five percent of these patients had X-rays and 22% had magnetic resonance imaging (MRI). Thirty-eight percent had repeated prescriptions of opioids, 61% got non-steroidal anti-inflammatories, and only 6% had acetaminophen (paracetamol). Sixty-two percent were referred for physiotherapy and 47% were prescribed exercises: but in contrast, 26% were prescribed heat treatment, 27% ultrasound, and 21% a corset. Ninety-three percent were advised to have lighter duties at work. Thirty-six percent saw a surgeon, at a median of 13 days after

Table 20.8 Treatment prescribed by emergency room physicians in 1991

	Acute back pain <1 week without sciatica (%)	Chronic back pain without sciatica (%)
Bed rest	76	57
CT	4	8
MRI	9	16
Refer to surgical specialist	41	52

CT, computed tomography; MRI, magnetic resonance imaging.
Based on data from Elam et al (1995).

Table 20.9 Treatment received by patients with severe chronic low back pain and disability in 1992

Treatment	Percentage of patients in past year
Pain medication	92
Bed rest	65
Back exercises	64
Massage	42
Corset or brace	35
Back injections	32
Ultrasound	27
Physical therapy	26
Spinal manipulation	22
TENS	18
Traction	8

TENS, transcutaneous electrical nerve stimulation.
From Carey et al (1995a), with permission.

injury, though only 2% required surgery. Clearly, management of these patients in 1995 did not match the AHCPR guidelines.

Carey et al (1995a) investigated the care received by 269 people with chronic disabling low back pain in North Carolina in 1991 (Table 20.9). These were the most severe cases. Fifty-three percent felt that their general health was poor, and 34% were permanently disabled from working. The number of days spent in bed varied widely, with a median of 3 days but a mean of over 25 days. Three people said they had spent all or nearly all of the previous 365 days in bed because of back pain. So most people, even those with chronic low back pain, had only brief spells in bed but a very few were more or less bed-bound. Many of these patients had seen multiple health care providers in the previous year, and most had three or four treatments in that time.

There was high use of imaging. Seventeen percent of these chronic patients had another X-ray, 37% had a computed tomography (CT) scan, and 25% had an MRI scan during the previous year. Nineteen percent had a myelogram or diskogram. Ten percent had back surgery, which is slightly higher than the true surgery rate in North Carolina, so there may be some selection bias and overreporting in this sample. Nevertheless, this study shows the extensive use of medical technology and passive treatment modalities in these chronic patients.

Webster et al (2002) provide the most recent information on US medical care in 1999. They surveyed 720 physicians in family practice, internal medicine, emergency medicine, and occupational health. They gave them two case scenarios:

- *case 1*: a patient with a first episode of acute low back pain without sciatica, normal physical examination, and no red flags.

- *case 2*: a patient with a previous history of nonspecific low back pain, presenting with an acute episode of back pain and first episode of sciatica. There were positive neurologic findings but no red flags.

Table 20.10 shows the results. Almost all physicians prescribed medication, gave some form of education about back pain and ordered exercises for both patients. However, we do not have any information from this survey or elsewhere about the usual content of current information and advice.

A majority of physicians broadly followed the AHCPR guidelines for the patient with acute low back pain. However, between a quarter and a half continued to overuse X-ray, opioids and muscle relaxants, and bed rest. For the patient with acute sciatica, there was considerable overuse of early investigation, specialist referral, and consideration of surgery.

- Physicians with <10 years in practice were more likely to practice according to the guidelines. However, they still ordered unnecessary tests and treatments for the patient with sciatica. General practitioners and those in practice >30 years were least likely to practice according to the guidelines.

- Emergency medicine physicians were least likely to order diagnostic studies. However, they most often prescribed treatment likely to promote inactivity (e.g., bed rest, opioid narcotics).

- Occupational medicine physicians were less likely to order diagnostic studies. They were also more likely to prescribe treatments likely to promote activity (e.g., less bed rest, less opioids and muscle relaxants, and more exercise).

At least up to 1999, primary medical care in the US appears to have been slow to change.

Table 20.10 Percentage of physicians prescribing treatment for different case scenarios in 1999

Treatment	Case 1 Acute back pain	Case 2 Acute sciatica	Agreement with AHCPR (1994) guidelines
X-ray	23	62	–
CT/MRI/myelogram	6	81	–
Medication: Acetaminophen (paracetamol)	49	46	+
NSAIDs	93	87	+
Short-course opioids	39	69	–
Muscle relaxants	83	67	–
Bed rest ≤3 days	59	52	–
>3 days	7	25	–
Refer physical therapy	33	55	+
Refer for manipulation	6	3	–
Refer to a specialist for	16	83	–
consideration of surgery	1.3	49	–

CT, computed tomography; MRI, magnetic resonance imaging; NSAIDs, non-steroidal anti-inflammatory drugs.
Based on data from Webster et al (2002).

Summary

"Who you see is what you get"
The choice of investigations and treatments for back pain depends more on the specialty of the doctor than the condition of the patient's back.

Individual doctors vary even more within each specialty:

• individual *diagnostic signature*
• individual *treatment signature*

Physical therapy

Hart et al (1995) found that physical therapy was ordered at 21% of medical visits for back pain in 1990. That would mean about 1.5 million people with back pain get physical therapy each year in the US. About 25% of all physical therapy is for low back pain. Jette et al (1994) found that 99% of physical therapy patients with back pain were referred by a doctor. At least until 1990, hardly any Americans went directly to physical therapy. About half the patients attended within 1 month of onset of pain but about 40% had chronic pain for more than

3 months. They were mainly white and middle-aged, and there were equal numbers of men and women. The average course of physical therapy was 10–11 visits over about 5 weeks. That compares with an average chiropractic course of 12–14 visits, though the median in both cases is closer to 7.

Mielenz et al (1997) found that patients were more likely to be referred for physical therapy if they had pain radiating below the knee and more disability. Orthopedic surgeons were more likely and chiropractors least likely to refer patients for physical therapy.

Battie et al (1994) gave Cherkin's three patient vignettes to physical therapists in 1990. They found striking professional differences in beliefs about the cause of non-specific low back pain. Physicians believed the most common cause was muscle strain. Chiropractors believed it was vertebral subluxation. And physical therapists believed it was disk problems and muscle strain. When it comes to diagnostic coding, however, they all used "sprains and strains" (ICD 846 and 847: WHO 1992–1994). Presumably that is because these are the codes for which they are most likely to get paid!

Physical therapists believed the goals of treatment for back pain are to reduce pain (90%), improve range of movement (57%), increase strength (35%), reduce muscle spasm (22%), and improve posture (22%) (Jette et al 1994). For Cherkin's three patients, therapists usually gave a combination of education, passive modalities, and some form of back exercises.

Jette et al (1994) reported actual practice from a national survey of physical therapists in 1989–1990. Seventy-six percent of patients with back pain were prescribed back exercises, 76% got modalities, 34% got manual therapy, and only 6% got functional training. The McKenzie system was most popular and 85% of its practitioners believed it to be effective. Mielenz et al (1997) had similar findings in 1992–1993.

Jette & Jette (1996) and Jette & Delitto (1997) carried out a further survey in 1993–1994 (Table 20.11). Ninety-six percent of patients got a combination of treatments – most often flexibility exercises, strengthening exercises, and heat. Many therapists started at the acute stage with mainly passive modalities and manual therapy to relieve pain. Then, as pain became less, they progressed to more active treatment such as aerobic exercises. However, the data from this study suggest that may have had more to do with the therapist's routine of treatment than with the clinical course of the individual patient.

Jette & Jette (1996) also related treatments to outcome. Patients who received passive treatments with heat or cold had worse outcomes. Flexibility and strengthening exercises made no difference to outcomes. Patients who were prescribed endurance exercises had better outcomes. These findings all

agree with the scientific evidence. Manual therapy made no difference to outcomes, which is contrary to the scientific evidence. However, at the acute stage, 27% of these patients received "mobilization" while only 3.7% received "manipulation". The lack of effect on outcomes may raise questions about the form of mobilization given by physical therapists.

There are limitations to this type of survey, and we should not overinterpret these results. There are no data on patient characteristics or on which patients received different treatments. Obviously, the therapist had some reason for giving different treatments to different patients and the patients may not have been comparable. Most patients got multiple treatments, which makes it difficult to disentangle the effect of each treatment. Nevertheless, it does appear that a great deal of physical therapy for back pain in 1993–1994 was still educational advice, passive modalities, and specific back exercises. More encouraging was the fact that there was increasing use of endurance exercises, and the survey confirmed the value of that approach on a national scale.

Li & Bombardier (2001) tried to assess the impact of the AHCPR (1994) guidelines in a survey of Canadian physical therapists in 1998. They presented three vignettes: a healthy young woman with acute low back pain for 1 week; the same patient if she did not respond after 4 weeks' physical therapy; and a 35-year-old man with severe low back pain and sciatica for 4 days. Almost all physical therapists said they would give all three patients education on back care and back exercises, including exercises to do at home. Eighty percent would give advice on work modifications. About a third would use spinal mobilization but only 3–5% manipulation. A quarter would advise the patient with sciatica to have a few days' bed rest but very few would advise bed rest for back pain alone. Up to 80% would use passive modalities and up to 30% would use traction. After 4 weeks, 80% would use mobilization, 50% would refer to a community exercise program, and 40% to a back school. But 65% would also continue modalities and 30% traction. By 1998, Canadian physical therapists' responses seemed to be broadly in line with the guidelines. However, they were also still using a lot of passive therapy and still had a lot of faith in it, contrary to the scientific evidence. And 48% of these therapists

Table 20.11 Treatments recorded by physical therapists for back pain in 1993–1994

Treatment	Percentage of patients with back pain
Flexibility exercises	84
Strengthening exercises	81
Heat modalities	81
Endurance exercises	52
Manual therapy	39
Cold modalities	19

Based on data from Jette & Jette (1996).

did not think guidelines were helpful for low back problems.

Physician beliefs and patient satisfaction

Bush et al (1993) found that primary care physicians in the late 1980s had little confidence in their ability to treat back pain. "I lack the diagnostic tools or knowledge to effectively assess patients with back pain." "There is little I can do to prevent patients with acute back pain from developing chronic back pain." "I am very uncomfortable treating patients with low back pain."

Chiropractors at that time were much more confident about their training and their ability to help patients with back pain (Cherkin et al 1988). They were more comfortable and less frustrated by spinal pain, which is just as well as it is two-thirds of their practice! Despite the philosophic basis of chiropractic medicine, the chiropractors in this study firmly believed that back pain depends on physical factors that they can and should diagnose. Family doctors (MDs) were less certain about the physical basis of back pain and their ability to assess it. Medical doctors and physical therapists placed more emphasis on the role of psychosocial factors in chronic pain and disability. Most practitioners agreed that job factors are also important, although DOs and DCs rated them less highly.

Battie et al (1994) found that only 8% of physical therapists in 1990 felt well prepared and ready to manage low back pain when they first entered practice. Even experienced therapists had doubts about their ability to affect recovery. Seventy-five percent felt that they could help patients with acute sciatica. Only 50–65% felt that they could help patients with acute, recurrent, or chronic low back pain without sciatica. Half the therapists agreed that: "Patients with low back pain often have unrealistic expectations about what therapists can do for them". "I often feel frustrated by patients with low back pain who want me to fix them."

Deyo & Diehl (1986) found that about one-third of patients with acute low back pain felt they did not get an adequate explanation of their problem. They still did not understand what was wrong. These patients remained more worried about serious illness and felt they should have had more tests. They were less satisfied with their doctor and less likely to want to see the same doctor again.

Bush et al (1993) found that patients in the late 1980s were reasonably satisfied with their health providers and treatment but less satisfied with the information they received. When physicians were more confident, their patients were more satisfied with the information they gave. Bush et al suggested that the main reason for consulting a physician with back pain might be to seek information and reassurance. These patients may not expect a cure and have little need for empathy. Rather, they wanted to learn about their low back pain, what to expect and what they could do about it. If they got the information they wanted, they were more satisfied with their care. Whatever its biologic basis, chiropractic patients were more satisfied with the chiropractor's explanations and with their care. Perhaps that is why a higher proportion of chiropractic patients continue to attend the same practitioner. Whatever the effect on better communication, Smucker et al (1998) found that greater practitioner confidence made no difference to clinical outcomes.

Von Korff et al (1994) studied 44 primary care physicians and how they managed patients with low back pain in 1989–1990. Practice style varied in the amount and intensity of medical intervention (Table 20.12). Some physicians ordered less medication on a time-contingent basis, advised patients to stay active, and put more emphasis on self-care. Others ordered more opioids and sedatives on a pain-contingent basis, and more and longer bed

Table 20.12 Physician practice styles

Percentage of patients receiving:	Low interven- tionist (%)	Moderate interven- tionist (%)	High interven- tionist (%)
Sedatives or hypnotics	22	27	44
Extended use	3	5	8
Opioids	17	31	43
Extended use	2	4	6
Multiple medications	3	11	20
Bed rest	16	29	40
Extended use	4	8	15

Based on 1989–1990 data from Von Korff et al (1994).

rest. They were also more likely to raise the question of further investigation and possible surgery.

Von Korff et al then looked at how physician practice style affected patient outcomes. Patients of low-interventionist physicians were more satisfied with the information they received. Despite getting fewer analgesics, they had similar pain relief. They returned to daily activities faster and had less activity limitation at 1 month, although there was no significant difference by 1 year. They had lower health care costs for back pain over the next year. The benefits are clear. A low-interventionist practice style can give faster return to normal activity at lower cost, with no difference in pain relief, patient satisfaction, or long-term outcomes.

Hospitalization

Back problems are the seventh leading cause for hospitalization in the US. In 1988, non-surgical hospitalization for back pain was the fourth most common medical reason after heart failure and shock, angina, and psychoses.

The total number of Americans admitted to hospital with back problems fell from 728 000 in 1979 to 544 500 in 1990. The latest figures for 2000–2001 show that it has continued to fall slightly to just over 500 000. Taylor et al (1994) analyzed the National Hospital Discharge Surveys and found that non-surgical hospitalizations fell from 580 500 in 1979 to 265 500 in 1990. They considered this reflected change in medical practice. There was some change from inpatient myelography to non-invasive imaging and outpatient investigation, but most of the change was probably due to insurers introducing review criteria for payment.

Cherkin & Deyo (1993) studied non-surgical hospitalizations for back pain in 1988. The mean age of these patients was 50 years, and 23% were over 65 years. There were equal numbers of males and females. Thirty-one percent were admitted from the emergency room. Eleven percent had pain for less than 1 day, 27% for 1–7 days, 30% for 1–6 weeks, and 32% for more than 6 weeks. The median length of stay was 4 days but a quarter stayed in hospital more than 1 week. Forty-three percent were under the care of a family physician or internist, 30% were under an orthopedic surgeon, 10% a neurosurgeon, and 17% other specialties. The discharge diagnosis

was non-specific back pain in 35%, a herniated disk in 31%, and degenerative changes in 15%.

In 1988, about half were admitted for imaging studies, a quarter for pain control, and a quarter for both reasons. While in hospital, 72% were prescribed bed rest and 22% received traction. Eighty-three percent were given narcotics and 71% were given sedatives: 55% of patients got these by the parenteral route. Forty-nine percent of these patients had previous hospitalization for back pain and 30% had previous back surgery. Twenty percent were subsequently readmitted for surgery and 8% for further non-surgical hospitalization within the next year. Psychosocial problems were very common: 20% of records noted psychological problems and a further 28% of patients had no one at home to care for them. The circumstances of admission and discharge diagnoses suggest that 70–80% of these patients had no clear medical indication for hospitalization. Rather, it reflected psychosocial pressure on physicians and the lack of adequate outpatient alternatives for acute pain relief.

Cherkin & Deyo (1993) suggested the need for a new medical and social consensus on the role of hospitalization for back pain. Valid medical reasons for hospitalization might include severe or increasing neurology, major trauma, and serious spinal pathology. Non-medical reasons might include difficulty ambulating and lack of a carer at home, especially for elderly patients. Rural patients living long distances from medical care and investigations might need accommodation, but that need not be in hospital. There was already a trend to outpatient investigations. There was also a need for alternative methods of providing outpatient acute pain relief.

I have not been able to find any more recent data on non-surgical hospitalization. However, the number of hospital admissions is now almost the same as the number who have surgery. That suggests non-surgical hospitalization has almost disappeared. So it seems that Cherkin & Deyo's recommendations may have come to pass.

Low back surgery

Back and neck operations are the third most common form of surgery in the US. Only cesarean section and tubal ligation are more common.

Table 20.13 US spinal procedures in 2001

Inpatient procedures	Number	Increase on previous year (%)
Disk excision	339 700	0.8
Laminectomy	244 100	4.5
Fusion	298 500	7.5
Average number of procedures	1.68	
Total number of people having surgery	522 900	2.1

Based on data from Mendenhall (2002).

Table 20.14 International back surgery rates compared with the US in 1988

	Ratio to US rate
US	1.0
Netherlands	0.73
Denmark	0.64
Finland	0.56
Norway	0.49
Canada	0.49
Australia	0.44
New Zealand	0.40
Sweden	0.33
UK	0.19

Based on data from Cherkin et al (1994b).

National Hospital Discharge Surveys show that low back operations increased from 147 500 in 1979 to 279 000 in 1990 (Taylor et al 1994). Surgery rates rose in all age groups, but the greatest rise was in the elderly. For those under age 65, the rate rose from 113 to 152 per 100 000. For older patients, it rose from 51 to 188 per 100 000 – nearly fourfold. The rate of fusion doubled, for no clear reason. The greatest increase was in surgery for spinal stenosis, which rose eightfold from 7.8 to 61.4 per 100 000. This was probably due to greater awareness of the condition and greater availability of imaging and surgery.

By 2001, the number of people having inpatient spinal surgery rose to 522 900. That included all parts of the spine, so it is not directly comparable to Taylor's figures, but most were to the lower back. The average patient received 1.68 procedures, so the total number of procedures rose to 882 300 (Table 20.13). And that does not include the increasing number of outpatient procedures. Nor does it include epidural, facet, and other spinal injections. These increased from 498 693 in 1993 to 637 294 in 1999 (Carrino 2002) – in elderly Medicare patients alone! So we can speculate that more than a million Americans now have some form of "procedure" performed on their back each year.

Several other sources confirm the continuing growth of fusion surgery in particular. Vitale (2002) analyzed California data and found an increase of 39% between 1995 and 1999. Anterior fusion more than doubled. Fusion also had a disturbingly high mortality of 0.4%. In a different data set, fusions increased 55% between 1997 and 2000, compared with 4% for hip replacement (R Deyo, personal communication). The majority of lumbar fusions now appear to use some form of fusion technology (Mendenhall 2002).

Spinal surgery seems to be unusual (Mendenhall 2002). With most health care, new technology coming on to the market *replaces* old technologies. This does not seem to be happening with spinal surgery. Here, established procedures continue or even increase alongside the new technology.

The US has always had the highest rate of spinal surgery in the world (Table 20.14). The latest figures suggest this has not changed.

REGIONAL VARIATION

By the early to mid-1990s there was great debate about regional variation in US health care for back pain. "Marked regional variations ... imply a lack of consensus about appropriate assessment and treatment of low back problems, suggesting that some patients may be receiving inappropriate or sub-optimal care" (AHCPR 1994). Much of the concern was about the escalating cost of health care. "Health care reform has assumed an aura of inevitability, with cost containment a major goal of the reform movement" (Volinn et al 1994).

There is little evidence of any regional variation in back pain. There is a great deal of regional variation in health care for back pain. Shekelle et al

Table 20.15 Regional variation in hospital treatment in 1990; annual rates per 100 000 adults

	Non-surgical hospitalization	Spinal surgery
West	104	113
North-east	162	131
Mid-west	191	157
South	204	171

Based on data from Taylor et al (1994).

(1995a) found that the numbers seeking health care for back pain each year varied between 4.5 and 7.5% in different centers. People with back pain in the north-east are least likely to consult a physician. There is also regional variation in whom they consult. Those in the north-east are more likely to go to family doctors and orthopedic surgeons. There is more use of chiropractic in the west and less in the north-east.

In 1990, there was nearly twofold variation in hospitalization and surgery rates in different regions of the country. Non-surgical hospitalization, investigation, and surgery rates were all highest in the south and lowest in the west and north-east (Table 20.15). Sixteen percent of spinal operations involved fusion in the mid-west, but only 11% in the north-east. There is still wide variation in spine surgery techniques and rates across the US (AAOS 2000).

The smaller the areas we compare, the greater the variations in health care for back pain. It varies up to twofold between the main regions of the country, up to about 10-fold between different centers, and most of all between individual practitioners. Volinn et al (1992) found nearly 15-fold variation in spinal surgical rates between Washington state countries in 1985. By 1990, after much professional education, non-surgical hospitalization rates varied from 38 to 97/100 000 and surgery rates from 153 to 300/100 000 in the same areas (Taylor et al 1995). Those centers with the highest surgery rates also had the highest non-surgical hospitalization rates. So non-surgical hospitalization is not a substitute for surgery. Rather, both hospital admission and surgery appear to reflect a more interventionist practice style.

Lurie et al (2003) found a similar association between high rates of imaging and high surgery rates. Some critics claim this shows that greater use of imaging "explains" or produces more surgery. Alternatively, both may simply reflect a more interventionist style.

We should keep this regional variation in perspective. Back pain is no different from any other medical condition. The variation in health care for back pain is actually less than for many other common health conditions. Nevertheless, as AHCPR pointed out, the amount of variation does imply lack of consensus. Patients and physicians may feel that they have to "do something" but they are unsure what to do. Volinn et al (1992) tried to analyze 28 possible influences on this variation, with little success. Occupational factors and the number of surgeons in each area did affect surgical rates, but to a limited extent. They could only suggest once more that the variation depends mainly on "physician practice style." Local medical cultures also seem to play a role, particularly in the medical specialties. Some of the more extreme local variations in treatment are difficult to explain in any other way.

If there is so much variation, how do we decide what is appropriate or "correct" care? Is medical care rationed in low-rate areas, or overused in high-rate areas, or both? We simply do not have the data at present to answer this. There is little evidence whether too little or too much health care for back pain produces better or worse outcomes, or affects the amount of pain and disability in the population. (Though out of interest, see Keller et al (1999).) If we cannot show what kind of care is effective, it is tempting to ask if expensive interventions are justified. If all regions had the same rates of hospitalization and surgery for back pain as those with the lowest rates, that might save $500 million in health care costs each year. That is certainly true, but it does not mean it is right.

We might also compare current practice with agreed standards or guidelines, and that can produce impressive figures. By this argument, we might reduce X-rays and imaging by 50%, most conservative treatments by 80%, disk surgery by 50%, and fusion by up to 90%. But are these figures real, and do they mean anything? It depends on who sets the standards, and how well they reflect scientific evidence, or simply consensus, or vested interests.

Guidelines and health care use are quite different things. The supporters of most of these procedures produce clinical evidence to suggest that current rates are actually too low. At present, we simply do not have the information to decide what should be the "correct" level of health care for back pain.

The answers to these dilemmas depend on research in three areas (Volinn et al 1994):

1. outcomes of treatment for low back pain, effectiveness, and cost-effectiveness
2. patient preferences
3. doctor and patient decision-making, practice style, and how to change practice to achieve the first two goals.

A decade later, we still do not have answers.

HEALTH CARE FOR BACK PAIN IN THE US

Let me try to summarize health care for back pain in the US.

About 70 million US adults have some low back pain each year and about 24 million have back pain lasting 2 weeks or more. There is no evidence that the prevalence of back pain in the US is changing or much different from that in Europe.

Health care for back pain in the US is a curious mixture of dramatic contrasts. It is easy to forget that most Americans still deal with back pain themselves most of the time and get on with their lives more or less normally.

Back pain is now the fifth most common reason for visiting a physician in the US and accounts for 2.8% of physician office visits. That is a total of about 16 million visits each year. The number of visits has remained fairly steady over the past decade.

Conventional medical care includes two very different patterns. Two-thirds of patients with back pain get their treatment mainly in primary care. But about a third get treatment from medical specialists with a great deal of high-tech and high-cost investigations and interventions. Half a million patients are now hospitalized each year for back disorders, but non-surgical hospitalization has fallen dramatically over the past 20 years. Something like half a million patients now have a low back operation each year and that number is doubling each decade.

Some 6 million Americans now make about 60 million visits to chiropractors each year. This has doubled over the last 15 years. There are also about 15 million visits to physical therapists. But recent surveys show there is even greater use of other alternative therapies, particularly massage, yoga, relaxation therapies, and energy healing.

Remember, the scientific evidence shows that many of the treatments still in common use for back pain are ineffective. The evidence suggests that medical and chiropractic care are more or less equally effective. So it is no surprise that the choice of provider makes little difference to clinical outcomes. And despite enormous and rising costs of health care for back pain, we have no clear evidence on the cost-effectiveness of different kinds of care.

There are no good figures for the cost of back pain in the US, though there is no doubt it is very expensive. Costs are difficult to estimate because of the way health care is organized and funded and the lack of national data. It is also difficult to estimate trends. There is increasing use of high-tech and high-cost investigations and interventions, but we do not know the impact of managed care. Frymoyer & Durett (1997) estimated direct medical costs to be $33 billion in 1994, but they based this on data that were already badly out of date. Indirect costs are likely to be at least two to four times the direct costs, but Frymoyer & Durett were unable to reach any definite figure.

CURRENT TRENDS IN THE US

What has happened to health care for back pain in the US since AHCPR (1994)? This would seem to be one of the most important questions about back pain today, but we have no clear answer. We have data on trends of health care visits, hospitalizations, and operations. But there is a lack of up-to-date information on current professional practice and the care patients with back pain receive.

In the absence of hard facts, all I can offer are my impressions. Schoene (2003) offers an independent view on the contemporary US scene.

I suspect there has been little change in the overall pattern of US health care for back pain since 1994 and the same trends continue. There is certainly no evidence of any major shift. It is more a question of continuing expansion in the types and numbers of all conservative and surgical treatments. And increasingly sophisticated marketing of medical technologies and products.

Evidence-based medicine suffered a major setback in the US with the political defeat of AHCPR (Waddell 2002). There is no strong guideline movement in the US, comparable to the UK and Europe. Despite that, or perhaps instead, most health care organizations are making some effort at managed care. Most have some kind of informal guideline, many of which are loosely based on AHCPR (1994). Most are at least trying to track what physicians are doing. Some are trying to influence the way primary care and, less frequently, specialist physicians evaluate and treat non-specific back pain, e.g., by feedback about X-rays, drug prescription, and referrals. However, there is no clear evidence whether this has much impact on practice.

I would guess that with all the publicity there is now less use of bed rest, but we do not really know. The latest data from 1999 are not encouraging (Table 20.10).

Hopefully, physicians are giving better information and advice to reassure patients and counter fears about returning to ordinary activities. So far, there is no convincing evidence of this. The same applies to advice about work.

There is very heavy use of analgesics. Forty-five percent of Americans say they take prescription analgesics for some form of pain (CBS News Poll 2003). Amazingly, 87% of all adults say they take over-the-counter analgesics (Harris Interactive 2003). Fifteen percent take them every day, 14% several times a week, and 27% several times a month. There is particular concern about increasing use of opioids. Hunkele & Vogt (2002) studied analgesic use in a Pittsburgh area Health Maintenance Organization in 2001. Fifty-six percent of 17 228 patients with back pain received an average of 4.6 prescriptions for analgesics. A third were for narcotics, 26% for narcotics and non-selective opioids, 9% for narcotics and other analgesics, and 27% for non-steroidal anti-inflammatories alone.

Chiropractic seems to be as popular as ever, and has probably overtaken conventional medicine in the number of patients it treats for back pain. However, patients also now seem to use a much wider range of alternative therapies such as massage and relaxation techniques.

We used to think that patients used *either* conventional *or* alternative health care. Recent surveys show this is no longer true. About half the patients who seek any health care for back pain use both conventional medical care and some form of alternative therapy. Many of them also use some form of self-treatment. However, it is not clear whether these are new trends or we simply did not recognize them before.

The central issue remains the battle of health care ideologies both in the market place and in the media. There is a proliferation of new, unproven, high-tech gadgets – all of which seem to be getting some market share. The surgical industries form a powerful political lobby to promote invasive, expensive care. The drug industry – with 80 000 reps in the US – spent $15.7 billion in 2000 to promote its products. Occupational Safety and Health Administration, the National Institute for Occupational Safety and Health (NIOSH) and the unions argue that back pain is an occupational disorder that should be solved by legislation. Disability insurers promote active case management. There are flourishing functional capacity evaluation, disability evaluation, and legal industries. Chiropractic continues its very effective campaign for market share. There is now a host of competing forms of alternative therapies ranging from the respectable to the lunatic. And this whole brew ferments in the hot house of unfettered, free-market enterprise.

US vs UK

I previously tried to compare health care for back pain in the US with that in the UK (Waddell 1996). I am less sure of this comparison now. There is emerging evidence of a major shift in the UK (Ch. 19), but it is not at all clear whether there is any comparable change in the US. We do not have data to make an accurate up-to-date comparison, so again let me simply try to give some impressions.

Perhaps surprisingly, it appears that people with back pain in the UK are more likely to seek medical care, which probably reflects free access to the National Health Service (NHS). The RAND Health Insurance Experiment in the US showed that free access can increase use of health care for back pain by up to 28%.

In the UK, 98% of all health care is by the NHS, and access to investigations, therapy, and specialists is via the family doctor. In the US, health care is a market place. More US patients with back pain see a medical specialist and many patients self-refer directly to a specialist. In the US there are many more chiropractors than in the UK and they now provide more health care for back pain than MDs. There are fewer chiropractors in the UK, but the numbers are growing.

Medical care for back pain in the UK is mainly in primary care and consists of analgesics, reassurance, and advice. If patients continue to attend, they get plain X-rays and physical therapy. It is high-volume, low-tech, and low-cost. It is still often delayed because of waiting lists. Dissatisfaction with NHS services for back pain is so high that 55% of patients seek private therapy instead. Primary medical care and treatment for back pain in the US are very similar to those in the UK. But more American patients see medical specialists, with much higher rates of MRI and surgery. This specialist care is high-tech and high-cost. Orthopedics is the main medical specialty in both countries, but US and UK orthopedic surgeons do different things for back pain. In the US, more than a quarter of the patients who go to see an orthopedic or neurosurgeon will sooner or later have surgery. In the UK, fewer than 3% of those who see a surgeon will ever have an operation. British patients go to an orthopedic surgeon for a second opinion and advice, and orthopedic principles then influence their management. American patients go to a surgeon for a procedure, and receive the most invasive treatment in the world.

The amazing thing is that it does not seem to make much difference. We do not have any evidence that more or less or different health care improves clinical outcomes. Health care seems to have little direct effect on the enormous social impact of back pain.

Summary

US vs UK – a caricature
- US medical care for back pain is fragmented, too specialized, too invasive, and too expensive
- NHS care for back pain in the UK is more cohesive, but underfunded, too little, and too late
- Despite the very different health care systems, there is little evidence that they make much difference to the social impact of back pain in the two countries

ACKNOWLEDGMENT

I am grateful to Mark Schoene for help in obtaining up-to-date US material for this chapter, though he bears no responsibility for my presentation and interpretation of the data.

References

AAOS 2000 The Dartmouth atlas of musculoskeletal health care. American Academy of Orthopedic Surgeons, Rosemont, IL

AHCPR 1994 Clinical practice guideline number 14. Acute low back problems in adults. Agency for Health Care Policy and Research, US Department of Health and Human Services, Rockville, MD

Baldwin M L, Cote P, Frank J W, Johnson W G 2001 Cost-effectiveness studies of medical and chiropractic care for occupational low back pain: a critical review of the literature. Spine Journal 1: 138–147

Battie M C, Cherkin D C, Dunn R, Clol M A, Wheeler K J 1994 Managing low back pain: attitudes and treatment preferences of physical therapists. Physical Therapy 74: 219–226

Bush T, Cherkin D, Barlow W 1993 The impact of physician attitudes on patient satisfaction with care for low back pain. Archives of Family Medicine 2: 301 305

Carey T S, Evans A, Hadler N, Kalsbeek W, McLaughlin C, Fryer J 1995a Care-seeking among individuals with chronic low back pain. Spine 20: 312–317

Carey T S, Garrett J, Jackman A, McLaughlin C, Fryer J, Smuckler D R 1995b The outcomes and costs of care for acute low back pain among patients seen by primary care practitioners, chiropractors and orthopaedic surgeons. New England Journal of Medicine 333: 913–917

Carrino J A 2002 Spinal injection procedures: volume, provider distribution and reimbursement in the United States Medicare population from 1993 to 1999. Radiology 225: 723–729

CBS News Poll 2003 Ouch! We're a hurting group. Available online at: www.cbsnews.com/stories/2003/01/28/opinion/polls/main538259.shtml

Cherkin D C, Deyo R A 1993 Non-surgical hospitalization for low-back pain: is it necessary? Spine 18: 1728–1735

Cherkin D C, MacCornack F A, Berg A O 1988 Managing low back pain – a comparison of the beliefs and behaviors of family physicians and chiropractors. Western Journal of Medicine 149: 475–480

Cherkin D C, Deyo R A, Wheeler K, Ciol M A 1994a Physician variation in diagnostic testing for low back pain. Arthritis and Rheumatism 37: 15–22

Cherkin D C, Deyo R A, Loeser J D, Bush T, Waddell G 1994b An international comparison of back surgery rates. Spine 19: 1201–1206

Cherkin D C, Deyo R A, Wheeler K, Ciol M A 1995 Physician views about treating low back pain. The results of a national survey. Spine 20: 1–10

Cherkin D C, Deyo R A, Battie M, Astreet J, Barlow W 1998 A comparison of physical therapy, chiropractic manipulation, and provision of an educational booklet for the treatment of patients with low back pain. New England Journal of Medicine 339: 1021–1029

Cherkin D C, Deyo R A, Sherman K J et al 2002 Characteristics of visits to licensed acupuncturists, chiropractors, massage therapists and physicians. Journal of the American Board of Family Practice 15: 463–472

Coulter I D, Hurwitz E L, Adams A H, Geneovese B J, Hays R, Shekelle P G 2002 Patients using chiropractors in North America: who are they and why are they in chiropractic care? Spine 27: 291–298

Cypress B K 1983 Characteristics of physician visits for back symptoms: a national perspective. American Journal of Public Health 73: 389–395

Deyo R A 1998 Low back pain. Scientific American August: 29–33

Deyo R A, Diehl A K 1986 Patient satisfaction with medical care for low back pain. Spine 11: 28–30

Deyo R A, Tsui-Wu Y-J 1987 Descriptive epidemiology of low back pain and its related medical care in the United States. Spine 12: 264–268

Deyo R A, Taylor V M, Diehr P et al 1994 Analysis of automated administrative and survey databases to study patterns and outcomes of care. Spine 19: 2083S–2091S

Druss B G, Marcus S C, Olfson M, Tanielian T, Pincus H A 2003 Trends in care by non-physicians clinicians in the United States. New England Journal of Medicine 348: 130–137

Eisenberg D M, Kessler R C, Foster C et al 1993 Unconventional medicine in the United States. New England Journal of Medicine 328: 246–252

Eisenberg D M, Davis R B, Ettner S L et al 1998 Trends in alternative medicine use in the United States, 1990–1997: results of a follow-up national survey. Journal of the American Medical Association 280: 1569–1575

Elam K C, Cherkin D C, Deyo R 1995 How emergency physicians approach low back pain: choosing costly options. Journal of Emergency Medicine 13: 143–150

Frymoyer J W, Durett C L 1997 The economics of spinal disorders. In: Frymoyer J W (ed.) The adult spine, 2nd edn. Lippincott-Raven, Philadelphia, pp 143–150

Harris Interactive 2003 National Consumers League over-the-counter pain medication study. Available online at: www.nclnet.org/otcpain/harrisesummary.htm

Hart L G, Deyo R A, Cherkin D C 1995 Physician office visits for low back pain. Frequency, clinical evaluation, and treatment patterns from a US national survey. Spine 20: 11–19

Hunkele J, Vogt M 2002 Use of narcotics and NSAIDs for low back pain: impact on medication costs. Presented to the Annual Meeting of the American College of Rheumatology, New Orleans

Hurwitz E L, Coulter I D, Adams A H et al 1998 Utilization of chiropractic services from 1985 through 1991 in the United States and Canada. American Journal of Public Health 88: 771–776

Hurwitz E L, Morgenstern H, Harber P et al 2002 A randomized trial of medical care with and without physical therapy and chiropractic care with and without physical modalities for patients with low back pain: 6-month follow-up outcomes from the UCLA low back pain study. Spine 27: 2193–2204

Jette A M, Delitto A 1997 Physical therapy treatment choices for musculoskeletal impairments. Physical Therapy 77: 145–154

Jette D U, Jette A M 1996 Physical therapy and health outcomes in patients with spinal impairments. Physical Therapy 76: 930–945

Jette A M, Smith K, Haley S M, Davis K D 1994 Physical therapy episodes of care for patients with low back pain. Physical Therapy 74: 101–110

Keller R B, Atlas S J, Soule D N, Singer D E, Deyo R A 1999 Relationship between rates and outcomes of operative treatment for lumbar disc herniation and spinal stenosis. Journal of Bone and Joint Surgery 81-A: 752–762

Li L C, Bombardier C 2001 Physical therapy management of low back pain: an exploratory survey of therapist approaches. Physical Therapy 81: 1018–1027

Lurie J D, Birkmeyer N J, Weinstein J N 2003 Rates of advanced imaging and spine surgery. Spine 28: 616–620

Meade T W, Dyer S, Browne W, Townsend J, Frank A O 1990 Low back pain of mechanical origin: randomized comparison of chiropractic and hospital outpatient treatment. British Medical Journal 300: 1431–1437

Mendenhall S 2002 Spinal surgery update. Orthopedic Network News 13: 1–20

Mielenz T J, Carey T S, Dyrek D A et al 1997 Physical therapy utilization by patients with acute low back pain. Physical Therapy 77: 1040–1051

Nyiendo J, Haas M, Goldberg B 1996 Cost-effectiveness of chiropractic and medical treatment for acute and chronic recurrent low back pain. Proceedings of the FCER International Conference on Spinal Manipulation, Bournemouth, England. Foundation for Chiropractic Education and Research, Des Maines, IA, pp 87–88

Saunders K W, Von Korff M, Pruitt S D, Moore J E 1999 Prediction of physician visits and prescription medicine use for back pain. Pain 83: 369–377

Schoene M 2003 The treatment of back and neck pain: a new pattern of care? Back Letter 18 (3): 25–36

Shekelle P G, Markovich M, Louie R 1995a An epidemiologic study of episodes of back pain care. Spine 20: 1668–1673

Shekelle P G, Markovich M, Louie R 1995b Comparing the costs between provider types of episodes of back pain care. Spine 20: 221–227

Skargren E I, Carlsson P G, Oberg B E 1998 One-year follow-up comparison of the cost-effectiveness of chiropractic and physiotherapy as primary management for back pain: sub-group analysis, recurrence, and additional health care utilization. Spine 23: 1875–1884

Smucker D R, Konrad T R, Curtis P, Carey T S 1998 Practitioner self-confidence and patient outcomes in acute low back pain. Archives of Family Medicine 7: 223–228

Tacci J A, Webster B S, Hashemi L, Christiani D C 1998 Healthcare utilization and referral patterns in the initial management of new onset, uncomplicated, low back workers' compensation disability claims. Journal of Occupational and Environmental Medicine 40: 958–963

Tacci J A, Webster B S, Hashemi L, Christiani D C 1999 Clinical practices in the management of new-onset, uncomplicated, low back workers compensation claims. Journal of Occupational and Environmental Medicine 41: 397–404

Taylor H, Curran N M 1985 The Nuprin pain report. Louis Harris, New York

Taylor V M, Deyo R A, Cherkin D C, Kreuter W 1994 Low back pain hospitalization. Recent United States trends and regional variations. Spine 19: 1207–1213

Taylor V M, Deyo R A, Goldberg H, Ciol M, Kreuter W, Spunt B 1995 Low back pain hospitalizations in Washington state: recent trends and geographical variations. Journal of Spinal Disorders 8: 1–7

Vitale M 2002 An analysis of all spinal fusions in the state of California from 1995 to 1999. Presented to the annual meeting of the North American Spine Society, Montreal

Volinn E, Mayer J, Diehr P, Van Koevering D, Connell F A, Loeser J D 1992 Small area analysis of surgery for low back pain. Spine 17: 575–581

Volinn E, Turczyn K M, Loeser J D 1994 Patterns in low back pain hospitalizations: implications for the treatment of low back pain in an era of health care reform. Clinical Journal of Pain 10: 64–70

Von Korff M, Barlow W, Cherkin D, Deyo R A 1994 Effects of practice style in managing back pain. Annals of Internal Medicine 121: 187–195

Waddell G 1996 Low back pain: a twentieth century health care enigma. Spine 21: 2820–2825

Waddell G 2002 Recent developments in low back pain. In: Giamberardino M A (ed.) Pain 2002 – an updated review: refresher course syllabus. IASP Press, Seattle

Waddell G, Aylward M, Sawney P 2002 Back pain, incapacity for work and social security benefits: an international literature review and analysis. Royal Society of Medicine Press, London

Webster B, Mahmud M, Courtney T, Matz M, Christiani D 2002 Physicians' knowledge and practice approach in the initial management of acute work-related low back pain. Presented at International Forum V for Primary Care Research on Low Back Pain. Montreal, 10–11 May

WHO 1992–1994 International classification of diseases and related health problems, 10th revision, vols 1–3. World Health Organization, London

Wolsko P M, Eisenberg D M, Davis R B, Kessler R, Phillips R S 2003 Patterns and perceptions of care for treatment of back and neck pain: results of a national survey. Spine 28: 292–298

Chapter 21

Future health care for back pain

This book has tried to chart recent developments and trends. It has presented the argument and the evidence for a new approach to back pain. To conclude, let me gaze in my crystal ball to see the future. This is a very personal view, though I have used ideas and material from many sources. I am particularly grateful to the Clinical Standards Advisory Group (CSAG) report on NHS services for back pain (CSAG 1994). A decade later, it is still one of the few attempts to consider how we should organize health care for back pain. I am well aware this is not the final answer, but simply offer it as a starting point for further research and development.

We now have a much more solid evidence base for what does (and, equally important, what does not) work. I believe we are already seeing a revolution in the clinical management of acute back pain. We are still struggling to find a better answer for those patients who develop chronic pain and disability. And we are slow to accept that if we are going to put this new approach into practice we must also change the health care delivery system to make it possible.

You may disagree with these suggestions, and some of them will surely turn out to be wrong. But it is not enough to argue that you have always practiced a certain way and you just know that you are right. These proposals are based on the best evidence that we have at present. If you want to justify your different way of practice, you will need to have a convincing argument and in due course produce the evidence that your way works. None of us can simply defend the status quo or evade the need to improve health care for back pain.

THE PROBLEMS WITH PRESENT HEALTH CARE FOR BACK PAIN

An epidemiologic perspective

Let us put this discussion into perspective with a dose of epidemiologic reality (Croft et al 1997).

- *Primary prevention* of back pain would be ideal, but there is little evidence that we can prevent most back pain. General health measures should include stopping smoking, regular exercise, and physical fitness, although it is doubtful how much impact that would have on back pain. It may be possible to reduce the risk for certain occupational groups, but there is little evidence that an ergonomic approach has much impact in modern work.

- *Secondary prevention*: concentrate on active treatment of episodes to reduce recurrences and chronicity. There is good evidence this can produce short-term benefits, but little evidence on its long-term benefits or effect on the natural history of back pain. As a corollary, concentrate services on those at high risk of chronic pain and disability, though this is limited by our ability to identify those patients. Croft et al (1997) gave secondary prevention cautious support but felt that it needs further research.

- *Tertiary prevention*: rehabilitation to reduce the impact of back pain on life and work. There is reasonable evidence this can improve clinical outcomes, but limited evidence that it improves capacity for work. In a sense, this approach also admits defeat, that it is not possible to prevent persistent or recurrent pain.

Health care for ordinary backache?

The major constraint is that patients can only get the health care that is available. When we presented the draft CSAG report to a group of British family doctors, one of them accosted us angrily with his dilemma:

> These proposals on how to treat back pain are all very well. I agree with most of them. But I can't do that. My local physiotherapy department has a 3-month waiting list. The only place I can refer patients with back pain is to the orthopedic clinic. I know these patients don't have a surgical problem, and the orthopedic surgeon won't do anything for them, but I don't have any alternative!

I heard a different version of the same dilemma at a meeting in the US:

> I agree we do too many MRI scans for back pain. But my patients all know about scans and they want to find out what's wrong. They expect to go and see a surgeon, and if I don't refer them they will just go themselves. The surgeons don't want to miss anything and are afraid they might be sued if they do. Then if the scan shows the slightest bulge, both patient and surgeon are hooked. You say that scans don't help the management of ordinary back pain, but how can I stop them? I sometimes feel as if these ******* scans drive my whole clinical practice!

Leave aside the rights or wrongs of these two examples. The common message is that treatment will always be constrained by the services available. As Cherkin et al (1994) showed, who you see is what you get. The basic problem is the mismatch between what patients with back pain need and the health care that we provide for them.

Patients with ordinary backache have very different needs from those with serious spinal disease. I believe that many of our present problems come from our failure to distinguish and provide for these different needs. We refer them all to the same specialists and clinics. We do not separate patients with non-specific low back pain from those with serious spinal pathology or nerve root problems. Most medical specialists rightly focus on the investigation and treatment of serious spinal pathology and neurologic problems. That is their expertise, and it is a vital service for those patients with such problems. But these patients are a small minority in the multitude of patients with back pain. The problem is that the present medical system simply does not provide appropriate resources or services for patients with ordinary backache. At the same time, patients with ordinary backache may swamp specialist services. In some countries, this may cause delay for those who need and can benefit from specialist investigation and treatment. More often, patients with ordinary backache receive inappropriate and even harmful investigations and treatment that are really designed for different problems. Even when such treatment is simply ineffective rather than directly harmful, it may cause more subtle harm. It perpetuates the focus on disease and on passive, mechanical treatment. It creates unrealistic expectations of symptomatic cure. Delays and protracted treatment also defer more effective management and lead directly to chronic pain and disability. In some cases it may have been better not to have that referral or treatment at all.

Expensive specialist and hospital investigations and treatments also consume a large portion of the health care dollars spent on back pain. There is much ineffective and wasteful use of health care resources for back pain, and we could spend that money much better in other ways.

The relative balance of these difficulties varies in each health care system. They all share the basic flaw of failing to separate ordinary backache from specific pathology.

First, do no harm

I am still haunted by too many patients who would probably have been better if they had never had any of our health care for their back pain. Failed treatment may be worse than no treatment at all.

An ideal world

So, if we want to put this new approach into practice, we must change the health care system to provide the resources and referral patterns required for the new management. All we need to do is change the world!

You may say that is Utopia, and Utopia is only a dream. It may be an ideal world, we wish it could be like that, but we know it can never be. It is unrealistic. But we need dreams. Utopia gives us a glimpse of what might be possible, a holy grail to drive us ever onwards. Perhaps we can never fully realize the ideal. In the real world, we must relax and adapt ideals to match reality. But our goal should be the best possible health care for our patients, and we should not settle for less before we even start. So let us dream (Box 21.1).

Box 21.1   Imagine

- Everyone gets back pain, but serious disease is rare
- Health care designed to suit the needs of patients, not what health professionals can deliver
- No financial restraint on health care resources; but payment according to outcomes rather than delivery of services
- Financial support to help patients rehabilitate, rather than for disability
- Everyone gets back pain, but no one is crippled by it

A NEW HEALTH CARE SYSTEM FOR BACK PAIN

How should we change professional practice and the health care system to deliver the new approach? It seems logical to start by thinking how we would need to reorganize the health care system to deliver the kind of care recommended in current guidelines. This should let us find common principles of a good back pain service, even if we will always need to adapt the system to suit different circumstances and priorities in each country.

Most specialist services for serious spinal pathology and nerve root problems are reasonably satisfactory, *if* patients are referred and seen without delay. The problem is to provide a better service for the large number of patients with ordinary backache. The aim is to deliver better health care for these patients, but these proposals should also lead to more efficient and cost-effective use of resources.

First, let us consider the basic principles for such a service. Then let us apply these principles to the primary care services needed to manage ordinary backache, and to a back pain rehabilitation service for those patients who do not settle with primary care management.

Principles of services for back pain

Diagnostic triage

Diagnostic triage forms the basis of appropriate referral and the division of responsibility between primary care and specialist services.

Diagnostic triage and decisions about referral occur at the point of first contact in primary care. Primary care clinicians must detect the few patients with specific pathology among the vast majority with ordinary backache. Deyo & Phillips (1996) compared this to searching for the proverbial needle in a haystack. Because of the primary care filter, specialists have a much easier task to search for the needles in a smaller stack of hay.

Primary care clinicians must also distinguish between what sometimes seem to be two very different groups of patients with non-specific back pain. Most patients seem to get better no matter what we do, and need little more than reassurance and advice. We need to identify as early as possible the few who are at risk of chronic pain and disability.

Diagnostic triage is generally accurate, but it is so fundamental to all these proposals that continuing education is essential.

Division of responsibility between primary care and medical specialist services

There should be a much clearer division of responsibility between primary care and specialist services. This applies both to clinical management and to the provision of services.

Most management of non-specific low back pain is, and should be, in primary care (Box 21.2). The main responsibility of specialist services is to investigate and treat patients with serious spinal pathology, nerve root problems that do not settle, and those who require consideration of surgery.

Primary care   The aim should be to manage, investigate, and treat patients with ordinary backache as far as possible in primary care. The facilities these patients require are most appropriate to primary care. They do not need medical specialist or hospital facilities. The family doctor or occupational health

Box 21.2   Primary care
• Family medicine • Osteopathic medicine • Chiropractic medicine • Physical therapy • Occupational health

professional should be aware of the patient's family and work background and can adjust advice and management to suit. We need professional and patient education to change attitudes and accept that back pain really is a primary care problem.

Better primary care management of back pain depends on a shift of resources from medical specialist services to primary care. It also requires better undergraduate training and continuing education of primary care health professionals who look after patients with back pain.

Specialist services   Specialists provide two distinct services to patients with back pain. Their main role is the investigation and treatment of patients with specific pathology. They may also provide a secondary service for those patients with ordinary backache who fail to settle with routine primary care. These two services should be quite distinct, with separate referral patterns, resources, and funding.

The main spinal disorders specialties are orthopedic surgery, rheumatology, neurology, and neurosurgery. The first priority of these acute specialties should be to provide a rapid and efficient service for those patients who need their expertise and facilities. Acute orthopedic services should focus on patients who need investigation of possible serious spinal pathology, and nerve root problems that are not settling in 3–6 weeks. Acute rheumatology services should focus on patients who need investigation of possible serious spinal pathology or inflammatory disorders. Neurology and neurosurgery should provide a service to patients who need investigation and management of neurologic problems or spinal surgery.

The other role is to provide a secondary service for patients with ordinary backache who do not get better with primary care management. Some specialists and departments do at present provide a very good service for such patients, incorporating many of the present ideas. However, most routine visits to medical specialists do not meet these needs, which is why many patients and family doctors are dissatisfied.

The reasons why patients go to a specialist are often different from what actually happens to them. Any referral of a patient with ordinary backache to a specialist should have clear and explicit goals. The referring doctor, patient, and specialist should all agree these goals, which may include excluding more serious problems, pain control, or rehabilitation. The choice of specialist, the facilities they provide, and the outcome measures should reflect these goals. There is no point referring a patient to a surgeon and judging success in surgical terms if what that patient really needs is rehabilitation.

Timing

Timing is vital. I know that I have repeated this ad nauseam about clinical management, but it is so fundamental that we must apply it one last time to health care delivery. Design of the system must also take account of the passage of time and the risks of chronic pain and disability. The natural history of back pain is of a persistent or recurrent problem, and recovery may not mean the complete absence of pain. The key issue is the duration of sickness absence. There are three stages (Fig. 21.1) in which health care needs are very different.

In the first few weeks most people have a very good chance of recovering rapidly. Indeed, most people with back pain do not seek any professional health care. Most of those who do seek help only need very basic care:

- reassurance that they do not have any serious disease
- simple, safe, symptomatic measures such as medication
- advice and support to stay as active as possible.

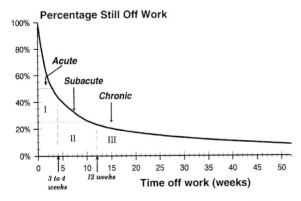

Figure 21.1 Time is of the essence. Health care delivery, just like clinical management, must take account of time. From Frank et al (1996), with permission.

A few patients with more severe pain and distress may require additional symptomatic measures such as manipulation. In view of the good natural history, however, the most important principle at this stage is: "First, do no harm." Do not turn a benign bodily symptom into a medical disaster. Avoid iatrogenic disability. The strategy at this stage should be to keep professional intervention to a minimum. There is even an argument that we should gently discourage any health care for most back pain and instead encourage people to deal with it themselves. If we are going to provide any health care at this stage, we must audit its impact critically.

For the 10% of patients who do not recover sufficient to return to ordinary activities and work within a few weeks, the needs of health care change rapidly. Now, time is of the essence. Waiting indefinitely for natural recovery may let the patient slide passively and unobtrusively into chronic pain and disability. All the evidence suggests that the first 3–6 weeks are crucial. Too much current health care for back pain is way beyond that time frame. There should be a major shift in resources to provide effective management at the subacute stage. Secondary prevention at this stage is much better and easier than the present relatively ineffective and wasteful treatment of chronic pain and disability.

Summary

Once someone is off work for 3–6 weeks with nonspecific low back pain:

- Time is of the essence
- They are at rapidly increasing risk of chronic pain and disability
- The priority of health care must be to get them back to normal activity and work as fast as possible

At the chronic stage, health care resources should be redirected to rehabilitation.

Equal emphasis on pain and disability

At present, most health care resources for back pain are designed for symptomatic treatment. We need equal emphasis on rehabilitation.

Pain and disability are equally important, and we must manage them both simultaneously. We cannot wait until treatment is complete and pain has gone before starting rehabilitation. The best method of achieving lasting relief of pain is to get the patient back to normal activity as soon as possible. We should devote much more effort and resources to the assessment and management of disability and to rehabilitation. We must reorganize the service so that access to these resources is readily available to every patient with back pain.

- Low back pain and disability are closely linked and equally important
- Too much current treatment for back pain is purely symptomatic
- Rehabilitation is equally important, from the very beginning

---

Shared responsibility

Back pain is a common bodily symptom that most people deal with themselves most of the time. Health care can help to control symptoms and aid recovery, but the natural history remains. Patients rightly have rising expectations of health care, but they must also be realistic. Some will always need help with acute symptoms, and a minority may need more prolonged periods of care. But health care can never be the permanent solution to a symptom like back pain. Patients must share responsibility with the doctor or therapist for their own recovery. People must take responsibility for their own continued management. In most cases, the sooner they do this, the better.

- Most back pain is an everyday bodily symptom
- There is no magic medical answer for ordinary backache
- Patients must share responsibility for dealing with their back pain

---

Audit and outcome measures

The twin aims of clinical management and of health care are to provide symptomatic relief and prevent disability. Effectiveness depends on the extent to which we achieve both these aims. Clinical outcome measures include pain, distress, activities of daily living, capacity for work, and health care use. But the most important measure of successful health care for back pain, for the patient and for society, is capacity for work. We do now have evidence on the effectiveness of various therapies for back pain. However, the epidemiology of low back disability raises serious doubts about the social impact of health care for back pain. All our professions need much more rigorous audit of health care delivery and social outcomes for patients with back pain.

Sick certification

The aim of health care is to control pain and restore the patient to normal activity. That is quite different from, and sometimes in direct conflict with, the need for medical certification for sickness benefits or compensation. Responsibility for clinical management should perhaps be separate from decisions about compensation, in which case the doctor who is caring for the patient should not be the one to decide about sick certification.

Key elements for a primary care service for back pain

If we are going to manage non-specific low back pain in primary care, we must provide the necessary health care facilities to make this possible (Box 21.3). These support services should be in primary care or provided by direct access to specialists or hospital services. The key issue is that they should be under the direct control and remain the responsibility of the primary health care provider. The exact form of such a service will vary in each health care system, and will depend on local needs and resources, and patient preferences.

The primary health care provider

I know it is not currently politically correct, but I am sufficiently old-fashioned to believe that patients still get the best care if one health professional takes final responsibility for their management. Other members of the health care team may

Box 21.3   A primary care service for back pain

- A primary health care provider
- Radiologic services
- Symptomatic control of pain
- Rehabilitation
- An acute pain relief service
- A second opinion
- *A multidisciplinary back pain rehabilitation service*

play vital roles, but the primary health care provider should take personal responsibility for:

- clinical assessment; investigation if appropriate
- diagnostic triage and referral to the appropriate specialist if required
- providing or arranging symptomatic relief
- providing accurate and up-to-date information and advice
- arranging rehabilitation and coordinating return to work or vocational rehabilitation if required.

Radiologic services

The place of radiology is in diagnostic triage and the work-up of patients with possible serious pathology or nerve root problems under consideration of surgery. It has little place in ordinary backache. There should be direct primary care access to plain X-rays and bone scans, provided we are always conscious of the role and limitations of these tests. They provide little information about ordinary backache. There is a strong argument that imaging is inappropriate to the primary care management of ordinary backache. Computed tomography (CT) and magnetic resonance imaging (MRI) have high false-positive rates in asymptomatic people, particularly with increasing age, which makes them unsuitable for screening tests. There is a logical argument that these are specialist investigations that should be used for patients with possible serious spinal pathology or those who are being worked up for surgery. There is less debate that we should order both plain X-rays and imaging on clear clinical indications according to radiologic guidelines. There is considerable concern on both sides of the

Atlantic about the overuse of these investigations in non-specific low back pain. X-rays of the spine involve high doses of irradiation. Overimaging leads directly to overtreatment. We should audit the use of radiology in non-specific low back pain.

Symptomatic measures

One of the primary roles of health care is the relief or at least control of pain, and patients will always need symptomatic measures. Simple, safe measures such as temporary modification of activities, medication, and the application of heat or cold are sufficient for most acute patients. In view of the evidence that is now available, we should orga-nize services to make manipulation available as an option for all patients who need additional symptomatic relief. Osteopathic physicians, chiropractors, osteopaths, and an increasing number of physical therapists have professional training and expertise in manipulation. A few medical practitioners also have some training. Some forms of manipulation or mobilization are now widely available, but the techniques used and levels of skills vary widely. We need further research on which forms of manual therapy are most effective for which patients. We also need to audit levels of education, skills, and the delivery of manual therapy. There is a wide range of other symptomatic options, but there is little scientific evidence that they are effective. There is now debate about whether there should be provision and funding of these services. Symptomatic modalities are not an end in themselves, and probably have little effect on the long-term natural history of back pain. Their main purpose is to provide temporary control of pain, thus allowing patients to increase their activity level and rehabilitate. Both patients and health professionals need re-education on the purpose and limitations of symptomatic treatment.

Summary

- Patients need symptomatic measures to relieve or control their pain
- Symptomatic measures do not cure the problem
- The main aim of symptomatic measures is to let patients get active

An acute pain relief service

Most patients with ordinary backache get adequate relief of pain from medication or manipulative therapy. Some patients with nerve root pain or, more rarely, ordinary backache may require further help for the control of acute pain and distress.

There are a few pilot schemes for acute pain relief for back pain, often linked to chronic pain services or an acute postoperative pain service. This type of service should be more generally available. It would be a much more appropriate and cost-effective service for these patients than hospitalization or inappropriate surgical consultations. Such an acute pain service would require specific resources and referral arrangements. Patients should be seen within 48 hours of telephone referral to a locally agreed, named contact. The acute pain service is most likely at present to be provided from hospital resources on an outpatient or day-case basis.

Second opinion

Some patients and primary care providers may feel the need for a second opinion, particularly if pain and disability do not settle as quickly as they wish. This may reassure both patient and provider and give extra support on:

- assessment, diagnostic triage, and psychosocial assessment
- further symptomatic control
- active exercise, rehabilitation, and return to work.

On the principle of managing back pain in primary care, this second opinion should ideally remain in the primary care setting. There are at least two ways of providing this:

1. *A family doctor with a special interest and expertise in back pain or musculoskeletal disorders.* A family doctor has the ideal skills and is in the ideal situation to provide this service. It is important that family doctors retain a broad clinical practice, but many also develop a special interest. Back pain is such a common problem that some family doctors do now have such a special interest in back pain, musculoskeletal medicine, or manipulative medicine. Some run special clinics, particularly in large group practices or health maintenance organizations.

2. *A chiropractor, osteopath, or physical therapist with specialist training and expertise in the assessment and management of back pain.* Many patients find this more satisfactory than a visit to a medical specialist. However, in some health care systems, the role and status of the practitioner or therapist must change if they are to fulfill this need. Every specialist must record and report their assessment, opinion, and advice on management, which might be a condition of contract and payment. Responsibility for overall clinical management might remain with the primary care provider, but the practitioner offering a second opinion would take professional responsibility for the treatment he or she gave. Perhaps most importantly, everyone must accept that this practitioner has the status of an expert or specialist. Some practitioners do now fulfill these criteria and there is emerging acceptance of this role.

A back pain rehabilitation service

Better early management and better primary care services should greatly reduce the number of patients who need further referral. Ideally, we should be able to manage all patients with ordinary backache in primary care. However, no matter how much we improve management and services, there will always be some patients with persistent pain and disability. There is a point at which we must accept that primary care management is failing and that some patients need further help. And because of the enormous number with back pain, even a small proportion of failure will still create a large demand.

Rehabilitation facilities should be available for all patients who are still off work after 3–6 weeks and at risk of chronic pain and disability. Physical therapy has a key role in rehabilitation. Referral patterns, physical therapy facilities, and organization should reflect this. At present, rehabilitation is often regarded as a tertiary service after medical treatment is complete or has failed. That must change.

CSAG (1994) considered how to reorganize these secondary services to best meet the needs of these patients. We got wide support for the idea of a back pain rehabilitation service (Box 21.4). This should be a dedicated service because of the number of patients and the resources it requires. These are

Box 21.4   A dedicated, multidisciplinary, back pain rehabilitation service

- Led by a specialist with expertise in back pain rehabilitation
- Distinct referral patterns
- Organization, staffing, and resources focusing on pain management and rehabilitation
- Facilities for:
  - diagnostic triage and investigation
  - clinical, psychological, and occupational assessment
  - pain control
  - manipulative therapy
  - an active exercise, functional restoration, and rehabilitation program
  - counseling
  - occupational or vocational rehabilitation

multidisciplinary in nature and cut across specialty and organizational boundaries. The service should have completely separate aims, resources, and referral patterns from medical specialty services for patients with serious spinal pathology or nerve root problems. The service should be clearly identified and named as a back pain rehabilitation service.

In principle, we could locate the service wherever the resources are available. Ideally, on the principle of managing back pain in primary care, we should locate it in primary care. To get patients back to work, it might be best in the workplace as part of an occupational health service. These options should be the subject of future research. However, the multidisciplinary resources that such a service needs are rarely available at present in either primary care or occupational health. The staff, resources, and organization may at present be most available and supplied most efficiently from a specialist or hospital service. The service should be multidisciplinary in nature and approach, although the exact range of staff might vary with local needs and resources. Ideally, the service should have the facilities to provide: diagnostic triage and investigation; clinical, psychological, and occupational assessment; pain control facilities; manipulative therapy; an active exercise, functional restoration, and

rehabilitation program; counseling; and occupational or vocational rehabilitation.

The major emphasis of the service should be on pain management and rehabilitation. The choice of staff should match this aim. These needs are mainly low-tech, low-cost, and high-volume in nature, and the organization, staffing, and resources should reflect that. CSAG did not recommend a multidisciplinary group of high-tech medical specialties.

The service should be led by an experienced clinician. Both patients and family doctors expect and demand a high-quality, expert service. This clinician should be able to take final professional responsibility for the service. Their contract should specify that responsibility and they should have adequate time in their job description. At present, they are most likely to be medical specialists from orthopedic surgery, rheumatology, rehabilitation medicine, pain management, orthopedic or musculoskeletal medicine. However, in future they might better come from family medicine, osteopathic medicine, chiropractic medicine, behavioral medicine, or physical therapy. Whatever the clinician's background, their main commitment and responsibility must be to the overall management and rehabilitation of back pain. Their job is not to provide individual specialty skills or techniques. Many of the resources required for such a service already exist, and are already provided piecemeal to patients with back pain. It is largely a matter of more efficient organization of these resources. This is also likely to be more cost-effective. Medical specialty input to the service should be on a sessional basis, e.g., pain relief techniques. Primary care staff of family doctors, chiropractors, osteopaths, physical therapists, and counselors can and should do much of the work.

The back pain rehabilitation service should work closely with local primary care services and contribute to continuing professional education. Close links will also facilitate referral and coordination with primary care management. There should be a major emphasis on self-help to prepare patients for their own continued management. Group therapy and support groups are useful in principle and cost-effective. The service should liaise with employers and occupational health services to help patients return to work as soon as possible. There may be links and shared resources with an acute pain service or pain management program.

The main physical resources are clinic space, physical and manual therapy and occupational therapy facilities, and low-cost rehabilitation equipment.

Conclusion

To change clinical management for back pain, we must reorganize the health care system to provide the necessary services. We must change referral patterns to suit the needs of patients rather than to suit professional interests. We need different numbers of different kinds of health professionals for back pain. We must shift health care resources and change how we spend health care dollars for back pain. Unless we change the system, we will not achieve real change in the health care that we deliver to patients with back pain.

CHANGE IN PROFESSIONAL PRACTICE

New clinical management and a new health care system for back pain mean that we must all change our professional practice. We must change what we do and how we use our time with patients with back pain. This applies to physicians, chiropractors, physical therapists, and osteopaths alike.

A biopsychosocial approach

We all share common philosophic ideals for health care. Despite that, most orthodox and alternative health professionals still think and practice according to an outdated biomedical model:

- pain as a signal of injury and tissue damage
- search for a structural cause and cure
- purely symptomatic treatment
- a mechanical "fix"
- taking over responsibility and control from the patient.

Too often, we focus too much on pain and the search for a biologic cause and cure, to the exclusion of all else.

A biopsychosocial approach offers the tools to put our common philosophic ideals into practice.

It demands a whole new way of thinking. We must assess and deal with:

- the biologic basis of low back pain and disability
- the patient's attitudes and beliefs, emotions, and behavior
- social, work, and economic influences and interactions.

These are all equally important to planning management. This is a much more difficult and challenging type of professional practice, but it opens a whole new vista on back pain.

Triage

One of our first priorities is to make sure there is no serious disease. The primary health care provider usually carries out initial assessment and triage. In some countries and situations, a physical therapist may do this.

Once we rule out serious disease, we should stop the frenzied search for structural pathology. Once we are sure this is non-specific low back pain, we must approach it more as a matter of disturbed function.

One of the major implications of triage is referral to appropriate care. All health professionals must have a clear idea about which patients for whom our care is appropriate. More important and more difficult, we must recognize and admit that there are patients for whom our care is not appropriate and refer them to someone else. This is particularly true of ordinary backache.

Information and advice

Too often, we all give patients the wrong message about back pain. Most of what we say and do – our investigations and diagnosis, and our information and advice to patients – reflects and reinforces the biomedical model. It is about:

- anatomy, disks, trapped nerves, degeneration, and mechanical dysfunction
- injury and fear of reinjury
- biomechanics, ergonomics
- physical treatment.

Too often, we label back pain patients with a serious disease, and at the same time offer unconvincing platitudes and unrealistic advice. Too often, patients get conflicting information and advice. Patients need accurate and honest information, in line with the biopsychosocial model and current guidelines. We should think about how our information and advice affect not only patients' backs but also their beliefs and what they do about their pain. We must direct our advice to the goals of rehabilitation and helping patients to take over the care of their own backs.

Printed and visual educational material should be available that is in line with current guidelines. All members of the primary health care team should give the same information and advice.

Symptomatic modalities

We must provide the best pain control that we can, in whatever way is most effective. But we must be realistic and honest that it can only provide relief and that it should be used to facilitate rehabilitation. Many health professionals need to reduce the amount of time, effort, and resources they put into passive modalities.

Rehabilitation

Every health professional who treats back pain must be interested in rehabilitation. Patients who do not recover sufficient to return to work by the subacute stage may need specialist rehabilitation services. But all clinical management of back pain should incorporate rehabilitation principles from the very start. Too often, in the name of symptomatic treatment, we actually prescribe disability. Instead, our treatment should support patients to continue their normal activities and to stay at work, or return to work as soon as possible. Our aim must be to help patients get on with their lives, and that is also the measure of our success. We must consider how all that we say and do, our advice, every treatment, and our whole management will promote rehabilitation. This is a very different agenda from just dealing with physical disease.

All health professionals dealing with back pain must understand rehabilitation principles. For some of us, this may mean learning new skills and further training. Liebenson (1996), in his book *Rehabilitation of the Spine*, showed how to integrate rehabilitation into chiropractic. He pointed out that manual

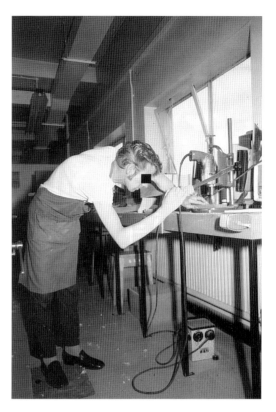

Figure 21.2   "Work for all, for those with low back pain as well". Return to normal activities and work is the ultimate measure of successful health care for back pain.

medicine and rehabilitation make natural partners in musculoskeletal health care.

The importance of work

At present, most health professionals regard their job as health care. We assume that if we make patients better, they will automatically return to normal activity and work. As a result, we pay little direct attention to work issues. Few of us have much knowledge of, or any contact with, our patient's workplace (Fig. 21.2).

If we are to put equal emphasis on rehabilitation, however, work is of paramount importance. We must all think about, ask about, and understand our patient's work situation and demands. We must try to keep patients at work or get them back to work as rapidly as possible. We should more readily and more often pick up the phone and contact their employers or supervisors or the occupational health service to coordinate return to work. Most of all, we should always be conscious of the impact of sickness absence on our patients and the risk of long-term incapacity.

Health care is not complete or wholly successful, and we have not fulfilled our professional responsibility, until we get our patients back to work.

> **The longer someone is off work with back pain, the lower their chance of returning to work**
> - The minute someone stops work with back pain, there is a risk of 1–10% that they will go on to long-term incapacity
> - Once they are off work for 3–6 months, the risk is 50%
> - By 1–2 years, they are virtually unemployable, irrespective of the physical state of their back or further health care

Sharing responsibility

Too often, health professionals are guilty of taking over control. Occasional patients with back pain continue to attend for months or even years. All our specialties are guilty of this. If patients are to take responsibility for their own backs, we must be willing to relinquish control.

That means one of the measures of success is when patients do take over their own management and no longer need our health care. I am not suggesting that we should deny treatment or set any arbitrary time limit. But in one sense, as long as patients continue to attend, our management has not been wholly successful. There is no evidence that regular maintenance therapy is of any value in the natural history of back pain. It goes against the basic principle that patients should take a large measure of responsibility for their own back pain. Whatever the claimed symptomatic benefit, continuing to attend a health professional may simply perpetuate the illness.

Change in practice

This all means a very different kind of professional practice. It means that we must change how we assess patients, what we say to them, and how we treat them.

All of us may argue defensively that we are already making these changes. I agree. Some physicians, chiropractors, physical therapists, and osteopaths are now putting these principles into practice. But too often these are isolated examples, or the change is only cosmetic. Different professions commit different sins and need to make different changes. You should recognize what applies to you. All our professions still have a long way to go to put the new management for back pain into routine practice.

This may mean major and fundamental change in our professional practice. At best, it is a challenge. At worst, it is a threat. It can exact a heavy price. I know, perhaps better than most, what that means. I spent most of my professional life as an orthopedic surgeon. It has been a good life, and I am proud of what I have done. But I have to admit that surgery is not the answer for back pain, and change what I do. The needs of our patients must override our professional pride.

Knowing what we need to change is one thing. Actually changing professional practice and patient behavior is quite another. There is a great deal of inertia and resistance to change and I can hear some howls of professional anguish.

There is also sometimes an element of vested interest in maintaining the professional status quo. I had a sudden wicked impulse during the opening ceremony of the Eighth World Congress on Pain. I wanted to jump up and address the 4300 pain professionals who had gathered from around the world:

> We have wonderful news. Someone has just discovered the cure for pain. It is 100% effective, has no side-effects and only costs a cent. Isn't that wonderful? Human beings need never suffer any more pain. So we might as well cancel this congress. Oh – and you are all out of a job.

I resisted the temptation. I do not know if I would have been lynched or crucified. Of course, health professionals do genuinely have the best interests of their patients at heart. It is just that sometimes we assume that our interests are the same as those of our patients and we lose sight of what is actually happening to them. We have so much faith and commitment to our own professional activities that we just assume they *must* be doing our patients good. There is an old saying that health professionals need patients more than patients need us. With back pain, that may be true.

Most health professionals do genuinely believe in most of these ideas for better patient care. The problem is putting these philosophic principles into daily practice. Too often, it is easier just to get

---

Box 21.5   Barriers to implementing guidelines and changing professional practice (reproduced with permission from COST B13 2002)

Practice environment
- Limitations of time
- Practice organization, e.g., lack of disease registers or mechanisms to monitor repeat prescribing

Educational environment
- Inappropriate continuing education and failure to link up with programs to promote quality of care
- Lack of incentives to participate in effective educational activities

Health care environment
- Lack of financial resources
- Lack of defined practice populations
- Health policies which promote ineffective or unproven activities
- Failure to provide practitioners with access to appropriate information

Social environment
- Influence of media on patients in creating demands/beliefs
- Impact of disadvantage on patients' access to care

Practitioner factors
- Obsolete knowledge
- Influence of opinion leaders
- Beliefs and attitudes (for example, related to previous adverse experience of innovation)

Patient factors
- Demands for care
- Perceptions/cultural beliefs about appropriate care

---

on with the job of mechanics. It is much more difficult and threatening to try to change what we do. It is much easier for me as a surgeon to deal with disks and scans and surgical techniques than to struggle with the complex biopsychosocial problems of chronic low back pain and disability. Yet to serve our patients best, we must all escape from our professional shackles.

There is now an extensive literature on changing professional practice (Oxman et al 1995, Haines & Donald 1998, Silagy & Haines 1998, Thorsen & Mäkelä 1999). There are many barriers (Box 21.5). There are many possible interventions, but their effectiveness is limited (Box 21.6).

Perhaps the problem is that is too much of a mechanical, methodologic approach imposed from without. This is the age of evidence-based medicine and I am a disciple. I am even a member of the Back Review Group Editorial Board of the Cochrane Collaboration. But I am a doubting disciple. Yes, I believe that health care for back pain should have a solid scientific base. Yes, I believe that methodologists can teach us a lot about how to develop and assess the evidence. Yes, I believe that guidelines are a convenient method of making that evidence easily available. But that is not enough. That very evidence shows that evidence alone has little direct effect on professional or patient behavior.

Real change comes from within and depends on new ideas that fire our imagination and change the way we think. Men fight and die for ideas, not evidence, as we all saw in Gulf War II. Ideally, these ideas should be firmly based on the evidence, but it is ideas that change the world. Optimistically, I believe the time for that revolution in thinking may have come for back pain.

FUTURE RESEARCH AND DEVELOPMENT

Priorities for health research should match patients' and society's needs. Back pain is now a major cause of human suffering and disability, health care use and cost to society. By any criteria, back pain should be a high priority for research funding.

Box 21.7 lists the main areas of biomedical research from a 1980 symposium on idiopathic back pain. These priorities are equally valid today. Continued research is vital. It is the hope for better

Box 21.6   Interventions to change professional practice (adapted from COST B13 2002)

Most consistently effective
- Interactive educational meetings, e.g., participation of health care providers in workshops that include discussions of practice
- Educational outreach visits
- Reminders (manual or computerized)
- Multifaceted interventions
- A combination that includes two or more of the following: audit and feedback, reminders, local consensus process, and marketing

Variable effect
- Audit and feedback: any summary of clinical performance
- Local opinion leaders: use of providers nominated by their colleagues as "educationally influential"
- Local consensus process: inclusion of providers in discussion to ensure that they agreed the chosen

clinical problem was important and that the approach to managing the problem was appropriate
- Patient-mediated interventions: any intervention aimed at changing the performance of health care providers where specific information was sought from or given to patients

Limited or no effect
- Educational materials: distribution of published or printed recommendations for clinical care, including clinical practice guidelines, audiovisual materials, and electronic publications
- Didactic educational meetings and lectures

The more cynical would suggest that health professionals, just like donkeys, may also respond to the carrots and sticks of financial incentives

Box 21.7   Research priorities from the 1980 symposium on idiopathic low back pain (LBP) sponsored by the National Institute of Arthritis, the American Academy of Orthopedic Surgeons, and the Orthopaedic Research Society (White & Gordon 1982). This list has changed remarkably little since that time (from Borkan & Cherkin 1996, with permission)

Epidemiology, natural course, and psychologic and psychiatric aspects
- Identification of risk factors that initiate or perpetuate LBP
- Identification of characteristics of patients without LBP
- Evaluation of strength testing and training techniques as preventive measures
- Evaluation of the role of smoking, drinking, and other off-the-job activities on LBP

Anatomy and ultrastructure of the lumbosacral spine
- Study of elderly asymptomatic individuals with degenerated disks
- Investigation of regional inflammation
- Use of animal models to study a number of variables, such as intraosseous pressure, on nociceptive nerve endings and intraspinal pathways

Biomechanics
- Study of the effect of different variables on the mechanical behavior of the spine
- Development of validated mathematical models of the spine, its components, and the whole trunk
- Complete analysis of the spine's material properties

Biochemistry of the supporting structures
- Investigation of the relationships between biochemical structure and mechanical function of components of the spinal unit
- Study whether biochemical breakdown products have the capacity to stimulate nociceptive nerve endings
- Anatomic, ultrastructural, radiographic, and biochemical analysis of lumbar disks

Neuromechanisms
- Investigation of nociceptors and nociceptive stimuli in bone, ligaments, and other deep tissues of the spinal unit
- Examination of the effects of various chemical substances present in lesions resulting from LBP injuries on the mediation of nociceptors

Development of animal models
- Study of mechanical and biologic variables in chemically or mechanically damaged nerves and ganglia
- Study of the role of endorphins, particularly in the placebo response
- Study of the trunk muscle activity and trigger points

understanding of the cause and treatment of back pain.

We need much more basic research into the physical basis of non-specific low back pain. We must relate this to clinical findings in the individual patient, and differentiate syndromes within non-specific low back pain. We must find which treatments are effective for which types of back pain, and develop a rational basis for choosing the best treatment for each patient. We must develop effective methods of dealing with the important psychosocial issues. We must develop more effective and cost-effective methods of rehabilitation for back pain, and ways of delivering them in primary care.

However, that is only one kind of research, which reflects the interests of basic scientists and medical specialists. But there are other kinds of research that are just as important. We also need health services research into how we can actually deliver better care. How can we provide the most effective and cost-effective health care with finite resources in the trenches of daily practice? How well does our health care actually meet the needs of our patients with non-specific low back pain?

Until recently, there was little primary care research into back pain, but that situation has now changed. In the last decade of the 20th century, there was an explosion of chiropractic research, mainly in the US. Even more recently, flourishing primary care research has emerged, particularly in the US, the UK, the Netherlands and Israel. The first international forum for primary care research on low back pain was in Seattle in October 1995. Sixty leading researchers in the field came from nine countries. One of the main goals of the forum was to draft an agenda for primary care research. All those coming to the meeting had to submit a written list of their most important research questions. At the end of the two-day meeting we discussed these issues, and then each cast five votes to those we felt were most important. Box 21.8 lists the top 20 research questions (Borkan & Cherkin 1996).

The forum felt that much traditional research on back pain has little relevance to primary health care. This list is very different. It does not include any strictly biomedical questions. It shows the very different interests and concerns of patients and providers in primary care, where most back pain

is treated. It places back pain in a much broader, clinical and psychosocial context. Borkan & Cherkin (1996) summarized these areas:

- the daily challenges facing patients with back pain and their providers
- providing effective and cost-effective health care for back pain
- more effective methods of routine assessment and management
- changing knowledge and behaviors in patients, providers, and society
- radical change in how we view low back pain – a new paradigm.

The forum hoped that this list would help to shift the focus of future research and encourage funding agencies to give priority to these areas.

CSAG (1994) listed areas for future research and development into health service delivery:

- diagnostic triage and referral systems
- an integrated service for the management of non-specific low back pain in primary care
- physical therapy and manipulative therapy
- a dedicated rehabilitation service for patients with non-specific low back pain who do not recover with routine primary care management and who fail to return to work by about 6 weeks
- audit of health care delivery and outcomes for patients with back pain.

CONCLUSION

I am well aware that these are the bare bones of a future back service. We still have many uncertainties about the best way to provide health care for patients with non-specific low back pain. The answer will vary with local circumstances and resources and needs. We may now have more questions than answers, but at least we can see some of the issues more clearly. The urgent need is research and development to test these and other ideas in different settings. There is wide scope for pilot schemes and experiment. What is not in any doubt is that we must provide better health care for patients with non-specific low back pain. The starting point is to recognize the need and a willingness to try to meet that need. I have a dream ….

Box 21.8 Research priorities from the first international forum for primary care research on low back pain (LBP) (with the number of votes in brackets) (from Borkan & Cherkin 1996, with permission)

1. Can different varieties or subgroups of LBP (including chronic LBP) be identified and, if they can, what criteria can be used to differentiate among them? (30)
2. What can be done to contain and reverse the epidemic of LBP disability and cost in developed countries? (17)
3. What psychosocial interventions are effective in LBP? (15)
4. What are the most effective ways of changing the way primary care practitioners deal with LBP? (15)
5. What are the "best" (i.e., most cost-effective, most satisfying, least iatrogenic) strategies for treating LBP? (14)
6. What can be done to improve the quality and value of LBP research? (13)
7. Is there a need for a new paradigm for thinking about LBP? (13)
8. How can we improve self-care strategies and stimulate self-reliance among persons with chronic or recurrent LBP? (11)
9. How do patient and provider beliefs and expectations influence outcomes of care for LBP? (9)
10. Can the development and dissemination of guidelines improve outcomes and reduce costs of care for LBP? (7)
11. What are the best strategies for diagnosis? In particular, what is the reliability, predictive value, and clinical utility of common symptoms and diagnostic tests? Can "gold standards" be developed? (6)
12. What is the role of patient preferences in treatment outcomes? (6)
13. What are the predictors, determinants, and risk factors for chronic disability in LBP patients, including physical, psychosocial, mental health, and behavioral factors? Can subgroups at high risk for chronic LBP or therapeutic failure be identified? (5)
14. What are the most pertinent LBP outcome measures for researchers, clinicians, and patients, and how can better measurement scales be created and validated? (5)
15. What strategies are effective in educating physicians about various aspects of LBP and reinforcing physician effectiveness in communicating and counseling? (4)
16. What impact do benefit systems (such as workers' compensation or social security disability) have on LBP? (3)
17. How do persons who seek care for LBP differ from those who manage their problem without professional care? (3)
18. What can individuals do to prevent LBP? (3)
19. What are the appropriate relationships between manual therapists (such as chiropractors) and primary care physicians? (3)
20. Should primary care physicians treat LBP in all its presentations or would it make more sense if some segment of these patients was seen instead by back care specialists (e.g., orthopedists, chiropractors, physical therapists)? (3)

Bibliography

Borkan J M, Cherkin D C 1996 An agenda for primary care research on low back pain. Spine 21: 2880–2884

Borkan J, Van Tulder M, Reis S, Schoene M L, Croft P, Hermoni D 2002 Advances in the field of low back pain in primary care: a report from the Fourth International Forum. Spine 27: E128–E132

Cherkin D C, Deyo R A, Wheeler K, Ciol M A 1994 Physician variation in diagnostic testing for low back pain. Arthritis and Rheumatism 37: 15–22

COST B13 (2002) Draft European guidelines for the management of acute non-specific low back pain in primary care. Appendix III. Dissemination and implementation. Available online at: www.backpaineurope.org

Coulter A, Bradlow J, Martin-Bates C 1991 Outcome of general practitioner referrals to specialist out-patient clinics for back pain. British Journal of Geneal Practice 41: 450–453

Croft P, Papageorgiou A, McNally R 1997 Low back pain. In: Stevens A, Rafferty J (eds) Health care needs assessment, 2nd series. Radcliffe Medical Press, Oxford, pp. 129–182

CSAG 1994 Report on back pain. Clinical Standards Advisory Group. HMSO, London

Deyo R A, Phillips W R 1996 Low back pain: a primary care challenge. Spine 21: 2826–2832

Deyo R A, Cherkin D, Conrad D, Volinn E 1991 Cost, controversy, crisis; low back pain and the health of the public. Annual Review of Public Health 12: 141–156

Evans R G, Barer M L, Marmor T R (eds) 1994 Why are some people healthy and others not? The determinants of the health of populations. Aldini de Gruyter, New York

Fordyce W E 1995 Back pain in the workplace: management of disability in non-specific conditions. IASP Press, Seattle

Frank J W, Brooker A-S, Demaio S E et al 1996 Disability resulting from occupational low back pain. Part II: What do we know about secondary prevention? A review of the scientific evidence on prevention after disability begins. Spine 21: 2918–2929

Haines A, Donald A (eds) 1998 Getting research findings into practice. BMJ Books, London

Klein B J, Radecki R T, Foris M P, Feil E I, Hickey M E 2000 Bridging the gap between science and practice in managing low back pain. Spine 25: 738–740

Korr I M 1974 Andrew Taylor Still memorial lecture: research and practice – a century later. Journal of the American Osteopathic Association 73: 362–370

Liebenson C 1996 Rehabilitation of the spine. Williams & Wilkins, Baltimore

Nachemson A 1983 Work for all: for those with low back pain as well. Clinical Orthopaedics and Related Research 179: 77–85

Oxman A D, Thomson M A, Davis D A, Haynes R B 1995 No magic bullets: a systematic review of 102 trials of interventions to improve professional practice. Canadian Medical Association Journal 153: 1423–1431

Robertson J T 1993 The rape of the spine. Surgical Neurology 39: 5–12

Silagy C, Haines A 1998 Evidence based practice in primary care. BMJ Books, London

Thorsen T, Mäkelä M 1999 Changing professional practice. Theory and practice of clinical guidelines implementation. Danish Institute for Health Services Research and Development, Copenhagen

White A A, Gordon S L (eds) 1982 American Academy of Orthopaedic Surgeons symposium on idiopathic low back pain. Mosby, St Louis

Chapter 22

Epilogue

We have come a long way from where we started. Or perhaps in a sense we have come full circle. And we still have a long way to go.

Summary

Back pain was a 20th-century health care disaster

- Human beings have had back pain throughout recorded history
- Back pain has not changed: it is no different, no more severe, and no more common than it has always been
- What has changed is how we think about back pain and what we do about it
- We have turned a benign bodily symptom into one of the most common causes of chronic disability in western society today
- But if we can create that epidemic, we can also reverse it

Back pain is a paradox. Our ability to prevent or treat serious spinal disease is part of the success story of 20th-century medicine. Tragically, much more often, chronic disability due to ordinary backache illustrates the failure of 20th-century western health care. The dilemma is that back pain can be the presenting symptom of many spinal diseases, but most back pain is not due to any serious disease. We get into trouble when we confuse symptoms and disease. The biomedical approach has not solved

that problem, and there is strong circumstantial evidence that much low back disability is iatrogenic. The fault lies not in our backs, my friends, but in ourselves and how we treat our patients.

I warned you that some of the issues discussed in this book might challenge your deeply felt professional convictions and practice. Perhaps they have disturbed your professional status quo. I hope they have, and I do not apologize, because we should all be ashamed of what health care has done to back pain. Of course, we can each claim that we have achieved a great deal for individual patients. But you are blind if you cannot see that we have also done a great deal of harm to many patients with ordinary backache.

If we simply continue our present biomedical approach, which has failed, or just try to do more and bigger and better of the same, this epidemic will continue. That is not acceptable. We need to face up to the real and difficult questions of back pain, and to meet our patients' and society's demands that we do better. Nor can we turn back the clock, or try to return to some mythologic state of low back innocence. But we can learn from our past mistakes.

All health professionals share a common philosophy of caring for sick people. Medicine has an ancient heritage of philosophy and ethics. It is a humanistic philosophy: treating the body and the mind; healer when possible, but also comforter during life's sickness. During the past century or more, as the practice of orthodox medicine has become more mechanistic, osteopathic medicine, and chiropractic have developed their own

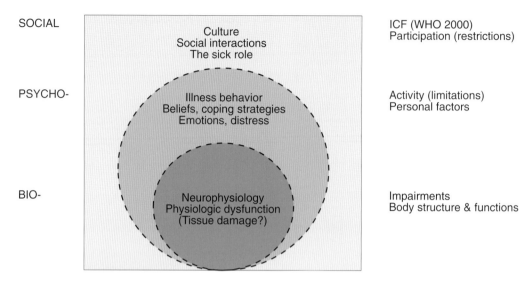

SOCIAL

PSYCHO-

BIO-

Culture
Social interactions
The sick role

Illness behavior
Beliefs, coping strategies
Emotions, distress

Neurophysiology
Physiologic dysfunction
(Tissue damage?)

ICF (WHO 2000)
Participation (restrictions)

Activity (limitations)
Personal factors

Impairments
Body structure & functions

Figure 22.1   The biopsychosocial model.

distinct versions of that ancient philosophy. The roots and traditions of physical and occupational therapy lie in helping patients to return to normal activities and work. All health professionals spend much of their day working with patients. Physical therapy, osteopathic medicine, and chiropractic are very much hands-on, with direct human contact between therapist and patient. We all, physicians, chiropractors, physical therapists, and osteopaths alike, believe that we should treat the whole person. The problem is that these ideals are abstract, and we get little guidance on how to turn them into practical reality in our daily practice. We are also limited by our human nature. As we have devoted more time, training, and effort to physical disease, so we have tended to neglect these more human aspects. It is all very well to say that we use science and mechanical treatment within a holistic framework, but it is too easy for that framework to dissolve in the starry mists of idealism. We all agree in principle that we should treat people and not spines, but then in daily practice we get on with the business of mechanics.

The biopsychosocial model (Fig. 22.1) is not a new philosophy. Rather, it is a method, or a set of tools, to apply that ancient philosophy to our daily practice. It helps us to a fuller understanding of pain and disability. That allows us to combine the

role of healer with the more ancient role of counselor, helping patients to cope with their problem (Fig. 22.2). The patient's role must also change from passive recipient of treatment to more active sharing of responsibility for their own progress.

Some doctors and therapists seem to be uncomfortable with this whole approach. They prefer to stick to nice, mechanical problems that they can understand and deal with. Some actually seem to feel threatened by these new ideas. It is no longer enough to know about anatomy and pathology. The biopsychosocial approach opens a whole new perspective on how people behave and cope with illness. It reveals the limitations of our treatment and of our professional skills. It exposes us to the difficulties and stress of dealing with emotions. We must accept that patients are not neat packages of mechanics or pathology, but suffering human beings. Professional life may be much simpler if we stick to physical treatment of mechanical problems, but health care demands that we treat people.

Some readers may argue that I have played down the physical problem of back pain. I would deny that. I have stressed again and again that I believe that back pain starts with a physical problem in the back. Back pain is very real, it causes a great deal of human suffering and disability, and at times it needs health care. Basic science and biomedical research

Hopefully, the pendulum will swing back. At the same time, I hope that we will continue to treat patients as well as their backs.

Summary

We must also change the health care system
- Clear and accurate diagnostic triage, and appropriate referral
- Most medical specialist services are designed for patients who need investigation and treatment of serious spinal pathology or nerve root problems that fail to resolve. They are inappropriate and may be harmful for patients with ordinary backache
- Most patients with ordinary backache should be mainly managed in primary care. We should design that service to meet the needs of these patients
- This requires a fundamental change in professional practice and a shift of resources

We really are talking about a revolution in health care for back pain. Health professionals, patients, and society must all adopt a new approach. All health professionals must face radical change in their practice. Patients and society must change their ideas and what they do about back pain. But health professionals cannot escape the final responsibility. We provide the health care. We must also give patients and society a new understanding of low back pain and disability, which alone makes real change possible.

I am now more optimistic than when I started writing the first edition of this book in 1996. There are still a lot of dinosaurs and sacred cows to be shot. We still need much research and development. But I believe that we can now glimpse a better way ahead, even if much of the detail is still obscure. The back pain revolution *is* beginning. Clinical management *is* changing. We do now have the first hints that the epidemic may have peaked, at least in some countries in some settings. Back pain is a challenge and an opportunity. The lessons of back pain may even serve as an example and test-bed of a new health care approach for many benign, non-specific symptoms. That is the challenge and the excitement of back pain at the start of a new millennium.

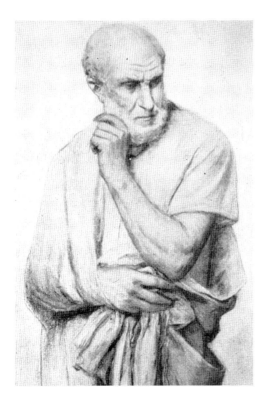

Figure 22.2 Hippocrates. Health care is about helping suffering human beings. The challenge is to combine treatment of their physical disorder with care of the whole person.

are the foundation for better understanding and treatment of that physical problem in the future. But they are only half the story. Back pain and disability also involve these equally important psychosocial issues that we ignore at our patients' peril.

- Back pain arises from a physical problem in the back
- The problem is how we react and what we do about it

I do agree that at the end of the 20th century the balance of back pain research perhaps swung too far towards psychological and then social issues, to the neglect of the physical. We need much more and better research into the physical basis of non-specific low back pain, though I would argue this should focus more on dysfunction than on anatomic and structural lesions. Of course we need better physical understanding and treatment.

Index